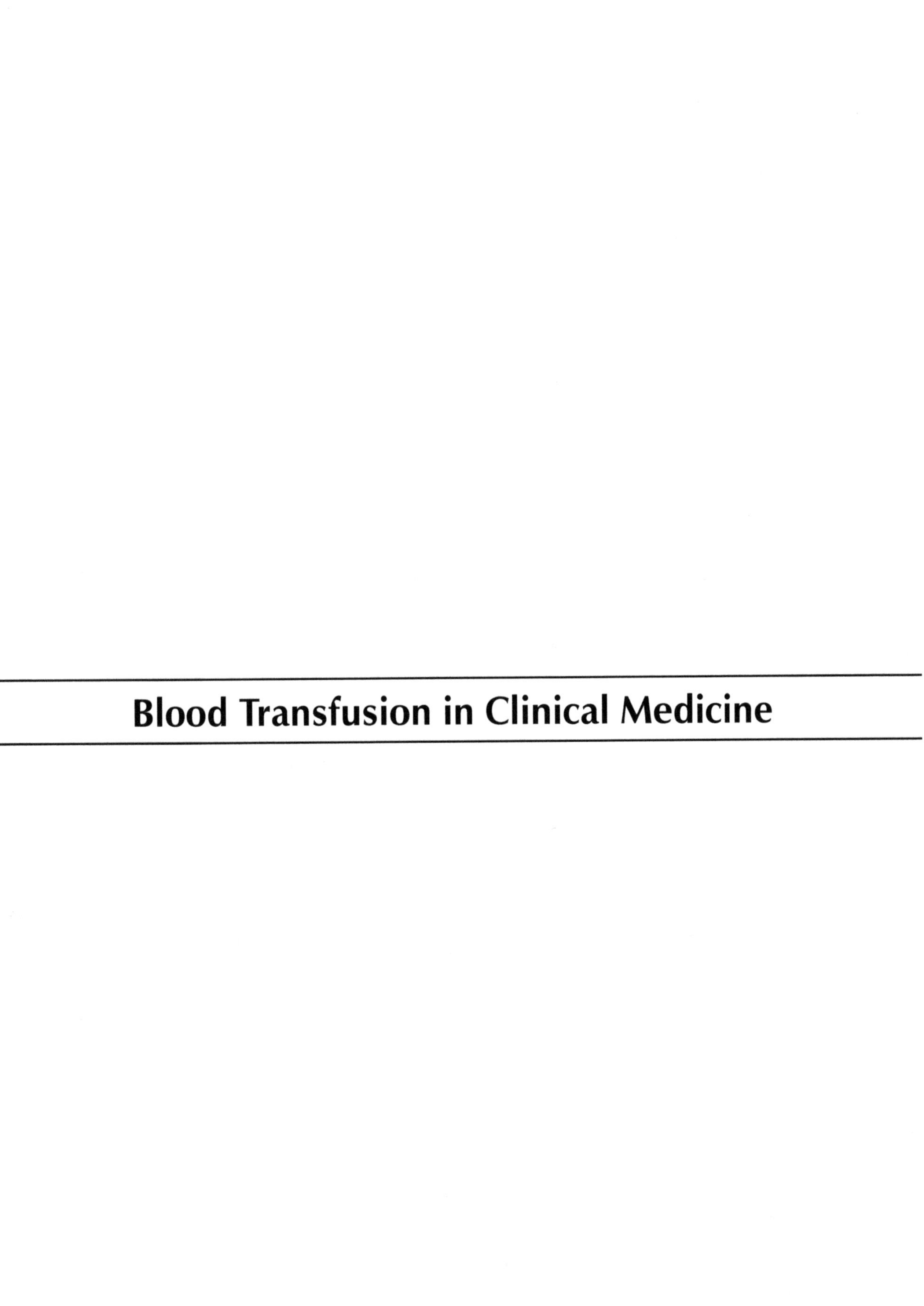

Blood Transfusion in Clinical Medicine

Blood Transfusion in Clinical Medicine

Editor: Albert Collins

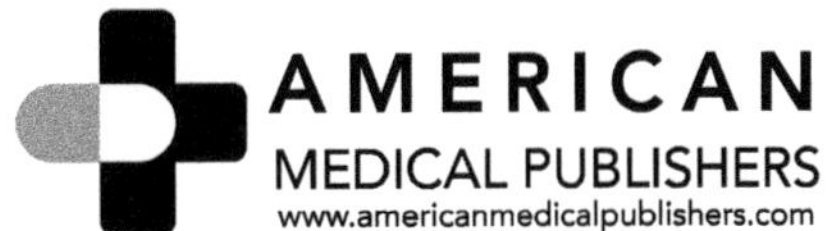

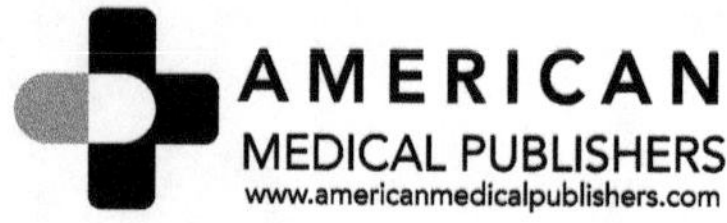

Cataloging-in-Publication Data

Blood transfusion in clinical medicine / edited by Albert Collins.
p. cm.
Includes bibliographical references and index.
ISBN 978-1-63927-937-1
1. Blood--Transfusion. 2. Blood--Transfusion--Complications. 3. Blood groups.
4. Clinical medicine. 5. Hematology. I. Collins, Albert.
RM171 .B56 2023
615.39--dc23

American Medical Publishers,
41 Flatbush Avenue,
1st Floor, New York,
NY 11217, USA

ISBN 978-1-63927-937-1 (Hardback)

Contents

Preface

This book aims to highlight the current researches and provides a platform to further the scope of innovations in this area. This book is a product of the combined efforts of many researchers and scientists, after going through thorough studies and analysis from different parts of the world. The objective of this book is to provide the readers with the latest information of the field.

Blood transfusion is the process of transferring blood into the vein of a patient. It is a therapeutic treatment used to restore blood or plasma volume after substantial bleeding, burns or trauma. Transfusion increases the quantity and concentration of red blood cells in anemic patients for improving the oxygen-carrying potential of the patient's blood. It is also used frequently as an important adjunct in various surgical operations where patients lose considerable volumes of whole blood that must be restored. Some of the important advancements in transfusion therapy include blood typing, pathogen screening and blood substitutes. Blood typing is a method of classifying blood in accordance with the distinctive inherited characteristics, related to the presence and absence of antibodies and antigens located on the surface of erythrocytes. There are various blood groups found in humans including ABO, Rh, Kidd, Kell, Duffy, MNS, and Lewis group. The receiver and donor must have the same or compatible blood types. Therefore, identification of these variables has become critical in the context of blood transfusion. This book strives to provide a fair idea about blood transfusion and help develop a better understanding of the latest advances within this area. Its extensive content provides the readers with a thorough understanding of the subject.

I would like to express my sincere thanks to the authors for their dedicated efforts in the completion of this book. I acknowledge the efforts of the publisher for providing constant support. Lastly, I would like to thank my family for their support in all academic endeavors.

Editor

1

Metabolism of Citrate and Other Carboxylic Acids in Erythrocytes As a Function of Oxygen Saturation and Refrigerated Storage

*Travis Nemkov[1], Kaiqi Sun[2], Julie A. Reisz[1], Tatsuro Yoshida[3], Andrew Dunham[3], Edward Y. Wen[2,4], Alexander Q. Wen[2], Rob C. Roach[1], Kirk C. Hansen[1], Yang Xia[2] and Angelo D'Alessandro[1]**

[1] Department of Biochemistry and Molecular Genetics, University of Colorado Denver – Anschutz Medical Campus, Aurora, CO, United States, [2] University of Texas Houston – McGovern Medical School, Houston, TX, United States, [3] New Health Sciences Inc., Boston, MA, United States, [4] University of California Berkeley, Berkeley, CA, United States

***Correspondence:**
Angelo D'Alessandro
angelo.dalessandro@ucdenver.edu

State-of-the-art proteomics technologies have recently helped to elucidate the unanticipated complexity of red blood cell metabolism. One recent example is citrate metabolism, which is catalyzed by cytosolic isoforms of Krebs cycle enzymes that are present and active in mature erythrocytes and was determined using quantitative metabolic flux analysis. In previous studies, we reported significant increases in glycolytic fluxes in red blood cells exposed to hypoxia *in vitro* or *in vivo*, an observation relevant to transfusion medicine owing to the potential benefits associated with hypoxic storage of packed red blood cells. Here, using a combination of steady state and quantitative tracing metabolomics experiments with $^{13}C_{1,2,3}$-glucose, $^{13}C_6$-citrate, $^{13}C_5{}^{15}N_2$-glutamine, and $^{13}C_1$-aspartate *via* ultra-high performance liquid chromatography coupled on line with mass spectrometry, we observed that hypoxia *in vivo* and *in vitro* promotes consumption of citrate and other carboxylates. These metabolic reactions are theoretically explained by the activity of cytosolic malate dehydrogenase 1 and isocitrate dehydrogenase 1 (abundantly represented in the red blood cell proteome), though moonlighting functions of additional enzymes cannot be ruled out. These observations enhance understanding of red blood cell metabolic responses to hypoxia, which could be relevant to understand systemic physiological and pathological responses to high altitude, ischemia, hemorrhage, sepsis, pulmonary hypertension, or hemoglobinopathies. Results from this study will also inform the design and testing of novel additive solutions that optimize red blood cell storage under oxygen-controlled conditions.

Keywords: hypoxia, metabolomics, mass spectrometry, tracing experiments, flux analysis

INTRODUCTION

Approximately 31,000 packed red blood cell (RBC) units are transfused every day in the US alone (1), thus illustrating the importance of RBC transfusion as a life-saving procedure for millions of people around the world. One hundred years of advancements in the field of transfusion medicine [as reviewed here (2, 3)] have tackled many of the issues associated with making ~110 million units/year available for transfusion all over the world. Though logistically inevitable, refrigerated storage of packed RBCs in the blood bank results in the progressive accumulation of a series of biochemical and morphological alterations, collectively termed the "storage lesion" (4–6). Hallmarks of the storage lesion include the early onset of an impaired energy and redox metabolism (7), which in turn affects redox homeostasis of proteins (8–10), lipids (11–13), and various small molecule metabolites (13–15). Reassuringly, evidence from randomized clinical trials [RCTs—extensively reviewed by Belpulsi and colleagues (16)] suggests that the general standard of care would not be improved by exclusively issuing fresh RBCs, at least for the clinical indications addressed by, and within the statistical power of, the completed RCTs. One tentative explanation reconciling the lack of correlation between the well-established storage lesion and the RCT results could involve the underappreciated role that donor and recipient biology plays in mediating transfusion safety and efficacy (17). In the last 7 years, such large-scale studies as the Recipient Epidemiology and Donor Evaluation Study-III have addressed the issue of biological variability and found that biological variability across donors (i.e., donor ethnicity, gender, and age) affects RBC storability and stress hemolysis (18). Such observations have been supported by smaller scale laboratory studies in humans (19, 20) that demonstrated heritability of the metabolic storage lesion (21–23), as well as studies performed in mice (24, 25) showing that post-transfusion recoveries are greatly variable across donors (26). Of note, Yoshida and colleagues have recently provided preliminary evidence suggesting that hemoglobin oxygen saturation (SO_2) at 8 h from donation and routine processing varies significantly across donors (27), potentially contributing to the donor-dependent development of the storage lesion. This is relevant in light of accumulating evidence suggesting that SO_2 significantly impacts RBC metabolism, as is the case in exposure to high-altitude hypoxia or hemorrhagic hypoxia (28, 29), as well as hypoxic storage in the blood bank (30–32). Hypoxic storage boosts energy metabolism and limits oxidative challenge to stored RBC proteins (10, 33), a phenomenon in part explained by the intracellular alkalinization accompanying the simultaneous removal of oxygen and carbon dioxide from the unit (34), as well as by the oxygen-dependent metabolic modulation of glycolytic enzyme activity (10, 35–37). Some of the benefits of anaerobic storage can indeed be phenocopied by alkaline additives (38, 39), which have been shown to boost glycolysis, Rapoport-Luebering shunt and pentose phosphate pathway activation (40) through a positive pH-dependent regulation of phosphofructokinase, bisphosphoglycerate mutase, and glucose 6-phosphate dehydrogenase (2). Because beneficial effects of metabolic interventions to attenuate the storage lesion have been demonstrated by washing and/or rejuvenating end-of-storage erythrocytes (41), boosting RBC metabolism through a combination of SO_2 control and novel additive solutions may represent a viable strategy to tackle the storability issue and further improve RBC storage quality in the future. Understanding how erythrocyte metabolism is affected by normoxia and hypoxia *in vivo* and *ex vivo* under refrigerated conditions is key to the development of novel additive solutions tailored to packed RBCs stored under oxygen-controlled conditions. In this view, it is worth considering how recent advancements in proteomics have expanded our understanding of the RBC proteome complexity, which was thought to include ~750 proteins just a decade ago (42) and is now known to enlist ~2,800 (43) and counting (44). While identification of trace levels of an enzyme in RBCs does not necessarily imply that the enzyme is functionally active, it has been recently demonstrated through flux experiments using stable isotope tracers that cytosolic isoforms of Krebs cycle enzymes are present and active in mitochondria-devoid human erythrocytes (44), an observation that is relevant for the RBC metabolism of citrate when stored in the most common additives in Europe [SAGM (45, 46)] and in the US [e.g., AS-3 (13)]. In these studies, it was shown that citrate metabolism can contribute to a varying percentage of lactate generation during storage progression (13, 45, 46). Since hypoxia promotes glycolysis and lactate generation in a SO_2-dependent fashion (10), we hypothesized that carboxylic acid metabolism (including citrate metabolism) in mature RBCs may be affected by hypoxia *in vivo* and *ex vivo* during short term (24 h) and prolonged refrigerated storage (up to 42 days) under SO_2-controlled conditions. To test this hypothesis, we re-analyzed RBCs from individuals exposed to high-altitude hypoxia to specifically look for carboxylates, as an expansion of the AltitudeOmics study (28). Moreover, we performed integrated metabolic tracing experiments in the presence of different stable isotope-labeled substrates (citrate, glucose, aspartate, and glutamine) in order to determine how hypoxia affected RBC metabolism of these substrates under normoxic and hypoxic conditions.

MATERIALS AND METHODS

Blood samples were collected from healthy donor volunteers upon receiving written informed consent and in conformity with the Declarations of Helsinki under protocol approved by the University of Texas Houston and University of Colorado Denver institutional review boards (no. AWC-14-0127 and 11-1581, respectively). Commercial reagents were purchased from Sigma-Aldrich (Saint Louis, MO, USA) unless otherwise noted.

Human RBCs, Stored under Normoxic or Hypoxic Conditions

Blood was collected from healthy donors at the Bonfils Blood Center (Denver, CO, USA) according to the Declaration of Helsinki. Filter leukocyte-reduced (>99.95% WBC depleted—Pall Medical, Braintree, MA, USA) packed RBCs were stored in CP2D-AS-3 ($n = 4$; Haemonetics Corp., Braintree, MA, USA). Units were sterilely sampled (0.1 mL per time point) on a weekly basis until storage day 42, and cells and supernatants were separated by centrifugation at 2,000 × g for 10 min at 4°C.

High-Altitude Studies

Whole blood was collected from 12 male and 9 female healthy human volunteers at sea level or after 3 h (ALT1 am), >8 h (ALT1 pm), or 7 days (ALT7) of exposure to high-altitude hypoxia (5,260 m) in Mt. Chacaltaya, Bolivia, within the framework of the AltitudeOmics study (28). RBCs were separated from whole blood through gentle centrifugation (~99% WBC depleted), as described (28).

Labeling Experiments

$^{13}C_{1,2,3}$-Glucose and RBC Storage under Controlled Oxygen Saturation Conditions

Filter leukocyte-reduced (>99.95% WBC depleted—Pall Medical, Braintree, MA, USA) packed red blood cells (n = 4) were collected, processed, and stored in CP2D-AS-3, as described above, supplemented with additional 11 mM $^{13}C_{1,2,3}$-glucose (no. CLM-4673-PK—Cambridge Isotope Laboratories Inc.—Tewksbury, MA, USA) prior to storage at six different oxygen saturation conditions, monitored throughout storage duration—including controls (untreated—averaging SO_2 = 47 ± 20), hyperoxic (SO_2 > 95%), and hypoxic (SO_2 = 20%, 10%, 5%, or <3%), as previously described (10, 27).

Tracing Experiments from Heavy Citrate, Glutamine Aspartate, and Glucose in Hypoxia and Normoxia for 24 h

Filter leukocyte-reduced (>99.95% WBC depleted—Pall Medical, Braintree, MA, USA) RBCs (n = 3) were stored for up to 24 h under normoxia (PO_2 = 21%) or hypoxia (PO_2 = 8%) in CP2D-AS-3 prepared in house (four independent experiments) in the presence of U-^{13}C-glucose (55 mM—Sigma-Aldrich Catalog no. 389374), $^{13}C_6$-citric acid (Sigma-Aldrich Catalog no. 606081—2.2 mM), $^{13}C_1$-aspartate (Sigma-Aldrich Catalog no. 489972—1 mM), or $^{13}C_5{}^{15}N_2$-glutamine (Sigma-Aldrich Catalog no. 607983—4 mM).

Sample Processing

Packed RBCs and supernatants were extracted in ice cold extraction solution (Optima LC-MS grade methanol:acetonitrile:water 5:3:2 v/v) at 1:10 or 1:25 dilutions, prior to vortexing for 30 min at 4°C. Insoluble proteins were pelleted by centrifugation at 4°C for 10 min at 10,000 × g and supernatants were collected and stored at −80°C until subsequent analysis.

UHPLC-MS Metabolomics Analysis

Sample extracts were analyzed by UHPLC-MS, as previously reported (47). Briefly, analyses were performed on a Vanquish UHPLC system (Thermo Fisher Scientific, San Jose, CA, USA) coupled online to a Q Exactive mass spectrometer (Thermo Fisher Scientific, Bremen, Germany). Samples were resolved over a Kinetex C18 column, 2.1 mm × 150 mm, 1.7 µm particle size (Phenomenex, Torrance, CA, USA) at 25°C using an isocratic runs with 5% B for 3 min at 250 µl/min or a 9 min method from 5 to 95% B flowed at 450 µl/min and 30°C, where mobile phase A consisted of water + 0.1% formic acid (for positive mode) or 5 mM ammonium acetate (for negative mode) and mobile phase B consisted of acetonitrile water + 0.1% formic acid (for positive mode) or 5 mM ammonium acetate (for negative mode). The mass spectrometer was operated independently in positive or negative ion mode scanning in Full MS mode (2 µscans) at 70,000 resolution from 60 to 900 m/z, with electrospray ionization operating at 4 kV spray voltage, 15 shealth gas, 5 auxiliary gas. Calibration was performed prior to analysis using the Pierce™ Positive and Negative Ion Calibration Solutions (Thermo Fisher Scientific). Acquired data was converted from .raw to .mzXML file format using Mass Matrix (Cleveland, OH, USA). Metabolite assignments, isotopologue distributions and correction for expected natural abundance of 13C and 15N isotopes were performed using MAVEN (Princeton, NJ, USA) (48).

Graphs were plotted and statistical analyses (either T-test or repeated measures ANOVA) performed with GraphPad Prism 5.0 (GraphPad Software, Inc., La Jolla, CA, USA). Significance was assessed through repeated measure ANOVA (time course), two way-ANOVA (SO_2 conditions), and T-test (% isotopologue enrichment)—threshold being $p < 0.05$.

RESULTS

High-Altitude Hypoxia Affects Steady-State Levels of Carboxylates in Human RBCs

Red blood cells were collected from 21 healthy volunteers (12 male and 9 female) at sea level (SL—Oregon) or within <3 h (ALT1 noon), 8–12 h (ALT1 pm), 7, or 16 days (ALT7 and ALT16, respectively) of exposure to high-altitude hypoxia in Bolivia (Mt. Chacaltaya, >5,260 m) (**Figure 1A**), within the framework of the AltitudeOmics study (28, 29). Even though previous metabolomics analyses of these RBCs did not cover carboxylic acids (28), new analyses were performed in light of the recent appreciation of carboxylic acid metabolism in mitochondria-deficient mature erythrocytes (13, 45, 46). Exposure to high-altitude hypoxia resulted in a progressive decrease in the RBC levels of carboxylic acids citrate, alpha-ketoglutarate, and 2-hydroxyglutarate from baseline levels at SL, and proportionally to the duration of stay at high altitude (**Figure 1B**). Transient decreases within hours after exposure to high altitude and progressive increases after 8–12 h during altitude acclimatization were observed for RBC fumarate and malate (**Figure 1B**). In parallel, elevated ratios of pyruvate/lactate [a proxy for NADH/NAD + ratios according to the mass action law (49)] and reduced/oxidized glutathione (GSH/GSSG) (**Figure 1B**) were observed, representing markers of a progressively increased reducing environment in the cytosol of RBCs from individuals acclimatizing to high-altitude hypoxia.

Ex Vivo Preservation of Packed RBCs under Controlled SO_2 Conditions Promotes Citrate Consumption and Accumulation of Fumarate, Malate, and Alpha-Ketoglutarate

To determine whether the observations in RBCs from individuals exposed to high-altitude hypoxia would be translatable to RBCs stored under oxygen-controlled conditions, we stored RBCs under normoxia (untreated—SO_2 = 47% ± 21, mean ± SD), hyperoxia (SO_2 > 95%), or four hypoxic conditions (SO_2 = 20, 10, 5, or <3%—**Figure 2**). Citrate consumption proportional to the degree of hypoxia was observed in supernatants and, most

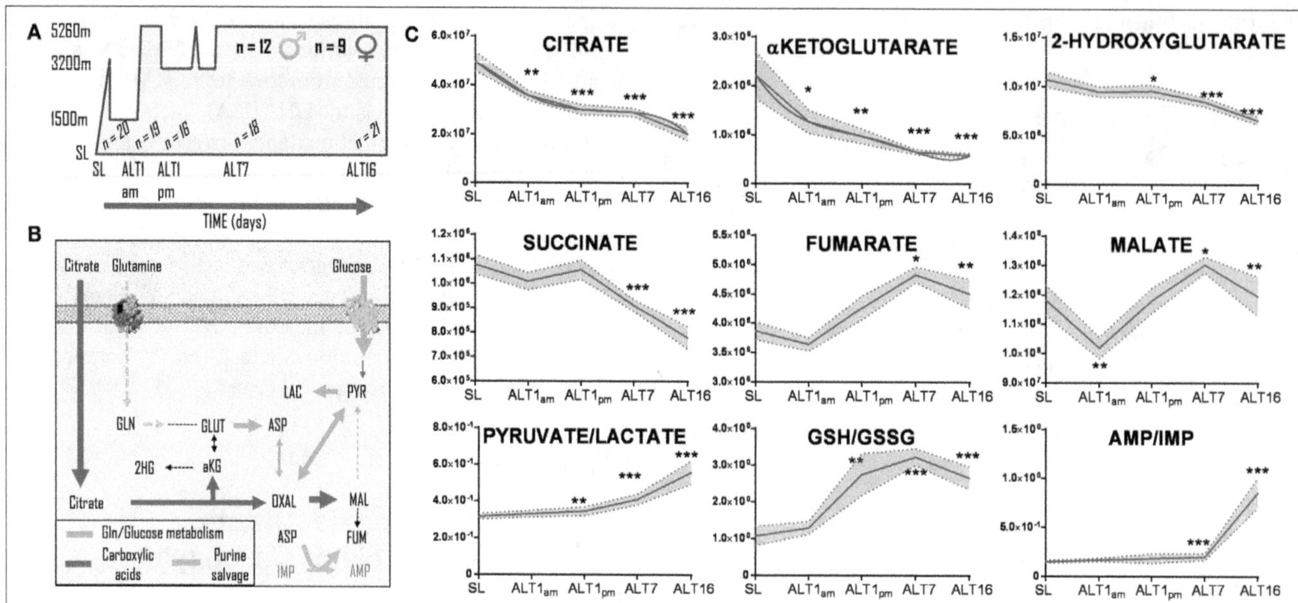

FIGURE 1 | Acclimatization to high-altitude hypoxia decreases steady-state levels of carboxylic acids in human red blood cells. Twenty-one healthy volunteers (12 male and 9 female) were flown from sea level (Oregon) to Bolivia (>5,260 m) for up to 16 days **(A)**, within the framework of the AltitudeOmics study (28, 29). While all of them successfully acclimatized to high-altitude hypoxia (28, 29), red blood cell (RBC) levels **(B)** of citrate, alpha-ketoglutarate, hydroxyglutarate, and succinate decrease from sea level to high altitude, proportionally to the duration of stay at over 5,000 m. Transient decrease and progressive increases in fumarate and malate were observed, paralleled by increases in the pyruvate/lactate ratios and reduced/oxidized glutathione (GSH/GSSG) ratios, suggestive of a progressively more reducing environment in the cytosol of RBCs from individuals acclimatizing to high-altitude hypoxia. $^{*}p < 0.05$; $^{**}p < 0.01$; $^{***}p < 0.001$ (repeated measures ANOVA). All data points on *x* axis were tested [*n* for each data point is reported in panel **(C)**].

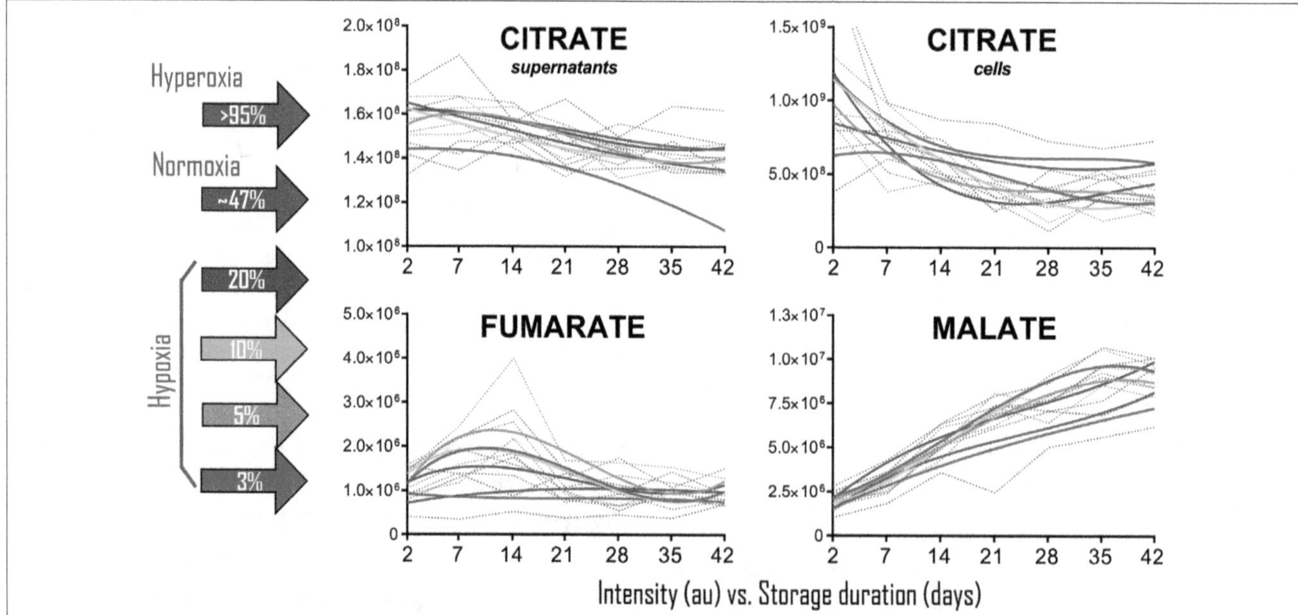

FIGURE 2 | Packed red blood cell (RBC) storage under controlled hemoglobin oxygen saturation conditions recapitulates high-altitude hypoxia-induced decreases in citrate and accumulation of fumarate/malate. RBCs were stored under normoxic conditions (untreated–SO_2 = 47 ± 21, mean ± SD—solid blue line), hyperoxia (SO_2 > 95%—solid purple line), or four hypoxic conditions (SO_2 = 20, 10, 5, or <3%—solid purple, green, orange, and red lines, respectively). Supernatant citrate was significantly lower than controls ($p < 0.05$) in SO_2 < 3% hypoxic RBCs at all tested time points. Fumarate was significantly higher than controls ($p < 0.05$) at storage day 7 and 14, while malate at day 14 onward in all hypoxic RBCs when compared to controls and hyperoxic counterparts. Dotted lines indicate ranges (same color-code—lighter tone). All data points on *x* axis were tested (n = 4).

notably, in cells during storage in AS-3, therefore suggesting increased consumption of citrate in hypoxic RBCs (**Figure 2**). In parallel, hypoxic RBCs generated more fumarate for the first 3 weeks of storage, and malate through the whole storage period (**Figure 2**). Recent proteomics (43, 44), metabolomics (13, 45), and computational evidence (46) has suggested that carboxylate metabolism in mature RBCs can be regulated by enzymatic reactions that are downstream to glucose-derived pyruvate by cytosolic isoforms of Krebs cycle enzymes such as acetyl-coA ligase, phosphoenolpyruvate carboxylase—PEPCK [or PEPCK-like activity of hemoglobin (50)], fumarate hydratase, isocitrate dehydrogenase 1, and malate dehydrogenase 1. To determine whether such reactions were affected by the degree of hypoxia, we incubated RBCs with $^{13}C_{1,2,3}$-glucose under varying SO_2 conditions (from <3% to >95%) and monitored ^{13}C distribution in downstream metabolites according to the reactions summarized in **Figure 3**. While generation of ^{13}C-fumarate from $^{13}C_{1,2,3}$-glucose was not observed, accumulation of $^{13}C_3$-malate and $^{13}C_3$-alpha-ketoglutarate isotopologues was observed during storage and followed a trend that was inversely proportional to SO_2 (i.e., higher generation of these compounds from heavy glucose was observed with hypoxia—**Figure 3**).

Determination of Isotopologue Distributions upon RBC Exposure to Hypoxia *Ex Vivo* in Presence of Stable Isotope-Labeled Citrate, Glutamine, and Aspartate

Our previous results showed encouraging evidence suggesting that the generation of malate and alpha-ketoglutarate from glucose could indeed occur in mature erythrocytes proportional to hypoxia. However, the amount of isotope-contribution was not sufficient to explain the observed increases in steady-state levels of these compounds during hypoxic refrigerated storage (<10% of which were derived from glucose oxidation in both cases of malate and alpha-ketoglutarate). Therefore, we hypothesized that hypoxia-induced catabolism of substrates other than glucose could more completely explain the observed increase in malate and altered metabolism of RBC carboxylic acids. To test this hypothesis, we incubated RBCs for 24 h under normoxic and hypoxic conditions using an in-house generated AS-3 supplemented with U-^{13}C-glucose or $^{13}C_6$-citratic acid (thereby replacing the unlabeled components in the formulation), $^{13}C_1$-aspartate, or $^{13}C_5{}^{15}N_2$-glutamine in four independent experiments ($n = 3$ for each). Heavy isotopologues derived from the catabolism of these substrates were quantified as a percentage of the total levels of the compound of interest, and included carboxylic acids (citrate, malate, and alpha-ketoglutarate), amino acids derived from transmination/oxidation of alpha-ketoglutarate (glutamate, 5-oxoproline), and lactate (**Figure 4**). In **Figures 4** and **5**, we provide a bar graph representation of the percent contribution to the generation of the aforementioned compounds from each of the heavy tracers in normoxia and hypoxia. Of note, >60% of RBC citrate was labeled independently from hypoxia, suggesting that the majority of this metabolite is uptaken from the media (**Figures 4** and **5**). Notably, citrate catabolism to malate was significant under normoxic conditions (~40% of the total) and reduced by hypoxia (<15%), which in turn promoted oxidative citrate metabolism to glutamate and 5-oxoproline (**Figure 4**). Minimal contribution of citrate catabolism to lactate generation (**Figures 4** and **5**) was observed under either normoxic or hypoxic

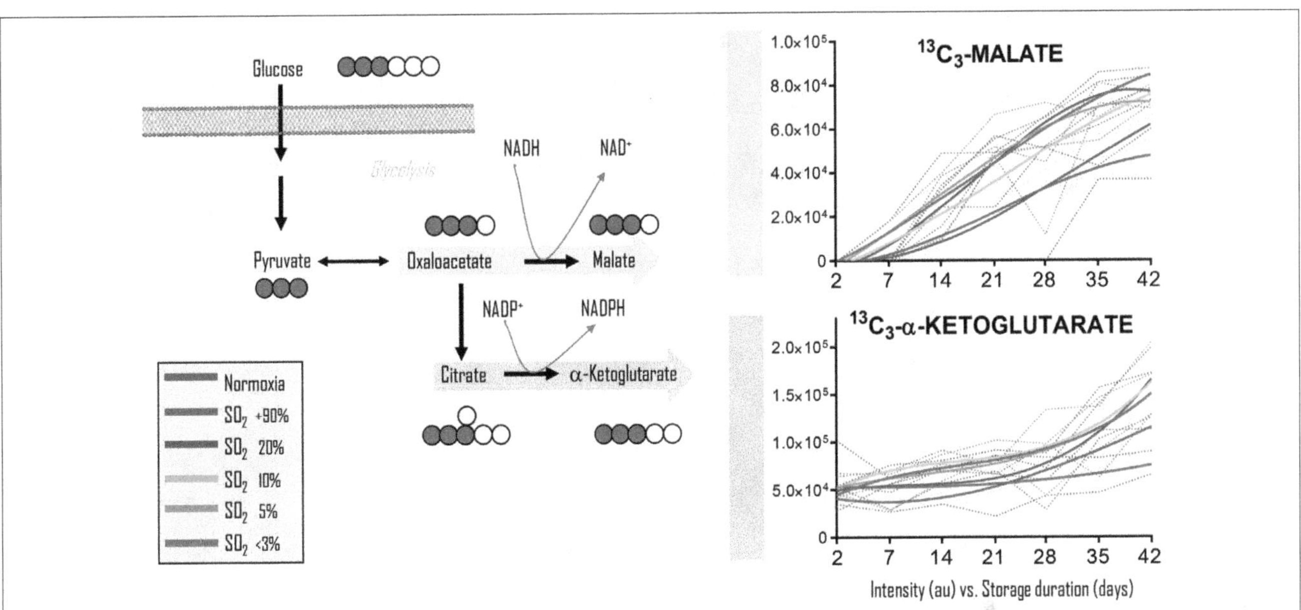

FIGURE 3 | Glucose tracing experiments indicate hypoxia-induced increases in carboxylic acids deriving from glucose. Cytosolic isoforms of Krebs cycle enzymes are present in mature red blood cells (RBCs) and can theoretically catalyze the reactions graphed here, reactions that could contribute to RBC reducing equivalent homeostasis. Heavy fumarate and malate accumulation in hypoxic RBCs was significantly higher ($p < 0.05$) than controls at all tested storage days after day 7. Hyperoxic RBCs had significantly ($p < 0.05$) lower heavy fumarate than control RBCs only at storage day 42. All data points on x axis were tested ($n = 4$).

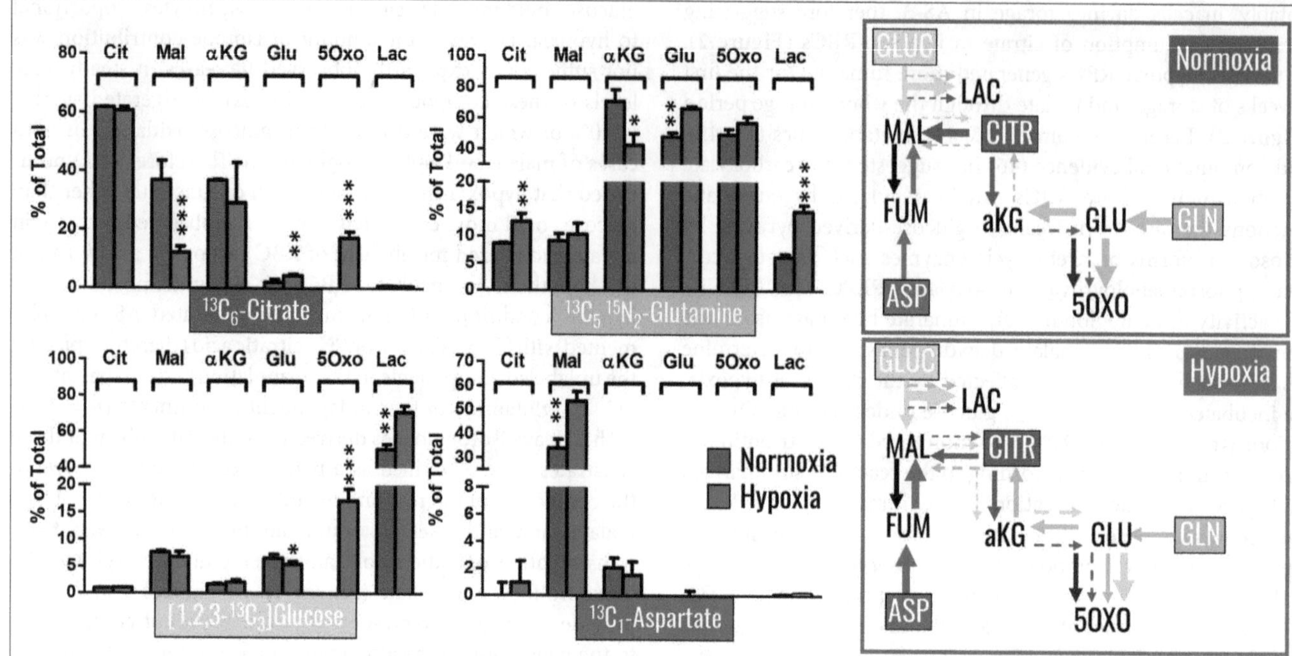

FIGURE 4 | Isotopologue distribution of heavy carbon atoms from heavy citrate, glutamine, glucose, and aspartate indicate a complex rewiring of red blood cell carboxylic acid metabolism in response to hypoxia, as summarized in the panels to the right. Bars indicate median (± SD)% accumulation of heavy isotopologues vs the total levels of the compound, as measured in three independent experiments per each condition (normoxia vs 24 h hypoxia—blue and red bars, respectively). Arrows in the panels to the right indicate metabolic rewiring in normoxia and hypoxia and color-code are consistent with the colors used to identify stable isotope tracers indicated in the four panels to the left. *$p < 0.05$; **$p < 0.01$; ***$p < 0.001$ (*T*-test to normoxic control).

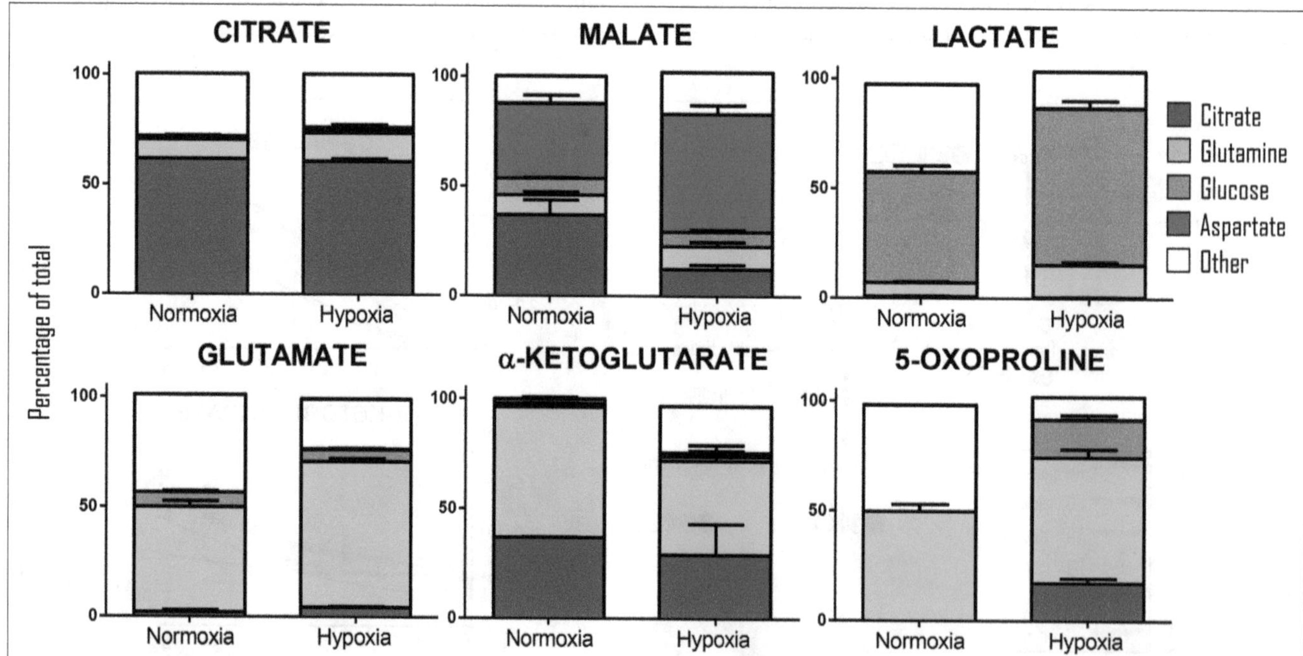

FIGURE 5 | Relative contribution of metabolic substrates (citrate, glutamine, glucoose, aspartate, other) to the generation of citrate, malate, lactate, glutamate, alpha-ketoglutarate, and 5-oxoproline under normoxic or hypoxic conditions (24 h). Mean ± SD are shown from three independent experiments per condition. Other here indicates either endogenous levels of the metabolite or derivation from other sources than the stable isotope tracers used here. Significant increases in glucose-derived lactate and glutamine-derived glutamate, but not ketoglutarate were observed under hypoxic conditions. Citrate and glucose-derived 5-oxoproline increased significantly ($p < 0.05$) under hypoxic conditions.

conditions for 24 h (<2.5%), suggesting that previous observations in AS-3 (13) may be explained by a metabolic switch only occurring later on during storage. Glutaminolysis mostly fueled the generation of alpha-ketoglutarate and its transamination byproducts glutamate and 5-oxoproline, a phenomenon that was exacerbated by exposure to hypoxia for 24 h (**Figure 4**). Metabolism of heavy glutamine contributed in part (<10%) to lactate generation under normoxia, and increased under hypoxia (up to 15%) where the contribution of glutamine to citrate reservoirs increased to ~13% of the total (**Figures 4** and **5**). Glucose catabolism mostly fueled lactate generation (55 to >70% of total lactate after 24 h in normoxia and hypoxia, respectively) and ~18% generation of 5-oxoproline under hypoxic conditions (**Figures 4** and **5**). Limited glucose incorporation into malate is consistent with tracing experiments with glucose during storage (**Figure 3**), though hypoxia-triggered increases in glucose metabolism to malate only became apparent after 1 week of storage rather than 24 h (**Figures 3** and **4**). This is important because we have previously shown that hypoxic RBCs may use glucose-derived carbons to synthesize amino acid moieties necessary for the synthesis of the tripeptide glutathione during hypoxic storage (27). Finally, aspartate catabolism was identified to influence malate generation (<40% under normoxia and up to 60% under hypoxia—**Figure 4**), making it the main source of hypoxic malate in human RBCs in this study (**Figure 5**).

DISCUSSION

Red blood cells are by far the most abundant host cell in the human body, accounting for nearly 80% of the 30 trillion host cells that make up the body of a 175 cm tall 70 kg man (44). Although loaded with hemoglobin (98% of the cytosolic proteome) and devoid of nuclei and organelles, RBCs are far more complex than previously believed (until the last decade or so). Appreciation through proteomics of the presence of cytosolic isoforms of Krebs cycle enzymes in mature erythrocytes has prompted the field to reconsider whether these enzymes are actually active and, if so, whether they actually influence RBC metabolism during routine storage in the blood bank. Indeed, tracing experiments in packed RBCs have suggested that citrate can be metabolized into lactate when stored in SAGM (45) and AS-3 (13); the latter being more directly relevant due to its elevated concentration of citrate (>20 mM) that compensates for the removal of the osmolite mannitol from its formulation. In light of these tracing experiments, it has been suggested that reactions catalyzed by cytosolic isoforms of Krebs cycle enzymes may contribute to the homeostasis of RBC reducing equivalents NADH and NADPH through reactions alternative to glycolysis, pentose phosphate pathway, and methemoglobin reductase, thereby expanding well-established understanding of RBC metabolic networks (51). Refinement of such networks is indeed important for the development of new storage additives, as *in silico* elaboration of quantitative metabolic information of metabolic markers of the storage lesion (52) would help in predicting the metabolic state of RBCs exposed to novel additives (53). In this study, we provide additional information to refine such models by determining the metabolic effect of RBC SO_2 modulation on carboxylate metabolism. Decreased RBC levels of 2-hydroxyglutarate and succinate in response to high-altitude acclimatization are relevant in that these metabolites are well-established markers of tissue hypoxia [e.g., ischemic (54) and hemorrhagic hypoxia (55)]. In nucleated cells, succinate accumulation is interesting given that it promotes the stabilization of hypoxia inducible factor 1α by inhibiting prolyl hydroxylase, therefore promoting acclimatization responses to hypoxia (56). Since all the subjects enrolled in the AltitudeOmics study effectively acclimatized to high-altitude hypoxia (57), it is interesting to note that declining levels of RBC succinate may be a marker of decreased tissue hypoxia as the subjects acclimatized.

For the first time, we provide evidence that exposure to hypoxia *in vivo* or *ex vivo* affects RBC capacity to metabolize (consume or generate) carboxylic acids. Through a combination of metabolic flux experiments using different stable isotope tracers, we confirm that RBCs can uptake carboxylic acids such as citrate and metabolize them into di-carboxylates (e.g., malate) or transamination intermediates (e.g., alpha-ketoglutarate, glutamate, 5-oxoproline) in an SO_2-dependent fashion. Most notably, we show that malate accumulation during storage and the exacerbation of this phenomenon under hypoxia are potentially explained by varying metabolic mechanisms, in that aspartate catabolism predominantly contributes to malate generation under hypoxia, rather than glucose or citrate catabolism. In this view, it is interesting to speculate that purine catabolism [deamination of purines to hypoxanthine and xanthine, a well-documented phenomenon in stored erythrocytes (7, 14, 15, 25, 52, 58)] may be influenced by hypoxia. Indeed, aspartate consumption *via* purine salvage reactions would explain increased fumarate accumulation, which in turn would become a substrate for fumarate hydratase [present and active in mature RBCs (46)] for the generation of malate. Future studies will investigate this interesting corollary to the observations reported here. Alternatively, aspartate may represent an eligible substrate (amino group donor) for transamination reactions. This hypothesis is consistent with the observed decrease in the level of alpha-ketoglutarate and increased glutamate isotopologues (both M + 5 and M + 5 + 1). Such observation can only be explained by combined glutamine metabolism to alpha-ketoglutarate (carbon backbone + 5), which is turn transaminated back to glutamate *via* glutamate oxaloacetate transaminases, previously identified in mature RBC proteomics datasets (43, 44).

Finally, though merely observational, the present study provides interesting hypothesis-generating evidence to investigate why carboxylic acid metabolism may be affected by hypoxia in an enucleated cell incapable of *de novo* protein synthesis, as is the case with RBCs. It is fascinating to speculate that, in similar fashion to the oxygen-dependent metabolic modulation model (28, 29, 35–37), post-translational modifications such as phosphorylation mediated by adenosine/AMPK-dependent signaling (59)—recently identified to contribute to hypoxic adaptations in eukaryotes as simple as *S. cervisiae* (60)—may influence enzyme sub-cellular compartmentalization, formation of multi-protein complexes, and activity. RBC multi-enzyme protein complexes have been preliminarily described in mature RBCs and reported to be susceptible to the storage lesion (61). Therefore, it remains to be assessed whether some of the observations reported here could be attributed to factors other than hypoxia-driven intracellular alkalinization that affects the activities of many RBC cytosolic enzymes, such as sub-cellular compartmentalization (e.g., membrane vs cytosol) or oligomerization of Krebs cycle enzymes into alternative multi-protein complexes under hypoxic conditions. Last but not least, the results presented here may be also interpreted as a result of as of yet uncharacterized reactions involving alternative to Krebs cycle cytosolic isoforms. A paradigmatic example of this notion is the conversion of late glycolytic trioses to oxaloacetate, an intermediate in malate/citrate generation/consumption in mature erythrocytes and a reaction that could be catalyzed by hemoglobin (50) through moonlighting functions (62). Similar considerations could be made for other carboxylates such as 2-hydroxyglutarate, which could be generated by lactate dehydrogenase under hypoxic conditions (63). Therefore, future studies will be necessary to disentangle and possibly identify new metabolic networks that are modulated by oxygen level in RBCs.

ETHICS STATEMENT

The AltitudeOmics study has been approved by the University of Colorado Institutional Review Board, Protocol no. 11-1581.

AUTHOR CONTRIBUTIONS

TN, JR, KH, and ADa performed metabolomics analyses and plotted the results. KS, EW, AW, and YX generated samples for *ex vivo* tracing experiments. RR designed, performed, and provided samples for high-altitude studies. TY and ADu generated technology and samples for *ex vivo* oxygen-controlled preservation of packed RBCs. ADa wrote the first draft of the manuscript, and all the authors critically contributed to its finalization.

REFERENCES

1. Ellingson KD, Sapiano MRP, Haass KA, Savinkina AA, Baker ML, Chung K-W, et al. Continued decline in blood collection and transfusion in the United States-2015. *Transfusion* (2017) 57(Suppl 2):1588–98. doi:10.1111/trf.14165
2. Nemkov T, Hansen KC, Dumont LJ, D'Alessandro A. Metabolomics in transfusion medicine. *Transfusion* (2016) 56:980–93. doi:10.1111/trf.13442
3. Hess JR. An update on solutions for red cell storage. *Vox Sang* (2006) 91:13–9. doi:10.1111/j.1423-0410.2006.00778.x
4. Zimring JC. Widening our gaze of red blood storage haze: a role for metabolomics. *Transfusion* (2015) 55:1139–42. doi:10.1111/trf.13071
5. Hod EA, Zhang N, Sokol SA, Wojczyk BS, Francis RO, Ansaldi D, et al. Transfusion of red blood cells after prolonged storage produces harmful effects that are mediated by iron and inflammation. *Blood* (2010) 115:4284–92. doi:10.1182/blood-2009-10-245001
6. D'Alessandro A, Kriebardis AG, Rinalducci S, Antonelou MH, Hansen KC, Papassideri IS, et al. An update on red blood cell storage lesions, as gleaned through biochemistry and omics technologies. *Transfusion* (2015) 55:205–19. doi:10.1111/trf.12804
7. D'Alessandro A, D'Amici GM, Vaglio S, Zolla L. Time-course investigation of SAGM-stored leukocyte-filtered red bood cell concentrates: from metabolism to proteomics. *Haematologica* (2012) 97:107–15. doi:10.3324/haematol.2011.051789
8. Harper VM, Oh JY, Stapley R, Marques MB, Wilson L, Barnes S, et al. Peroxiredoxin-2 recycling is inhibited during erythrocyte storage. *Antioxid Redox Signal* (2015) 22:294–307. doi:10.1089/ars.2014.5950
9. Rinalducci S, D'Amici GM, Blasi B, Vaglio S, Grazzini G, Zolla L. Peroxiredoxin-2 as a candidate biomarker to test oxidative stress levels of stored red blood cells under blood bank conditions. *Transfusion* (2011) 51:1439–49. doi:10.1111/j.1537-2995.2010.03032.x
10. Reisz JA, Wither MJ, Dzieciatkowska M, Nemkov T, Issaian A, Yoshida T, et al. Oxidative modifications of glyceraldehyde 3-phosphate dehydrogenase regulate metabolic reprogramming of stored red blood cells. *Blood* (2016) 128:e32–42. doi:10.1182/blood-2016-05-714816
11. Fu X, Felcyn JR, Zimring JC. Bioactive lipids are generated to micromolar levels during RBC storage, even in leukoreduced units. *Blood* (2015) 126:2344–2344.
12. Silliman CC, Moore EE, Kelher MR, Khan SY, Gellar L, Elzi DJ. Identification of lipids that accumulate during the routine storage of prestorage leukoreduced red blood cells and cause acute lung injury. *Transfusion* (2011) 51:2549–54. doi:10.1111/j.1537-2995.2011.03186.x
13. D'Alessandro A, Nemkov T, Yoshida T, Bordbar A, Palsson BO, Hansen KC. Citrate metabolism in red blood cells stored in additive solution-3. *Transfusion* (2017) 57:325–36. doi:10.1111/trf.13892
14. Roback JD, Josephson CD, Waller EK, Newman JL, Karatela S, Uppal K, et al. Metabolomics of ADSOL (AS-1) red blood cell storage. *Transfus Med Rev* (2014) 28:41–55. doi:10.1016/j.tmrv.2014.01.003
15. Bordbar A, Johansson PI, Paglia G, Harrison SJ, Wichuk K, Magnusdottir M, et al. Identified metabolic signature for assessing red blood cell unit quality is associated with endothelial damage markers and clinical outcomes. *Transfusion* (2016) 56:852–62. doi:10.1111/trf.13460
16. Belpulsi D, Spitalnik SL, Hod EA. The controversy over the age of blood: what do the clinical trials really teach us? *Blood Transfus* (2017) 15:112–5. doi:10.2450/2017.0328-16
17. Kanias T, Gladwin MT. Nitric oxide, hemolysis, and the red blood cell storage lesion: interactions between transfusion, donor, and recipient. *Transfusion* (2012) 52:1388–92. doi:10.1111/j.1537-2995.2012.03748.x
18. Kanias T, Lanteri MC, Page GP, Guo Y, Endres SM, Stone M, et al. Ethnicity, sex, and age are determinants of red blood cell storage and stress hemolysis: results of the REDS-III RBC-Omics study. *Blood Adv* (2017) 1:1132–41. doi:10.1182/bloodadvances.2017004820
19. Tzounakas VL, Kriebardis AG, Georgatzakou HT, Foudoulaki-Paparizos LE, Dzieciatkowska M, Wither MJ, et al. Glucose 6-phosphate dehydrogenase deficient subjects may be better "storers" than donors of red blood cells. *Free Radic Biol Med* (2016) 96:152–65. doi:10.1016/j.freeradbiomed.2016.04.005
20. Tzounakas VL, Kriebardis AG, Papassideri IS, Antonelou MH. Donor-variation effect on red blood cell storage lesion: a close relationship emerges. *Proteomics Clin Appl* (2016) 10:791–804. doi:10.1002/prca.201500128
21. Weisenhorn EMM, van T Erve TJ, Riley NM, Hess JR, Raife TJ, Coon JJ. Multi-omics evidence for inheritance of energy pathways in red blood cells. *Mol Cell Proteomics* (2016) 15:3614–23. doi:10.1074/mcp.M116.062349
22. van't Erve TJ, Wagner BA, Martin SM, Knudson CM, Blendowski R, Keaton M, et al. The heritability of hemolysis in stored human red blood cells. *Transfusion* (2015) 55:1178–85. doi:10.1111/trf.12992
23. van't Erve TJ, Wagner BA, Martin SM, Knudson CM, Blendowski R, Keaton M, et al. The heritability of metabolite concentrations in stored human red blood cells. *Transfusion* (2014) 54:2055–63. doi:10.1111/trf.12605
24. de Wolski K, Fu X, Dumont LJ, Roback JD, Waterman H, Odem-Davis K, et al. Metabolic pathways that correlate with post-transfusion circulation of stored murine red blood cells. *Haematologica* (2016) 101:578–86. doi:10.3324/haematol.2015.139139
25. Zimring JC, Smith N, Stowell SR, Johnsen JM, Bell LN, Francis RO, et al. Strain-specific red blood cell storage, metabolism, and eicosanoid generation in a mouse model. *Transfusion* (2014) 54:137–48. doi:10.1111/trf.12264
26. Dumont LJ, AuBuchon JP. Evaluation of proposed FDA criteria for the evaluation of radiolabeled red cell recovery trials. *Transfusion* (2008) 48: 1053–60. doi:10.1111/j.1537-2995.2008.01642.x

27. Yoshida T, Blair A, D'Alessandro A, Nemkov T, Dioguardi M, Silliman CC, et al. Enhancing uniformity and overall quality of red cell concentrate with anaerobic storage. *Blood Transfus* (2017) 15:172–81. doi:10.2450/2017.0325-16
28. D'Alessandro A, Nemkov T, Sun K, Liu H, Song A, Monte AA, et al. AltitudeOmics: red blood cell metabolic adaptation to high altitude hypoxia. *J Proteome Res* (2016) 15:3883–95. doi:10.1021/acs.jproteome.6b00733
29. Sun K, Zhang Y, D'Alessandro A, Nemkov T, Song A, Wu H, et al. Sphingosine-1-phosphate promotes erythrocyte glycolysis and oxygen release for adaptation to high-altitude hypoxia. *Nat Commun* (2016) 7:12086. doi:10.1038/ncomms12086
30. D'Alessandro A, Gevi F, Zolla L. Red blood cell metabolism under prolonged anaerobic storage. *Mol Biosyst* (2013) 9:1196–209. doi:10.1039/c3mb25575a
31. Prudent M, Stauber F, Rapin A, Hallen S, Pham N, Abonnenc M, et al. Small-scale perfusion bioreactor of red blood cells for dynamic studies of cellular pathways: proof-of-concept. *Front Mol Biosci* (2016) 3:11. doi:10.3389/fmolb.2016.00011
32. Kinoshita A, Tsukada K, Soga T, Hishiki T, Ueno Y, Nakayama Y, et al. Roles of hemoglobin allostery in hypoxia-induced metabolic alterations in erythrocytes: simulation and its verification by metabolome analysis. *J Biol Chem* (2007) 282:10731–41. doi:10.1074/jbc.M610717200
33. Yoshida T, Shevkoplyas SS. Anaerobic storage of red blood cells. *Blood Transfus* (2010) 8:220–36. doi:10.2450/2010.0022-10
34. Dumont LJ, D'Alessandro A, Szczepiorkowski ZM, Yoshida T. CO_2-dependent metabolic modulation in red blood cells stored under anaerobic conditions. *Transfusion* (2016) 56:392–403. doi:10.1111/trf.13364
35. Puchulu-Campanella E, Chu H, Anstee DJ, Galan JA, Tao WA, Low PS. Identification of the components of a glycolytic enzyme metabolon on the human red blood cell membrane. *J Biol Chem* (2013) 288:848–58. doi:10.1074/jbc.M112.428573
36. Rogers SC, Said A, Corcuera D, McLaughlin D, Kell P, Doctor A. Hypoxia limits antioxidant capacity in red blood cells by altering glycolytic pathway dominance. *FASEB J* (2009) 23:3159–70. doi:10.1096/fj.09-130666
37. Castagnola M, Messana I, Sanna MT, Giardina B. Oxygen-linked modulation of erythrocyte metabolism: state of the art. *Blood Transfus* (2010) 8:s53–8. doi:10.2450/2010.009S
38. de Korte D. New additive solutions for red cells. *ISBT Sci Ser* (2016) 11:165–70. doi:10.1111/voxs.12186
39. Hess JR, Hill HR, Oliver CK, Lippert LE, Greenwalt TJ. Alkaline CPD and the preservation of RBC 2,3-DPG. *Transfusion* (2002) 42:747–52. doi:10.1046/j.1537-2995.2002.00115.x
40. D'Alessandro A, Nemkov T, Hansen KC, Szczepiorkowski ZM, Dumont LJ. Red blood cell storage in additive solution-7 preserves energy and redox metabolism: a metabolomics approach. *Transfusion* (2015) 55:2955–66. doi:10.1111/trf.13253
41. D'Alessandro A, Gray AD, Szczepiorkowski ZM, Hansen K, Herschel LH, Dumont LJ. Red blood cell metabolic responses to refrigerated storage, rejuvenation, and frozen storage. *Transfusion* (2017) 57:1019–30. doi:10.1111/trf.14034
42. Goodman SR, Kurdia A, Ammann L, Kakhniashvili D, Daescu O. The human red blood cell proteome and interactome. *Exp Biol Med* (2007) 232:1391–408. doi:10.3181/0706-MR-156
43. Wilson MC, Trakarnsanga K, Heesom KJ, Cogan N, Green C, Toye AM, et al. Comparison of the proteome of adult and cord erythroid cells, and changes in the proteome following reticulocyte maturation. *Mol Cell Proteomics* (2016) 15:1938–46. doi:10.1074/mcp.M115.057315
44. D'Alessandro A, Dzieciatkowska M, Nemkov T, Hansen KC. Red blood cell proteomics update: is there more to discover? *Blood Transfus* (2017) 15:182–7. doi:10.2450/2017.0293-16
45. Rolfsson Ó, Sigurjonsson ÓE, Magnusdottir M, Johannsson F, Paglia G, Guðmundsson S, et al. Metabolomics comparison of red cells stored in four additive solutions reveals differences in citrate anticoagulant permeability and metabolism. *Vox Sang* (2017) 112:326–35. doi:10.1111/vox.12506
46. Bordbar A, Yurkovich JT, Paglia G, Rolfsson O, Sigurjónsson ÓE, Palsson BO. Elucidating dynamic metabolic physiology through network integration of quantitative time-course metabolomics. *Sci Rep* (2017) 7:46249. doi:10.1038/srep46249
47. Nemkov T, Hansen KC, D'Alessandro A. A three-minute method for high-throughput quantitative metabolomics and quantitative tracing experiments of central carbon and nitrogen pathways. *Rapid Commun Mass Spectrom* (2017) 31:663–73. doi:10.1002/rcm.7834
48. Melamud E, Vastag L, Rabinowitz JD. Metabolomic analysis and visualization engine for LC–MS data. *Anal Chem* (2010) 82:9818–26. doi:10.1021/ac1021166
49. Li M, Riddle S, Zhang H, D'Alessandro A, Flockton A, Serkova NJ, et al. Metabolic reprogramming regulates the proliferative and inflammatory phenotype of adventitial fibroblasts in pulmonary hypertension through the transcriptional co-repressor C-terminal binding protein-1. *Circulation* (2016) 134:1105–21. doi:10.1161/CIRCULATIONAHA.116.023171
50. Simpson RJ, Brindle KM, Campbell ID. Spin echo proton NMR studies of the metabolism of malate and fumarate in human erythrocytes. *Biochim Biophys Acta* (1982) 721:191–200. doi:10.1016/0167-4889(82)90068-4
51. Bordbar A, Jamshidi N, Palsson BO. iAB-RBC-283: a proteomically derived knowledge-base of erythrocyte metabolism that can be used to simulate its physiological and patho-physiological states. *BMC Syst Biol* (2011) 5:110. doi:10.1186/1752-0509-5-110
52. Paglia G, D'Alessandro A, Rolfsson Ó, Sigurjónsson ÓE, Bordbar A, Palsson S, et al. Biomarkers defining the metabolic age of red blood cells during cold storage. *Blood* (2016) 128:e43–50. doi:10.1182/blood-2016-06-721688
53. Yurkovich JT, Yang L, Palsson BO. Biomarkers are used to predict quantitative metabolite concentration profiles in human red blood cells. *PLoS Comput Biol* (2017) 13:e1005424. doi:10.1371/journal.pcbi.1005424
54. Chouchani ET, Pell VR, Gaude E, Aksentijević D, Sundier SY, Robb EL, et al. Ischaemic accumulation of succinate controls reperfusion injury through mitochondrial ROS. *Nature* (2014) 515:431–5. doi:10.1038/nature13909
55. D'Alessandro A, Moore HB, Moore EE, Reisz JA, Wither MJ, Ghasabyan A, et al. Plasma succinate is a predictor of mortality in critically injured patients. *J Trauma Acute Care Surg* (2017) 83:491–5. doi:10.1097/TA.0000000000001565
56. Tannahill GM, Curtis AM, Adamik J, Palsson-McDermott EM, McGettrick AF, Goel G, et al. Succinate is an inflammatory signal that induces IL-1β through HIF-1α. *Nature* (2013) 496:238–42. doi:10.1038/nature11986
57. Subudhi AW, Bourdillon N, Bucher J, Davis C, Elliott JE, Eutermoster M, et al. AltitudeOmics: the integrative physiology of human acclimatization to hypobaric hypoxia and its retention upon reascent. *PLoS One* (2014) 9:e92191. doi:10.1371/journal.pone.0092191
58. Casali E, Berni P, Spisni A, Baricchi R, Pertinhez TA. Hypoxanthine: a new paradigm to interpret the origin of transfusion toxicity. *Blood Transfus* (2015) 14:555–6. doi:10.2450/2015.0177-15
59. Liu H, Zhang Y, Wu H, D'Alessandro A, Yegutkin GG, Song A, et al. Beneficial role of erythrocyte adenosine A2B receptor-mediated AMP-activated protein kinase activation in high-altitude hypoxia. *Circulation* (2016) 134:405–21. doi:10.1161/CIRCULATIONAHA.116.021311
60. Jin M, Fuller GG, Han T, Yao Y, Alessi AF, Freeberg MA, et al. Glycolytic enzymes coalesce in G bodies under hypoxic stress. *Cell Rep* (2017) 20:895–908. doi:10.1016/j.celrep.2017.06.082
61. Pallotta V, Rinalducci S, Zolla L. Red blood cell storage affects the stability of cytosolic native protein complexes. *Transfusion* (2015) 55:1927–36. doi:10.1111/trf.13079
62. Huberts DHEW, van der Klei IJ. Moonlighting proteins: an intriguing mode of multitasking. *Biochim Biophys Acta* (2010) 1803:520–5. doi:10.1016/j.bbamcr.2010.01.022
63. Intlekofer AM, Dematteo RG, Venneti S, Finley LWS, Lu C, Judkins AR, et al. Hypoxia induces production of L-2-hydroxyglutarate. *Cell Metab* (2015) 22:304–11. doi:10.1016/j.cmet.2015.06.023

2

Redox Status, Procoagulant Activity and Metabolome of Fresh Frozen Plasma in Glucose 6-Phosphate Dehydrogenase Deficiency

Vassilis L. Tzounakas[1], Federica Gevi[2], Hara T. Georgatzakou[1], Lello Zolla[3], Issidora S. Papassideri[1], Anastasios G. Kriebardis[4]*, Sara Rinalducci[2]* and Marianna H. Antonelou[1]

[1] Department of Biology, School of Science, National and Kapodistrian University of Athens, Athens, Greece, [2] Department of Ecological and Biological Sciences, University of Tuscia, Viterbo, Italy, [3] Department of Science and Technology for Agriculture, Forestry, Nature and Energy, University of Tuscia, Viterbo, Italy, [4] Department of Medical Laboratories, Faculty of Health and Caring Professions, Technological and Educational Institute of Athens, Athens, Greece

***Correspondence:**
Anastasios G. Kriebardis
akrieb@biol.uoa.gr;
Sara Rinalducci
sara.r@unitus.it

Objective: Transfusion of fresh frozen plasma (FFP) helps in maintaining the coagulation parameters in patients with acquired multiple coagulation factor deficiencies and severe bleeding. However, along with coagulation factors and procoagulant extracellular vesicles (EVs), numerous bioactive and probably donor-related factors (metabolites, oxidized components, etc.) are also carried to the recipient. The X-linked glucose 6-phosphate dehydrogenase deficiency (G6PD$^-$), the most common human enzyme genetic defect, mainly affects males. By undermining the redox metabolism, the G6PD$^-$ cells are susceptible to the deleterious effects of oxidants. Considering the preferential transfusion of FFP from male donors, this study aimed at the assessment of FFP units derived from G6PD$^-$ males compared with control, to show whether they are comparable at physiological, metabolic and redox homeostasis levels.

Methods: The quality of $n = 12$ G6PD$^-$ and control FFP units was tested after 12 months of storage, by using hemolysis, redox, and procoagulant activity-targeted biochemical assays, flow cytometry for EV enumeration and phenotyping, untargeted metabolomics, in addition to statistical and bioinformatics tools.

Results: Higher procoagulant activity, phosphatidylserine positive EVs, RBC-vesiculation, and antioxidant capacity but lower oxidative modifications in lipids and proteins were detected in G6PD$^-$ FFP compared with controls. The FFP EVs varied in number, cell origin, and lipid/protein composition. Pathway analysis highlighted the riboflavin, purine, and glycerolipid/glycerophospholipid metabolisms as the most altered pathways with high impact in G6PD$^-$. Multivariate and univariate analysis of FFP metabolomes showed excess of diacylglycerols, glycerophosphoinositol, aconitate, and ornithine but a deficiency in riboflavin, flavin mononucleotide, adenine, and arginine, among others, levels in G6PD$^-$ FFPs compared with control.

Conclusion: Our results point toward a different redox, lipid metabolism, and EV profile in the G6PD$^-$ FFP units. Certain FFP-needed patients may be at greatest benefit of receiving FFP intrinsically endowed by both procoagulant and antioxidant activities. However, the clinical outcome of G6PD⁻ FFP transfusion would likely be affected by various other factors, including the signaling potential of the differentially expressed metabolites and EVs, the degree of G6PD⁻, the redox status in the recipient, the amount of FFP units transfused, and probably, the storage interval of the FFP, which deserve further investigation by future studies.

Keywords: transfusion medicine, fresh frozen plasma, G6PD⁻ donors, donor variation, metabolomics, extracellular vesicles, antioxidant capacity, interactome

INTRODUCTION

Fresh frozen plasma (FFP) is commonly used in transfusion therapy to maintain the coagulation status in patients with acquired multiple coagulation factor deficiencies and severe bleeding after injury (1). In addition, FFP units can be used as a pool for biopharmaceutical fractionation in order to manufacture medicinal products (2). Practically, FFP is used for its ability to generate thrombin and form a clot as a result of intrinsic components, including coagulation factors, calcium and procoagulant phospholipid surfaces, involved in the assembly of coagulation complexes, and coagulation activation (3). However, apart from coagulation factors and procoagulant extracellular vesicles (EVs), numerous bioactive signaling factors and oxidized lipids and proteins (4) pass to the FFP recipient.

The extent of this risk is partly related to inter-individual donor characteristics. Indeed, several studies have recently reported significant donor-to-donor variation in numerous blood properties *in vivo* and in labile blood products. In the case of red-cell concentrates, apart from in-bag hemolysis and 24-h posttransfusion recovery, units from different donors might have substantial variation in antioxidant capacity (5, 6), cellular fragility (6, 7), or surface removal signals (8). Extracellularly, the uric-acid-dependent antioxidant capacity of the supernatant (that influence the storage lesion, and thus, the quality of the blood component) significantly varies among donors (9–11). In the same context, and since the plasma reflects the physiological state of donor's cells and tissues (12), significant variation has been observed among FFP units used for transfusion, in terms of EV characteristics and lipid peroxidation (4, 13).

Certain aspects of the so-called "donor variation effect" are attributed to genetic factors that dictate subclinical inter-donor differences in blood physiology as clearly exemplified by the distinct blood profile of beta thalassemia trait and glucose-6-phosphate dehydrogenase (G6PD)-deficient donors (14). In the last case, the subjects are characterized by extremely low levels of G6PD activity that catalyzes the first reaction in the pentose phosphate pathway converting glucose 6-phosphate to gluconolactone-6-phosphate. Pentose phosphate pathway feeds cells with reducing equivalents (like nicotinamide dinucleotide hydrogen phosphate, NADPH) needed for the maintenance of redox equilibrium. In cases of oxidative stress, NADPH helps in the regeneration of reduced glutathione, in the detoxification of hydrogen peroxide and in the prevention of oxidative damage in membrane lipids and proteins. G6PD deficiency (G6PD⁻) affects the energy and redox status of cells and consequently, a range of energy-dependent cellular activities, including the transport properties of cell membrane, a feature that might link changes in cell metabolomes to those of plasma (15).

Genetic factors may determine the quality of stored blood and probably, its posttransfusion performance and effects. Thus, a study of donors carrying the most common human enzyme genetic defect might be highly relevant to blood transfusion. Moreover, since G6PD⁻ is an X-linked defect, males are more commonly affected than females. Considering that G6PD activity influences both the cellular and plasma homeostases and that a typical transfusion practice is the use of FFP units donated exclusively by male donors, the study of G6PD⁻ male donors is especially relevant to FFP transfusion. However, and despite this intrinsic clinical interest, little is known about the physiological properties and the metabolome of FFP donated by eligible, G6PD⁻ donors. This study aimed at the comparative assessment of FFP units produced by whole blood donations from G6PD-deficient and -sufficient male donors, by using a number of biochemical measurements, flow cytometry and mass spectrometry, in addition to statistical and bioinformatics tools.

MATERIALS AND METHODS

Blood Donors and Fresh Frozen Plasma (FFP) Preparation

Blood from 12 eligible male regular donors was used for the production of FFP units. G6PD⁻ donors under study (n = 6) carried the common Mediterranean variant of G6PD⁻ (16). After donation of approximately 465 mL of blood and addition of 63 mL of CPDA-1 (citrate–phosphate–dextrose–adenine) anticoagulant, clinical-grade FFP was prepared according to the standard blood banking procedures (17), directly from whole blood units at 4°C. Briefly, after centrifugation at 4,500× g for 15 min, the supernatant plasma was squeezed off by a plasma expressor (Fenwall Laboratories, Deerfield, IL, USA) and frozen for 12 months at −20°C. For analysis, FFP samples were rapidly thawed for 15–20 min at 30–37°C to avoid precipitation of cold-precipitating proteins, consistent with the blood banking procedure for the thawing of clinical FFP for transfusion and the standard AABB operating procedures. The study was approved by the Ethics Committee of the Department of Biology, School of Science, NKUA. Investigations were carried out upon signing of written consent, in accordance with the principles of the Declaration of Helsinki.

Free Hemoglobin, Redox Parameters, and Protein Analysis

Free hemoglobin was calculated by using the Harboe method as previously described (10). Total (TAC) and uric-acid-dependent antioxidant capacity (UA/AC) of FFP samples were determined in the absence or presence of uricase (Sigma-Aldrich, Munich, Germany) treatment, respectively (18), by using the ferric reducing antioxidant power assay (19). Lipid peroxidation of FFP units was assessed by measuring the levels of malondialdehyde (MDA), a natural by-product of lipid peroxidation. Briefly, after deproteinization of each sample with 15% trichloroacetic acid, thiobarbituric acid was added (all chemicals by Sigma-Aldrich, Munich, Germany). After heating of the samples for 50 min at 95°C, the absorption of the produced chromogenic MDA–thiobarbituric acid complex was measured at 532 nm. Measurements were plotted against a standard curve of known MDA concentration.

For the FFP protein characterization, 20 μg of FFP samples were separated in homogeneous 10% sodium dodecyl sulfate polyacrylamide gels, transferred onto nitrocellulose membranes, and probed with primary antibodies against advanced glycated end products (AGEs, 1:1,000 Millipore AB9890), soluble clusterin (sCLU, 1:1,000 Santa Cruz Biotechnology), human hemoglobin (Hb, 1:15,000, Europa Bioproducts), IgGs (1:1,000; Sigma I-2011), and horseradish peroxidase-conjugated secondary antibodies. Immunoblots were developed using a standard enhanced chemiluminescence reagent kit and the relative amount of each protein was quantified by scanning densitometry (Gel Analyzer v.1.0 image-processing program, Athens, Greece). In addition, FFP samples were processed for the detection of protein carbonylation using the Oxyblot detection kit as per manufacturer's specifications (20).

Extracellular Vesicles (EV) Profiling

Extracellular vesicle-associated procoagulant activity was estimated by using a functional Elisa assay kit (Zymuphen MP-activity, Hyphen BioMed, Neuville-sur-Oise, France) as per manufacturer's instructions. All FFP samples were supplemented with calcium, Factor Xa, and thrombin inhibitors before addition into microplate wells precoated with streptavidin and biotinylated Annexin V (AnnV). Subsequently, samples were incubated at 37°C before introduction of factor Xa-Va and prothrombin. After addition of the chromogenic substrate, thrombin activation induced by the AnnV positivity ($AnnV^+$) EVs was detected at 405 nm and expressed as nM of phosphatidylserine (PS) equivalents.

Enumeration and phenotyping of FFP EVs was performed by flow cytometry within 15 min from units' thawing, as previously described (13). Briefly, EVs were identified by size (<1 μm), exposure of cell-specific markers, and $AnnV^+$. All samples were double stained with AnnV-phycoerythrin (PE Annexin V Apoptosis Detection Kit I, 559763) and CD235a-fluorescein isothiocyanate (clone GA-R2, HIR2, 559943) or integrin-α2b-FITC (CD41a, clone HIP8, 555466) or CD45-fluorescein isothiocyanate (clone HI30, 555482) from BD Biosciences to identify $AnnV^+$ red-cell-derived, platelet-derived, or leukocyte-derived vesicles, respectively. After addition of phycoerythrin-AnnV and a cell-specific and fluorescein isothiocyanate-conjugated monoclonal antibody in AnnV buffer environment, samples were incubated in the dark for 15 min at room temperature. The samples run within 30 min in a FACScan flow cytometer (Beckton Dickinson) using CELL Quest Software (Becton Dickinson, San Jose, CA, USA). TruCount™ tubes (340334, BD Pharmingen) were used to calculate the absolute EVs count/μL.

The protein composition of EVs isolated by FFP units was estimated by immunoblotting analysis. To this purpose, EVs were precipitated with high-speed centrifugation of 1-mL FFP at 30,000× *g* for 1 h at 4°C. The produced pellet was resuspended in saline buffer and washed twice under the same conditions. The EV proteins were separated in homogeneous 10% sodium dodecyl sulfate polyacrylamide gels, and transferred onto nitrocellulose membranes. Membranes were probed with primary antibodies against vesicular proteins [anti-Hb 1:15,000, Europa Bioproducts; anti-IgGs 1:1,000 Sigma; anti-Hsp70 (K-20) 1:300 Santa Cruz Biotechnology; anti-sCLU 1:1,000 Santa Cruz Biotechnology; anti-Alix 1:1,000 Cell Signaling Technology; and monoclonal antibody against stomatin, kindly provided by Prof. R. Prohaska, Institute of Medical Biochemistry, University of Vienna, Austria] diluted in 5% non-fat milk for 1 h at room temperature. After incubation with the appropriate horseradish peroxidase-conjugated secondary antibody (1:8,000–1:14,000), the immunoreactivity was visualized by enhanced chemiluminescence.

Statistical and Biological Network Analyses

For statistical analysis, the Statistical Package for Social Sciences (SPSS, IBM) was used. After checking all variables for normal distribution profile and presence of outliers (by using the Shapiro–Wilk test and detrended normal $Q - Q$ plots), inter-groups differences were evaluated through independent *t*-test or Mann–Whitney test as appropriate. In addition, and according to the outcome of the normal distribution and outliers' analyses, correlations between parameters that subsequently used for the construction of biological networks were evaluated by the Pearson's and Spearman's tests. The statistically significant correlations between biochemical, metabolomics, and physiological parameters collected from $G6PD^-$ and control FFP samples were used for the construction of undirected biological networks. The topological representation was processed by the Cytoscape version 3.2.0 application, as previously described (6). The length of each edge was inversely proportional to the r value (the shortest the edge, the higher the r value). Significance for both network and inter-group analyses was accepted at $p < 0.05$.

Metabolite Extraction and LC–MS Analysis

Metabolites were extracted by adding 200 μL of plasma sample (control: $n = 5$; G6PD: $n = 6$) to 200 μL of chloroform/methanol/water (1:3:1 ratio) solvent mixture stored at −20°C. Samples were vortexed for 1 min and left on ice for

2 h for complete protein precipitation. The solutions were then centrifuged for 15 min at 15,000× *g*. Twenty microliters of supernatants (two technical replicates) were injected into an ultra high-performance liquid chromatography (UHPLC) system (Ultimate 3000, Thermo) and run in positive ion mode. A Reprosil C18 column (2.0 mm × 150 mm, 2.5 µm—Dr Maisch, Germany) was used for metabolite separation. Chromatographic separations were achieved at a column temperature of 30°C and flow rate of 0.2 mL/min. A 0–100% linear gradient of solvent A (ddH2O, 0.1% formic acid) to B (acetonitrile, 0.1% formic acid) was employed over 20 min, returning to 100% A in 2 min and a 6-min post-time solvent A hold. The UHPLC system was coupled online with a mass spectrometer Q Exactive (Thermo) scanning in full MS mode (2 µscans) at 70,000 resolution in the 67–1,000 *m*/*z* range, target of 1×10^6 ions, and a maximum ion injection time (IT) of 35 ms. Source ionization parameters were as follows: spray voltage, 3.8 kV; capillary temperature, 300°C; sheath gas, 40; auxiliary gas, 25; S-Lens level, 45. Calibration was performed before each analysis against positive ion mode calibration mixes (Piercenet, Thermo Fisher, Rockford, IL, USA) to ensure subppm error of the intact mass.

Metabolomic Data Processing and Statistical Analysis

Raw files of replicates were exported and converted into mzXML format through MassMatrix (Cleveland, OH, USA), then processed by MAVEN software[1] (21). Mass spectrometry chromatograms were elaborated for peak alignment, matching and comparison of parent and fragment ions, and tentative metabolite identification (within a 2-ppm mass-deviation range between observed and expected results against the imported KEGG database). Univariate (two-sample *t*-test, Volcano plot) and multivariate (PCA, PLS-DA) statistical analyses were performed on the entire metabolomics data set using the MetaboAnalyst 3.0 software[2]. Before the analysis, raw data were normalized by sum and pareto scaled in order to increase the importance of low-abundance ions without significant amplification of noise. False discovery rate (FDR) and Holm–Bonferroni method were used for controlling multiple testing. The web-based tools MSEA (metabolite set enrichment analysis) and MetPA (metabolic pathway analysis), which are incorporated into MetaboAnalyst platform, were used to perform metabolite enrichment and pathway analyses, respectively. Data for identified metabolites detected in all samples were submitted into MSEA and MetPA with annotation based on common chemical names. Verification of accepted metabolites was conducted manually using HMDB, KEGG, and PubChem DBs. *Homo sapiens* pathway library was used for pathway analysis. Global test was the selected pathway enrichment analysis method, whereas the node importance measure for topological analysis was the relative betweenness centrality.

[1] http://maven.princeton.edu/.
[2] http://metpa.metabolomics.ca/.

RESULTS

High-Antioxidant Capacity and Low-Oxidative Defects to Plasma Lipids and Proteins in FFP Units from G6PD$^-$ Donors

Oxidative stress and antioxidant capacity are donor-related factors that may contribute to the quality of FFP products. Biochemical analysis of FFP units stored for 12 months at −20°C revealed substantial differences in the oxidant/antioxidant equilibrium and the extent of oxidative defects between the two groups. Both TAC and UA/AC were significantly higher in G6PD$^-$ FFP units vs. control (TAC: 698 ± 92 vs. 574 ± 52 µM Fe^{2+}, UA/AC: 466 ± 89 vs. 360 ± 46 µM Fe^{2+}, respectively, mean ± SD, $p < 0.05$, $n = 12$) (**Figures 1A,B**). In addition, the levels of lipid peroxidation, as measured by the production of malonyldialdehyde (MDA), formed during the breakdown of peroxidized fatty-acid side chains of the phospholipids (TBARS assay), was lower in the G6PD$^-$ units as compared with control FFPs (0.175 ± 0.113 vs. 0.597 ± 0.219-µM MDA, $p < 0.01$, respectively, mean ± SD, $n = 12$), as shown in **Figure 1C**. To analyze the FFP proteins for probable oxidative defects, we performed immunoblotting analysis of an equal quantity of plasma proteins (20 µg per sample, **Figure 1D**). Substantially lower levels of albumin carbonylation ($p < 0.05$, $n = 12$) along with a trend for decreased levels of advanced glycation end-products (AGEs) and sCLU were detected in G6PD$^-$ FFP units compared with controls. Only traces of soluble Hb were detected in some units, signifying low pre-donation levels of autohemolysis and high-quality level of the FFP preparation procedure followed, which resulted in minimal lysis of RBCs. IgG immunodetection was used for loading control.

The EV Component of the FFP Units Differed between the Two Groups of Donors

In large consistence with the results of the immunoblotting analysis of FFP proteins (**Figure 1D**), extremely low levels of free hemoglobin (<5 mg/dL) were detected by the Harboe method in all the FFP samples ($n = 12$) under study, without any inter-group difference (**Figure 2A**). On the contrary, the EV-associated procoagulant activity of the FFP (**Figure 2B**), which stands for the total concentration of PS exposed on EVs' surface, was significantly higher in G6PD$^-$ units vs. control units (33.93 ± 8.98 vs. 19.03 ± 11.76 nM PS, respectively, $p < 0.05$, mean ± SD).

To further characterize the EV part of the FFP units, we proceeded to enumeration and phenotyping analysis by flow cytometry. There was no statistically significant difference in the concentration of total EV populations between the two groups under examination; however, the concentration of AnnV$^+$ EVs was higher in G6PD$^-$ FFPs (**Figure 2C**), verifying the finding of high procoagulant activity of G6PD$^-$ FFP. The platelet-derived EVs (CD41$^+$) were the most abundant, followed by the red-cell-derived (CD235$^+$) and the leukocyte-derived (CD45$^+$) vesicles. The G6PD$^-$ FFP units contained more red-cell EVs and more AnnV$^+$ red-cell EVs ($p < 0.05$) compared with controls. Moreover, while similar concentrations of platelet EVs and leukocyte EVs

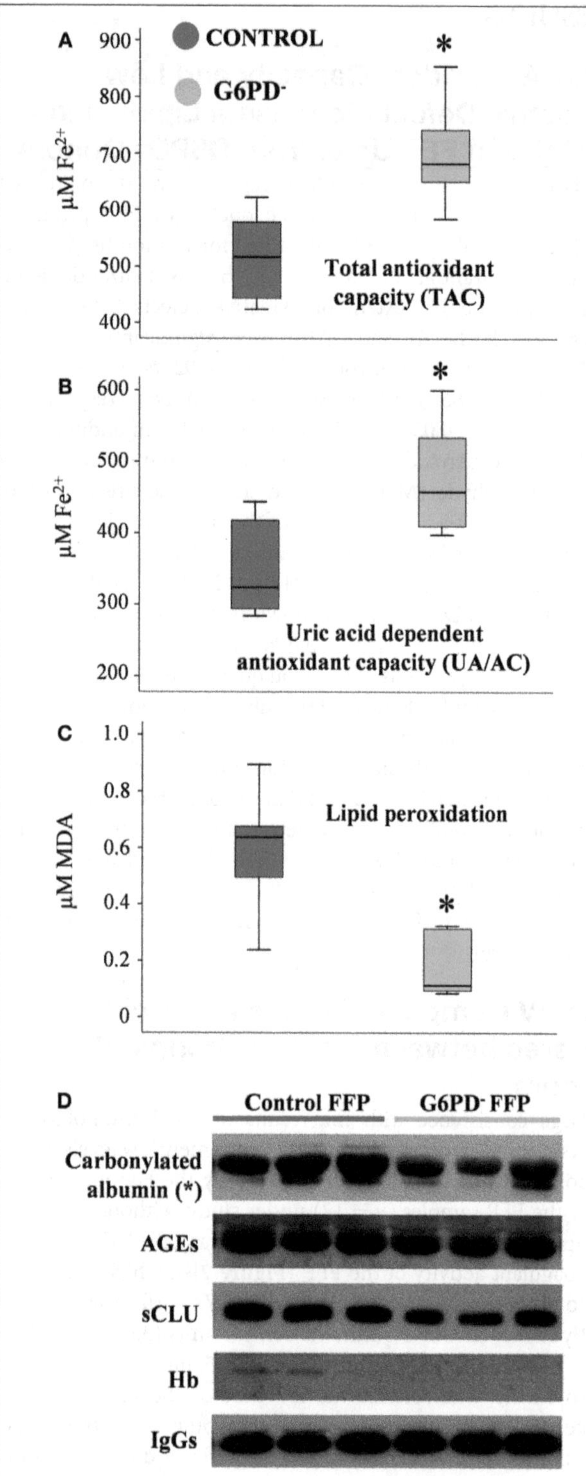

FIGURE 1 | Redox status of fresh frozen plasma (FFP) units prepared from G6PD deficient (G6PD⁻) and control donors. Levels of total antioxidant capacity **(A)**, uric-acid-dependent antioxidant capacity **(B)**, and lipid peroxidation **(C)** in FFP units from G6PD⁻ donors ($n = 6$) compared with control ($n = 6$). MDA: malondialdehyde. **(D)** Representative immunoblots showing variation in the expression of stress protein markers in the two groups of FFP. AGEs: advanced glycation end-products. sCLU, soluble clusterin (apolipoprotein J). *$p < 0.05$, G6PD⁻ vs. control FFPs.

were measured in the two FFP groups, the platelet EVs from G6PD⁻ FFP units demonstrated a higher percentage of AnnV⁺ as compared with the control group (96.5 ± 4.1 vs. 88.6 ± 5.4%, respectively, $p < 0.05$, mean ± SD).

The above-mentioned differences in the PS exposure and cell origin between the otherwise similar EV pools of G6PD⁻ and control FFPs prompted us to a rough examination of their protein composition by immunoprobing of selected components typically associated with the microvesicles or the exosomes (**Figure 2D**). Indeed, the vesicles precipitated by high-speed centrifugation of an equal volume (1 mL) of G6PD⁻ and control FFPs differed significantly between them in protein expression, by showing lower levels of oxidized Hb, IgGs, Hsp70, sCLU, and the red-cell lipid raft marker stomatin in the G6PD⁻ samples. As a component of the late endosomal machinery, the Alix protein has been considered a marker of endosome-derived EVs, namely of exosomes (22). Of note, traces of Alix were detected in some control samples, but not in G6PD⁻ FFP EVs.

Metabolome FFP

Metabolites were extracted from plasma samples of five healthy and six G6PD⁻ donors and were analyzed by LC–MS (two technical replicates). More than 2,000 peaks per sample were obtained referring to the KEGG database; among them, 195 metabolites were analyzed more precisely and identified. To compare the metabolomes between control and G6PD⁻ donors, both multi- and univariate statistical analyses were performed. For unsupervised multivariate analysis, principal component analysis (PCA) showed that the 70.6% of variance was captured by the first three principal components and sample groups could be clearly distinguished in the 3D-PCA score plot (**Figure 3A**). However, to maximize the separation achieved by PCA, partial least square discriminant analysis (PLS-DA) was subsequently performed and the obtained 3D score plots are shown in **Figure 3B**. The prediction accuracies were assessed by cross-validation and the best performance was obtained with three PCs (accuracy 1, $R2 > 0.94$, $Q2 > 0.87$; Figure S1 in Supplementary Material). As a supervised method, PLS-DA also enables the identification of the metabolites most contributing to the segregation of the diagnostic groups, thus variable importance in the projection (VIP) scores were calculated to rank the significance of these metabolites as potential biomarkers. Considering that variables having a VIP score of ≥1 are interpreted as being highly influential (23), 15 metabolites were considered as significant important features to differentiate control from G6PD⁻ FFP (**Figure 4A**). These changed plasma metabolites were mainly lipids (including 1,2-diacylglycerol, DAG), amino acids, nucleotides, and organic acids. To further confirm the specificity and significance of potentially discriminating metabolites identified from PLS-DA, univariate analysis of each metabolite was performed by combining statistical significance (Student's *t*-test) with fold-change (FC) variations. The generated Volcano plot (FDR adjusted $p < 0.05$; $FC > 2$) is displayed in **Figure 4B** where additional metabolites included riboflavin, FMN, ornithine, D-glucono-lattone-6-phosphate, and acylglycerophosphoinositol, among others. Quantitative variations

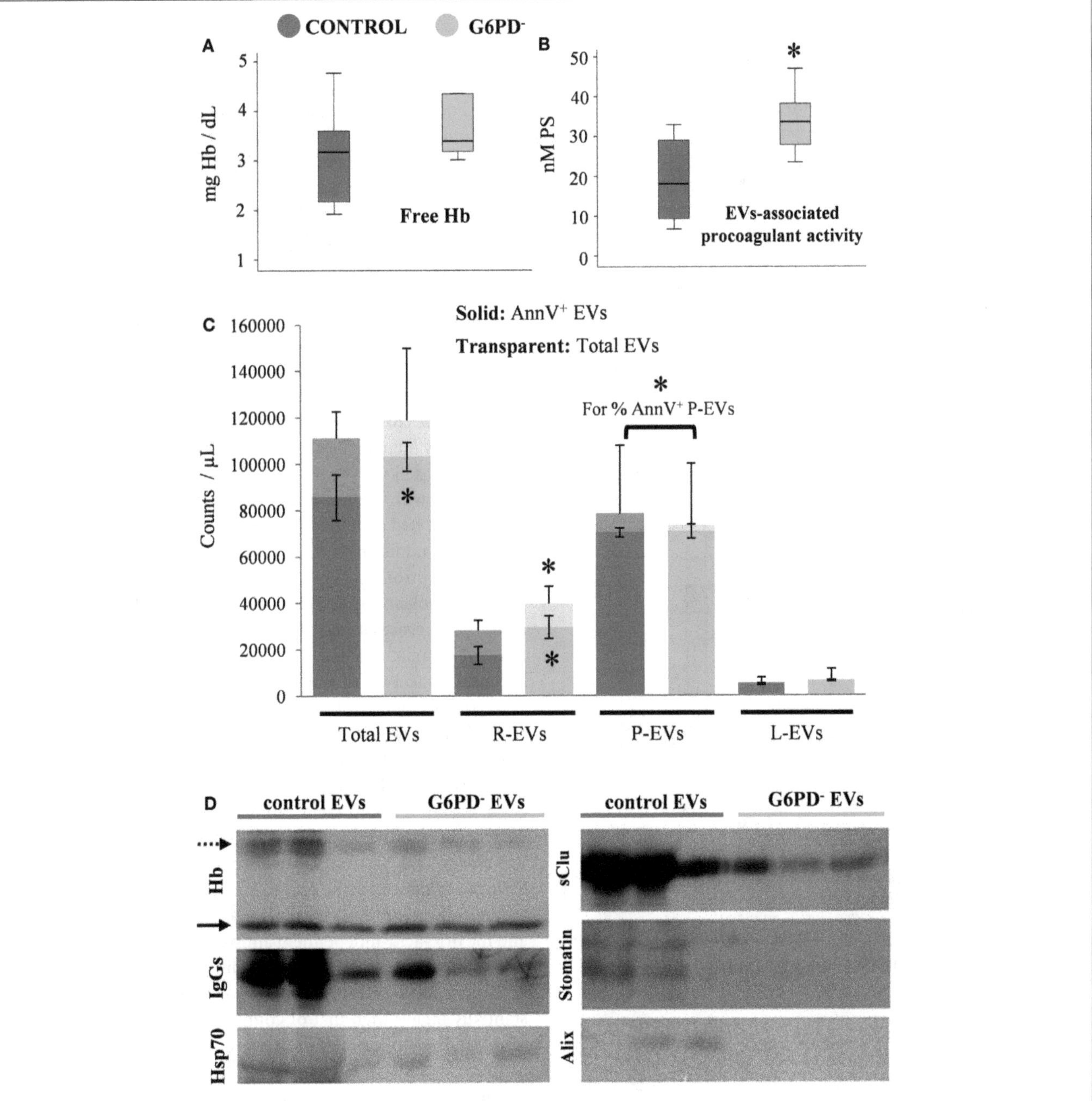

FIGURE 2 | Hemolysis and extracellular vesicles (EV) analyses in fresh frozen plasma (FFP) units prepared from G6PD-deficient ($G6PD^-$) and control donors. Free hemoglobin (Hb). **(A)** and EV-associated procoagulant activity **(B)** levels in the $G6PD^-$ and control FFP units. **(C)** Enumeration and phenotyping of total and annexin V positive ($AnnV^+$) EVs by flow cytometry. R-, P-, L-EVs stand for red cell-, platelet-, and leukocyte-derived EVs, respectively. $^*p < 0.05$, $G6PD^-$ vs. control FFPs; error bars: mean ± SD. **(D)** Representative immunoblots showing similar Hb levels (solid arrows) but variable expression of other protein components in EVs precipitated by high-speed centrifugation of equal volumes of $G6PD^-$ and control FFP. Dashed arrow: oxidized Hb bands.

for a number of important metabolites are shown in **Figure 5**. Nevertheless, by performing PLS-DA or Volcano-plot analysis, the potential to identify subtle but substantial changes among a group of related compounds could be weakened. To overcome this obstacle, an MSEA was performed on plasma metabolites along with their relative concentrations by using the web-based platform MetaboAnalyst (**Figure 6A**). Metabolomic data from control and $G6PD^-$ FFP showed that the pathways significantly enriched (FDR < 0.05) were as follows: (i) riboflavin metabolism, (ii) phospholipid biosynthesis, (iii) purine metabolism, (iv) tricarboxylic acid cycle, and (v) histidine metabolism. In parallel, we also utilized the MetPA module of MetaboAnalyst, which combines results from the pathway enrichment analysis with the pathway topology analysis. A graphical list of the pathways

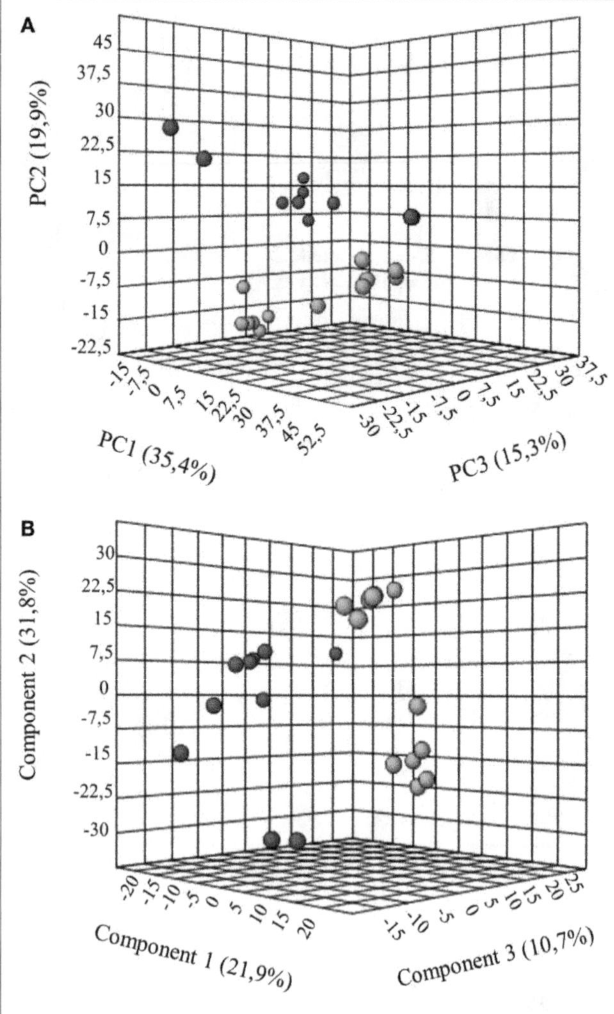

FIGURE 3 | Multivariate statistical analysis of metabolomics data from control and G6PD⁻ donors. Three-dimensional principal component analysis (PCA) and partial least squares-discriminate analysis (PLS-DA) score plots are shown in **(A)** and **(B)**, respectively. Control sample groups are in red; G6PD⁻ sample groups are in green.

identified and their relative impact is shown in **Figure 6B**. The most important ones (FDR < 0.05; impact values > 0.1) included tricarboxylic acid cycle and the metabolism of the following compounds: (i) glycerolipids, (ii) glycerophospholipids, (iii) purines, (iv) riboflavin, (v) glyoxylate/dicarboxylates, and (vi) inositol phosphate. Taken together, these results point out that both analyses concurred on most of the pathways, with MetPA being slightly more sensitive.

The Biological Networks of G6PD⁻ and Control FFP Were Different

More than 1,000 statistically significant correlations ($p < 0.05$) were detected between the biochemical, physiological, and metabolic variables in control FFP units. They were topologically arranged in an untargeted biological network according to the power of the correlation coefficient r (the shorter the edge, the higher the r value, small magnification network in **Figure 7**). A significant part of that network ($n = 266$ pairs) referred to connections between redox, EVs, and metabolic parameters (see Table S1 in Supplementary Material for code numbering and abbreviations). Focusing on that part of the control FFP network resulted in the interactome shown in **Figure 7**. In that subnetwork, uric acid and uric-acid-related physiological features and metabolites (antioxidant capacity, allantoin) exhibited the higher degree of connectivity, followed by the hub nodes of EVs, homocysteine, aconitate, and riboflavin. Half of the connections involved at least one of those variables. Worth to mention here, allantoin, the precursor of allantoate in serum, is a biomarker of oxidant generation *in vivo* (24). Uric acid may be oxidized non-enzymatically to allantoin by various ROS, leading to hydrogen peroxide generation. Uric-acid-related correlations included lactate, numerous amino acids, phosphoinositol, carnitine, creatinine, and NADP/NADPH. The concentration of the AnnV⁺ EVs in the control FFP was strongly interconnected with the levels of lipid peroxidation, uric acid, adenosine, glycerophospholipids, lactate, ornithine, and, again, with several amino acids. AnnV⁺ red-cell EVs and platelet EVs had a similar degree of interconnection, while both of them, in addition to the EV-associated procoagulant activity of the FFP, strongly correlated with the levels of amino acids, lipid metabolism, and redox state components (ascorbic, uric acid, lipid peroxidation). In fact, the procoagulant activity had negative correlations with several amino acids but positive correlations with acetylcarnitine. PS exposure on platelet-derived EVs seemed to be more influenced by lipid metabolites, and thus the relevant node was arranged out of the main core of the network. Homocysteine showed significant connections with adenine and citrulline, while aconitate with citrulline, lactate, purines, choline, and ascorbic acid, among others. Riboflavin and the correlated ascorbic acid localized to the center of the network. Riboflavin had correlations with adenine, acetylcarnitine, and lipid peroxidation, while ascorbic acid with several components (adenosine-monophosphate, glycerophosphocholine, ornithine) and the uric-acid-independent antioxidant capacity of the control FFP, along with vitamin B6 metabolites.

Regarding the biological network of G6PD⁻ FFP, it was substantially bigger than that of control FFP, with more than 2,000 statistically significant connections at total, and 434 connections in the relevant subnetwork shown in **Figure 8**. It was also different compared with the control network, in terms of pairing, topography, and hub nodes. While the uric-acid-related box and aconitate represented main hub nodes here too, they constructed along with the hubs of DAG, lipid peroxidation, and glutathione the extremely dense core of the network that included strongly interconnected variables. The degree of PS exposure on EVs was strongly interconnected with the levels of pyruvate, allantoin, adenosine, and inosine and, again, with several amino acids, similarly with the control network. In contrast, however, to the control FFP, the PS-exposing red-cell EVs had more connections compared with the other EV subtypes in the G6PD⁻ FFP, mostly with adenosine, amino acids, and purine metabolism variables. The platelet-EV node was again located away from the network's core, being linked, though, with it by the pyruvate–glutathione connection. The procoagulant activity of the G6PD⁻ FFP had positive

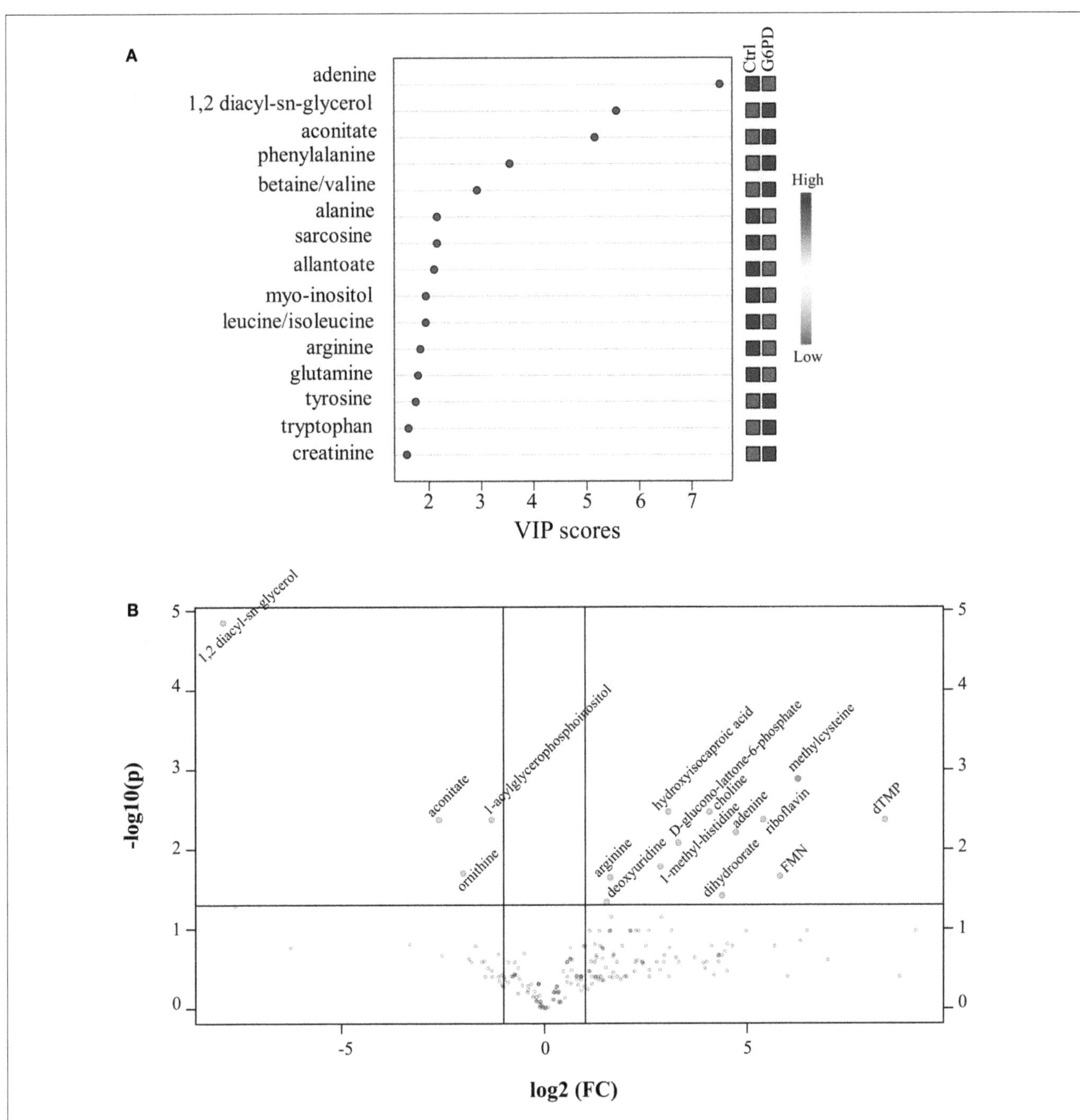

FIGURE 4 | Important features identified by uni- and multivariate analyses. **(A)** G6PD⁻ vs. control variable importance in projection (VIP) plot; colored boxes on the right indicate the relative concentrations of the corresponding metabolite in each group under current study. **(B)** Volcano plot showing the distribution of the fold changes in metabolite concentrations. Metabolites with absolute fold change >2 and adjusted *p*-value (FDR < 0.05) are indicated in pink. Comparisons were analyzed using Student's *t*-test.

correlations with pentose phosphate pathway intermediates and allantoin. Riboflavin and ascorbic acid were not connected with the core of the network, while the uric-acid-independent antioxidant capacity had no correlation with the levels of ascorbic acid, as occurred in the control FFP. Uric acid and related variables were connected with lipid biosynthesis, transfer, and metabolism, in addition to amino acids and arginine metabolism/urea cycle components. The newly appearing hub node of DAG was strongly connected to the other hub nodes of the network, namely, the lipid peroxidation (MDA), aconitate, glutathione, and allantoate, in addition to lactate and many lipid-related, amino acids, purine, and arginine metabolism components. The hub of MDA was further connected to those of glutathione and aconitate, in addition to adenine, purine metabolism components, glycerophospholipids,

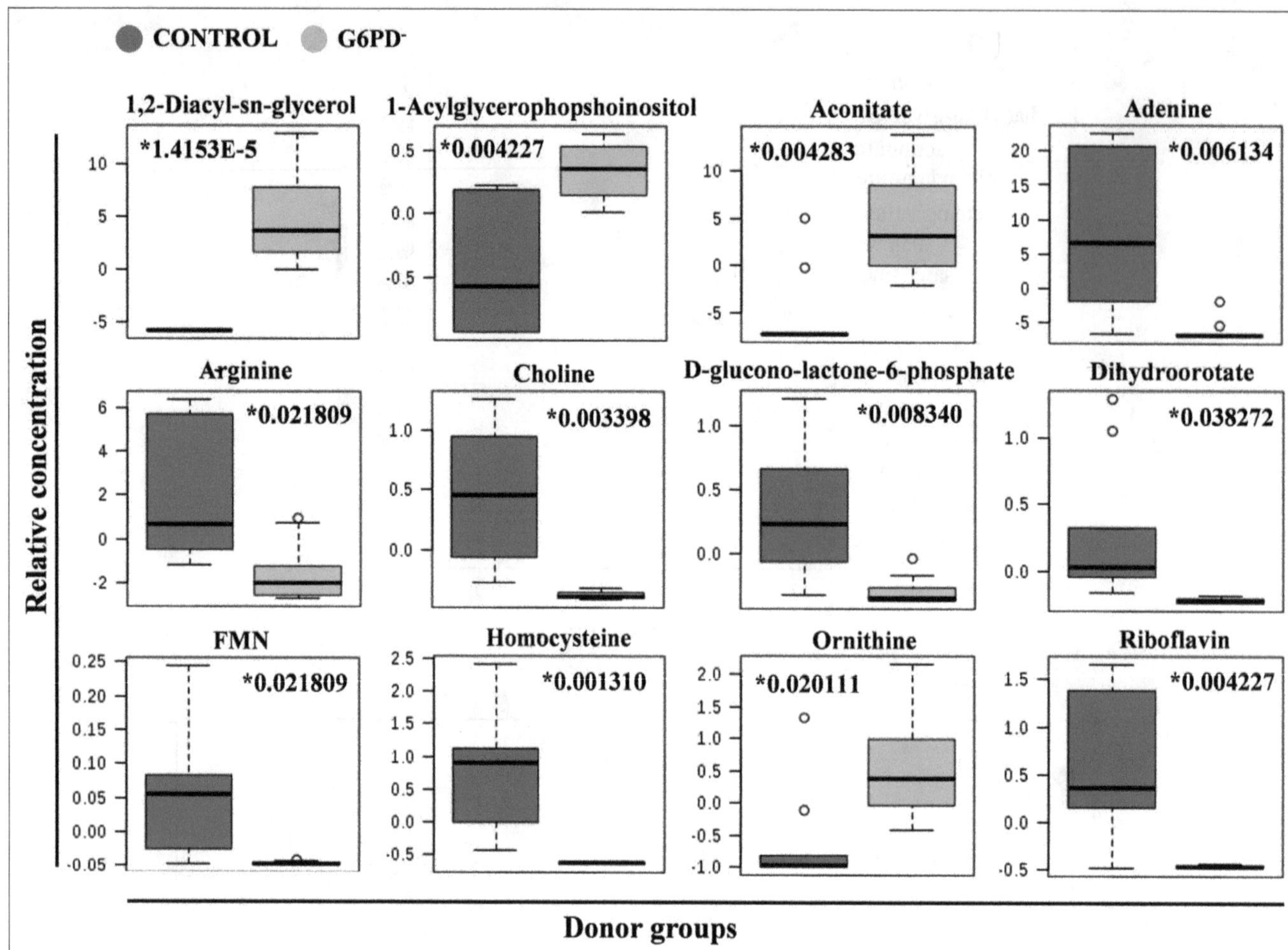

FIGURE 5 | Quantitative assessment of selected metabolites. Box and whisker plots for selected significantly altered metabolites in G6PD⁻ FFP compared with control (units in normalized and scaled concentrations). The *x*-axis shows the specific metabolite and the *y*-axis is the relative concentration. Medians are indicated by horizontal lines within each box. Outliers are plotted as individual points. Numbers with asterisks indicate adjusted *p*-values.

and aminoacids. Glutathione hub was related to glycolysis and arginine metabolism, glycerophospholipids, and aminoacids and finally, aconitate had connections with purine and arginine metabolism, lipids, and amino acids.

DISCUSSION

Human plasma has been often utilized in biomarker discovery studies because its molecular composition reflects the physiological state of donor's cells and tissues (12, 25). According to recent reports, inheritable omics variation among labile blood products, including FFP, may be associated with inter-donor differences observed in their quality, before and following transfusion (26). In similarity with the storage effect on blood components (27), G6PD$^-$ affects the glycolysis and the pentose phosphate pathways, and thus, the energy and redox status of cells. Since the "fluxome," namely, the transport properties of cell membrane, in G6PD$^-$ would interconnect the intracellular and plasma metabolomes (15), we used untargeted mass spectrometry-based metabolomics strategies to study the systemic metabolic effects of G6PD$^-$ on FFP used for transfusion in association with other physiological assessments, including the antioxidant capacity and the EV component, compared with G6PD$^+$ controls. To the best of our knowledge, this is the first study to show FFP metabolome and physiological changes related to G6PD$^-$.

Metabolomics and Physiological Analyses Supported the Low Level of Oxidative Defects Seen in G6PD$^-$ FFP Based on Uric Acid

G6PD$^-$ cells are extremely sensitive to the deleterious effects of oxidants. As a probable adaptation to this inherent danger, FFP from G6PD$^-$ donors was characterized by higher antioxidant capacity, which was mostly uric-acid-dependent. In fact, uric acid and its metabolic (allantoin, hypaxanthine) and physiological (antioxidant capacity) relatives constituted as high as 24% or 30% of the statistically significant correlations between the currently measured plasma variables in control and G6PD$^-$ FFPs, respectively, signifying the central role of purine

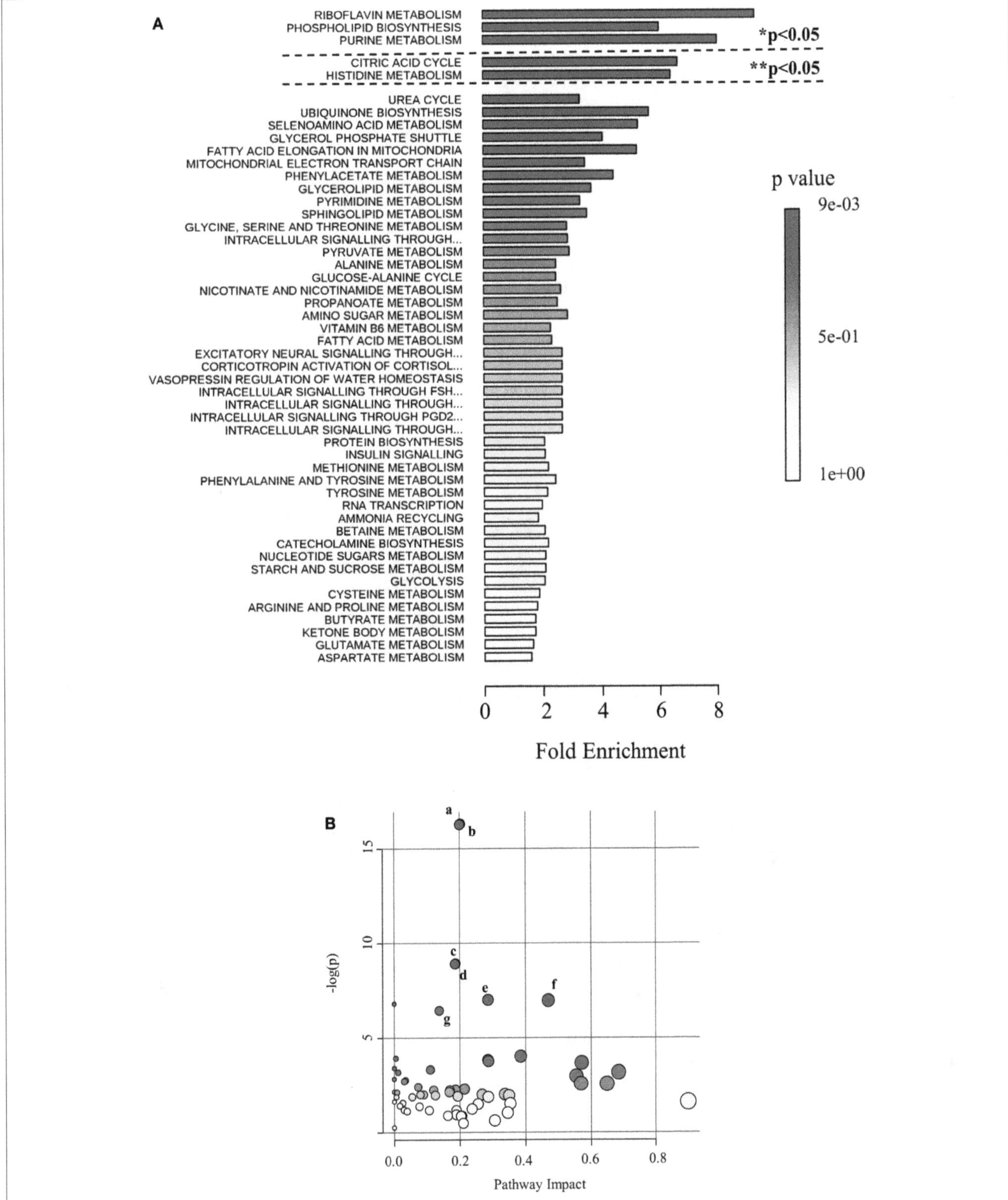

FIGURE 6 | Pathway analysis as generated by MetaboAnalyst software package. Identified metabolites and their relative quantity were used to calculate the enrichment and statistical significance. **(A)** Metabolite set enrichment analysis (MSEA). Top 50 perturbed pathways are shown. The dashed lines indicate the cutoff of the adjusted *p*-value (*Holm; ** FDR). **(B)** Metabolic pathway analysis (MetPA). All the matched pathways are displayed as circles. The color and size of each circle are based on *p*-value and pathway impact value, respectively. The most impacted pathways having high statistical significance scores are indicated with letters: a, glycerolipid metabolism; b, glycerophospholipid metabolism; c, purine metabolism; d, riboflavin metabolism; e, glyoxylate and dicarboxylate metabolism; f, tricarboxylic acid cycle; g, inositol phosphate metabolism.

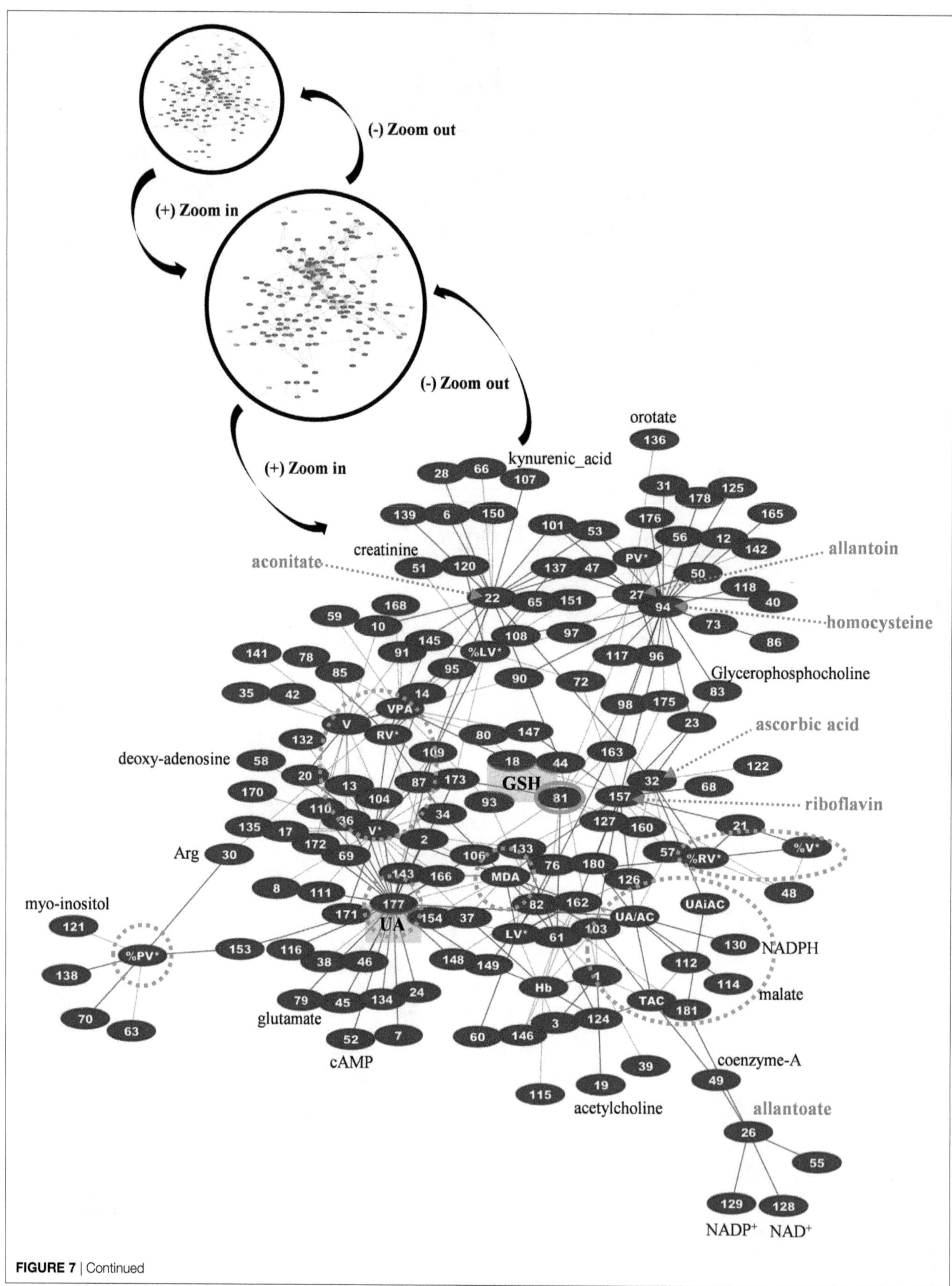

FIGURE 7 | Continued

FIGURE 7 | Network presentation of correlations among biochemical, physiological, and metabolomic variables in control FFP units. "Magnification" of a part of the total interactome of control fresh frozen plasma (FFP) units (networks in black circles) allowed focusing on the main connections between redox, EVs, and metabolic parameters. In the subnetwork of 266 connections (see Table S1 in Supplementary Material for code numbering and abbreviations), uric acid (UA), homocysteine, and reduced glutathione (GSH) constituted significant hub nodes, while ascorbic acid had correlations with the uric-acid-independent antioxidamt capacity of the FFP unit. Light blue dashed arrows indicate metabolites of high connectivity, and light blue circles stand for distinct groups of highly interconnected variables, or "boxes," corresponding to FFP EVs and antioxidant capacity. Only the statistical significant correlations at $p < 0.05$ are shown. The length of each line is inversely proportional to the *r* value of the correlation (the shorter the edge, the higher the *r* value). Red lines: positive correlations; gray lines: negative correlations.

metabolism in plasma homeostasis. The high-antioxidant capacity of FFP in G6PD⁻ is very reminiscent of the high small molecule antioxidant capacity found in the umbilical cord blood from G6PD⁻ newborns (28). Notably, the antioxidant capacity of fresh plasma in G6PD⁻ was found similar to that of G6PD⁺ plasma (29). Thus, our data suggest either a G6PD⁻ donor variation effect or an effect of preparation and storage manipulations on the antioxidant capacity, and likely on other features of the donated plasma, which renders it only in part analogous to the *in vivo* state.

G6PD⁻ FFP under investigation had normal levels of free hemoglobin (which otherwise might trigger oxidative reactions), and substantially lower oxidative modifications to both lipids and proteins. MDA units increase as a result of oxidative stress and according to previous studies (4), their levels are influenced by pre-analytical and donor-related factors. According to our results, G6PD⁻ represents a donor-related variable with significant effects on lipid peroxidation, protein carbonylation, membrane vesiculation, and metabolome of FFP, in addition to their "wiring" in biological networks. Lipid peroxidation had significant correlations with uric acid and riboflavin in control FFP samples and with glutathione, xanthine/hypoxanthine, adenine/adenosine, and DAG in G6PD⁻ samples.

The metabolomic assessment is in harmony with the substantially low lipid peroxidation in G6PD⁻ units. Underrepresentation of riboflavin in G6PD⁻ FFP, for instance, compared with the control FFP is likely the effect of its consumption in the context of a homeostatic antioxidant activity. This water-soluble vitamin is very effective in ameliorating oxidative stress, especially lipid peroxidation, through many molecular pathways, including reduction–oxidation reactions of the molecule itself and participation in the glutathione redox cycle (30). Riboflavin is a hub node in the network of control FFP, having strong correlation with lipid peroxidation, while in G6PD⁻ FFP it correlated with glycolysis metabolites and biotin, another vitamin involved in fatty-acid metabolism and amino-acid catabolism. In addition, riboflavin exhibits anti-inflammatory and neuroprotective effects and seems to be involved in immune-mediated clinical conditions like sepsis and multiple-organ failure (30). Apart from riboflavin, the high levels of aconitate may be associated with the redox homeostasis of G6PD⁻ FFP, since in both mouse model of human G6PD⁻ (31) and in Alzheimer's disease subjects (32) the activity of aconitase had correlations with the oxidative stress and the antioxidant protection. In our samples, aconitate was a hub node in both control and G6PD⁻ FFP networks, with significant correlations with the redox state of FFP (ascorbic acid, uric acid, lipid peroxidation), amino acids, lipids, and several metabolic pathways (glycolysis, purines, arginine). The increased antioxidant capacity but low riboflavin levels of G6PD⁻ FFP compared with control, which are reported for the first time, may be important for FFP recipients characterized by increased systemic oxidative stress, but this finding deserves further examination at clinical level.

Increased Red-Cell EVs and EV-Associated Procoagulant Activity in G6PD⁻ FFP

By affecting the redox potential, G6PD has a critical role in the development, cell survival, and apoptotic cell death (33). PS exposure and increased vesiculation rates characterize the surface of stressed, activated, or apoptotic cells (34). Indeed, higher concentration of circulating PS⁺ microparticles (both red-cell- and platelet-derived) was reported in G6PD⁻ subjects in close association with the severity of G6PD⁻ (35). In FFP, the population of EVs is a mixture of (ex-) circulating EVs and those produced during the preparation, storage, and thawing of the unit. In our study, their cellular origin was similar to that found in previous reports (4, 13). Despite the expected (13) profound donor-dependent variation in EV enumeration among FFP samples in both groups, the G6PD⁻ samples were characterized by invariably increased procoagulant activity and percentage of PS exposure mainly on red-cell- and platelet EVs, in consistence with previous studies showing enhanced PS exposure on circulating G6PD⁻ red cells (36). Moreover, these EVs were characterized by different protein composition compared with those isolated from control FFP, and probably by a different origin, as shown by the different pattern of Alix staining. The lower expression of stress protein markers in G6PD⁻ EVs, including oxidized Hb, heat shock protein 70, and clusterin (37), was in line with the higher antioxidant capacity of the G6PD⁻ FFP.

The PS- or tissue factor-exposing EVs are likely to have procoagulant activities (38) and of note, higher levels of coagulation cascade components have been detected by proteomics analyses in EVs released by G6PD⁻ stored RBCs in comparison to controls (36). Consequently, the FFP prepared by G6PD⁻ donors probably represents a unique case, where its EV-based hemostatic activity (38–40) is combined with a high-antioxidant capacity and low-oxidative defects. The baseline rate of EV generation is strongly modulated by the endogenous or exogenous oxidative stress levels and the capacity of the antioxidant machinery, under a wide variety of physiological and pathological conditions (41). Indeed, in both FFP groups, the extent of PS exposure on EVs had significant correlations with the levels of redox state components including lipid peroxidation, uric acid/allantoin, and ascorbic acid. Moreover, the concentration of PS⁺

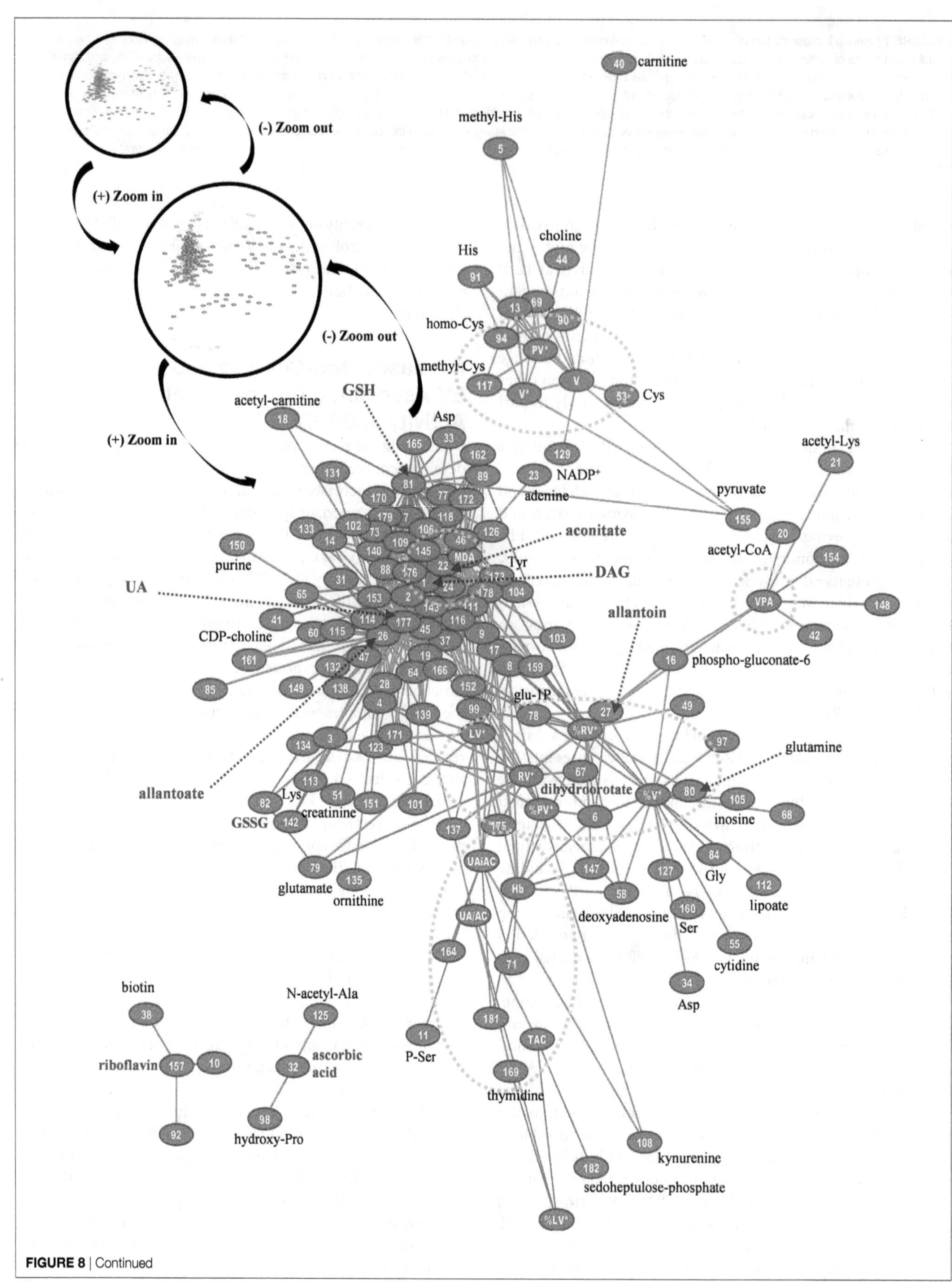

FIGURE 8 | Continued

FIGURE 8 | Topological presentation of correlations between biochemical, physiological and metabolomic variables in G6PD⁻ fresh frozen plasma (FFP) units. Starting from the total G6PD⁻ network (shown in black circles) and by using continuous "zoom in" tools we studied the main connections between redox, EVs, and metabolic parameters. This subnetwork was bigger and quite different compared with that of control FFP. It consisted of 434 connections (see Table S1 in Supplementary Material for code numbering and abbreviations), and while uric acid is also a hub node, diacylglycerol (DAG), lipid peroxidation (MDA), allantoate, aconitate, and reduced glutathione (GSH) have substantially more connections. The red dashed arrows indicate metabolites of high connectivity, and the yellow dashed circles stand for "boxes" of distinct groups of interconnected variables that correspond to the core of the network, FFP EVs, and antioxidant capacity. Only the statistical significant correlations at $p < 0.05$ are shown. The length of each line is inversely proportional to the *r* value of the correlation (the shorter the edge, the higher the *r* value). Green lines: positive correlations; Gray lines: negative correlations.

EVs seemed to have correlations with the levels of adenosine, amino acids, and energy metabolism, despite the fact that the individual components differed between the two groups (e.g., lactate instead of pyruvate). RBC vesiculation and EV-related procoagulant activity, which was assessed by thrombin generation *in vitro*, were found especially increased in G6PD⁻, in close association with adenosine, pentose phosphate pathway, and purine metabolism variants, showing a diverse pattern of wiring compared with the control FFP, in which ascorbic acid, lipids, and lipid modifications were more influential.

Main Metabolic Changes in G6PD⁻ FFP with Probable Impact on Signaling

The main metabolic profile of G6PD⁻ FFP reflects to some extent a systemic cellular response to G6PD⁻, as revealed, for example, by the deficiency in gluconolactone-6-phosphate. Favic response in G6PD⁻ mice includes alterations in a similar group of plasma (e.g., ornithine) and liver (e.g., phosphoglycerols and adenine) metabolites (42). Apart from riboflavin metabolism, purine metabolism, arginine metabolism/urea cycle components, and phospholipid biosynthesis constituted the most significant differences between the G6PD⁻ and G6PD⁺ FFP units. Indeed, increased levels of ornithine were found in G6PD⁻ FFP at the expense of L-arginine, suggesting increased energy consumption/waste by the G6PD⁻ cells (43).

The significantly low extracellular levels of the purine derivative adenine in the G6PD⁻ FFP verify the previously suggested strong positive correlation of plasma adenosine (adenine nucleoside) levels with glycolysis (44, 45). RBCs, in particular, use extracellular purines to maintain their intracellular nucleotide pool and to exploit the pentose moiety for energy production. More importantly, this finding suggested a different dynamics in purinergic signaling, since purinergic receptors are widely expressed in almost every cell type, including erythrocytes (46). Adenosine arising by the metabolism of extracellular nucleotides can transmit signals through G-protein-coupled receptors and anti-inflammatory adenosine (P1 purinergic) receptors (47). Extracellular adenosine signaling serves regulatory functions in inflammation, in acute lung injury (48) and in the O_2 delivery ability of red cell targets through boosting the production of 2,3-BPG (46). Nucleoside transporters assist in the control of plasma adenosine levels, and notably, decreased nucleoside transporter hENT1 [that also mediates hypoxanthine transport (49)] expression and activity was detected in G6PD⁻ RBCs (50). In G6PD⁻ FFP, adenosine was correlated with red-cell vesiculation, lipid peroxidation, hemolysis, DAG, oxidized glutathione, and uric acid/allantoate levels, suggesting more influential effects compared with the control FFP and a second level of intercellular signaling potential.

Aberrations in glycerolipid biosynthesis have been associated with G6PD⁻ from nematodes to humans (51). Increased activity of phospholipase A2 is observed during eryptosis which is enhanced in G6PD⁻ subjects (52). As a probable result of lower NAPDH, which is used in the reductive biosynthesis of fatty acids and cholesterol (53), lower cholesterol content (54), and clear differences in the lipid repertoire, biosynthesis and metabolism were detected between the Mediterranean type G6PD⁻ and control red cells both *in vivo* and during refrigerated storage (55). Notably, the levels of free fatty acids and oxidized derivatives were found significantly lower in stored G6PD⁻ compared with control red cells.

The presence of the highly hydrophobic DAG extracellularly was not expected. DAG has significant signaling potential that is exerted, however, at cell and subcellular membranes loci. Despite that, targeted lipidomics analysis revealed increased levels of DAG in the plasma of Alzheimer's disease patients (56), a clinical condition with indirect, however strong, pathophysiological connections with the G6PD activity. In fact, G6PD⁻ predisposes to a variety of chronic neurological diseases by undermining the defenses against the endogenous ROS-mediated neurodegeneration during aging (57). The high oxygen concentration and fatty acids levels but low antioxidant activity in brain tissue render it highly susceptible to peroxidation and oxidative damage (58). While DAG was a minor component of the control FFP network, it was the central hub node in the G6PD⁻ network, showing numerous direct connections with glycerophospholipid biosynthesis, amino acids, and components of glycolysis, glutathione, purine, glutamate, and arginine pathways, and indirect connections with the EVs through choline, purine, and glycolysis pathways metabolites.

Partitioning of DAG into the circulating vesicles may account for its detection in biological fluids in primary G6PD⁻ and in G6PD-related clinical conditions, principally characterized by enhanced release of EVs. While exosomes are not enriched in DAG compared with the cell membrane of origin (59), DAG is a component of urinary exosomes (60, 61), and of mesenchymal stem-cell-derived EVs (62). Of note, DAG and DAG-kinase have critical role in the polarized secretion of exosomes in T and B (and probably in other kinds of) cells (63). The putative DAG-bearing exosomes in G6PD⁻ FFP may transfer powerful signaling hits to target cells through fusion or endocytosis, especially in neuronal and immune tissues that principally express the targeting molecules (namely, the C1 domain-containing proteins) (64). FFP DAG may be arisen from the hydrolysis of phosphatidic acid produced by the activity of exosomal phospholipase D (65) on extracellular phosphatidylcholine, which is quite probable, since choline—the second product of phosphatidylcholine hydrolysis by phospholipase D—was extremely low in G6PD$^-$ FFP. In the same context, the levels of 1-acylglycerophosphoinositol (that is formed *via* cytidine diphosphate-DAG by reaction with inositol) were found substantially increased compared with control samples.

CONCLUSION

The metabolome and several physiological features of FFP units prepared from donors with G6PD$^-$ differ compared with control FFP. Higher EV-related procoagulant activity, PS concentration, red-cell vesiculation, and antioxidant capacity, along with lower oxidative modifications in lipids and proteins were detected in G6PD$^-$ FFP than in G6PD$^+$ units. The EVs of G6PD$^-$ FFP further varied in number, cell origin, lipid and protein composition, and probably, in generation pathway. Metabolomics analysis revealed that riboflavin metabolism, purine metabolism, and glycerolipid/glycerophospholipid biosynthesis constitute the most significant variances between the two groups of FFP. Units prepared from G6PD$^-$ donors had excess of DAGs, glycerophosphoinositol, aconitate, and ornithine but they were deficient in riboflavin, flavin mononucleotide, adenine, and arginine, among others. Certain FFP-needed patients may be at greatest benefit of receiving units from G6PD$^-$ donors, intrinsically endowed by both procoagulant and antioxidant activities and low oxidative defects. However, the clinical outcome is likely affected by various other preparation and donor/recipient-related factors (4), including the signaling potential of the differentially expressed metabolites and EVs, the degree of G6PD$^-$, the redox status in the recipient, the amount of FFP units transfused, the leukoreduction (66), and probably, the storage interval of the FFP (13). All these parameters deserve further investigation by large-scale laboratory and clinical studies.

ETHICS STATEMENT

The study was approved by the Ethics Committee of the Department of Biology, School of Science, NKUA. Investigations were carried out upon signing of written consent in accordance with the principles of the Declaration of Helsinki.

AUTHOR CONTRIBUTIONS

SR and MA designed the study. VT performed the biochemical and ELISA assays. HG performed the immunoblots. AK performed the flow cytometry analysis. FG and SR performed the UHPLC-MS analyses. VT, FG, SR, and MA analyzed the results, prepared the figures, and wrote the manuscript. LZ and IP critically commented on the interpretation of data and drafting of the manuscript. All the authors contributed to the final version.

ACKNOWLEDGMENTS

The authors thank Dr Leontini E. Foudoulaki-Paparizos MD pathologist, former Director of the "Agios Panteleimon" General Hospital of Nikea Blood Transfusion Center, for the recruitment of the G6PD-deficient volunteers. Dr Giuseppina Fanelli is acknowledged for her support in LC-MS runs. The authors also thank Ms Artemis Voulgaridou, MSc, for the valuable assistance in the network analysis, as well as the MSc student Alkmini Anastasiadi and the graduate students Tzeni Krespa and Zafeirios Kardaras for their kind contribution in the gel electrophoresis and immunoblotting experiments.

REFERENCES

1. O'Shaughnessy DF, Atterbury C, Bolton Maggs P, Murphy M, Thomas D, Yates S, et al. Guidelines for the use of fresh-frozen plasma, cryoprecipitate and cryosupernatant. *Br J Haematol* (2004) 126(1):11–28. doi:10.1111/j.1365-2141.2004.04972.x
2. Farrugia A. Plasma for fractionation: safety and quality issues. *Haemophilia* (2004) 10(4):334–40. doi:10.1111/j.1365-2516.2004.00911.x
3. Lawrie AS, Harrison P, Cardigan RA, Mackie IJ. The characterization and impact of microparticles on haemostasis within fresh-frozen plasma. *Vox Sang* (2008) 95(3):197–204. doi:10.1111/j.1423-0410.2008.01081.x
4. Sparrow RL, Chan KS. Microparticle content of plasma for transfusion is influenced by the whole blood hold conditions: pre-analytical considerations for proteomic investigations. *J Proteomics* (2012) 76:SecNo:211–9. doi:10.1016/j.jprot.2012.07.013
5. van 't Erve TJ, Doskey CM, Wagner BA, Hess JR, Darbro BW, Ryckman KK, et al. Heritability of glutathione and related metabolites in stored red blood cells. *Free Radic Biol Med* (2014) 76:107–13. doi:10.1016/j.freeradbiomed.2014.07.040
6. Tzounakas VL, Georgatzakou HT, Kriebardis AG, Voulgaridou AI, Stamoulis KE, Foudoulaki-Paparizos LE, et al. Donor variation effect on red blood cell storage lesion: a multivariable, yet consistent, story. *Transfusion* (2016) 56(6):1274–86. doi:10.1111/trf.13582
7. Tzounakas VL, Anastasiadi AT, Karadimas DG, Zeqo RA, Georgatzakou HT, Pappa OD, et al. Temperature-dependent haemolytic propensity of CPDA-1 stored red blood cells vs whole blood—red cell fragility as donor signature on blood units. *Blood Transfus* (2017) 15(5):447–55. doi:10.2450/2017.0332-16
8. Dinkla S, Peppelman M, Van Der Raadt J, Atsma F, Novotny VM, Van Kraaij MG, et al. Phosphatidylserine exposure on stored red blood cells as a parameter for donor-dependent variation in product quality. *Blood Transfus* (2014) 12(2):204–9. doi:10.2450/2013.0106-13
9. Tzounakas VL, Karadimas DG, Anastasiadi AT, Georgatzakou HT, Kazepidou E, Moschovas D, et al. Donor-specific individuality of red blood cell performance during storage is partly a function of serum uric acid levels. *Transfusion* (2018) 58(1):34–40. doi:10.1111/trf.14379
10. Tzounakas VL, Georgatzakou HT, Kriebardis AG, Papageorgiou EG, Stamoulis KE, Foudoulaki-Paparizos LE, et al. Uric acid variation among regular blood donors is indicative of red blood cell susceptibility to storage lesion markers: a new hypothesis tested. *Transfusion* (2015) 55(11):2659–71. doi:10.1111/trf.13211
11. Bardyn M, Maye S, Lesch A, Delobel J, Tissot JD, Cortes-Salazar F, et al. The antioxidant capacity of erythrocyte concentrates is increased during the first week of storage and correlated with the uric acid level. *Vox Sang* (2017) 112(7):638–47. doi:10.1111/vox.12563
12. Bowler RP, Jacobson S, Cruickshank C, Hughes GJ, Siska C, Ory DS, et al. Plasma sphingolipids associated with chronic obstructive pulmonary disease

phenotypes. *Am J Respir Crit Care Med* (2015) 191(3):275–84. doi:10.1164/rccm.201410-1771OC

13. Kriebardis AG, Antonelou MH, Georgatzakou HT, Tzounakas VL, Stamoulis KE, Papassideri IS. Microparticles variability in fresh frozen plasma: preparation protocol and storage time effects. *Blood Transfus* (2016) 14(2):228–37. doi:10.2450/2016.0179-15
14. Tzounakas VL, Kriebardis AG, Papassideri IS, Antonelou MH. Donor-variation effect on red blood cell storage lesion: a close relationship emerges. *Proteomics Clin Appl* (2016) 10(8):791–804. doi:10.1002/prca.201500128
15. Bosman GJ. The involvement of erythrocyte metabolism in organismal homeostasis in health and disease. *Proteomics Clin Appl* (2016) 10(8):774–7. doi:10.1002/prca.201500129
16. Pamba A, Richardson ND, Carter N, Duparc S, Premji Z, Tiono AB, et al. Clinical spectrum and severity of hemolytic anemia in glucose 6-phosphate dehydrogenase-deficient children receiving dapsone. *Blood* (2012) 120(20):4123–33. doi:10.1182/blood-2012-03-416032
17. Roback JD, Grossman BJ, Harris T, Hillyer CD. *AABB Technical Manual*. 17th ed. Bethesda, MD: AABB (2011).
18. Duplancic D, Kukoc-Modun L, Modun D, Radic N. Simple and rapid method for the determination of uric acid-independent antioxidant capacity. *Molecules* (2011) 16(8):7058–68. doi:10.3390/molecules16087058
19. Benzie IF, Strain JJ. The ferric reducing ability of plasma (FRAP) as a measure of "antioxidant power": the FRAP assay. *Anal Biochem* (1996) 239(1):70–6. doi:10.1006/abio.1996.0292
20. Antonelou MH, Tzounakas VL, Velentzas AD, Stamoulis KE, Kriebardis AG, Papassideri IS. Effects of pre-storage leukoreduction on stored red blood cells signaling: a time-course evaluation from shape to proteome. *J Proteomics* (2012) 76:SecNo:220–38. doi:10.1016/j.jprot.2012.06.032
21. Melamud E, Vastag L, Rabinowitz JD. Metabolomic analysis and visualization engine for LC-MS data. *Anal Chem* (2010) 82(23):9818–26. doi:10.1021/ac1021166
22. Raposo G, Stoorvogel W. Extracellular vesicles: exosomes, microvesicles, and friends. *J Cell Biol* (2013) 200(4):373–83. doi:10.1083/jcb.201211138
23. Giulivi C, Napoli E, Tassone F, Halmai J, Hagerman R. Plasma metabolic profile delineates roles for neurodegeneration, pro-inflammatory damage and mitochondrial dysfunction in the FMR1 premutation. *Biochem J* (2016) 473(21):3871–88. doi:10.1042/BCJ20160585
24. Chung WY, Benzie IF. Plasma allantoin measurement by isocratic liquid chromatography with tandem mass spectrometry: method evaluation and application in oxidative stress biomonitoring. *Clin Chim Acta* (2013) 424:237–44. doi:10.1016/j.cca.2013.06.015
25. Patti GJ, Yanes O, Siuzdak G. Innovation: metabolomics: the apogee of the omics trilogy. *Nat Rev Mol Cell Biol* (2012) 13(4):263–9. doi:10.1038/nrm3314
26. Weisenhorn EM, van T Erve TJ, Riley NM, Hess JR, Raife TJ, Coon JJ. Multi-omics evidence for inheritance of energy pathways in red blood cells. *Mol Cell Proteomics* (2016) 15(12):3614–23. doi:10.1074/mcp.M116.062349
27. D'Alessandro A, Nemkov T, Kelher M, West FB, Schwindt RK, Banerjee A, et al. Routine storage of red blood cell (RBC) units in additive solution-3: a comprehensive investigation of the RBC metabolome. *Transfusion* (2015) 55(6):1155–68. doi:10.1111/trf.12975
28. Stadem PS, Hilgers MV, Bengo D, Cusick SE, Ndidde S, Slusher TM, et al. Markers of oxidative stress in umbilical cord blood from G6PD deficient African newborns. *PLoS One* (2017) 12(2):e0172980. doi:10.1371/journal.pone.0172980
29. Tzounakas VL, Kriebardis AG, Georgatzakou HT, Foudoulaki-Paparizos LE, Dzieciatkowska M, Wither MJ, et al. Data on how several physiological parameters of stored red blood cells are similar in glucose 6-phosphate dehydrogenase deficient and sufficient donors. *Data Brief* (2016) 8:618–27. doi:10.1016/j.dib.2016.06.018
30. Marashly ET, Bohlega SA. Riboflavin has neuroprotective potential: focus on Parkinson's disease and migraine. *Front Neurol* (2017) 8:333. doi:10.3389/fneur.2017.00333
31. Hecker PA, Lionetti V, Ribeiro RF Jr, Rastogi S, Brown BH, O'Connell KA, et al. Glucose 6-phosphate dehydrogenase deficiency increases redox stress and moderately accelerates the development of heart failure. *Circ Heart Fail* (2013) 6(1):118–26. doi:10.1161/CIRCHEARTFAILURE.112.969576
32. Mangialasche F, Baglioni M, Cecchetti R, Kivipelto M, Ruggiero C, Piobbico D, et al. Lymphocytic mitochondrial aconitase activity is reduced in Alzheimer's disease and mild cognitive impairment. *J Alzheimers Dis* (2015) 44(2):649–60. doi:10.3233/JAD-142052
33. Tian WN, Braunstein LD, Apse K, Pang J, Rose M, Tian X, et al. Importance of glucose-6-phosphate dehydrogenase activity in cell death. *Am J Physiol* (1999) 276(5 Pt 1):C1121–31. doi:10.1152/ajpcell.1999.276.5.C1121
34. Zwaal RF, Comfurius P, Bevers EM. Surface exposure of phosphatidylserine in pathological cells. *Cell Mol Life Sci* (2005) 62(9):971–88. doi:10.1007/s00018-005-4527-3
35. Nantakomol D, Palasuwan A, Chaowanathikhom M, Soogarun S, Imwong M. Red cell and platelet-derived microparticles are increased in G6PD-deficient subjects. *Eur J Haematol* (2012) 89(5):423–9. doi:10.1111/ejh.12010
36. Tzounakas VL, Kriebardis AG, Georgatzakou HT, Foudoulaki-Paparizos LE, Dzieciatkowska M, Wither MJ, et al. Glucose 6-phosphate dehydrogenase deficient subjects may be better "storers" than donors of red blood cells. *Free Radic Biol Med* (2016) 96:152–65. doi:10.1016/j.freeradbiomed.2016.04.005
37. Antonelou MH, Kriebardis AG, Stamoulis KE, Trougakos IP, Papassideri IS. Apolipoprotein J/clusterin in human erythrocytes is involved in the molecular process of defected material disposal during vesiculation. *PLoS One* (2011) 6(10):e26033. doi:10.1371/journal.pone.0026033
38. Kriebardis A, Antonelou M, Stamoulis K, Papassideri I. Cell-derived microparticles in stored blood products: innocent-bystanders or effective mediators of post-transfusion reactions? *Blood Transfus* (2012) 10(Suppl 2):s25–38. doi:10.2450/2012.006S
39. Jy W, Johansen ME, Bidot C Jr, Horstman LL, Ahn YS. Red cell-derived microparticles (RMP) as haemostatic agent. *Thromb Haemost* (2013) 110(4):751–60. doi:10.1160/TH12-12-0941
40. Matijevic N, Kostousov V, Wang YW, Wade CE, Wang W, Letourneau P, et al. Multiple levels of degradation diminish hemostatic potential of thawed plasma. *J Trauma* (2011) 70(1):71–9; discussion 9–80. doi:10.1097/TA.0b013e318207abec
41. Rinalducci S, Zolla L. Biochemistry of storage lesions of red cell and platelet concentrates: a continuous fight implying oxidative/nitrosative/phosphorylative stress and signaling. *Transfus Apher Sci* (2015) 52(3):262–9. doi:10.1016/j.transci.2015.04.005
42. Xiao M, Du G, Zhong G, Yan D, Zeng H, Cai W. Gas chromatography/mass spectrometry-based metabolomic profiling reveals alterations in mouse plasma and liver in response to Fava Beans. *PLoS One* (2016) 11(3):e0151103. doi:10.1371/journal.pone.0151103
43. Brosnan JT, Brosnan ME. Creatine metabolism and the urea cycle. *Mol Genet Metab* (2010) 100(Suppl 1):S49–52. doi:10.1016/j.ymgme.2010.02.020
44. D'Alessandro A, Nemkov T, Sun K, Liu H, Song A, Monte AA, et al. AltitudeOmics: red blood cell metabolic adaptation to high altitude hypoxia. *J Proteome Res* (2016) 15(10):3883–95. doi:10.1021/acs.jproteome.6b00733
45. Liu H, Zhang Y, Wu H, D'Alessandro A, Yegutkin GG, Song A, et al. Beneficial role of erythrocyte adenosine A2B receptor-mediated AMP-activated protein kinase activation in high-altitude hypoxia. *Circulation* (2016) 134(5):405–21. doi:10.1161/CIRCULATIONAHA.116.021311
46. Sun K, D'Alessandro A, Xia Y. Purinergic control of red blood cell metabolism: novel strategies to improve red cell storage quality. *Blood Transfus* (2017) 15(6):535–42. doi:10.2450/2017.0366-16
47. Cekic C, Linden J. Purinergic regulation of the immune system. *Nat Rev Immunol* (2016) 16(3):177–92. doi:10.1038/nri.2016.4
48. Eckle T, Koeppen M, Eltzschig HK. Role of extracellular adenosine in acute lung injury. *Physiology (Bethesda)* (2009) 24:298–306. doi:10.1152/physiol.00022.2009
49. Young JD, Yao SY, Sun L, Cass CE, Baldwin SA. Human equilibrative nucleoside transporter (ENT) family of nucleoside and nucleobase transporter proteins. *Xenobiotica* (2008) 38(7–8):995–1021. doi:10.1080/00498250801927427
50. Al-Ansari M, Craik JD. Decreased erythrocyte nucleoside transport and hENT1 transporter expression in glucose 6-phosphate dehydrogenase deficiency. *BMC Hematol* (2015) 15:17. doi:10.1186/s12878-015-0038-0
51. Chen TL, Yang HC, Hung CY, Ou MH, Pan YY, Cheng ML, et al. Impaired embryonic development in glucose-6-phosphate dehydrogenase-deficient *Caenorhabditis elegans* due to abnormal redox homeostasis induced activation of calcium-independent phospholipase and alteration of glycerophospholipid metabolism. *Cell Death Dis* (2017) 8(1):e2545. doi:10.1038/cddis.2016.463

52. Briglia M, Antonia Rossi M, Faggio C. Eryptosis: ally or enemy. *Curr Med Chem* (2017) 24(9):937–42. doi:10.2174/0929867324666161118142425.
53. Park J, Rho HK, Kim KH, Choe SS, Lee YS, Kim JB. Overexpression of glucose-6-phosphate dehydrogenase is associated with lipid dysregulation and insulin resistance in obesity. *Mol Cell Biol* (2005) 25(12):5146–57. doi:10.1128/MCB.25.12.5146-5157.2005
54. Rice-Evans C, Rush J, Omorphos SC, Flynn DM. Erythrocyte membrane abnormalities in glucose-6-phosphate dehydrogenase deficiency of the Mediterranean and A-types. *FEBS Lett* (1981) 136(1):148–52. doi:10.1016/0014-5793(81)81235-5
55. Reisz JA, Tzounakas VL, Nemkov T, Voulgaridou AI, Papassideri IS, Kriebardis AG, et al. Metabolic linkage and correlations to storage capacity in erythrocytes from glucose 6-phosphate dehydrogenase-deficient donors. *Front. Med* (2018). doi:10.3389/fmed.2017.00248
56. Wood PL, Medicherla S, Sheikh N, Terry B, Phillipps A, Kaye JA, et al. Targeted lipidomics of fontal cortex and plasma diacylglycerols (DAG) in mild cognitive impairment and Alzheimer's disease: validation of DAG accumulation early in the pathophysiology of Alzheimer's disease. *J Alzheimers Dis* (2015) 48(2):537–46. doi:10.3233/JAD-150336
57. Jeng W, Loniewska MM, Wells PG. Brain glucose-6-phosphate dehydrogenase protects against endogenous oxidative DNA damage and neurodegeneration in aged mice. *ACS Chem Neurosci* (2013) 4(7):1123–32. doi:10.1021/cn400079y
58. Uttara B, Singh AV, Zamboni P, Mahajan RT. Oxidative stress and neurodegenerative diseases: a review of upstream and downstream antioxidant therapeutic options. *Curr Neuropharmacol* (2009) 7(1):65–74. doi:10.2174/157015909787602823
59. Laulagnier K, Motta C, Hamdi S, Roy S, Fauvelle F, Pageaux JF, et al. Mast cell- and dendritic cell-derived exosomes display a specific lipid composition and an unusual membrane organization. *Biochem J* (2004) 380(Pt 1):161–71. doi:10.1042/BJ20031594
60. Skotland T, Ekroos K, Kauhanen D, Simolin H, Seierstad T, Berge V, et al. Molecular lipid species in urinary exosomes as potential prostate cancer biomarkers. *Eur J Cancer* (2017) 70:122–32. doi:10.1016/j.ejca.2016.10.011
61. Yang JS, Lee JC, Byeon SK, Rha KH, Moon MH. Size dependent lipidomic analysis of urinary exosomes from patients with prostate cancer by flow field-flow fractionation and nanoflow liquid chromatography-tandem mass spectrometry. *Anal Chem* (2017) 89(4):2488–96. doi:10.1021/acs.analchem.6b04634
62. Zhang X, Tu H, Yang Y, Fang L, Wu Q, Li J. Mesenchymal stem cell-derived extracellular vesicles: roles in tumor growth, progression, and drug resistance. *Stem Cells Int* (2017) 2017:1758139. doi:10.1155/2017/1758139
63. Alonso R, Mazzeo C, Rodriguez MC, Marsh M, Fraile-Ramos A, Calvo V, et al. Diacylglycerol kinase alpha regulates the formation and polarisation of mature multivesicular bodies involved in the secretion of Fas ligand-containing exosomes in T lymphocytes. *Cell Death Differ* (2011) 18(7):1161–73. doi:10.1038/cdd.2010.184
64. Almena M, Merida I. Shaping up the membrane: diacylglycerol coordinates spatial orientation of signaling. *Trends Biochem Sci* (2011) 36(11):593–603. doi:10.1016/j.tibs.2011.06.005
65. Laulagnier K, Grand D, Dujardin A, Hamdi S, Vincent-Schneider H, Lankar D, et al. PLD2 is enriched on exosomes and its activity is correlated to the release of exosomes. *FEBS Lett* (2004) 572(1–3):11–4. doi:10.1016/j.febslet.2004.06.082
66. Chan KS, Sparrow RL. Microparticle profile and procoagulant activity of fresh-frozen plasma is affected by whole blood leukoreduction rather than 24-hour room temperature hold. *Transfusion* (2014) 54(8):1935–44. doi:10.1111/trf.12602

3

Metabolic Linkage and Correlations to Storage Capacity in Erythrocytes from Glucose 6-Phosphate Dehydrogenase-Deficient Donors

Julie A. Reisz[1†], Vassilis L. Tzounakas[2†], Travis Nemkov[1], Artemis I. Voulgaridou[3], Issidora S. Papassideri[2], Anastasios G. Kriebardis[4], Angelo D'Alessandro[1*] and Marianna H. Antonelou[2]*

[1] Department of Biochemistry and Molecular Genetics, School of Medicine, University of Colorado, Aurora, CO, United States, [2] Department of Biology, School of Science, National and Kapodistrian University of Athens, Athens, Greece, [3] "Apostle Paul" Educational Institution, Thessaloniki, Greece, [4] Department of Medical Laboratories, Faculty of Health and Caring Professions, Technological and Educational Institute of Athens, Athens, Greece

***Correspondence:**
Anastasios G. Kriebardis
akrieb@biol.uoa.gr,
akrieb@teiath.gr;
Angelo D'Alessandro
angelo.dalessandro@ucdenver.edu

†These authors are equal first authors.

Objective: In glucose 6-phosphate dehydrogenase (G6PD) deficiency, decreased NADPH regeneration in the pentose phosphate pathway and subnormal levels of reduced glutathione result in insufficient antioxidant defense, increased susceptibility of red blood cells (RBCs) to oxidative stress, and acute hemolysis following exposure to pro-oxidant drugs and infections. Despite the fact that redox disequilibrium is a prominent feature of RBC storage lesion, it has been reported that the G6PD-deficient RBCs store well, at least in respect to energy metabolism, but their overall metabolic phenotypes and molecular linkages to the storability profile are scarcely investigated.

Methods: We performed UHPLC-MS metabolomics analyses of weekly sampled RBC concentrates from G6PD sufficient and deficient donors, stored in citrate phosphate dextrose/saline adenine glucose mannitol from day 0 to storage day 42, followed by statistical and bioinformatics integration of the data.

Results: Other than previously reported alterations in glycolysis, metabolomics analyses revealed bioactive lipids, free fatty acids, bile acids, amino acids, and purines as top variables discriminating RBC concentrates for G6PD-deficient donors. Two-way ANOVA showed significant changes in the storage-dependent variation in fumarate, one-carbon, and sulfur metabolism, glutathione homeostasis, and antioxidant defense (including urate) components in G6PD-deficient vs. sufficient donors. The levels of free fatty acids and their oxidized derivatives, as well as those of membrane-associated plasticizers were significantly lower in G6PD-deficient units in comparison to controls. By using the strongest correlations between *in vivo* and *ex vivo* metabolic and physiological parameters, consecutively present throughout the storage period, several interactomes were produced that revealed an interesting interplay between redox, energy, and hemolysis variables, which may be further associated with donor-specific differences in the post-transfusion performance of G6PD-deficient RBCs.

Conclusion: The metabolic phenotypes of G6PD-deficient donors recapitulate the basic storage lesion profile that leads to loss of metabolic linkage and rewiring. Donor-related issues affect the storability of RBCs even in the narrow context of this donor subgroup in a way likely relevant to transfusion medicine.

Keywords: glucose 6-phosphate dehydrogenase deficiency, transfusion medicine, red blood cell storage lesion, donor variation, mass spectrometry, metabolomics, interactome

INTRODUCTION

Routine storage of packed red blood cells (RBCs) in the blood bank is a logistic necessity that makes ~110 millions of units available for life-saving transfusions to millions of recipients worldwide every year. Storage in the blood bank is associated with the progressive accumulation of a series of biochemical and morphological alterations to RBCs collectively referred to as the storage lesion (1, 2). Deranged metabolic homeostasis of stored RBCs is a heritable trait, i.e., it is affected—like hemolysis—by the donor's genetic background (3–5). The metabolic storage lesion can be cursorily summarized in two main components, i.e., decreased energy metabolism and increased oxidative stress (6–10). Despite laboratory observations suggesting that old blood may be associated with poorer transfusion outcomes, reassuring evidence from randomized clinical trials has been generated to support the overall safety and efficacy of current transfusion practices (11). The apparent disconnect on the age of blood issue between laboratory observations and randomized clinical trials is in part reconciled by the appreciation of the many confounding factors affecting the interpretation of prospective clinical trials and limited size of cohorts tested in most basic science/laboratory studies. Introduction of high-throughput omics technologies and combination of omics results with functional outcomes (12) has fostered a new era in the field of transfusion medicine where the focus has been shifted from the final product to the donor (13–15) and the intrinsic variability across the donor population. Animal studies further strengthened this conclusion, reporting that while not all (mouse strain) donor RBCs store similarly (16), transfusion of RBCs from different (mouse strain) donors may result in a "good apple/bad apple" effect (17), further increasing the complexity of the donor/recipient system and increasing the noise of clinical studies where exclusively and consistently young or old blood is hardly ever transfused to the same recipient (18). In humans, factors such as donor age, ethnicity, and gender ultimately affect RBC storability (influencing parameters such as hemolysis or oxidative stress-induced hemolysis) (12). Gender in particular may be an underestimated confounder (19).

Glucose 6-phosphate dehydrogenase (G6PD) deficiency is an X-linked (20) recessive inborn error of metabolism that affects ~400 million individuals worldwide and results in impaired antioxidant capacity. Indeed, carriers of G6PD-deficient traits are characterized by a reduced capacity to generate antioxidant equivalents (i.e., NADPH) through the pentose phosphate pathway (PPP), which in turn results in an increased susceptibility to hemolysis. As oxidative stress has been considered an etiological contributor to the RBC storage lesion, it has been anticipated that RBCs from G6PD-deficient donors may suffer from exacerbated alterations during storage in the blood bank (21). While clinical evidence on the issue is still missing, preliminary omics studies have revealed that RBCs from G6PD-deficient donors unexpectedly better preserve energy homeostasis and morphology during storage in the blood bank though they are increasingly more susceptible to temperature and oxidative stress-induced hemolysis than stored RBCs from G6PD sufficient donors (22, 23). In that preliminary study, we focused specifically on glycolysis and the PPP. However, Tang and colleagues (24) recently showed that RBCs from G6PD-deficient donors challenged with pro-oxidant stimuli such as diamide are characterized by a wide series of alterations, including alterations of purine homeostasis which in turn result in activation of AMP protein kinase. Other pathways, such as fatty acid metabolism, are significant correlates to post-transfusion recoveries in mouse models (25, 26). In this study, we expand on our previous observation on the metabolic phenotypes of RBCs from G6PD-deficient vs. sufficient donors. Results are correlated to physiological measurements of potential clinical impact, such as extracellular potassium, oxidative lesions, RBC fragility, and susceptibility to hemolysis *in situ* or at post-storage mimicking conditions (e.g., incubation at 37°C).

MATERIALS AND METHODS

Subjects, Blood Collection, and Processing

Six male, 22–30 years old G6PD-deficient (G6PD$^-$, Mediterranean variant, <10% residual activity of the enzyme) and three gender- and age-matched G6PD-normal (G6PD$^+$) regular blood donors were recruited. Venous blood was collected into EDTA or citrate vacutainers just before blood donation and preparation of packed RBCs. RBC storage quality was evaluated in citrate phosphate dextrose (CPD)/saline adenine glucose mannitol (SAGM) log4 leukofiltered units (Haemonetics Corp., MA, USA) stored for 42 days at 4–6°C. Samples were collected aseptically at weekly intervals of the storage period (days 7, 14, 21, 28, 35, and 42). The study was approved by the Ethics Committee of the Department of Biology, School of Science, NKUA. Investigations were carried out upon signing of written consent, in accordance with the principles of the Declaration of Helsinki.

Hematological, Biochemical, and Physiological Measurements

Pre-donation blood and RBC concentrates of G6PD-deficient donors were further evaluated for almost 45 hematological, biochemical, and physiological parameters before and throughout the storage period in CPD/SAGM, as described in the previously published study (22, 23). Shortly, Hb concentration and RBC indexes (RBC and reticulocyte counts, hematocrit, mean corpuscular volume, mean corpuscular Hb, mean corpuscular Hb concentration, and RBC distribution width) were measured using the Sysmex K-4500 automatic blood cell counter (Roche), while serum biochemical analysis (triglycerides, cholesterol, low density lipoproteins, high density lipoproteins, iron, ferritin, total billirubin, uric acid, aspartate transaminase, alanine aminotransferase, potassium, and sodium) was performed using the analyzers Hitachi 902, 9180 and Elecsys Systems Analyzer (Roche). Levels of glycated Hb (HbA1c) and G6PD activity were measured in fresh blood and in packed RBCs on the last day of storage. Levels of extracellular (free) Hb, total or uric acid-dependent/independent antioxidant activities, total and RBC-derived microparticles (MPs), and MP-associated pro-coagulant activity were evaluated in plasma/supernatant by standard biochemical assays, flow cytometry, or ELISA approaches. Fresh and stored RBCs were finally evaluated for shape modifications (scanning electron microscopy), osmotic and mechanical fragility, membrane protein carbonylation, and accumulation of intracellular reactive oxygen species (ROS) and calcium. Measurements of RBC fragilities and ROS accumulation were performed before and after 24 h incubation at 37°C, while ROS accumulation was estimated before and after treatment with the oxidative agents diamide (dROS) and *tert*-butyl hydroperoxide (tBHP, tROS). All measurements were run in triplicate.

Metabolomics Analyses

Metabolomics analyses were performed as previously reported (22). Briefly, 100 μL of stored RBCs were collected on a weekly basis and extracted at 1:6 dilutions in methanol:acetonitrile:water (5:3:2), vortexed, and centrifuged to pellet proteins, prior to analysis by UHPLC-MS (Ultimate 3000 RSLC-Q Exactive, Thermo Fisher). Sample extracts (10 μL) were loaded onto a Kinetex XB-C18 column (150 mm × 2.1 mm × 1.7 μm—Phenomenex, Torrance, CA, USA). A 9-min gradient from 5 to 95% B (phase A: water + 0.1% formic acid and B: acetonitrile + 0.1% formic acid) eluted metabolites into a Q Exactive system (Thermo, Bremen, Germany), scanning in full MS mode (3 min method) or performing acquisition independent fragmentation (MS/MS analysis—9 min method) at 70,000 resolution in the 60–900 *m/z* range, 4 kV spray voltage, 15 sheath gas, and 5 auxiliary gas, operated in negative and then positive ion mode (separate runs). Metabolite assignment was performed against an in house standard library, as reported (27), through the freely available software Maven (Princeton University, USA) (28). No data pre-processing (neither normalization nor log-transformation) was performed. In our previous study (22, 23), only glycolysis, ribose phosphate, glutathione, and NADH/NAD+ ratios were reported. Here, we expanded the analysis to amino acids, lipids, purines, and other metabolites, as extensively reported in Table S1 in Supplementary Material.

Statistics

For statistical analysis, the Statistical Package for Social Sciences (SPSS, IBM) was used. Correlations between parameters were evaluated by the Pearson's and Spearman's tests after checking out the variables for normal distribution profile (by using the Shapiro–Wilk test) and presence of outliers. Briefly, in the absence of normal distribution, Spearman test was performed. In addition, and since Pearson's test is sensitive to extreme outliers, in the presence of such an outlier the value was excluded and the analysis was performed again, to minimize the possibility of false results likely associated with the small size of the cohort. If the outcome of the subsequent Pearson analysis was not modified compared to the first one, the outlier was included back to the cohort. If not, Spearman analysis was preferred. Outliers (any measurement outside the range of mean $\pm 2 \times$ SD) were identified by using both the Shapiro–Wilk test and detrended normal Q–Q plots. Significance was accepted at a p value of less than 0.01.

Network Analysis

All hematological, biochemical, omics, and physiological parameters collected from G6PD-deficient donors (for abbreviations, see Table S2 in Supplementary Material) were used for the construction of biological networks connecting variables of fresh donor's blood (*in vivo* state) with those of packed RBCs (*ex vivo* state) by significant and repeated correlations that existed throughout (namely, at every time point of) the storage period (with the exception of the G6PD activity and percentage of HbA1c, for which only end-of-storage measurements were available). The reasoning behind selection of correlations that were repeatedly evident at all time points of storage (namely, fresh blood vs. 7th and 14th and so on until the 42nd day) was to find out sound links between variables regardless of storage duration and in parallel, to minimize the false discovery rate that is intrinsically connected to any small sized sample. To increase the confidence level, the outputs of that analysis were further analyzed by a Bonferroni-like correction for multiple comparisons. The multiply checked and thus, most probably true, correlations were topologically represented in undirected biological networks by using Cytoscape version 3.2.0 application, as previously described (15). The length of each edge was inversely proportional to the r value (the shortest the edge, the higher r value).

RESULTS AND DISCUSSION

Metabolic Phenotypes of G6PD-Deficient Donors Recapitulate the Storage Lesion Observed in G6PD Sufficient Donors

Overall, a total of 293 metabolites were monitored in this study, as extensively reported in Table S1 in Supplementary Material. Recently, Palsson's group (29, 30) recognized three stages identifying the metabolic age of blood (18). Multivariate analysis of metabolomics data from RBC concentrates stored in different additives (29–31) results in a U-shaped graph which is indicative of three time-dependent metabolic phases as RBCs age during storage. Consistently, Paglia et al. have reported that transition from phase 2 to phase 3 occurs after storage day 18 (29). Here, multivariate analysis of metabolomics data from SAGM-stored RBCs from G6PD-deficient donors suggests that such transition may occur earlier in this population (storage day 14—**Figure 1A**),

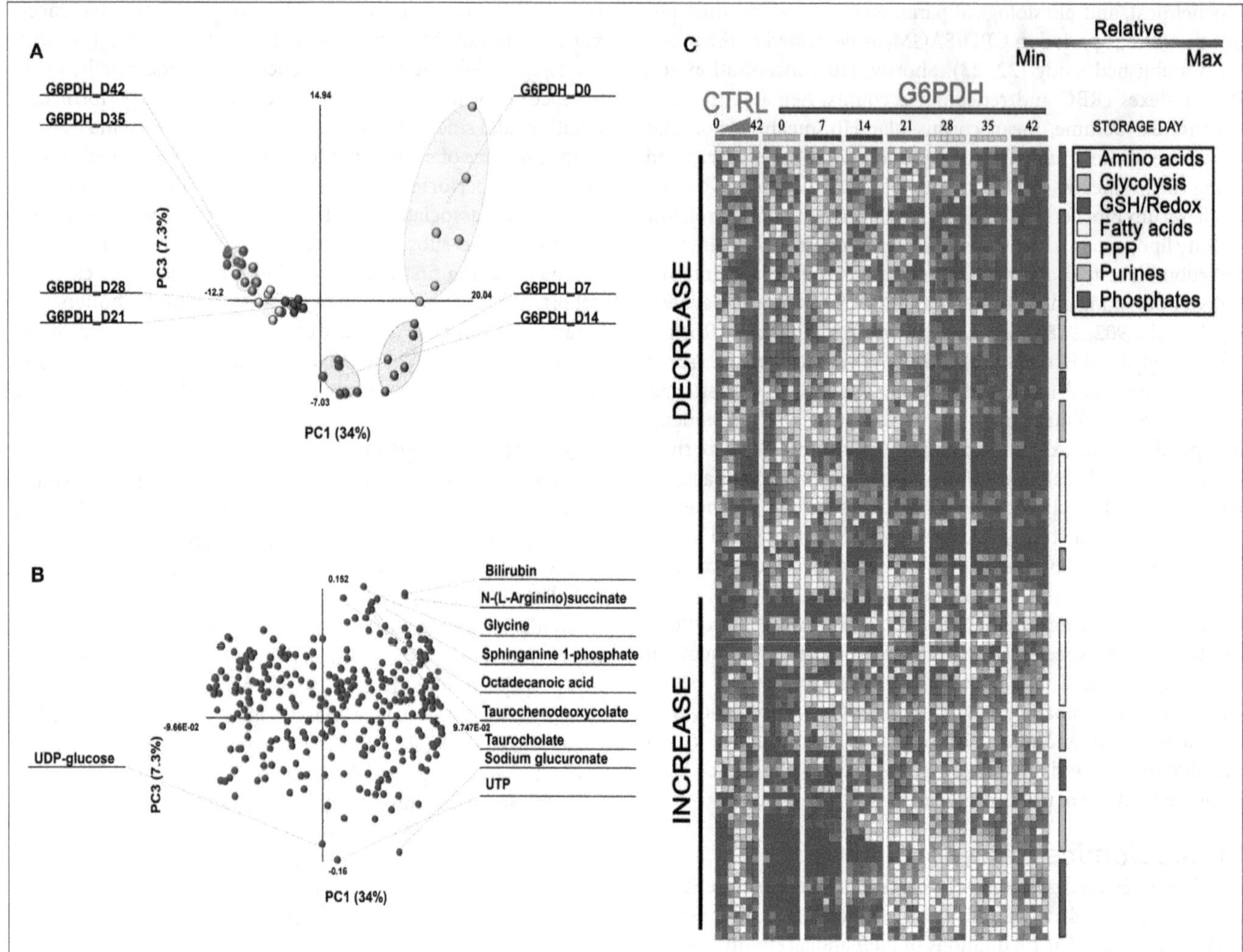

FIGURE 1 | Multivariate analysis of metabolic phenotypes of stored red blood cells (RBCs) from glucose 6-phosphate dehydrogenase (G6PD)-deficient donors. Partial least square discriminant analysis [PLS-DA—panel **(A)**] revealed a U-shaped distribution of packed RBC samples from G6PD-deficient donors over storage in the blood bank, consistent with previous reports from Palsson's lab (29, 30) and our group (9, 31). A loading plot for most significant variables informing the PLS-DA discrimination is shown in panel **(B)**, and includes bioactive lipids and bile acids. In panel **(C)**, a heat map of time course metabolic changes in RBCs from G6PD sufficient (median) or deficient ($n = 6$) donors, divided by pathway as specified by color codes in the top right corner of the panel.

though greater temporal resolution in the 10–18 storage day range would be necessary to further support this conclusion. Overall, the top variables discriminating RBC concentrates for G6PD-deficient donors include bioactive lipids and free fatty acids, bile acids, glycolytic metabolites, purines, and amino acids, as reported in the loading plot and heat maps in **Figures 1B,C**, respectively. A vectorial version of the heat map with hierarchical clustering is provided as Figure S1 in Supplementary Material.

G6PD-Deficient Donors Are Characterized by Alterations in One-Carbon Metabolism, Glutathione/Urate Homeostasis, and Fatty Acid Metabolism Compared to G6PD Sufficient Donors

Two-way ANOVA comparing storage-dependent trends in G6PD-deficient vs. sufficient donors revealed significant changes in metabolites involved in one-carbon and sulfur metabolism (including cystathionine, methionine, S-adenosyl-L-methionine, methylenetetrahydrofolate, and homocysteine—**Figures 2A–E**), metabolites involved in glutathione homeostasis and antioxidant defenses (urate, glutamine, glutathionylcysteine—**Figures 2F–H**), and the carboxylic acid fumarate (**Figure 2I**), all significantly lower in the G6PD-deficient group except for cystathionine and homocysteine.

Consistent with a better preserved morphology (22) and a trend of decreased storage vesiculation degree (23), the levels of free fatty acids and oxidized derivatives (e.g., HPETE/LTB4 or isobaric isomers) were significantly lower in G6PD-deficient donors in comparison to control RBCs, with the exception of oleate and linoleate (**Figure 3**). Previous proteomics analyses revealed increased oxidation and stress markers accumulation but also increased levels of antioxidant enzymes in the plasma membrane and the extracellular vesicles released by the stored G6PD^{-} RBCs (22). Of note, the levels of several polyunsaturated fatty acids, including the linoleate, were found to be both

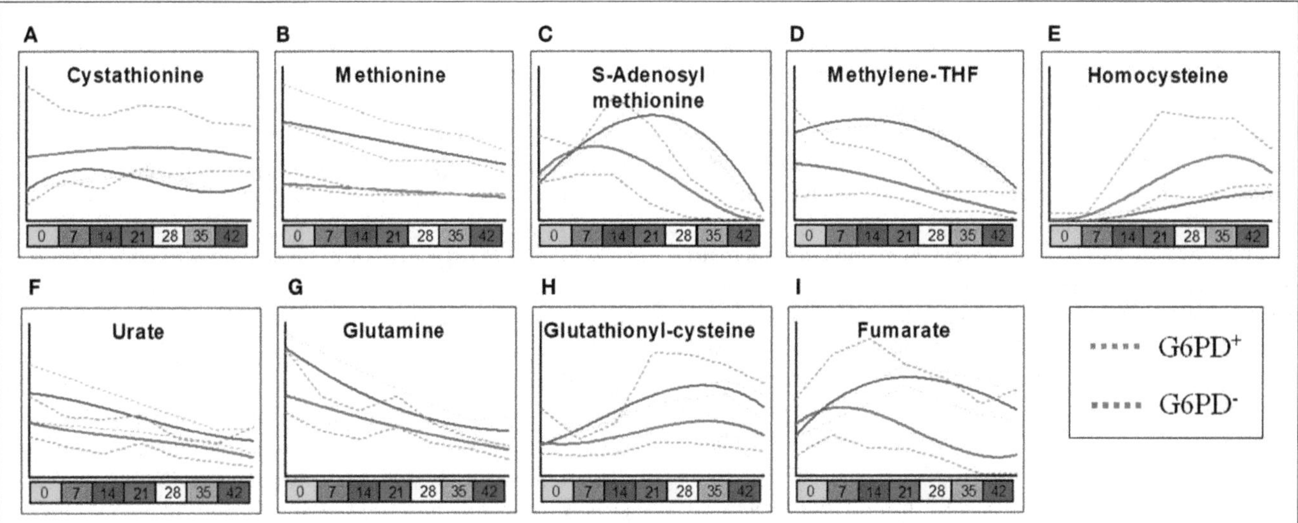

FIGURE 2 | Most significant metabolic differences between glucose 6-phosphate dehydrogenase (G6PD) sufficient and deficient red blood cells (RBCs). Panels indicate alterations to sulfur/one-carbon metabolism **(A–E)**, purine oxidation **(F)**, glutathione homeostasis **(G,H)**, and carboxylates **(I)** in G6PD sufficient (blue line) and deficient (red line) RBCs during storage in the blood bank (median + ranges are shown in light blue or red for both G6PD sufficient and deficient groups, respectively).

Eicosatrienoate (C20:3)
Arachidonate (C20:4)
Eicosapentanoate (C20:5)
Docosapentanoate (C22:5)
Glycerol phosphate
Thromboxane B2
Lipid (DAGs, TAGs, Phospholipids
(Phospho)lipases
Lipid heads (e.g. glycerol phosphate)
Free fatty acids
Palmitate (C16:0)
Prostaglandin D2/E2 Thromboxane A2 (isobars)
Eicosatrienoate (C20:3)
Prostaglandins
Thromboxanes
Palmitate (C16:0)
Oleate (C18:1)
Arachidonate (C20:4)
HPETE
LTC_4
Palmitoleate (C16:1)
Linoleate (C18:2)
LTB_4
Palm itoleate (C16:1)
Eicosapentanoate (C20:5)
Leukotriene C4
Octadecatrienoate (C18:3)
Docoosapentanoate (C22:5)
Oleate (C18:1)
Linoleate (C18:2)
Octadecatrienoate (C18:3)
HPETE/ Leukotriene B4 (isobars)
0 7 14 21 28 35 42

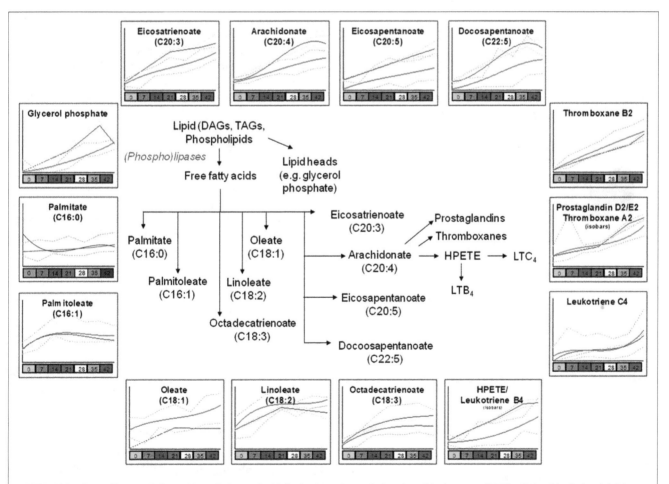

FIGURE 3 | Significant differences in fatty acid metabolism and oxidation between glucose 6-phosphate dehydrogenase (G6PD) sufficient (blue line) and deficient (red line) red blood cells during storage in the blood bank (median + ranges are shown in light blue or red for both G6PD sufficient and deficient groups, respectively).

heritable and associated with ATP levels in AS-3 stored RBCs (4), while in this study, the linoleate concentration in G6PD⁻ donors at donation time had a strong negative correlation with the 2,3-biphosphoglycerate (2,3-BPG) levels in stored RBCs (see below). The different concentration of oleate in fresh and stored G6PD⁻ blood compared to control blood may be associated with a different rate of incorporation into phosphatidylcholine that significantly decreases during storage (32).

Similarly, lower levels of plasticizers monoethyl-hexylphthalate and phthalate were detected in RBC concentrates from G6PD-deficient donors (**Figure 4**). Approximately 28% of the available bis(2-ethylhexyl) phthalate (DEHP) is taken up by stored RBCs where it exerts a protective effect on membrane stability and flexibility similar to that of mannitol (33). Since NADPH is indispensable for the synthesis of fatty acids and cholesterol, the RBC membrane in G6PD deficiency of Mediterranean type is characterized by increased fluidity and decreased cholesterol-to-phospholipid ratio (34). Considering that RBCs from both donor cohorts were processed and stored through comparable manufacturing processes, and that the DEHP levels in G6PD⁻ units were equal to the control levels, it is plausible to speculate that the lipid remodeling in G6PD deficiency may favor incorporation of DEHP in the membrane, preventing thus its hydrolysis to MEHP and phthalate. This kind

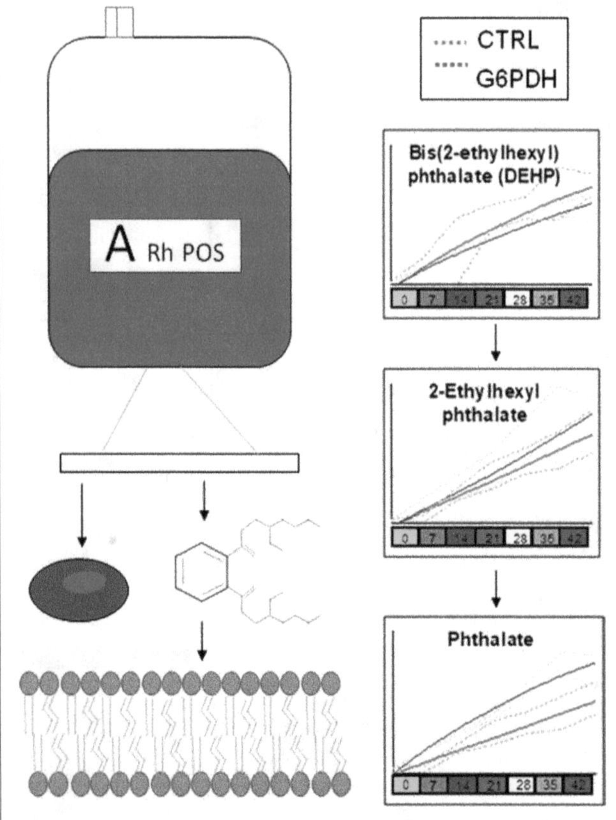

FIGURE 4 | Different levels of phthalate plasticizers and breakdown products are observed in red blood cells from glucose 6-phosphate dehydrogenase (G6PD) sufficient (blue line) and deficient (red line) during storage in the blood bank (median + ranges are shown in light blue or red for both G6PD sufficient and deficient groups, respectively).

of protective effect is consistent with the previously reported trend of stored G6PD⁻ RBCs to reduced mechanical fragility compared to that of control RBCs at body temperature (23).

Loss of Metabolic Linkage and Metabolic Rewiring in G6PD-Deficient Donors

Though correlations do not necessarily imply causation, in the field of metabolomics, a high degree of correlation is observed among the levels of metabolites from pathways that are linked by biochemical constraints of enzymatic reactions (35). The identification of such correlates under physiological conditions and the disruption of such correlations under pathological conditions (e.g., here G6PD deficiency, **Figure 5**) are indicative of metabolic rewiring. Here, for example, we identify alterations between the correlates of pyruvate/lactate ratios, suggestive of disrupted NADH/NAD+ homeostasis in G6PD-deficient subjects. This observation confirms and expands upon our previous report about increased levels (and potentially increased activity) of methemoglobin reductase in RBCs from G6DP⁻ donors (22). On the other hand, we also noted a disruption in the correlation between acetylcarnitine and fructose. Of note, RBC levels of carnitine and acetylcarnitine are, respectively, comparable and higher to the levels observed in plasma (36). Indeed, RBCs are equipped with a functional ATP-citrate lyase, as we (31, 37) and others (38) have shown with tracing experiments with ^{13}C-glucose and other stable isotope tracers. Disruption of correlation between acetylcarnitine and fructose levels in G6DP⁻ donors is suggestive that, in normal RBCs, at least part of the acetylcarnitine pool is derived from fructose sugar and that this metabolic route is dysregulated in G6DP⁻ donors. Follow-up tracing experiments with ^{13}C-fructose will be necessary to expand on this observation.

In addition, apart from the intrametabolic correlates, several couples of correlations involving metabolites and physiological RBC/plasma characteristics can be identified in G6PD⁻ donors, physically linked to each other by exhibiting the same variation profile in fresh blood (non-stored, NS) and throughout storage in CPD/SAGM (**Figure 6**). Results are indicative of a correlation between the energy state of the stored RBC (as gleaned by 2,3-DPG, glucose, and lactate levels) and the preservation of a discocytic phenotype, while MPs release and phosphatidylserine exposure correlated with markers of impaired glutathione homeostasis and (maybe merely spuriously) with the total levels of phthalates measured at any given time point. Of note, correlations between AMP levels and gamma-glutamyl-cycle end-product 5-oxoproline (in oxoprolinase-deficient mature RBCs) is suggestive of an intertwinement between energy and redox metabolism, further confirming our recent reports on the role of oxidative stress in stored RBC energy impairment secondary to AMP deaminase activation (39).

The Metabolic and Biopreservation Profiles of G6PD⁻ Packed RBCs Were Closely Related to the Biological Profile of the Donor: Intra-Parameter Relationships

Several metabolites and physiological characteristics of G6PD⁻ packed RBCs fluctuate throughout the storage period

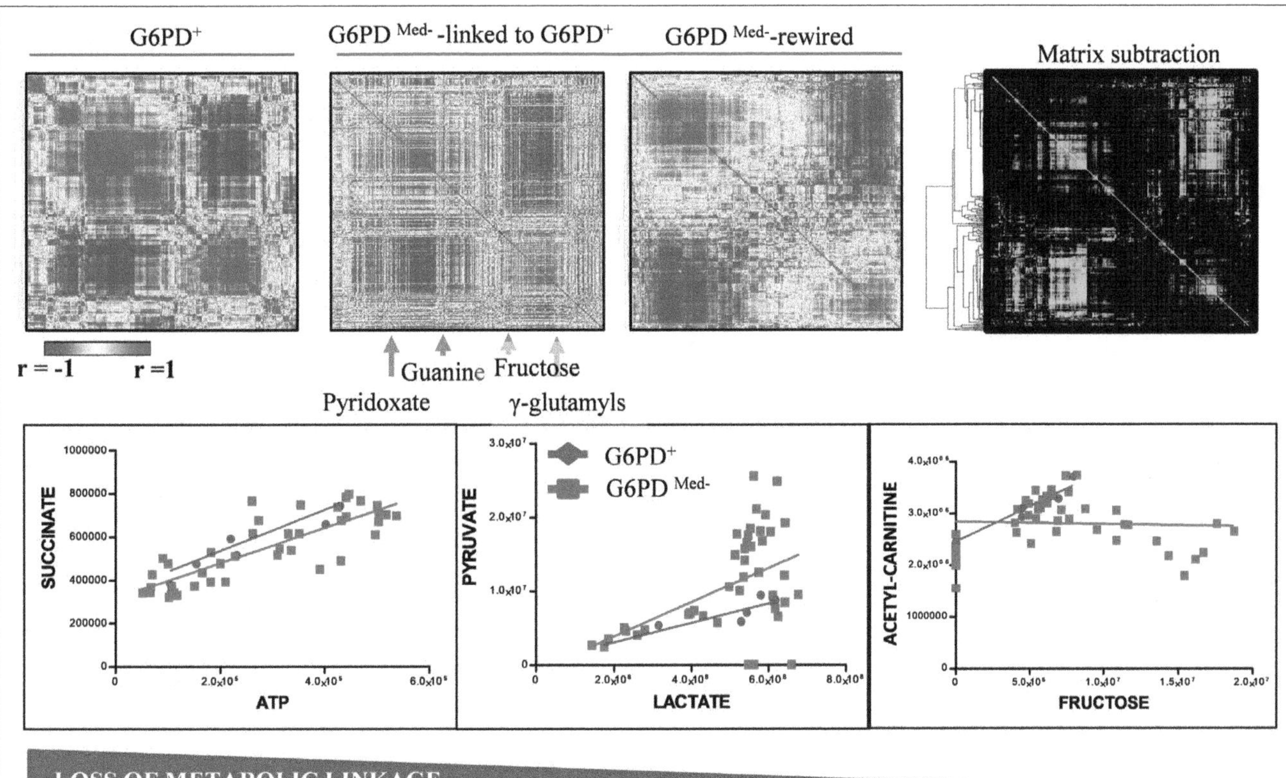

FIGURE 5 | Metabolic linkage (35) analyses in glucose 6-phosphate dehydrogenase (G6PD)-deficient and sufficient red blood cells (RBCs). Metabolite levels were correlated to each other in both groups (independently of storage age), to identify variations ($\Delta|r| > 30\%$) in metabolite levels secondary to metabolic rewiring in G6PD-deficient donors when compared to G6PD sufficient controls. Phenotypic alterations that disrupted this fine tuning of the kinetics of specific metabolic pathways would be highlighted by a differential analysis of correlation of metabolites across conditions. Blue to red = $-1 < r < +1$. A highlight of correlations varying >30% between these two conditions is shown in green. For example, significant alteration of the linkage between lactate and pyruvate or acetyl carnitines and fructose, but not succinate and ATP, was observed in G6PD-deficient RBCs (red line and squares) vs. G6PD sufficient counterparts (blue lines and rhomboids).

proportionally to their own baseline levels *in vivo*, as shown in Table S3 in Supplementary Material (whole storage) and in the representative scatter plots of **Figure 7** (end-of-storage). Among these, the decreasing over storage (22, 40) G6PD activity, reducing power (NADPH) and antioxidant capacity (23), along with the increasing glycated Hb (HbA1c) (41) and osmotic hemolysis levels (23) were included. Similar findings regarding the donor-dependent resistance of RBCs to osmotic lysis and the antioxidant capacity of the supernatant have been previously detected in packed RBCs from G6PD$^+$ donors (14, 15, 42, 43), signifying a "donor-signature effect" on storage. Indeed, while their absolute values vary following variations in storage duration, mediums, and strategies, or in the genetic background (current study), their overall storage profile is steadily a function of donor levels. In other words, the blood banking affects them equally and by a "stable factor" of effect.

Inter-Parameter Relationships and Networking

In addition to those "intra-parameter" relationships, more than 900 repeatable correlations observed between variables in fresh and stored RBCs, as shown in the G6PD$^-$ specific *in vivo*-vs. *-ex vivo* biological network of Figure S2 in Supplementary Material. This complex structure is a correlation-based, strict assessment of distinct and multifarious experimental metrics, designed to minimize the unreliable interrelations, as each connection is statistically significant at 6 different time points of the storage period (a total of 36 replicates in the 6 G6PD$^-$ units). Certain hub nodes represented specific storability variables that correlated to a large number of donor entities (and *vice versa*). The higher density of connections is observed at the upper right area of the network (I), where in-bag hemolysis and susceptibility to hemolysis (I-A) clustered with the 2,3-BPG (I-B) and dehydroascorbate (DHA, I-C) hub nodes. In a clockwise way, the areas of bile acids (II), extracellular K$^+$ (III), G6PD activity (IV), redox (including ROS, urate, and antioxidant capacity, V), hematological (MCV, MCH, HbA_{1c}, VI), and fatty/bile acids (VII) can be observed (Figure S2 in Supplementary Material). To focus on entities intrinsically related to the G6PD deficiency, the progress of storage lesion (e.g., redox status) and the quality of RBC concentrates (e.g., hemolysis-related variables) fragmentary analyses of sub-networks were subsequently performed.

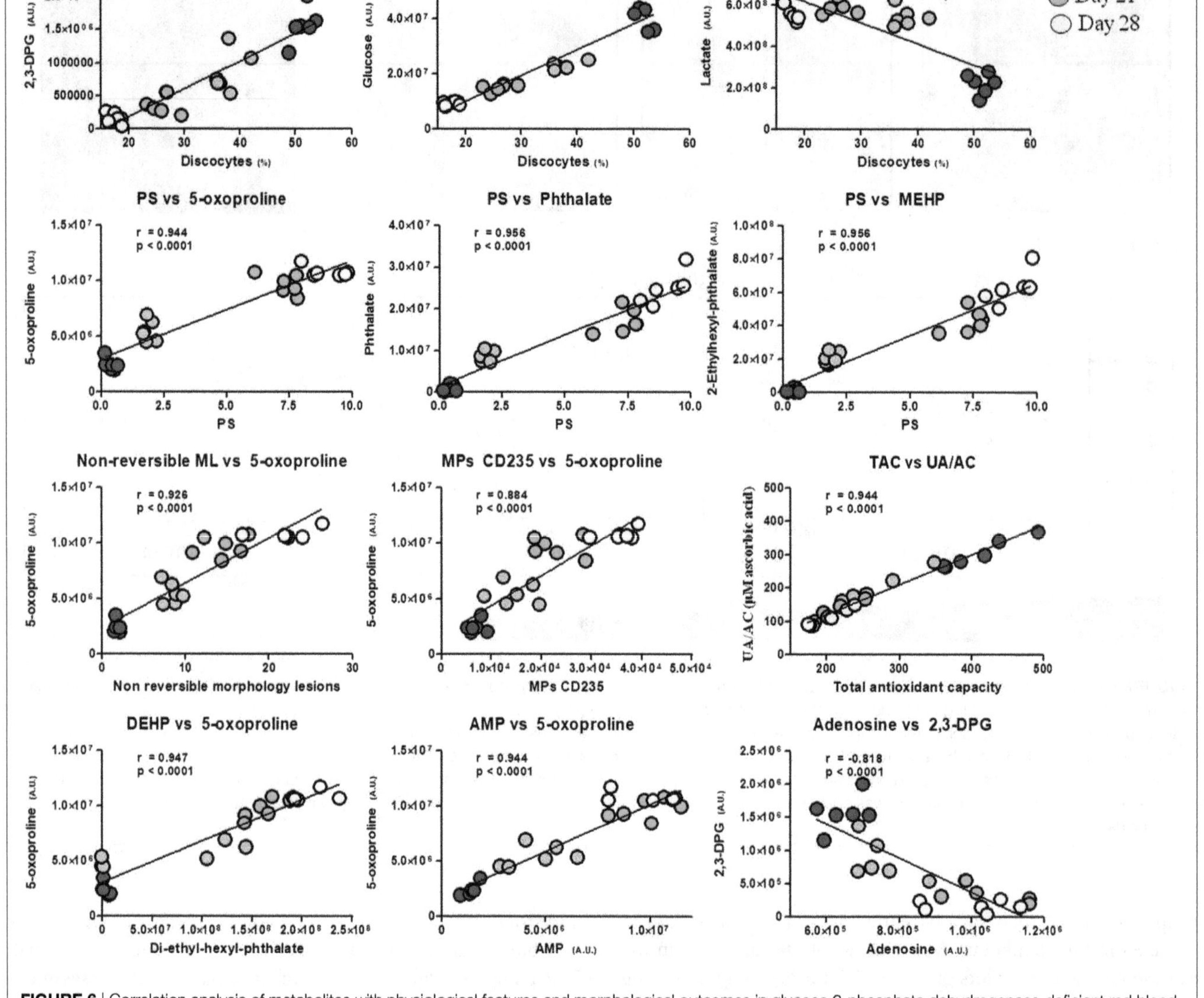

FIGURE 6 | Correlation analysis of metabolites with physiological features and morphological outcomes in glucose 6-phosphate dehydrogenase-deficient red blood cells at different storage days (non-stored/fresh blood: dark blue; day 14: light blue; day 21: green; day 28: yellow dots).

G6PD and Metabolic Networking Revealed that RBC Storage Biology Is Physically Related to Donor Biology, though at a Broader Level of Interwoven Underlying Pathways

In the G6PD activity network (**Figure 8**), the baseline levels had positive correlations with the in-bag levels of amino acids and 2-OH-glutarate. On the other side, in-bag G6PD activity had inverse correlations with metabolites of the PPP cycle, monounsaturated fatty acids, bile acids, and oxidized lipids in fresh blood.

Regarding the main metabolic pathways, the end-products of glycolysis (Figure S3 in Supplementary Material) *in vivo* had negative correlations with the levels of 2,3-BPG but opposite correlations with numerous hemolysis/fragility parameters of the RBC concentrates and supernatant K^+. In the same way, in the PPP and one-carbon metabolism pathways (Figure S4 in Supplementary Material), sedoheptulose-1-phosphate, and folate levels in fresh RBCs had positive correlations with in-bag levels of 2,3-BPG and redox variables (DHA) but inverse correlations with hemolysis-related metrics. An interesting link between *in vivo* levels of protein carbonylation and osmotic fragility with the reducing power of the packed RBCs was also noticed. In reverse, *in vivo* levels of glucono-1,5-lactone-6P had strong correlations with those of the UA-dependent antioxidant capacity of the supernatant and of the G6PD activity. In the glutathione cycle, transaminases, and malate-aspartate shuttle, the majority of connections concerned *in vivo* GSH/GSSG content, fumarate, and malate toward stored RBCs' amino acid and fatty acids metabolism, DHA, malate, 2,3-BPG, hemolysis, and extracellular K^+.

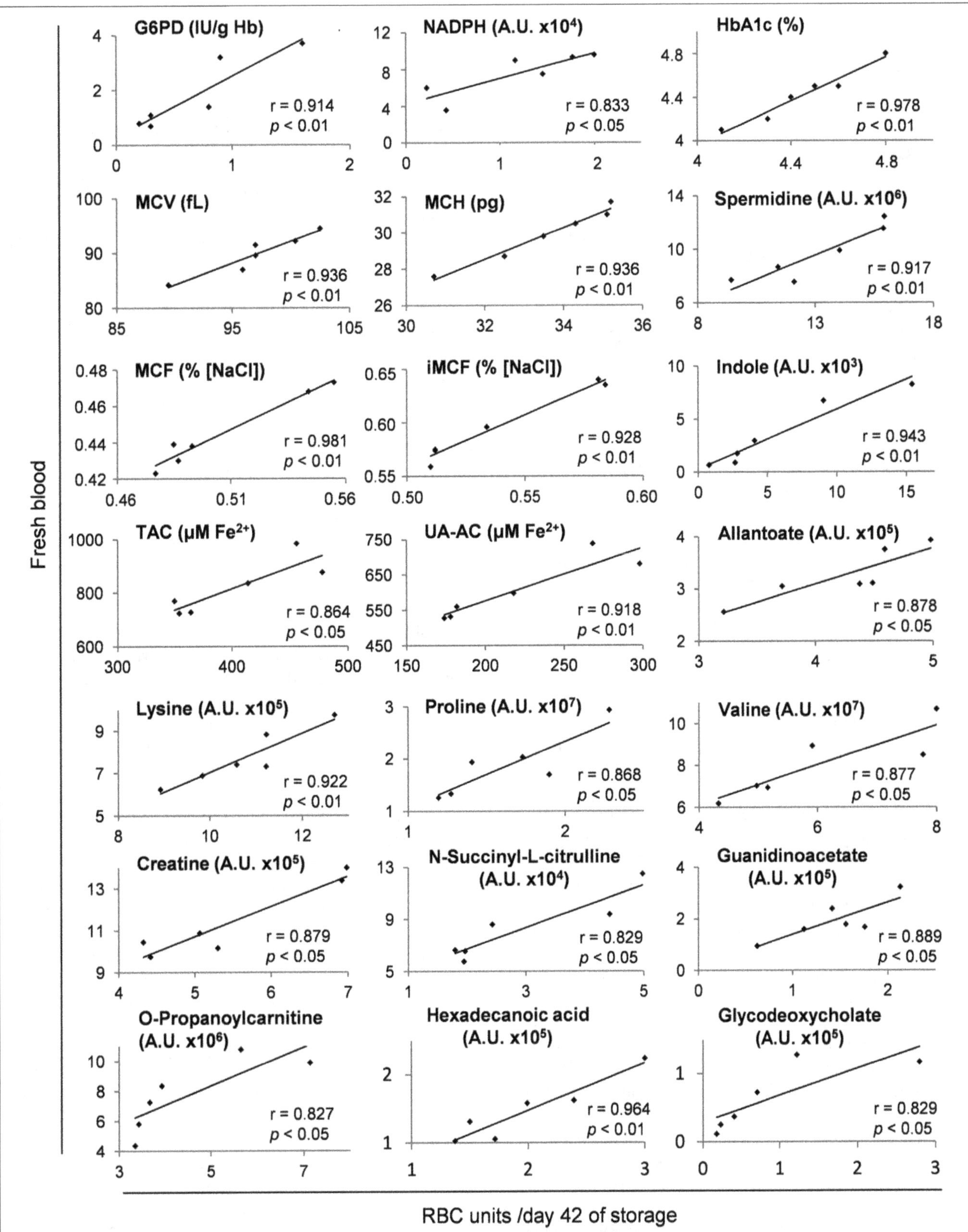

FIGURE 7 | Representative scatter plots of Pearson's correlations between hematological, physiological, and metabolism parameters in fresh donors' blood and packed red blood cells (RBCs) of the same donors after 42 days of storage. Apart from day 42 shown here, these fresh blood variables had statistically significant correlations (see Materials and Methods) with those of stored RBC units at every time point of the storage period, as shown in Table S3 in Supplementary Material.

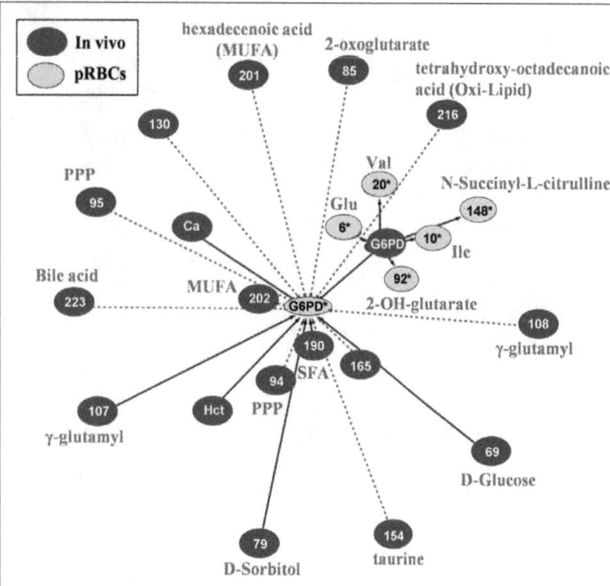

FIGURE 8 | *In vivo* (fresh blood) vs. *ex vivo* [packed red blood cells (RBCs)] network analysis of glucose 6-phosphate dehydrogenase (G6PD) activity in G6PD⁻ donors. The G6PD activity sub-network consists of 23 statistically significant and repeatable at any storage duration correlations (see Materials and Methods). Same as all networks currently reported, only the correlations of Day 42 with fresh blood measurements are shown; however, those pairs of statistically significant connections (with slightly different *r*) applied to all possible storage durations (Days 7, 14, 21, 28, 35, and 42). The length of each line is inversely proportional to the *r* value of the correlation (the shorter the edge, the higher *r* value). Continuous black lines: positive correlations; dashed red lines: negative correlations.

Consistent with the involvement of G6PD (through the production of NADPH) in the reductive biosynthesis of fatty acids and cholesterol (44), two-way ANOVA processing of the metabolomics analyses revealed clear differences in lipid content, biosynthesis, and metabolism between G6PD⁻ and control RBCs both *in vivo* (e.g., palmitate, oleate) and during storage (e.g., glycerol phosphate, eiosatrienoate, arachidonate) (**Figure 3**), in a way likely affecting recoveries, as shown in multiple mouse strains (16, 25). In those studies, lipid metabolism, degradation and oxidation emerged as the strongest correlates with poor 24-h recoveries. Moreover, in both animal and human transfusion contexts, bioactive lipid components of the transfusate are considered clinically relevant for the transfused recipients (45). Subsequent network analysis (Figure S5 in Supplementary Material) further verified the central role of lipids in defining the demanding membrane properties and thus, the quality of stored G6PD⁻ RBCs (5, 25). The levels of linoleate, thromboxane B2, and leukotriene C4 had inverse correlations with those of 2,3-BPG and DHA in the RBC unit, while those of eicosapentaenoic/eicosatetraenoic and hexadecanoic acids at donation correlated well (negatively) with the fragility of stored RBCs and the concentration of extracellular potassium in the supernatant.

The interesting interplay among the G6PD-affected metabolic pathways (e.g., NAD+/glucose-6-phosphate, GSH/2,3-BPG) before and during refrigerated storage, suggests that RBC storage biology reflects a part of donor biology, in a way hardly revealed by individual factor metrics. Lactate levels in the G6PD⁻ donors, for example, were not proportional to lactate levels in stored RBC units, but rather with those of the pathway-interconnected 2,3-BPG.

The Quality of the Biopreservation of the G6PD⁻ RBC Unit Is Linked by Biochemical and Cellular Pathways with the *In Vivo* State

The network analyses made clear that the redox and hemolysis-related parameters of the G6PD⁻ RBC unit are among those most correlated with the *in vivo* state. These variables characterize not only the storability of G6PD⁻ RBCs but also a part of their post-transfusion performance. The sub-interactome shown in **Figure 9** contains the sum of the *in vivo* physiological and omics variables having correlations with the in-bag levels of oxidant/antioxidant variables. According to this map, donor levels of RBC ROS had no correlation with those of stored RBCs, but they did have a strong inverse correlation with DHA levels, throughout the storage period. Reversely, susceptibility of stored RBCs to thermal- or oxidant-induced ROS generation had strong correlations with the levels of serum UA in fresh blood. In addition, the antioxidant capacity of the supernatant had positive correlations with the *in vivo* levels of UA/allantoin, PPP components, GSH, arachidonate, and fatty acid metabolism. It seemed that high levels of GSSG in fresh blood predispose the RBC unit to low levels of UA-dependent antioxidant activity throughout the storage period. Storage DHA was the most important hub nod in the redox network. It showed positive correlations with amino acids, nucleotides, GPLs such as sphingosine-1-phosphate, prostaglandin D3, leukotriene A4, and folate, but opposite correlations with the levels of intracellular ROS, fumarate, malate, and leukotriene C4 at donation.

Regarding the hemolytic variables of the RBC units in G6PD deficiency, an impressive polyparametric sub-network of 173 connections links them to the *in vivo* state (**Figure 10**). The network refers to in-bag levels of hemolysis and to the osmotic/mechanical fragility of stored RBCs *in situ* or in post-storage-simulating conditions. A few donor variables had individual correlations with in-bag hemolysis (e.g., AMP, 5-oxoproline, GSH), or osmotic hemolysis (e.g., NADPH, xanthine, citrulline), or mechanical hemolysis (e.g., homocysteine); however, the vast majority of them correlated (positively or negatively) with most of, or all, the hemolysis-related variables of packed RBCs (*r*-independent circular network in the upper panel of **Figure 10**). Thus, increased levels of amino acids, lipids, and lipid metabolism factors (including sphingosine-1-phosphate and prostaglandin D3), serine biosynthesis metabolites, NADPH, and GSH, among others *in vivo* predispose RBCs to better storability profiles (*r*-driven sub-network in the down panel of **Figure 10**). A clear opposite trend was seen for the protein carbonylation, osmotic fragility, AMP (see also purines involving network in Figure S6 in Supplementary Material), lactate, malate, 2-OH-glutarate (that is a marker of hypoxia), fumarate, and oxoproline. In the hemolysis network, certain donor metabolites are components of the one-carbon and sulfur metabolism (see also Figure S7

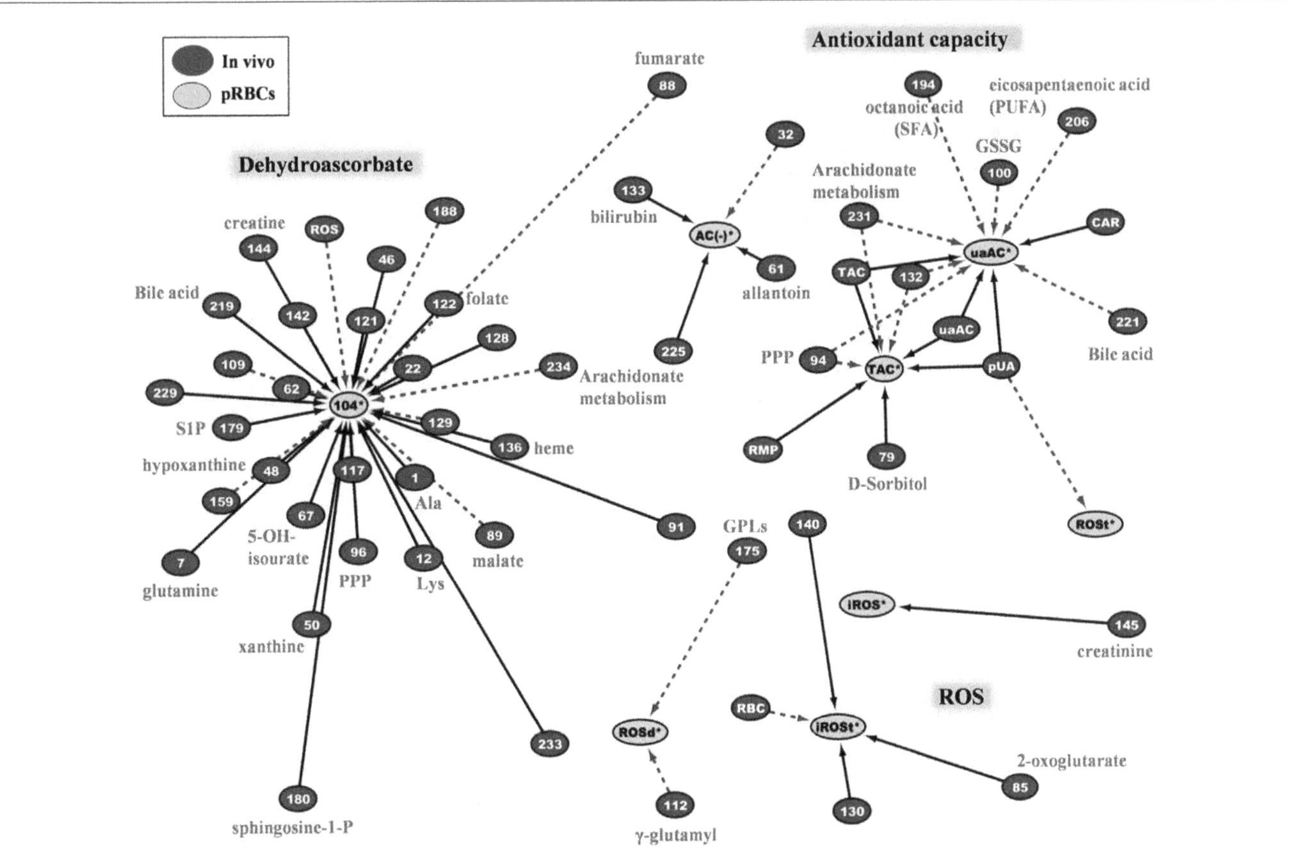

FIGURE 9 | Network analysis of donors' variables at time of donation that had significant correlations with the redox status of the packed red blood cells (RBCs) regardless of the storage duration. The sub-network consists of 62 connections involving intracellular reactive oxygen species (ROS) accumulation, antioxidant capacity of the supernatant, DHA, and other variables. In-bag DHA and ROS levels at post-storage-mimicking conditions represented the most important hub nods. Plasma uric acid and its attributed antioxidant capacity revealed their "intra-parameter" dynamics (see also **Figure 7**). Continuous black lines: positive correlations; dashed red lines: negative correlations.

in Supplementary Material) that were found at lower (e.g., methionine) or higher (e.g., homocysteine) levels in the G6PD$^-$ donors compared to controls (**Figure 2**). It is worth noting that while G6PD activity *in vivo* had no correlation itself with in-bag hemolysis or cellular fragilities, several G6PD-related metabolites (GSH, NADPH, etc.) had strong correlations with at least one hemolysis-related node, verifying the significantly higher analytical power of metabolomics compared to one-molecule-targeted biochemical approaches for probing cellular physiology (46).

The G6PD$^-$ RBCs are more susceptible than the G6PD$^+$ RBCs to K^+ leak (22), which potentially increases the risk of hyperkalemia-induced arrhythmia in susceptible recipients (47). End-of-storage extracellular potassium had numerous negative correlations with donor metabolites in fresh RBCs, most of which in the categories of fatty acids and lipid metabolism or metabolites potentially involved in lipid and protein oxidation (e.g., the highly expressed L-homocysteine) (**Figure 11**, *left panel*). As in the case of in-bag hemolysis and mechanical fragility, high *in vivo* levels of fumarate, phosphoenolopyruvate, and hydroxybutyrate correlated with high in-bag potassium concentration. The progressive degradation of RBC membrane with storage apparently leads to increasing levels of extracellular Hb (as both free Hb and extracellular vesicles) and potassium. Of note, donor levels of AMP were negatively associated with both variables. Finally, the phthalate-specific network support the above mentioned hypothesis that the distinct lipid composition and mechanical properties of the membrane in G6PD deficiency may drive the differential incorporation of DEHP in the bilayer of stored RBCs (**Figure 11**, *right panel*).

Hemolysis Is a Multivariate "Phenotype" of the RBC Storage Lesion, Functionally Connected to Donor Biology by More than One Tethers

Strikingly enough, donor levels of free Hb and RBC mechanical fragility did not correlate with any of the hemolysis-related variables of the RBC concentrates (**Figure 10**). According to a number of metabolomic studies, genetic factors contribute substantially to the degree of storage hemolysis (5), while several donor-specific "metabotypes" have been described in stored RBCs (48). Hemolysis, however, is a multivariate phenotype of the stored

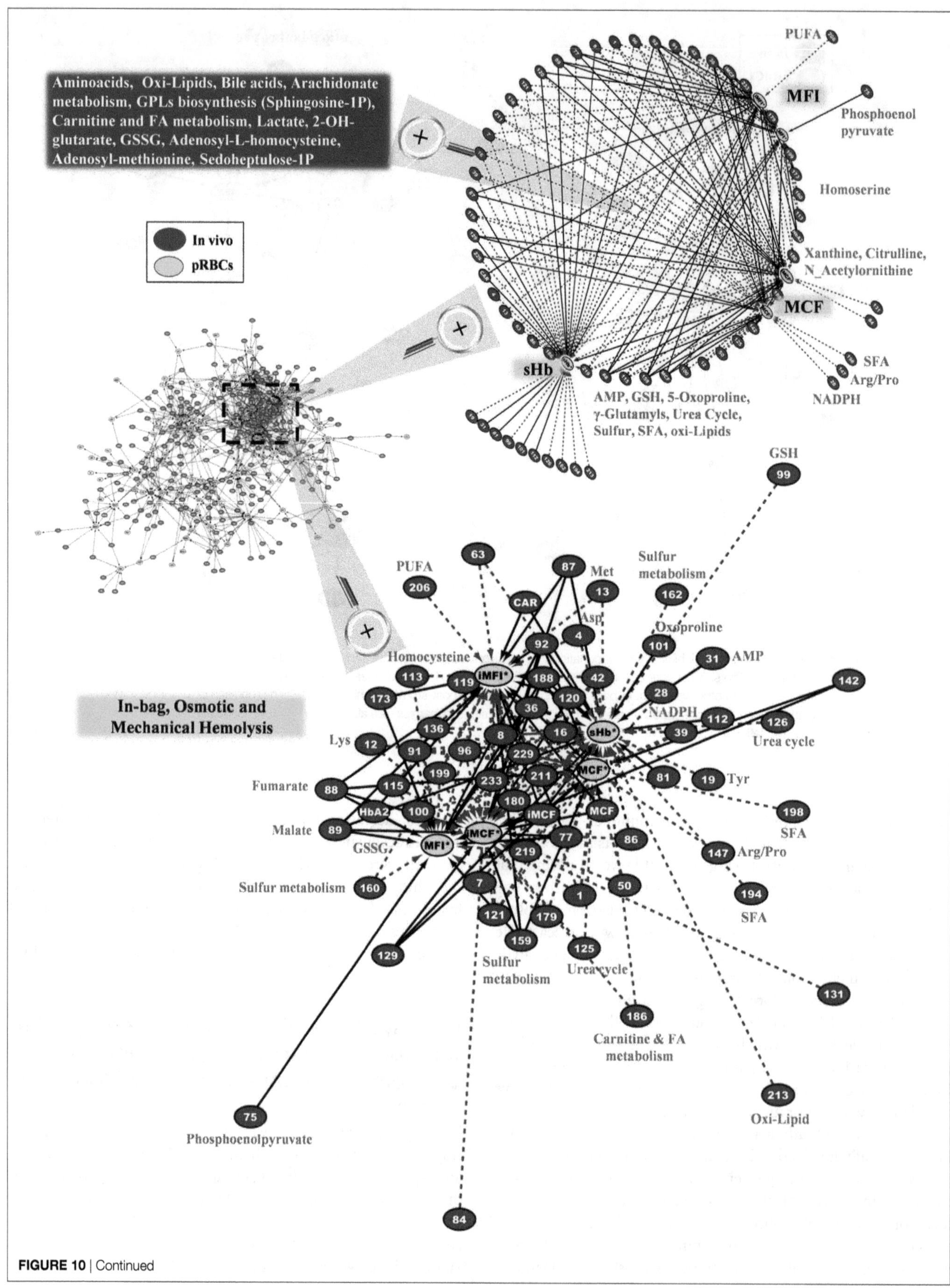

FIGURE 10 | Continued

FIGURE 10 | In-bag hemolysis (sHb) and the resistance of stored G6PD⁻ red blood cells (RBCs) to osmotic or mechanical lysis had several correlations with the *in vivo* state. Magnification of the most dense network cluster (dashed frame) that contains the hemolysis-related nodes of the packed RBCs. *Upper panel*: circle layout of the donor variables reveals that only few of them had correlations with individual hemolysis metrics in packed RBCs (right side of the map), as the majority are connected with at least two of them (blue box in the left side). In this layout, the length of the connections is unrelated to the correlation coefficient *r* value; however, the positive/negative correlations follow the color code shown in **Figure 8** (black-solid/red-dashed, respectively). *Down panel*: the interactome connecting hemolysis-related nodes by 173 repeatable correlations captures a part of the polyparametricity of the "hemolysis" phenotype and the "intra-parameter" dynamics of RBC osmotic fragility both *in situ* (MCF) and following incubation for 24 h at 37°C (iMCF). Continuous black lines: positive correlations; dashed red lines: negative correlations.

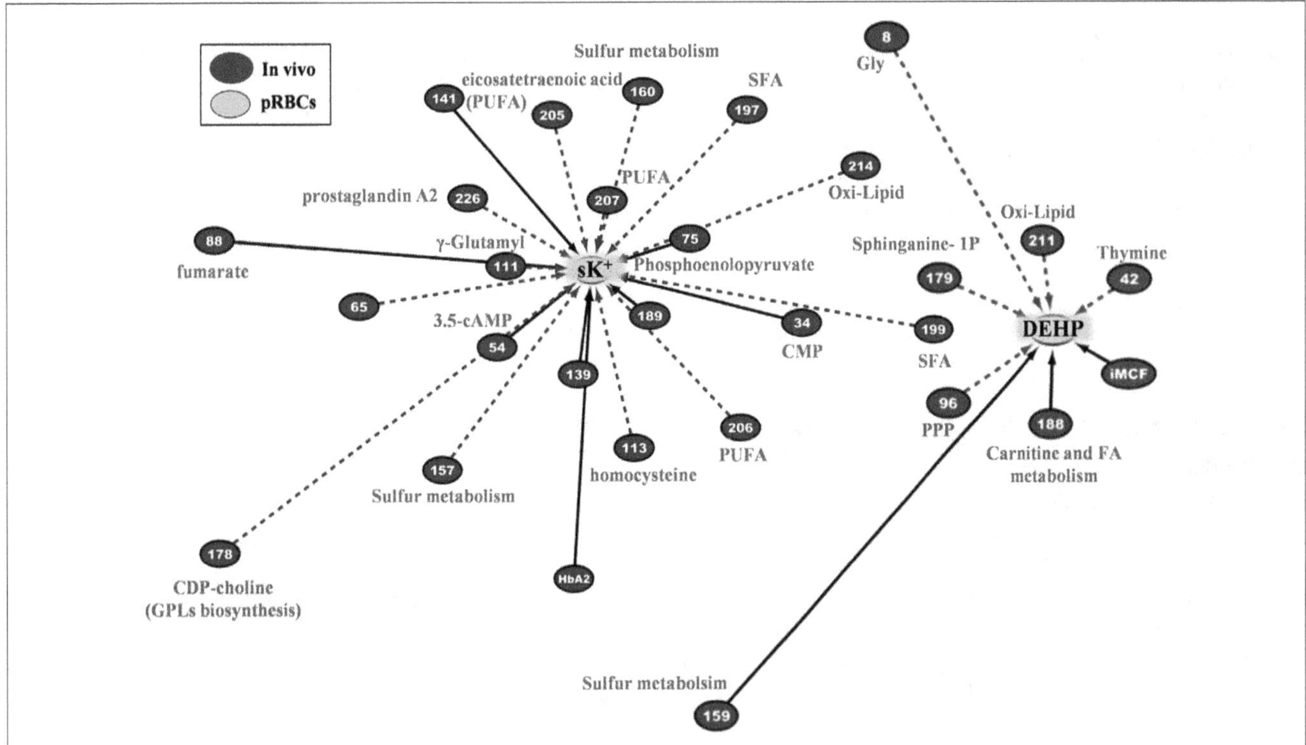

FIGURE 11 | Extracellular potassium and bis(2-ethylhexyl) phthalate (DEHP) connections in pRBCs donated by G6PD⁻ donors. Lipids and lipid metabolism constitute significant contributors in both networks. Continuous black lines: positive correlations; dashed red lines: negative correlations.

RBCs and our study revealed only a fraction of the multitude and the complexity of the donor factors that likely affect it. Without doubt, additional omics analyses (proteomics, lipidomics, etc.) would further elucidate the phenomenon. The biological complexity is too high and the *in vitro* system substantially different compared to the *in vivo* state where the homeostatic mechanisms of healthy RBCs were evolved to meet the cell integrity needs. In-bag hemolysis and post-transfusion recovery represent the overall effect of storage- and recipient-related stresses on distinct physiological characteristics of RBCs that might be donor related. For instance, the osmotic fragility of CPDA-stored RBCs has a correlation with the levels of in-bag hemolysis, but, in quantity terms, fragility can reveal no more than 11% of its variation (42). Moreover, stored RBCs from G6PD⁺ donors that repeatedly exhibit high in-bag hemolysis at outdate are also characterized by reduced ability to resist osmotic stress compared to those exhibiting normal hemolysis (49). In a similar way, in-bag hemolysis in G6PD⁻ units had a positive correlation with the baseline levels of osmotic hemolysis at body temperature (**Figure 10**).

Interplay of Redox, Energy, and Hemolysis-Related Factors before and during Storage

The hemolytic phenotype is likely based on changes in redox and energy metabolism that affect the deformability and stability of RBCs under physiological or pathologically levels of stress (50). The redox activity of RBCs, which contain a strongly oxidizing cytoplasm, governs their lifetime in circulation (51, 52), and thus, changes in the antioxidant activity during storage (53) may have a substantial effect on pre- and post-storage viability. Quantitative proteomics analyses have identified a number of proteins in the supernatant of RBC units showing linear correlations with the absolute levels of extracellular Hb (54), while the donor-related susceptibility of stored RBCs to hemolysis was associated with modifications in RBC membrane proteins involved in oxidative response pathways and decreased storage levels of 2,3-BPG (49). The present study in G6PD⁻ RBCs, which are more susceptible to metabolic changes and protein oxidation compared to normal cells (22, 24), further revealed the strong interplay of in-bag hemolysis and donor biology, since, for instance, RBC protein oxidation at baseline had positive correlations with both in-bag and mechanical hemolysis at body temperature (**Figure 10**).

Moreover, the levels of a relatively homogeneous panel of metabolites in fresh blood (including amino acids, carboxylic acids, GPLs, fatty acids, and purine metabolism components) strongly predispose RBCs to either good or poor storage. Previous studies in stored RBCs have identified some of them (e.g., amino acids) as having similar trend of correlations (negative) with the same-day hemolysis levels (5). In our study, sphingosine-1-phosphate showed positive correlation with the quality of the RBC unit. This bioactive signaling lysophospholipid, is functionally related to RBC (55, 56) and transfusion biology (57) as having critical roles in blood homeostasis and vascular permeability (58). The interconnections of redox, energy, and hemolysis parameters before and during storage (e.g., lactate/hemolysis, GSH/hemolysis, NADPH/osmotic fragility, ROS/2,3-BPG in fresh/stored samples, respectively), further highlight the usefulness of omics/bioinformatics analyses in revealing the complexity of the RBC storage lesion as a function of inter-donor variability and its underlying mechanisms.

Some Pieces of the Interactomes Might Be Related with the Post-Transfusion Performance of G6PD-Deficient RBCs

According to previous reports, the G6PD$^-$ RBCs exhibited normal levels of ROS and in-bag hemolysis; however, exposure to post-transfusion mimicking conditions, including recipient plasma, body temperature (37°C), and oxidants (24), promote hemolysis and ROS accumulation compared to control RBCs (22). The deformability of stored RBCs may determine their quality and post-transfusion performance (59), while *in vitro* testing of RBC responses in recipient-mimicking contexts would reveal clinically relevant sublethal injuries of transfused RBCs (2, 60, 61). In this context, it was interesting that the redox network of **Figure 9** includes several responses of stored RBCs to oxidants (tBHP, diamide) that may indeed interfere with the function of stored RBCs in recipients characterized by (medication- or infection-induced) redox disequilibrium. Moreover, variation in the RBC osmotic fragility throughout the storage period was found proportional to its baseline levels in G6PD$^-$ donors (**Figure 10**). In a similar way, numerous biochemical components *in vivo* (including S-adenosyl methionine that provides cysteine to support GSH synthesis) had significant correlations with the fragilities of stored G6PD$^-$ RBCs after 24 h staying at body temperature (iMCF, iMFI). Of note, alpha-tocopherol levels in fresh mouse RBCs were reported to correlate with recovery in animal studies (25) and its levels in G6PD$^-$ donors correlated not only with in-bag hemolysis but also with the pro-hemolytic features of the stored RBCs. Our findings may be functionally linked to the performance of G6PD$^-$ RBCs, which has been questioned at both laboratory (22) and clinical levels (21). To support, *in vivo* levels of aspartate, glutamine and thymine were indeed reported to correlate with recovery in mice (25). Despite the fact that these correlations should be confirmed by *in vivo* studies in human, they provide an insight into the pathophysiology of post-transfusion complications in therapies involving G6PD$^-$ donors.

CONCLUSION

This study showed for the first time that the metabolic phenotypes of G6PD-deficient donors recapitulate the basic storage lesion profile observed in G6PD sufficient donors, which is characterized by loss of metabolic linkage and rewiring, in spite of certain differences observed in one-carbon metabolism, glutathione/urate homeostasis, and fatty acid pathways. Moreover, it revealed that donor variability issues affect the storage quality even in the narrow context of this small donor subgroup characterized by an enzymatic genetic defect. We reported an interesting and informative interplay between redox, energy, and hemolysis parameters before and during storage, namely, between factors which differ among G6PD$^-$ donors at the time blood was harvested, and the storability of donated RBCs, a part of which may be related to their performance in the transfused patient. Our data provide mechanistic insight into the biology of RBC storage in G6PD deficiency and could guide future studies focusing on donor biology-related factors involved in the regulation of storage-induced hemolysis that is a multivariate phenotype of the RBC storage lesion. Development of reliable physiological and metabolic biomarkers of storage quality and post-transfusion performance (e.g., post-transfusion recovery, iron metabolism) in fresh or stored blood from G6PD sufficient or deficient donors would allow donor screening and thus improved management of both donor and RBC inventory at time of collection or prior to release of the RBC concentrates from the Blood Bank.

ETHICS STATEMENT

The study was approved by the Ethics Committee of the Department of Biology, School of Science, NKUA. Investigations were carried out upon signing of written consent, in accordance with the principles of the Declaration of Helsinki.

AUTHOR CONTRIBUTIONS

Each author has contributed to the submitted work as follows: AK, AD, and MA designed the study. JR, TN, and AD performed the UHPLC-MS analyses. VT, AK, and MA prepared the RBC units and performed the hematological and physiological analyses. AV performed the biological networks. VT, AD and MA analyzed the results, prepared the figures, and wrote the first draft of the manuscript. IP critically commented on the interpretation of data and drafting of the manuscript, and all the authors contributed to the final version.

ACKNOWLEDGMENTS

The authors would like to thank Leontini E. Foudoulaki-Paparizos MD pathologist, former Director of the "Agios Panteleimon" General Hospital of Nikea Blood Transfusion Center, for the recruitment of the G6PD-deficient volunteers.

REFERENCES

1. D'Alessandro A, Kriebardis AG, Rinalducci S, Antonelou MH, Hansen KC, Papassideri IS, et al. An update on red blood cell storage lesions, as gleaned through biochemistry and omics technologies. *Transfusion* (2015) 55(1):205–19. doi:10.1111/trf.12804
2. Tissot JD, Bardyn M, Sonego G, Abonnenc M, Prudent M. The storage lesions: from past to future. *Transfus Clin Biol* (2017) 24(3):277–84. doi:10.1016/j.tracli.2017.05.012
3. van 't Erve TJ, Doskey CM, Wagner BA, Hess JR, Darbro BW, Ryckman KK, et al. Heritability of glutathione and related metabolites in stored red blood cells. *Free Radic Biol Med* (2014) 76:107–13. doi:10.1016/j.freeradbiomed.2014.07.040
4. van 't Erve TJ, Wagner BA, Martin SM, Knudson CM, Blendowski R, Keaton M, et al. The heritability of metabolite concentrations in stored human red blood cells. *Transfusion* (2014) 54(8):2055–63. doi:10.1111/trf.12605
5. Van 't Erve TJ, Wagner BA, Martin SM, Knudson CM, Blendowski R, Keaton M, et al. The heritability of hemolysis in stored human red blood cells. *Transfusion* (2015) 55(6):1178–85. doi:10.1111/trf.12992
6. Bardyn M, Tissot JD, Prudent M. Oxidative stress and antioxidant defenses during blood processing and storage of erythrocyte concentrates. *Transfus Clin Biol* (2017). doi:10.1016/j.tracli.2017.08.001
7. Kriebardis AG, Antonelou MH, Stamoulis KE, Economou-Petersen E, Margaritis LH, Papassideri IS. Progressive oxidation of cytoskeletal proteins and accumulation of denatured hemoglobin in stored red cells. *J Cell Mol Med* (2007) 11(1):148–55. doi:10.1111/j.1582-4934.2007.00008.x
8. Reisz JA, Wither MJ, Dzieciatkowska M, Nemkov T, Issaian A, Yoshida T, et al. Oxidative modifications of glyceraldehyde 3-phosphate dehydrogenase regulate metabolic reprogramming of stored red blood cells. *Blood* (2016) 128(12):e32–42. doi:10.1182/blood-2016-05-714816
9. D'Alessandro A, Nemkov T, Kelher M, West FB, Schwindt RK, Banerjee A, et al. Routine storage of red blood cell (RBC) units in additive solution-3: a comprehensive investigation of the RBC metabolome. *Transfusion* (2015) 55(6):1155–68. doi:10.1111/trf.12975
10. Rolfsson O, Sigurjonsson OE, Magnusdottir M, Johannsson F, Paglia G, Guethmundsson S, et al. Metabolomics comparison of red cells stored in four additive solutions reveals differences in citrate anticoagulant permeability and metabolism. *Vox Sang* (2017) 112(4):326–35. doi:10.1111/vox.12506
11. Dhabangi A, Ainomugisha B, Cserti-Gazdewich C, Ddungu H, Kyeyune D, Musisi E, et al. Effect of transfusion of red blood cells with longer vs shorter storage duration on elevated blood lactate levels in children with severe anemia: the TOTAL randomized clinical trial. *JAMA* (2015) 314(23):2514–23. doi:10.1001/jama.2015.139772472941
12. Kanias T, Lanteri MC, Page GP, Guo Y, Endres SM, Stone M, et al. Ethnicity, sex, and age are determinants of red blood cell storage and stress hemolysis: results of the REDS-III RBC-Omics study. *Blood* (2017) 1(15):1132–41. doi:10.1182/bloodadvances.2017004820
13. Liumbruno G, D'Alessandro A, Grazzini G, Zolla L. Blood-related proteomics. *J Proteomics* (2010) 73(3):483–507. doi:10.1016/j.jprot.2009.06.010
14. Tzounakas VL, Georgatzakou HT, Kriebardis AG, Papageorgiou EG, Stamoulis KE, Foudoulaki-Paparizos LE, et al. Uric acid variation among regular blood donors is indicative of red blood cell susceptibility to storage lesion markers: a new hypothesis tested. *Transfusion* (2015) 55(11):2659–71. doi:10.1111/trf.13211
15. Tzounakas VL, Georgatzakou HT, Kriebardis AG, Voulgaridou AI, Stamoulis KE, Foudoulaki-Paparizos LE, et al. Donor variation effect on red blood cell storage lesion: a multivariable, yet consistent, story. *Transfusion* (2016) 56(6):1274–86. doi:10.1111/trf.13582
16. Zimring JC, Smith N, Stowell SR, Johnsen JM, Bell LN, Francis RO, et al. Strain-specific red blood cell storage, metabolism, and eicosanoid generation in a mouse model. *Transfusion* (2014) 54(1):137–48. doi:10.1111/trf.12264
17. Hay A, Howie HL, Waterman HR, de Wolski K, Zimring JC. Murine red blood cells from genetically distinct donors cross-regulate when stored together. *Transfusion* (2017) 57:2657–64. doi:10.1111/trf.14313
18. Prudent M, Tissot JD, Lion N. The 3-phase evolution of stored red blood cells and the clinical trials: an obvious relationship. *Blood Transfus* (2017) 15(2):188. doi:10.2450/2017.0317-16
19. Kanias T, Sinchar D, Osei-Hwedieh D, Baust JJ, Jordan A, Zimring JC, et al. Testosterone-dependent sex differences in red blood cell hemolysis in storage, stress, and disease. *Transfusion* (2016) 56:2571–83. doi:10.1111/trf.13745
20. Luzzatto L, Nannelli C, Notaro R. Glucose-6-phosphate dehydrogenase deficiency. *Hematol Oncol Clin North Am* (2016) 30(2):373–93. doi:10.1016/j.hoc.2015.11.006
21. Francis RO, Jhang JS, Pham HP, Hod EA, Zimring JC, Spitalnik SL. Glucose-6-phosphate dehydrogenase deficiency in transfusion medicine: the unknown risks. *Vox Sang* (2013) 105(4):271–82. doi:10.1111/vox.12068
22. Tzounakas VL, Kriebardis AG, Georgatzakou HT, Foudoulaki-Paparizos LE, Dzieciatkowska M, Wither MJ, et al. Glucose 6-phosphate dehydrogenase deficient subjects may be better "storers" than donors of red blood cells. *Free Radic Biol Med* (2016) 96:152–65. doi:10.1016/j.freeradbiomed.2016.04.005
23. Tzounakas VL, Kriebardis AG, Georgatzakou HT, Foudoulaki-Paparizos LE, Dzieciatkowska M, Wither MJ, et al. Data on how several physiological parameters of stored red blood cells are similar in glucose 6-phosphate dehydrogenase deficient and sufficient donors. *Data Brief* (2016) 8:618–27. doi:10.1016/j.dib.2016.06.018
24. Tang HY, Ho HY, Wu PR, Chen SH, Kuypers FA, Cheng ML, et al. Inability to maintain GSH pool in G6PD-deficient red cells causes futile AMPK activation and irreversible metabolic disturbance. *Antioxid Redox Signal* (2015) 22(9):744–59. doi:10.1089/ars.2014.6142
25. de Wolski K, Fu X, Dumont LJ, Roback JD, Waterman H, Odem-Davis K, et al. Metabolic pathways that correlate with post-transfusion circulation of stored murine red blood cells. *Haematologica* (2016) 101:578–86. doi:10.3324/haematol.2015.139139
26. Fu X, Felcyn JR, Odem-Davis K, Zimring JC. Bioactive lipids accumulate in stored red blood cells despite leukoreduction: a targeted metabolomics study. *Transfusion* (2016) 56(10):2560–70. doi:10.1111/trf.13748
27. Nemkov T, Hansen KC, D'Alessandro A. A three-minute method for high-throughput quantitative metabolomics and quantitative tracing experiments of central carbon and nitrogen pathways. *Rapid Commun Mass Spectrom* (2017) 31(8):663–73. doi:10.1002/rcm.7834
28. Clasquin MF, Melamud E, Rabinowitz JD. LC-MS data processing with MAVEN: a metabolomic analysis and visualization engine. *Curr Protoc Bioinformatics* (2012) Chapter 14:Unit 141. doi:10.1002/0471250953.bi1411s37
29. Paglia G, D'Alessandro A, Rolfsson O, Sigurjonsson OE, Bordbar A, Palsson S, et al. Biomarkers defining the metabolic age of red blood cells during cold storage. *Blood* (2016) 128:e43–50. doi:10.1182/blood-2016-06-721688
30. Bordbar A, Johansson PI, Paglia G, Harrison SJ, Wichuk K, Magnusdottir M, et al. Identified metabolic signature for assessing red blood cell unit quality is associated with endothelial damage markers and clinical outcomes. *Transfusion* (2016) 56(4):852–62. doi:10.1111/trf.13460
31. D'Alessandro A, Nemkov T, Yoshida T, Bordbar A, Palsson BO, Hansen KC. Citrate metabolism in red blood cells stored in additive solution-3. *Transfusion* (2017) 57(2):325–36. doi:10.1111/trf.13892
32. Rusnak A, Coghlan G, Zelinski T, Hatch GM. Incorporation of fatty acids into phosphatidylcholine is reduced during storage of human erythrocytes: evidence for distinct lysophosphatidylcholine acyltransferases. *Mol Cell Biochem* (2000) 213(1–2):137–43. doi:10.1023/A:1007128501636

33. Rock G, Tocchi M, Ganz PR, Tackaberry ES. Incorporation of plasticizer into red cells during storage. *Transfusion* (1984) 24(6):493–8. doi:10.1046/j.1537-2995.1984.24685066808.x
34. Rice-Evans C, Rush J, Omorphos SC, Flynn DM. Erythrocyte membrane abnormalities in glucose-6-phosphate dehydrogenase deficiency of the Mediterranean and A-types. *FEBS Lett* (1981) 136(1):148–52. doi:10.1016/0014-5793(81)81235-5
35. D'Alessandro A, Nemkov T, Reisz J, Dzieciatkowska M, Wither MJ, Hansen KC. Omics markers of the red cell storage lesion and metabolic linkage. *Blood Transfus* (2017) 15(2):137–44. doi:10.2450/2017.0341-16
36. Cooper MB, Forte CA, Jones DA. Carnitine and acetylcarnitine in red blood cells. *Biochim Biophys Acta* (1988) 959(2):100–5. doi:10.1016/0005-2760(88)90020-3
37. Nemkov T, Sun K, Reisz JA, Yoshida T, Dunham A, Wen EY, et al. Metabolism of citrate and other carboxylic acids in erythrocytes as a function of oxygen saturation and refrigerated storage. *Front Med* (2017) 4:175. doi:10.3389/fmed.2017.00175
38. Bordbar A, Yurkovich JT, Paglia G, Rolfsson O, Sigurjonsson OE, Palsson BO. Elucidating dynamic metabolic physiology through network integration of quantitative time-course metabolomics. *Sci Rep* (2017) 7:46249. doi:10.1038/srep46249
39. Nemkov T, Sun K, Reisz JA, Song A, Yoshida T, Dunham A, et al. Hypoxia modulates the purine salvage pathway and decreases red blood cell and supernatant levels of hypoxanthine during refrigerated storage. *Haematologica* (2017). doi:10.3324/haematol.2017.178608
40. Peters AL, van Bruggen R, de Korte D, Van Noorden CJ, Vlaar AP. Glucose-6-phosphate dehydrogenase activity decreases during storage of leukoreduced red blood cells. *Transfusion* (2016) 56(2):427–32. doi:10.1111/trf.13378
41. D'Alessandro A, Mirasole C, Zolla L. Haemoglobin glycation (Hb1Ac) increases during red blood cell storage: a MALDI-TOF mass-spectrometry-based investigation. *Vox Sang* (2013) 105(2):177–80. doi:10.1111/vox.12029
42. Tzounakas VL, Anastasiadi AT, Karadimas DG, Zeqo RA, Georgatzakou HT, Pappa OD, et al. Temperature-dependent haemolytic propensity of CPDA-1 stored red blood cells vs whole blood – red cell fragility as donor signature on blood units. *Blood Transfus* (2017) 15(5):447–55. doi:10.2450/2017.0332-16
43. Bardyn M, Maye S, Lesch A, Delobel J, Tissot JD, Cortes-Salazar F, et al. The antioxidant capacity of erythrocyte concentrates is increased during the first week of storage and correlated with the uric acid level. *Vox Sang* (2017) 112:638–47. doi:10.1111/vox.12563
44. Park J, Rho HK, Kim KH, Choe SS, Lee YS, Kim JB. Overexpression of glucose-6-phosphate dehydrogenase is associated with lipid dysregulation and insulin resistance in obesity. *Mol Cell Biol* (2005) 25(12):5146–57. doi:10.1128/MCB.25.12.5146-5157.2005
45. Silliman CC, Moore EE, Kelher MR, Khan SY, Gellar L, Elzi DJ. Identification of lipids that accumulate during the routine storage of prestorage leukoreduced red blood cells and cause acute lung injury. *Transfusion* (2011) 51(12):2549–54. doi:10.1111/j.1537-2995.2011.03186.x
46. Antonelou MH, Seghatchian J. Insights into red blood cell storage lesion: toward a new appreciation. *Transfus Apher Sci* (2016) 55(3):292–301. doi:10.1016/j.transci.2016.10.019
47. Vraets A, Lin Y, Callum JL. Transfusion-associated hyperkalemia. *Transfus Med Rev* (2011) 25(3):184–96. doi:10.1016/j.tmrv.2011.01.006
48. Roback JD, Josephson CD, Waller EK, Newman JL, Karatela S, Uppal K, et al. Metabolomics of ADSOL (AS-1) red blood cell storage. *Transfus Med Rev* (2014) 28(2):41–55. doi:10.1016/j.tmrv.2014.01.003
49. Chen D, Schubert P, Devine DV. Proteomic analysis of red blood cells from donors exhibiting high hemolysis demonstrates a reduction in membrane-associated proteins involved in the oxidative response. *Transfusion* (2017) 57(9):2248–56. doi:10.1111/trf.14188
50. Orbach A, Zelig O, Yedgar S, Barshtein G. Biophysical and biochemical markers of red blood cell fragility. *Transfus Med Hemother* (2017) 44(3):183–7. doi:10.1159/000452106
51. Welbourn EM, Wilson MT, Yusof A, Metodiev MV, Cooper CE. The mechanism of formation, structure and physiological relevance of covalent hemoglobin attachment to the erythrocyte membrane. *Free Radic Biol Med* (2017) 103:95–106. doi:10.1016/j.freeradbiomed.2016.12.024
52. Matte A, Pantaleo A, Ferru E, Turrini F, Bertoldi M, Lupo F, et al. The novel role of peroxiredoxin-2 in red cell membrane protein homeostasis and senescence. *Free Radic Biol Med* (2014) 76:80–8. doi:10.1016/j.freeradbiomed.2014.08.004
53. Rinalducci S, D'Amici GM, Blasi B, Vaglio S, Grazzini G, Zolla L. Peroxiredoxin-2 as a candidate biomarker to test oxidative stress levels of stored red blood cells under blood bank conditions. *Transfusion* (2011) 51:1439–49. doi:10.1111/j.1537-2995.2010.03032.x
54. D'Alessandro A, Dzieciatkowska M, Hill RC, Hansen KC. Supernatant protein biomarkers of red blood cell storage hemolysis as determined through an absolute quantification proteomics technology. *Transfusion* (2016) 56(6):1329–39. doi:10.1111/trf.13483
55. Ksiazek M, Chacinska M, Chabowski A, Baranowski M. Sources, metabolism, and regulation of circulating sphingosine-1-phosphate. *J Lipid Res* (2015) 56(7):1271–81. doi:10.1194/jlr.R059543
56. Sun K, Zhang Y, D'Alessandro A, Nemkov T, Song A, Wu H, et al. Sphingosine-1-phosphate promotes erythrocyte glycolysis and oxygen release for adaptation to high-altitude hypoxia. *Nat Commun* (2016) 7:12086. doi:10.1038/ncomms12086
57. Selim S, Sunkara M, Salous AK, Leung SW, Berdyshev EV, Bailey A, et al. Plasma levels of sphingosine 1-phosphate are strongly correlated with haematocrit, but variably restored by red blood cell transfusions. *Clin Sci (Lond)* (2011) 121(12):565–72. doi:10.1042/CS20110236
58. Camerer E, Regard JB, Cornelissen I, Srinivasan Y, Duong DN, Palmer D, et al. Sphingosine-1-phosphate in the plasma compartment regulates basal and inflammation-induced vascular leak in mice. *J Clin Invest* (2009) 119(7):1871–9. doi:10.1172/JCI38575
59. Barshtein G, Pries AR, Goldschmidt N, Zukerman A, Orbach A, Zelig O, et al. Deformability of transfused red blood cells is a potent determinant of transfusion-induced change in recipient's blood flow. *Microcirculation* (2016) 23(7):479–86. doi:10.1111/micc.12296
60. Bosman GJ. Survival of red blood cells after transfusion: processes and consequences. *Front Physiol* (2013) 4:376. doi:10.3389/fphys.2013.00376
61. Tzounakas VL, Kriebardis AG, Seghatchian J, Papassideri IS, Antonelou MH. Unraveling the Gordian knot: red blood cell storage lesion and transfusion outcomes. *Blood Transfus* (2017) 15(2):126–30. doi:10.2450/2017.0313-16

4

The Role of Plasma Transfusion in Massive Bleeding: Protecting the Endothelial Glycocalyx?

Stefano Barelli[1] *and Lorenzo Alberio*[1,2]*

[1] Division of Haematology and Central Haematology Laboratory, CHUV, Lausanne University Hospital, University of Lausanne, Lausanne, Switzerland, [2] Faculté de Biologie et Médecine, UNIL, University of Lausanne, Lausanne, Switzerland

***Correspondence:**
Lorenzo Alberio
lorenzo.alberio@chuv.ch

ORCID ID:
orcid.org/0000-0001-9686-9920

Massive hemorrhage is a leading cause of death worldwide. During the last decade several retrospective and some prospective clinical studies have suggested a beneficial effect of early plasma-based resuscitation on survival in trauma patients. The underlying mechanisms are unknown but appear to involve the ability of plasma to preserve the endothelial glycocalyx. In this mini-review, we summarize current knowledge on glycocalyx structure and function, and present data describing the impact of hemorrhagic shock and resuscitation fluids on glycocalyx. Animal studies show that hemorrhagic shock leads to glycocalyx shedding, endothelial inflammatory changes, and vascular hyper-permeability. In these animal models, plasma administration preserves glycocalyx integrity and functions better than resuscitation with crystalloids or colloids. In addition, we briefly present data on the possible plasma components responsible for these effects. The endothelial glycocalyx is increasingly recognized as a critical component for the physiological vasculo-endothelial function, which is destroyed in hemorrhagic shock. Interventions for preserving an intact glycocalyx shall improve survival of trauma patients.

Keywords: massive hemorrhage, shock, resuscitation, fresh frozen plasma, endothelium, glycocalyx

The aim of this mini-review is to give an overview on plasma treatment in massive bleeding. We will briefly describe current pathophysiological concepts of vascular damage in hemorrhagic shock, summarize data on the use of plasma as a resuscitation fluid, and report experimental data suggesting a protective role of plasma on endothelial integrity.

TRAUMA, MASSIVE HEMORRHAGE, AND TRAUMA-INDUCED COAGULOPATHY (TIC)

Epidemiology and Definition of Massive Hemorrhage

The World Health Organization estimates that in the year 2000, 5 million people died of injuries, accounting for 9% of global annual mortality (1). After central nervous injury, massive hemorrhage represents the second-leading cause of death, being responsible for 30–40% of trauma-related mortality (1). Death can occur within 3–6 h by exsanguination from uncontrolled hemorrhage and one-third to half of the deaths occur before reaching the hospital (1, 2). Modern transfusion practices and blood supply make massive hemorrhage a potentially preventable cause of death in different settings (e.g., civilian or military trauma, surgery, post-partum). The benefit of blood component transfusion in the context of trauma has been discussed for many years but it is only since the retrospective study of Borgmann published in 2007 (3) that plasma transfusion has been recognized as a probable positive factor for survival. However, "survival bias" remains an unsolved pitfall of retrospective studies, not only for interpreting potentially causative factors related to survival (i.e., did the patient "survive because she received plasma transfusion" *or* did she "get plasma transfusion because survived long enough to receive it"?) but also for defining massive hemorrhage. In fact, the classical definition of massive hemorrhage is based on the number of packed red blood cells (PRBC) units transfused during the first 24 h after admission. High mortality rates during the first 24 h and rapid time course of massive hemorrhage make transfusion rate (e.g., ≥3 PRBC units/60 min) a more appropriate definition (4). In addition, data analysis from the PROMMT study enabled Rahbar et al. to identify those patients most likely to develop massive hemorrhage based on emergency admission variables, such as systolic blood pressure, heart rate, pH, and hemoglobin (5). This prospective observational study showed that transfusion with higher ratio of plasma to PRBC early in resuscitation is associated with an improved survival at 24 h (6). Specifically, adult trauma patients surviving beyond 30 min from admission and transfused with ≥1 unit of PRBC in the first 6 h and ≥3 units of PRBC during the first 24 h showed a significantly higher survival at 6 and 24 h, and 30 days when receiving plasma units and PRBC at a ratio of at least 1:1 (6, 7). Of note, such high plasma to PRBC ratios beyond the first 24 h was not associated with survival by day 30.

Pathophysiological Concepts

The so-called acute trauma coagulopathy (ATC) (8) and TIC (9) have been conceptualized through different models, all converging to the key concept of «endothelial stress» (10–20), also named «endotheliopathy of trauma» (21, 22) or «shock-induced endotheliopathy» (23). The endothelium covering an area of about 5,000 m^2 is one of the frailest and initial victims of massive hemorrhage (24). For instance, severe hypo-perfusion is associated with increased levels of circulating heparan sulfate, a component of the endothelial surface with anticoagulatory properties similar to heparin (25). Moreover, the co-existence of severe tissue injury, leading to high *in vivo* thrombin generation, and severe hypo-perfusion, leading to endothelial sufferance and thrombomodulin shedding, is complicated by circulating thrombin–thrombomodulin complexes culminating in systemic protein C activation and fibrinolysis (8, 9).

Several factors drive the system into a vicious circle: (1) on the one side, endothelial injury with enhanced vascular permeability leads to further loss of intravascular volume, hypovolemia, tissue hypoxia, and exacerbated shock and (2) on the other side, resuscitation-related blood dilution with acidosis and hypothermia (the classical iatrogenic triad) further impair vasculo-endothelial functions. In sum, massive hemorrhage means perfusion, oxygenation, coagulation, and metabolic failures.

PLASMA AS A RESUSCITATION FLUID

Plasma Type, Delivery, and Supply

Plasma sources and plasma processing have been developed during these last decades (18). Each preparation addresses and mitigates particular risks related to transfusion hazards: single donor fresh frozen plasma (FFP) vs pooled plasma or quarantine FFP vs pathogen-inactivated FFP to diminish the risk of transfusion-transmitted infections; FP24 (frozen within 24 h after donation) instead of standard FFP (frozen within 8 h after donation) to enable HLA testing and remove high risk units for TRALI; frozen plasma vs liquid or thawed plasma to extend storage duration; lyophilization formulas for rapid reconstitution. Study of the variability of coagulation factors and natural anticoagulants levels in different plasma preparations are summarized elsewhere (26). Of note, the factor V and factor VIII, known to be «labile» and critical in the evaluation of manufacture practice, show heterogeneous decrease during storage, depending on formulas. Several studies reveal how processing conditions (whole blood hold-time, storage duration/temperature before freezing, freezing mode, leucodepletion, pathogen inactivation, lyophilization) specifically influence coagulation factor levels, microparticles content, clot generation capacity and protein composition in plasma (27–30) and clotting factor stability after thawing (31). In massive hemorrhage management, logistical concerns, besides biological aspects such as type of plasma, FFP to PRBC ratio or functional monitoring of clot generation, matters as well. Time between trauma and transfusion, transport of plasma from blood bank to the clinical unit, mode of checking plasma unit before transfusion and provision of thawed/liquid plasma are most critical aspects in massive transfusion protocols (32–34).

Hence, one logistical challenge for blood bankers is plasma supply. Benefit from plasma transfusion in massive hemorrhage lead to growing use of «universal» but scarce AB plasma (35). At the same time, implementation of the «male policy» (plasma donation from male donors only) to improve the transfusion safety regarding risk of TRALI significantly restricts plasma availability. This demand/supply imbalance led the American Red Cross to consider the use of group A plasma to adult trauma patients (36). Novak et al. reported the experience of 12 trauma centers participating in the PROPPR study in managing plasma inventory to meet new guidelines issued by the American College of Surgeons in 2013 for trauma resuscitation (37). Rapid delivery is made possible by the selection of group A plasma with low titer anti-B, in addition to plasma formulations and thawing systems with short turnaround time.

Benefit of Plasma Transfusion: Do Coagulation Factors Tell the Whole Story?

Since the time Borgman et al. demonstrated in 2007 that FFP transfusion in massive hemorrhage resulted in increased survival (3), researcher started to wonder which mechanisms may be responsible for this effect. The first hypothesis at hand would have been the correction of coagulopthy. However, plasma transfusion in the form of FFP cannot replace coagulation factor loss (38). Therefore, several publications aimed to investigate the benefit of plasma resuscitation on other pathophysiological variables, such as endothelial restoration (39–45).

ENDOTHELIAL GLYCOCALYX

The Endothelial Glycocalyx Structure and Function

The endothelial glycocalyx is a thick (about 0.2–3.0 μm *in vivo*) (46, 47), negatively charged carbohydrate-rich layer coating the vascular endothelium (48–52). The glycocalyx *sensu stricto* is formed by cell membrane-bound sulfated proteoglycans, consisting of a core protein (e.g., transmembrane syndecan, membrane-bound glypican, or basement matrix-associated perlecan) with glycosaminoglycans side chains (e.g., heparan sulfate, hyaluronic acid, and chondroitin sulfate) (53), and cell membrane glycoproteins bearing sialoproteins (50, 53). Syndecan-1 (CD 138), a heparan sulfate containing proteoglycan, is one of the major constituents ensuring endothelial integrity (51). Under physiological conditions, positively charged soluble components (such as plasma proteins, enzymes, growth factors, cytokines, amino acids, and cations) and water are trapped in the glycocalyx forming an extended endothelial surface layer. The mesh formed by the gylcocalyx contains ~1 to 1.5 l plasma, which are in dynamic equilibrium with the flowing blood (48, 54, 55).

The glycocalyx has several recognized functions (**Table 1**) (49–52). In particular, it forms a physical barrier between blood and vessel wall (48, 56–60); it maintains blood fluidity by modulating the interactions of the endothelium with blood cells and proteins (50, 61–63); it regulates cell adhesion and vascular permeability (64); it creates a high intravascular colloid-osmotic gradient (65, 66); and it acts as a mechano-transducer, e.g., by sensing shear stress and inducing endothelial release of nitric oxide (60, 63, 67, 68). As it may be expected from its many functions, the disruption of the glycocalyx leads to several clinically relevant pathologies (48, 52, 61). In the following paragraph, we will discuss the effect of hemorrhagic shock and type of resuscitation fluid on the glycocalyx.

TABLE 1 | Some recognized functions of the endothelial glycocalyx (48–50, 52, 69, 70).

Functions	Mechanisms	Reference
Barrier and filter	Protection from shear	(71)
	Exchange of water and solutes	(48)
	Sieve for plasma proteins	(57, 59)
	Uptake of low density lipoproteins	(63, 72)
	Repels red blood cells	(50)
Cell adhesion regulation	Prevents leukocyte adhesion	(56–58, 60, 73)
	Prevents platelet adhesion	(74)
Anticoagulation	Tissue factor pathway inhibitor	(48)
	Antithrombin	(50, 75)
	Thrombomodulin	(50)
Complement regulation	Complement factor H binding	(76)
Colloid-osmotic gradient	Absorption of albumin and smaller solutes	(65, 71)
Mechano-transducer	Nitric oxyde production	(50, 68, 77)
	Prostacyclin production	(48)
Inter-endothelial communication	Regulation of endothelial gap junctions	(78, 79)

Hemorrhagic Shock, Endothelial Glycocalyx, and Resuscitation Fluid

Shedding of endothelial glycocalyx components has been shown to occur in response to, e.g., ischemia and hypoxia (80), reactive oxygen species (81), inflammation and sepsis (82), and trauma-related sympatho-adrenal activation (83). As recently reviewed by Becker et al., loss of glycocalyx appears to be mediated by "sheddases," such as matrix metalloproteases, heparanases, hyaluronidases, and proteases (60) and to be responsible for endothelial inflammatory changes and vascular hyperpermeability (51, 64). In hemorrhagic shock, loss of the endothelial glycocalyx correlates with a dismal outcome. For instance, human studies indicate that in trauma patients with severe bleeding, high levels of syndecan-1 on admission (≥40 ng/ml) correlate with the extent of tissue damage, laboratory indicators of ATC and, in particular, mortality (84–86). Rahbar et al. showed that high circulating syndecan-1 levels correlate with increased vascular permeability (87). Since plasma-based resuscitation appears to exert a beneficial effect on survival (6, 7, 88), the question is whether plasma as a resuscitation fluid may have an impact on the endothelial glycocalyx and, therefore, potentially on vascular integrity and function.

Investigations in animal models may help framing a working concept (**Table 2**). Kozar et al. (40) employed a pressure-controlled model of hemorrhagic shock. Rats were bled to a mean arterial pressure of 30 mmHg for 90 min then resuscitated with either lactated Ringer's solution (LR) or fresh plasma to a mean arterial pressure of 80 mmHg. These animals were compared to shams (all procedures without bleeding) and positive controls (hemorrhagic shock without resuscitation). The authors found that (1) hemorrhagic shock is associated with a significant shedding of the endothelial glycocalyx, as indicated by circulating syndecan-1 levels, cell surface expression of syndecan-1, and electron microscopy imaging; (2) loss of the endothelial syndecan-1 correlates with the extent of lung injury, as assessed by alveolar wall thickness, capillary congestion, and cellularity; (3) resuscitation with plasma partially restores the endothelial glycocalyx while LR cannot, as assessed by electron microscopy on post-capillary venules obtained from the small bowel mesentery and by syndecan-1 expression in the lung; (4) the endothelial glycocalyx appears to be restored within 3 h after plasma resuscitation; (5) a clinically potential beneficial effect of plasma is suggested by the observations that plasma resuscitation required significantly less volume to maintain the mean arterial pressure at 80 mmHg compared to LR, and by the fact that plasma reduced lung injury while LR resuscitation increased it (40). These observations were expanded by the work of Torres et al. (42). In their model, a 40% blood volume hemorrhage was induced in rats. After 30 min of shock, animals were resuscitated with LR, hydroxyethyl starch (HES) or FFP, and compared to sham and hemorrhage without resuscitation. First, the authors confirmed that the endothelial glycocalyx is significantly damaged by the hemorrhagic shock and can be restored only with FFP, as assessed by circulating syndecan-1 levels and glycocalyx thickness. Second, a clinically beneficial effect of plasma-based resuscitation was

TABLE 2 | Studies[a] investigating endothelial integrity through plasma exposition in HS conditions.

Reference	Experimental models	Types of plasma	Main results
Pati et al. (39)	Studies on HUPECs monolayers (hypoxia-induced permeability) with assessment of EC permeability (FITC-Dextran) after FFP treatment, comparing FFP stored for 0 vs FFP stored for 5 days *In vivo* studies on rat model of HS for testing capacity of FFP (comparing FFP stored for 0 vs for 5 days) to restore MAP	Human FFP (ABO blood types, same donor or pooled from three donors, thawed-aliquoted-stored at 4°C for 0 or 5 days before use)	Day 0 FFP inhibits EC permeability; day 5 FFP demonstrated a diminished capacity to inhibit EC permeability Day 0 FFP, but not day 5 FFP, restores blood pressure to baseline
Kozar et al. (40)	Studies on a rat model of HS, comparing effect of LR vs fresh plasma resuscitation with assessment of endothelial glycocalyx on mesenteric vessels (electronic microscopy), relative expression level of syndecan-1 (QRT RT PCR) and cell surface expression of syndecan-1 (immunostaining) in lung tissue	Fresh plasma (not otherwise specified)	Glycocalyx is partially restored by plasma resuscitation Syndecan-1 expression in lung is enhanced by plasma Lung injury is lessened by plasma resuscitation
Haywood-Watson et al. (86)	Studies on HUVECs monolayers (hypoxia-induced permeability) with assessment of VE-cadherin and syndecan-1 expression (immunofluorescence), topographical properties (AFM), permeability (FITC-Dextran) after LR vs FFP treatment Patients admitted to ICU for shock, resuscitation with plasma, syndecan-1 and cytokines measurements	FFP (not otherwise specified)	Vascular integrity is disrupted by shock but mitigated by FFP FFP hastens syndecan-1 restoration compared to LR Injured patients in shock shed syndecan-1; syndecan-1 correlates with specific inflammatory cytokines
Torres et al. (42)	Studies on a rat HS models comparing effect of LR/HS vs fresh plasma resuscitation with studies on blood samples (including thromboelastometry) and on endothelium (glycocalyx thickness measurements by fluorescent dye-exclusion method)	FFP defined as plasma frozen within 6–8 h of collection and stored at −20°C, prepared by separation form whole blood collected on donor rats	Restoration of coagulation function by a small-volume resuscitation with FFP in contrast to resuscitation with LR/HS groups
Peng et al. (41)	Studies on HUPECs monolayers (VEGF-A165-induced permeability) with assessment of EC permeability (TEER/ECIS and FITC-Dextran) and leukocyte-endothelial binding Mouse model of HS and trauma comparing effect of LR vs FFP resuscitation with *in vivo* studies (MAP monitoring, measurement of syndecan-1 in plasma) and *in vitro* studies on harvested lungs: vascular permeability (intravenous fluorescent dye extravasation), infiltration of neutrophils (MPO immunofluorescence staining and activity), syndecan-1 detection (anti-syndecan-1 antibody)	Human FFP used in both *in vitro* and *in vivo* studies (frozen within 8 h after donation, kept frozen until the day of experiment and used within 1–2 h of thaw)	In HUPECs monolayers, FFP compared with LR reduces pulmonary endothelial hyper-permaeability and leukocyte binding In mouse HS models, FFP and LR similarly restore MAP. FFP mitigates lung hyper-permeability, reduces lung inflammation, increases lung syndecan-1, and reduces syndecan-1 shedding compared with LR resuscitation
Wataha et al. (44)	Studies on HUVECs and PECs monolayers (VEGF-A165-induced permeability) comparing effect of FFP, SD-FFP, SDP (controls: LR/HS) with assessment of EC permeability (FITC-Dextran), WBC binding assay (fluorescent labeling), surface adhesion molecules/integrin expression (flow cytometry) and VE-cadherin/β-catenin mobilization to cell surface (staining)	Human FFP (frozen at −20°C, thawed at 37°C and used on day 0–1 of thaw) SDP defined as pooled liquid plasma that has been dehydrated by means of spray drying and reconstituted citric acid and monobasic sodium phosphate (SD-FFP being the starting material)	FFP, SD-FFP, and SPD equivalently inhibit vascular permeability, ensures EC adherens junctions integrity and endothelial WBC binding Lack of difference between FFP and SD-FFP and between SD-FFP and SDP indicating that solvent-detergent treatment and spray drying do not affect the ability of plasma product to modulate endothelial function
Potter et al. (45)	Studies on HUVECs monolayers (VEGF-A165-induced permeability), comparing FFP and SDP (controls: LR) by testing endothelial permeability (TEER/ECIS), cytokine production in EC and gene expression Mouse model of HS comparing FFP and SDP (controls: LR) with *in vivo* studies (MAP and BE monitoring) and measurement of EC adherent junctions stability (immunofluorescence and histological staining) on harvested lungs	FFP obtained from human donors plasma by apheresis collection, used freshly thawed (same day of thaw) SDP from multidonor plasma (more than 150 type AB donors)	On HUVECs monolayers, FFP and SDP decrease endothelial permeability, induce similar patterns of gene expression and cytokines production in EC In mouse HS models, SDP and FFP equivalently correct MAP and BE, reduce pulmonary vascular leak, equivalently inhibit leukocyte infiltration and breakdown of endothelial adherens and tight junctions
Torres Filho et al. (90)	Rat model of HS for studying quantitatively the relationship between plasma biomarkers and changes in microvascular parameters, including glycocalyx thickness after resuscitation with FWB, PRBC, FFP, 5% albumin, or crystalloids (RL, NS, and HTS)	FWB (3.2% citrate, stored at 4°C, used with 24 h), PRBC (used within 48 h), and FFP (frozen within 6–8 h of collection, stored at −80°C for up to 1 year) all from donor rats	Changes in glycocalyx thickness (and microvascular permeability) negatively (positively) correlated with changes in plasma levels of syndecan-1 and heparane sulfate FWB and FFP, but neither colloid or crystalloid resuscitation, support vascular stabilization by reconstitution of the endothelia glycocalyx after HS

(Continued)

TABLE 2 | Continued

Reference	Experimental models	Types of plasma	Main results
Diebel et al. (91)	HUVEC lined microfluidics model for studying endothelial cell activation/injury and glycocalyx barrier function after simulation of HS by treatment with epinephrine and hypoxia reoxygenation	5% human plasma perfused immediately following treatment or after a 3 h delay	"Early" plasma mitigates glycocalyx degradation and inflammatory prothrombotic endothelial response
Pati et al. (92)	Studies on HUVECs monolayers (VEGF-A165-induced permeability), comparing FFP and LP (controls: LR or no treatment) by testing EC permeability (FITC-Dextran), EC resistance (TEER/ECIS), VE-cadherin/β-catenin mobilization to cell surface (staining), leukocyte-binding (fluorescent labeling) Mouse model of HS comparing FFP and LP (controls: LR or no treatment) with assessment of inflammation (MPO staining), vascular permeability (dye extravasation) and tissue edema (wet-to-dry weight ratio)	Human FFP (male donors O+) thawed and used freshly (day 0 of thaw) LP defined as lyophilized plasma (male O+) reconstituted in buffer	On HUVECs monolayers, FFP and LP decrease endothelial permeability, preserve EC adherens junctions, attenuate EC-leukocyte-binding In mouse HS models, LP and FFP reduce pulmonary vascular permeability, edema, and inflammation

AFM, atomic force microscopy; BE, base excess; EC, endothelial cell; ECIS, electric cell-substrate impedance system; FFP, fresh frozen plasma; FITC, fluorescein isothiocyanate-conjugated; FWB, fresh whole blood; HES, hydroxyethyl starch; HS, hemorrhagic shock; HTS, hypertonic (3%) sodium chloride; HUPEC, human pulmonary endothelial cell; HUVEC, human umbilical vein endothelial cell; LP, lyophilized plasma; LR, lactated ringers; MAP, mean arterial pressure; NS, normal saline; PEC, pulmonary endothelial cells; PRBC, packed red blood cells; QRT RT PCR, quantitative real-time reverse-transcription polymerase chain reaction; SD, solvent detergent; SDP, spray-dried plasma; TEER, trans-endothelial electrical resistance; VE-cadherin, vascular endothelial cadherin; WBC, white blood cell.

[a]*Studies identified by searching the terms "glycocalyx, haemorrhagic shock, plasma" on PubMed and secondary references.*

indicated by the fact that FFP corrected metabolic acidosis significantly better than LR and HES, as assessed by pH, base excess, and lactate. This was associated with an improved microcirculation and a lesser degree of hemodilution by FFP compared to LR and HES (42). This latter point was also observed by a recent publication of Nelson et al. (89), who demonstrated that resuscitation with FFP resulted in a circulating volume expansion equaling the volume of blood loss, while circulating volume expansion by Ringer's acetate was less effective.

The pulmonary effects of hemorrhagic shock and resuscitation fluids were addressed by Peng et al. (41). They investigated pulmonary endothelial inflammation and hyper-permeability employing a coagulopathic mouse model of hemorrhagic shock and trauma. Mice were bled to a mean arterial pressure of 35 ± 5 mmHg for 90 min (93) and subsequently resuscitated over 15 min with either LR (at 3× shed blood volume) or FFP (at 1× shed blood volume). Resuscitated animals were compared to shams (all procedures without shock) and positive controls (hemorrhagic shock without resuscitation). Major findings were as follows: (1) lung permeability, assessed *in vivo* by the extravasation of a fluorescent dextrane or Evan's blue, was significantly increased after hemorrhagic shock compared to shams, and FFP resuscitation was significantly more effective than LR in preventing/correcting shock-induced pulmonary hyper-permeability; (2) similarly, lung inflammation, assessed by detecting myeloperoxidase which reflects neutrophils infiltration, significantly increased after hemorrhagic shock and was lessened by FFP resuscitation; (3) shock-induced loss of pulmonary syndecan-1 was most efficiently prevented by resuscitation with FFP. Of note, similar results on pulmonary inflammation and permeability were reported by Potter et al. employing FFP and spray-dried plasma (SDP) (45).

A recent publication by Torres Filho et al. (90) employing a rat model of hemorrhagic shock showed that (1) syndecan-1 and heparan sulfate represent valuable biomarkers of glycocalyx shedding and (2) fresh whole blood and FFP support vascular stabilization by reconstitution of the endothelial glycocalyx (see **Table 2**).

Syndecan-1 as a Key Mediator of Plasma's Effect

A key question is which plasma component may exert a beneficial effect on the glycocalyx. *In vitro* experiments have shown that FFP enhances pulmonary endothelial syndecan-1 expression in a time- and dose-dependent manner (94). A key role for syndecan-1 is supported by *in vivo* experiments as well. Utilizing the model of trauma-hemorragic shock described by Peng (41), Wu et al. investigated the pulmonary response to the type of resuscitation fluid (FFP vs LR) in wild-type and *Syndecan* gene knock-out ($Sdc1^{-/-}$) mice (94). They found that the inability to synthesize syndecan-1 abrogated the protective effect observed with plasma. In particular, they demonstrated that in absence of syndecan-1 synthesis: (1) the ability of FFP to mitigate the increase in lung permeability induced by hemorrhagic shock was abrogated; (2) FFP lost its ability to dampen the shock-induced increase of pulmonary neutrophil infiltration; and (3) FFP lost its protective effect on histopathologic signs of lung injury. Similar results have been reported by Ban et al. with an animal model of gut injury and inflammation after hemorrhagic shock (95).

Plasma: Coagulation Factors or Other Components?

Intriguingly, a major plasma component that may play a role in preserving endothelial integrity appears to be albumin. While loss of circulating albumin correlated with loss of the glycocalyx and increased fluid extravasation (96), albumin supplementation attenuated glycocalyx shedding and reduced interstitial edema in a guinea pig heart model of cold ischemia (97). Kheirabadi et al. (98) studied the role of albumin in a model of uncontrolled hemorrhage. Rabbits were subjected to a splenic injury. Ten minutes after injury, at a mean arterial pressure less than 40 mmHg, the rabbits received equal volumes (15 ml/kg) of rabbit plasma, HES, or 5% human albumin, targeting a mean arterial pressure of 65 mmHg. The authors observed that: (1) onset of resuscitation initiated additional bleeding and total blood loss did not differ among the three groups; (2) thromboelastography revealed a faster and stronger clot formation in the plasma and albumin groups compared to HES; (3) shock indices were increased in all three groups but less in the albumin one; (4) the albumin group had the highest survival rate (8 out of 9 rabbits) compared to plasma and HES (both 4/10), and positive controls (1/9). This apparent beneficial role of albumin, if confirmed in further studies, may be related to its ability to attenuate neutrophil adhesion to the endothelium and other anti-inflammatory properties, its scavenging and buffering capacity, its potential to enhance nitric oxide production and stabilize glycocalyx (50, 60, 99). However, a recent publication showed that a four-factor prothrombin complex concentrate (containing vitamin K-dependent coagulation factors and several other plasma proteins) and FFP but not albumin inhibit vascular permeability in an *in vivo* mice model (100). Thus far, it is not known which soluble factor present in the factor concentrate might be responsible for its beneficial effect (100).

As of coagulation factors, despite a current of thought supporting the use of fibrinogen in massive bleeding, we are not aware of publications investigating its impact on glycocalyx and endothelial functions. A recent work observed a U-shaped association between initial fibrinogen concentration in major bleeding and in-hospital mortality, with similar rates of increased mortality for fibrinogen levels <1 g/l and >4 g/l (101). A possible explanation for the negative effect of higher fibrinogen levels is offered by *in vitro* data, suggesting that fibrin promotes endothelial transmigration of neutrophils and inflammation (102).

As of other plasma proteins, adiponectin is an interesting candidate (103). Adiponectin is produced in adipocytes and has been shown to have anti-inflammatory properties and to prevent cytokine-induced endothelial cell hyper-permeability (104–106). Employing a mouse model, Deng et al. demonstrated that (1) hemorrhagic shock leads to a significant decrease of adiponectin levels and a disruption of the lung vascular barrier function; (2) plasma resuscitation improves adiponectin levels and reverses lung injury; (3) the beneficial effect of plasma-based resuscitation is abolished by immunodepletion of adiponectin; and (4) it is restored when plasma was replenished with adiponectin (103). These findings suggest that adiponectin may be an important component contributing to a vasoprotective effect of plasma-based resuscitation.

In sum, several animal studies suggest that early use of plasma in hemorrhagic shock may exert a clinically significant beneficial effect by preserving or even restoring the glycocalyx layer and, therefore, maintaining critical endothelial functions. This appears to be due to the ability of a plasma component to lessen endothelial inflammatory response, possibly by limiting neutrophil adhesion. As of today, it is not known which plasma components are responsible for these effects, which impact plasma processing may exert on them, and which might be the dose–effect relationship.

Human Studies

From a clinical point of view, the key question is whether early resuscitation of hemorrhagic shock with plasma is truly able to improve vasculo-endothelial function and survival. As a proof of principle, a small study in non-bleeding critically ill patients demonstrated that plasma transfusion decreased syndecan-1 and factor VIII levels, suggesting an endothelial stabilizing effect (107). To our knowledge, the only human study prospectively investigating the effect of early plasma-based resuscitation in humans is the COMBAT study (108). In this prospective randomized trial, casualties are treated with 2 units of FFP (thawed in the ambulance) vs conventional crystalloids as initial pre-hospital resuscitation. The study aims to verify whether a "plasma first" resuscitation strategy might be able to (1) attenuate acute traumatic coagulopathy; (2) improve metabolic recovery; (3) decrease blood component transfusion; (4) reduce the incidence of acute lung injury and multiple organ failure; (5) decrease mortality at 24 h or 28 days. According to www.clinicaltrials.gov, the study has been closed after having enrolled 144 patients as per protocol. Results are eagerly awaited.

In conclusion, plasma as early resuscitation fluid for massive hemorrhage appears to exert beneficial effects improving patient survival. Experimental data suggest that this may be related to its ability to preserve endothelial glycocalyx structure and function. We think that these fascinating data shall be confirmed in prospective randomized clinical trials and the mechanisms underlying these effects shall be revealed in order to develop more targeted treatments.

AUTHOR CONTRIBUTIONS

Both authors discussed the literature, wrote the manuscript, and approved the final version.

REFERENCES

1. Kauvar DS, Lefering R, Wade CE. Impact of hemorrhage on trauma outcome: an overview of epidemiology, clinical presentations, and therapeutic considerations. *J Trauma* (2006) 60(6 Suppl):S3–11. doi:10.1097/01.ta.0000199961.02677.19
2. Seghatchian J, Samama MM. Massive transfusion: an overview of the main characteristics and potential risks associated with substances used for correction of a coagulopathy. *Transfus Apher Sci* (2012) 47(2):235–43. doi:10.1016/j.transci.2012.06.001
3. Borgman MA, Spinella PC, Perkins JG, Grathwohl KW, Repine T, Beekley AC, et al. The ratio of blood products transfused affects mortality in patients receiving massive transfusions at a combat support hospital. *J Trauma* (2007) 63(4):805–13. doi:10.1097/TA.0b013e3181271ba3
4. Savage SA, Zarzaur BL, Croce MA, Fabian TC. Redefining massive transfusion when every second counts. *J Trauma Acute Care Surg* (2013) 74(2):396–400. doi:10.1097/TA.0b013e31827a3639
5. Rahbar MH, del Junco DJ, Huang H, Ning J, Fox EE, Zhang X, et al. A latent class model for defining severe hemorrhage: experience from the PROMMTT study. *J Trauma Acute Care Surg* (2013) 75(1 Suppl 1):S82–8. doi:10.1097/TA.0b013e31828fa3d3
6. Holcomb JB, del Junco DJ, Fox EE, Wade CE, Cohen MJ, Schreiber MA, et al. The prospective, observational, multicenter, major trauma transfusion (PROMMTT) study: comparative effectiveness of a time-varying treatment with competing risks. *JAMA Surg* (2013) 148(2):127–36. doi:10.1001/2013.jamasurg.387
7. del Junco DJ, Holcomb JB, Fox EE, Brasel KJ, Phelan HA, Bulger EM, et al. Resuscitate early with plasma and platelets or balance blood products gradually: findings from the PROMMTT study. *J Trauma Acute Care Surg* (2013) 75(1 Suppl 1):S24–30. doi:10.1097/TA.0b013e31828fa3b9
8. Brohi K, Cohen MJ, Davenport RA. Acute coagulopathy of trauma: mechanism, identification and effect. *Curr Opin Crit Care* (2007) 13(6):680–5. doi:10.1097/MCC.0b013e3282f1e78f

9. Giordano S, Spiezia L, Campello E, Simioni P. The current understanding of trauma-induced coagulopathy (TIC): a focused review on pathophysiology. *Intern Emerg Med* (2017) 12(7):981–91. doi:10.1007/s11739-017-1674-0
10. Maegele M, Spinella PC, Schochl H. The acute coagulopathy of trauma: mechanisms and tools for risk stratification. *Shock* (2012) 38(5):450–8. doi:10.1097/SHK.0b013e31826dbd23
11. Hess JR, Lawson JH. The coagulopathy of trauma versus disseminated intravascular coagulation. *J Trauma* (2006) 60(6 Suppl):S12–9. doi:10.1097/01.ta.0000199545.06536.22
12. Cap A, Hunt BJ. The pathogenesis of traumatic coagulopathy. *Anaesthesia* (2015) 70(Suppl 1):e32–4. doi:10.1111/anae.12914
13. Bjerkvig CK, Strandenes G, Eliassen HS, Spinella PC, Fosse TK, Cap AP, et al. "Blood failure" time to view blood as an organ: how oxygen debt contributes to blood failure and its implications for remote damage control resuscitation. *Transfusion* (2016) 56(Suppl 2):S182–9. doi:10.1111/trf.13500
14. Chang R, Cardenas JC, Wade CE, Holcomb JB. Advances in the understanding of trauma-induced coagulopathy. *Blood* (2016) 128(8):1043–9. doi:10.1182/blood-2016-01-636423
15. Gando S, Hayakawa M. Pathophysiology of trauma-induced coagulopathy and management of critical bleeding requiring massive transfusion. *Semin Thromb Hemost* (2016) 42(2):155–65. doi:10.1055/s-0035-1564831
16. Poole D, Cortegiani A, Chieregato A, Russo E, Pellegrini C, De Blasio E, et al. Blood component therapy and coagulopathy in trauma: a systematic review of the literature from the trauma update group. *PLoS One* (2016) 11(10):e0164090. doi:10.1371/journal.pone.0164090
17. Stensballe J, Ostrowski SR, Johansson PI. Haemostatic resuscitation in trauma: the next generation. *Curr Opin Crit Care* (2016) 22(6):591–7. doi:10.1097/MCC.0000000000000359
18. Watson JJ, Pati S, Schreiber MA. Plasma transfusion: history, current realities, and novel improvements. *Shock* (2016) 46(5):468–79. doi:10.1097/SHK.0000000000000663
19. Wong H, Curry N, Stanworth SJ. Blood products and procoagulants in traumatic bleeding: use and evidence. *Curr Opin Crit Care* (2016) 22(6):598–606. doi:10.1097/MCC.0000000000000354
20. Jenkins DH, Rappold JF, Badloe JF, Berseus O, Blackbourne L, Brohi KH, et al. Trauma hemostasis and oxygenation research position paper on remote damage control resuscitation: definitions, current practice, and knowledge gaps. *Shock* (2014) 41(Suppl 1):3–12. doi:10.1097/SHK.0000000000000140
21. Naumann DN, Hazeldine J, Dinsdale RJ, Bishop JR, Midwinter MJ, Harrison P, et al. Endotheliopathy is associated with higher levels of cell-free DNA following major trauma: a prospective observational study. *PLoS One* (2017) 12(12):e0189870. doi:10.1371/journal.pone.0189870
22. Naumann DN, Hazeldine J, Davies DJ, Bishop J, Midwinter MJ, Belli A, et al. Endotheliopathy of trauma is an on-scene phenomenon, and is associated with multiple organ dysfunction syndrome: a prospective observational study. *Shock* (2018) 49(4):420–8. doi:10.1097/SHK.0000000000000999
23. Johansson P, Stensballe J, Ostrowski S. Shock induced endotheliopathy (SHINE) in acute critical illness – a unifying pathophysiologic mechanism. *Crit Care* (2017) 21(1):25. doi:10.1186/s13054-017-1605-5
24. Cannon JW. Hemorrhagic shock. *N Engl J Med* (2018) 378(4):370–9. doi:10.1056/NEJMra1705649
25. Ostrowski SR, Johansson PI. Endothelial glycocalyx degradation induces endogenous heparinization in patients with severe injury and early traumatic coagulopathy. *J Trauma Acute Care Surg* (2012) 73(1):60–6. doi:10.1097/TA.0b013e31825b5c10
26. Boyd TM, Lockhart E, Welsby I. Split blood products. In: Marcucci CE, Schoettker P, editors. *Perioperative Hemostasis*. Berlin Heidelberg: Springer (2015). p. 151–75.
27. Seltsam A, Muller TH. Update on the use of pathogen-reduced human plasma and platelet concentrates. *Br J Haematol* (2013) 162(4):442–54. doi:10.1111/bjh.12403
28. Chan KS, Sparrow RL. Microparticle profile and procoagulant activity of fresh-frozen plasma is affected by whole blood leukoreduction rather than 24-hour room temperature hold. *Transfusion* (2014) 54(8):1935–44. doi:10.1111/trf.12602
29. Runkel S, Hitzler WE, Hellstern P. The impact of whole blood processing and freezing conditions on the quality of therapeutic plasma prepared from whole blood. *Transfusion* (2015) 55(4):796–804. doi:10.1111/trf.12914
30. Steil L, Thiele T, Hammer E, Bux J, Kalus M, Volker U, et al. Proteomic characterization of freeze-dried human plasma: providing treatment of bleeding disorders without the need for a cold chain. *Transfusion* (2008) 48(11):2356–63. doi:10.1111/j.1537-2995.2008.01856.x
31. Thiele T, Kellner S, Hron G, Wasner C, Nauck M, Zimmermann K, et al. Storage of thawed plasma for a liquid plasma bank: impact of temperature and methylene blue pathogen inactivation. *Transfusion* (2012) 52(3):529–36. doi:10.1111/j.1537-2995.2011.03317.x
32. Holcomb JB, Pati S. Optimal trauma resuscitation with plasma as the primary resuscitative fluid: the surgeon's perspective. *Hematology Am Soc Hematol Educ Program* (2013) 2013:656–9. doi:10.1182/asheducation-2013.1.656
33. Etchill E, Sperry J, Zuckerbraun B, Alarcon L, Brown J, Schuster K, et al. The confusion continues: results from an American Association for the Surgery of Trauma survey on massive transfusion practices among United States trauma centers. *Transfusion* (2016) 56(10):2478–86. doi:10.1111/trf.13755
34. Treml AB, Gorlin JB, Dutton RP, Scavone BM. Massive transfusion protocols: a survey of academic medical centers in the United States. *Anesth Analg* (2017) 124(1):277–81. doi:10.1213/ANE.0000000000001610
35. Yazer M, Eder AF, Land KJ. How we manage AB plasma inventory in the blood center and transfusion service. *Transfusion* (2013) 53(8):1627–33. doi:10.1111/trf.12223
36. Dunbar NM, Yazer MH; Biomedical Excellence for Safer Transfusion Collabrative. A possible new paradigm? A survey-based assessment of the use of thawed group A plasma for trauma resuscitation in the United States. *Transfusion* (2016) 56(1):125–9. doi:10.1111/trf.13266
37. Novak DJ, Bai Y, Cooke RK, Marques MB, Fontaine MJ, Gottschall JL, et al. Making thawed universal donor plasma available rapidly for massively bleeding trauma patients: experience from the Pragmatic, Randomized Optimal Platelets and Plasma Ratios (PROPPR) trial. *Transfusion* (2015) 55(6):1331–9. doi:10.1111/trf.13098
38. Garrigue D, Godier A, Glacet A, Labreuche J, Kipnis E, Paris C, et al. French lyophilized plasma versus fresh frozen plasma for the initial management of trauma-induced coagulopathy: a randomized open-label trial. *J Thromb Haemost* (2018) 16(3):481–9. doi:10.1111/jth.13929
39. Pati S, Matijevic N, Doursout MF, Ko T, Cao Y, Deng X, et al. Protective effects of fresh frozen plasma on vascular endothelial permeability, coagulation, and resuscitation after hemorrhagic shock are time dependent and diminish between days 0 and 5 after thaw. *J Trauma* (2010) 69(Suppl 1):S55–63. doi:10.1097/TA.0b013e3181e453d4
40. Kozar RA, Peng Z, Zhang R, Holcomb JB, Pati S, Park P, et al. Plasma restoration of endothelial glycocalyx in a rodent model of hemorrhagic shock. *Anesth Analg* (2011) 112(6):1289–95. doi:10.1213/ANE.0b013e318210385c
41. Peng Z, Pati S, Potter D, Brown R, Holcomb JB, Grill R, et al. Fresh frozen plasma lessens pulmonary endothelial inflammation and hyperpermeability after hemorrhagic shock and is associated with loss of syndecan 1. *Shock* (2013) 40(3):195–202. doi:10.1097/SHK.0b013e31829f91fc
42. Torres LN, Sondeen JL, Ji L, Dubick MA, Torres Filho I. Evaluation of resuscitation fluids on endothelial glycocalyx, venular blood flow, and coagulation function after hemorrhagic shock in rats. *J Trauma Acute Care Surg* (2013) 75(5):759–66. doi:10.1097/TA.0b013e3182a92514
43. Matijevic N, Wang YW, Cotton BA, Hartwell E, Barbeau JM, Wade CE, et al. Better hemostatic profiles of never-frozen liquid plasma compared with thawed fresh frozen plasma. *J Trauma Acute Care Surg* (2013) 74(1):84–90. doi:10.1097/TA.0b013e3182788e32
44. Wataha K, Menge T, Deng X, Shah A, Bode A, Holcomb JB, et al. Spray-dried plasma and fresh frozen plasma modulate permeability and inflammation in vitro in vascular endothelial cells. *Transfusion* (2013) 53(Suppl 1):80S–90S. doi:10.1111/trf.12040
45. Potter DR, Baimukanova G, Keating SM, Deng X, Chu JA, Gibb SL, et al. Fresh frozen plasma and spray-dried plasma mitigate pulmonary vascular permeability and inflammation in hemorrhagic shock. *J Trauma Acute Care Surg* (2015) 78(6 Suppl 1):S7–17. doi:10.1097/TA.0000000000000630
46. Betteridge KB, Arkill KP, Neal CR, Harper SJ, Foster RR, Satchell SC, et al. Sialic acids regulate microvessel permeability, revealed by novel in vivo studies of endothelial glycocalyx structure and function. *J Physiol* (2017) 595(15):5015–35. doi:10.1113/JP274167
47. Ebong EE, Macaluso FP, Spray DC, Tarbell JM. Imaging the endothelial glycocalyx in vitro by rapid freezing/freeze substitution transmission

electron microscopy. *Arterioscler Thromb Vasc Biol* (2011) 31(8):1908–15. doi:10.1161/ATVBAHA.111.225268
48. Reitsma S, Slaaf DW, Vink H, van Zandvoort MA, Egbrink MG. The endothelial glycocalyx: composition, functions, and visualization. *Pflugers Arch* (2007) 454(3):345–59. doi:10.1007/s00424-007-0212-8
49. Weinbaum S, Tarbell JM, Damiano ER. The structure and function of the endothelial glycocalyx layer. *Annu Rev Biomed Eng* (2007) 9:121–67. doi:10.1146/annurev.bioeng.9.060906.151959
50. Alphonsus CS, Rodseth RN. The endothelial glycocalyx: a review of the vascular barrier. *Anaesthesia* (2014) 69(7):777–84. doi:10.1111/anae.12661
51. Ushiyama A, Kataoka H, Iijima T. Glycocalyx and its involvement in clinical pathophysiologies. *J Intensive Care* (2016) 4(1):59. doi:10.1186/s40560-016-0182-z
52. Schott U, Solomon C, Fries D, Bentzer P. The endothelial glycocalyx and its disruption, protection and regeneration: a narrative review. *Scand J Trauma Resusc Emerg Med* (2016) 24:48. doi:10.1186/s13049-016-0239-y
53. Li L, Ly M, Linhardt RJ. Proteoglycan sequence. *Mol Biosyst* (2012) 8(6):1613–25. doi:10.1039/c2mb25021g
54. Rehm M, Zahler S, Lotsch M, Welsch U, Conzen P, Jacob M, et al. Endothelial glycocalyx as an additional barrier determining extravasation of 6% hydroxyethyl starch or 5% albumin solutions in the coronary vascular bed. *Anesthesiology* (2004) 100(5):1211–23. doi:10.1097/00000542-200405000-00025
55. Nieuwdorp M, van Haeften TW, Gouverneur MC, Mooij HL, van Lieshout MH, Levi M, et al. Loss of endothelial glycocalyx during acute hyperglycemia coincides with endothelial dysfunction and coagulation activation in vivo. *Diabetes* (2006) 55(2):480–6. doi:10.2337/diabetes.55.02.06.db05-1103
56. Henry CB, Duling BR. Permeation of the luminal capillary glycocalyx is determined by hyaluronan. *Am J Physiol* (1999) 277(2 Pt 2):H508–14.
57. Lipowsky HH, Gao L, Lescanic A. Shedding of the endothelial glycocalyx in arterioles, capillaries, and venules and its effect on capillary hemodynamics during inflammation. *Am J Physiol Heart Circ Physiol* (2011) 301(6):H2235–45. doi:10.1152/ajpheart.00803.2011
58. Constantinescu AA, Vink H, Spaan JA. Endothelial cell glycocalyx modulates immobilization of leukocytes at the endothelial surface. *Arterioscler Thromb Vasc Biol* (2003) 23(9):1541–7. doi:10.1161/01.ATV.0000085630.24353.3D
59. Vink H, Duling BR. Capillary endothelial surface layer selectively reduces plasma solute distribution volume. *Am J Physiol Heart Circ Physiol* (2000) 278(1):H285–9. doi:10.1152/ajpheart.2000.278.1.H285
60. Becker BF, Jacob M, Leipert S, Salmon AH, Chappell D. Degradation of the endothelial glycocalyx in clinical settings: searching for the sheddases. *Br J Clin Pharmacol* (2015) 80(3):389–402. doi:10.1111/bcp.12629
61. Chelazzi C, Villa G, Mancinelli P, De Gaudio AR, Adembri C. Glycocalyx and sepsis-induced alterations in vascular permeability. *Crit Care* (2015) 19:26. doi:10.1186/s13054-015-0741-z
62. Bansch P, Nelson A, Ohlsson T, Bentzer P. Effect of charge on microvascular permeability in early experimental sepsis in the rat. *Microvasc Res* (2011) 82(3):339–45. doi:10.1016/j.mvr.2011.08.008
63. Kolarova H, Ambruzova B, Svihalkova Sindlerova L, Klinke A, Kubala L. Modulation of endothelial glycocalyx structure under inflammatory conditions. *Mediators Inflamm* (2014) 2014:694312. doi:10.1155/2014/694312
64. Schmidt EP, Lee WL, Zemans RL, Yamashita C, Downey GP. On, around, and through: neutrophil-endothelial interactions in innate immunity. *Physiology (Bethesda)* (2011) 26(5):334–47. doi:10.1152/physiol.00011.2011
65. Rehm M, Bruegger D, Christ F, Conzen P, Thiel M, Jacob M, et al. Shedding of the endothelial glycocalyx in patients undergoing major vascular surgery with global and regional ischemia. *Circulation* (2007) 116(17):1896–906. doi:10.1161/CIRCULATIONAHA.106.684852
66. Biddle C. Like a slippery fish, a little slime is a good thing: the glycocalyx revealed. *AANA J* (2013) 81(6):473–80.
67. Florian JA, Kosky JR, Ainslie K, Pang Z, Dull RO, Tarbell JM. Heparan sulfate proteoglycan is a mechanosensor on endothelial cells. *Circ Res* (2003) 93(10):e136–42. doi:10.1161/01.RES.0000101744.47866.D5
68. Yen W, Cai B, Yang J, Zhang L, Zeng M, Tarbell JM, et al. Endothelial surface glycocalyx can regulate flow-induced nitric oxide production in microvessels in vivo. *PLoS One* (2015) 10(1):e0117133. doi:10.1371/journal.pone.0117133
69. Mitra R, O'Neil GL, Harding IC, Cheng MJ, Mensah SA, Ebong EE. Glycocalyx in atherosclerosis-relevant endothelium function and as a therapeutic target. *Curr Atheroscler Rep* (2017) 19(12):63. doi:10.1007/s11883-017-0691-9
70. Sieve I, Munster-Kuhnel AK, Hilfiker-Kleiner D. Regulation and function of endothelial glycocalyx layer in vascular diseases. *Vascul Pharmacol* (2018) 100:26–33. doi:10.1016/j.vph.2017.09.002
71. Pries AR, Secomb TW, Gaehtgens P. The endothelial surface layer. *Pflugers Arch* (2000) 440(5):653–66. doi:10.1007/s004240000307
72. Segrest JP, Jones MK, De Loof H, Dashti N. Structure of apolipoprotein B-100 in low density lipoproteins. *J Lipid Res* (2001) 42(9):1346–67.
73. Mulivor AW, Lipowsky HH. Role of glycocalyx in leukocyte-endothelial cell adhesion. *Am J Physiol Heart Circ Physiol* (2002) 283(4):H1282–91. doi:10.1152/ajpheart.00117.2002
74. Chappell D, Brettner F, Doerfler N, Jacob M, Rehm M, Bruegger D, et al. Protection of glycocalyx decreases platelet adhesion after ischaemia/reperfusion: an animal study. *Eur J Anaesthesiol* (2014) 31(9):474–81. doi:10.1097/EJA.0000000000000085
75. Dimitrievska S, Gui L, Weyers A, Lin T, Cai C, Wu W, et al. New functional tools for antithrombogenic activity assessment of live surface glycocalyx. *Arterioscler Thromb Vasc Biol* (2016) 36(9):1847–53. doi:10.1161/ATVBAHA.116.308023
76. Boels MG, Lee DH, van den Berg BM, Dane MJ, van der Vlag J, Rabelink TJ. The endothelial glycocalyx as a potential modifier of the hemolytic uremic syndrome. *Eur J Intern Med* (2013) 24(6):503–9. doi:10.1016/j.ejim.2012.12.016
77. Jacob M, Rehm M, Loetsch M, Paul JO, Bruegger D, Welsch U, et al. The endothelial glycocalyx prefers albumin for evoking shear stress-induced, nitric oxide-mediated coronary dilatation. *J Vasc Res* (2007) 44(6):435–43. doi:10.1159/000104871
78. Ampey BC, Morschauser TJ, Lampe PD, Magness RR. Gap junction regulation of vascular tone: implications of modulatory intercellular communication during gestation. *Adv Exp Med Biol* (2014) 814:117–32. doi:10.1007/978-1-4939-1031-1_11
79. Radeva MY, Waschke J. Mind the gap: mechanisms regulating the endothelial barrier. *Acta Physiol (Oxf)* (2018) 222(1). doi:10.1111/apha.12860
80. Annecke T, Fischer J, Hartmann H, Tschoep J, Rehm M, Conzen P, et al. Shedding of the coronary endothelial glycocalyx: effects of hypoxia/reoxygenation vs ischaemia/reperfusion. *Br J Anaesth* (2011) 107(5):679–86. doi:10.1093/bja/aer269
81. van Golen RF, Reiniers MJ, Vrisekoop N, Zuurbier CJ, Olthof PB, van Rheenen J, et al. The mechanisms and physiological relevance of glycocalyx degradation in hepatic ischemia/reperfusion injury. *Antioxid Redox Signal* (2014) 21(7):1098–118. doi:10.1089/ars.2013.5751
82. Nieuwdorp M, Meuwese MC, Mooij HL, van Lieshout MH, Hayden A, Levi M, et al. Tumor necrosis factor-alpha inhibition protects against endotoxin-induced endothelial glycocalyx perturbation. *Atherosclerosis* (2009) 202(1):296–303. doi:10.1016/j.atherosclerosis.2008.03.024
83. Ostrowski SR, Henriksen HH, Stensballe J, Gybel-Brask M, Cardenas JC, Baer LA, et al. Sympathoadrenal activation and endotheliopathy are drivers of hypocoagulability and hyperfibrinolysis in trauma: a prospective observational study of 404 severely injured patients. *J Trauma Acute Care Surg* (2017) 82(2):293–301. doi:10.1097/TA.0000000000001304
84. Johansson PI, Stensballe J, Rasmussen LS, Ostrowski SR. A high admission syndecan-1 level, a marker of endothelial glycocalyx degradation, is associated with inflammation, protein C depletion, fibrinolysis, and increased mortality in trauma patients. *Ann Surg* (2011) 254(2):194–200. doi:10.1097/SLA.0b013e318226113d
85. Gonzalez Rodriguez E, Ostrowski SR, Cardenas JC, Baer LA, Tomasek JS, Henriksen HH, et al. Syndecan-1: a quantitative marker for the endotheliopathy of trauma. *J Am Coll Surg* (2017) 225(3):419–27. doi:10.1016/j.jamcollsurg.2017.05.012
86. Haywood-Watson RJ, Holcomb JB, Gonzalez EA, Peng Z, Pati S, Park PW, et al. Modulation of syndecan-1 shedding after hemorrhagic shock and resuscitation. *PLoS One* (2011) 6(8):e23530. doi:10.1371/journal.pone.0023530
87. Rahbar E, Cardenas JC, Baimukanova G, Usadi B, Bruhn R, Pati S, et al. Endothelial glycocalyx shedding and vascular permeability in severely

injured trauma patients. *J Transl Med* (2015) 13:117. doi:10.1186/s12967-015-0481-5

88. Holcomb JB, Wade CE, Michalek JE, Chisholm GB, Zarzabal LA, Schreiber MA, et al. Increased plasma and platelet to red blood cell ratios improves outcome in 466 massively transfused civilian trauma patients. *Ann Surg* (2008) 248(3):447–58. doi:10.1097/SLA.0b013e318185a9ad
89. Nelson A, Statkevicius S, Schott U, Johansson PI, Bentzer P. Effects of fresh frozen plasma, Ringer's acetate and albumin on plasma volume and on circulating glycocalyx components following haemorrhagic shock in rats. *Intensive Care Med Exp* (2016) 4(1):6. doi:10.1186/s40635-016-0080-7
90. Torres Filho IP, Torres LN, Salgado C, Dubick MA. Plasma syndecan-1 and heparan sulfate correlate with microvascular glycocalyx degradation in hemorrhaged rats after different resuscitation fluids. *Am J Physiol Heart Circ Physiol* (2016) 310(11):H1468–78. doi:10.1152/ajpheart.00006.2016
91. Diebel LN, Martin JV, Liberati DM. Microfluidics: a high throughput system for the assessment of the endotheliopathy of trauma and the effect of timing of plasma administration on ameliorating shock associated endothelial dysfunction. *J Trauma Acute Care Surg* (2017) 84(4):575–82. doi:10.1097/TA.0000000000001791
92. Pati S, Peng Z, Wataha K, Miyazawa B, Potter DR, Kozar RA. Lyophilized plasma attenuates vascular permeability, inflammation and lung injury in hemorrhagic shock. *PLoS One* (2018) 13(2):e0192363. doi:10.1371/journal.pone.0192363
93. Chesebro BB, Rahn P, Carles M, Esmon CT, Xu J, Brohi K, et al. Increase in activated protein C mediates acute traumatic coagulopathy in mice. *Shock* (2009) 32(6):659–65. doi:10.1097/SHK.0b013e3181a5a632
94. Wu F, Peng Z, Park PW, Kozar RA. Loss of syndecan-1 abrogates the pulmonary protective phenotype induced by plasma after hemorrhagic shock. *Shock* (2017) 48(3):340–5. doi:10.1097/SHK.0000000000000832
95. Ban K, Peng Z, Pati S, Witkov RB, Park PW, Kozar RA. Plasma-mediated gut protection after hemorrhagic shock is lessened in syndecan-1-/- mice. *Shock* (2015) 44(5):452–7. doi:10.1097/SHK.0000000000000452
96. Jacob M, Bruegger D, Rehm M, Welsch U, Conzen P, Becker BF. Contrasting effects of colloid and crystalloid resuscitation fluids on cardiac vascular permeability. *Anesthesiology* (2006) 104(6):1223–31. doi:10.1097/00000542-200606000-00018
97. Jacob M, Paul O, Mehringer L, Chappell D, Rehm M, Welsch U, et al. Albumin augmentation improves condition of guinea pig hearts after 4 hr of cold ischemia. *Transplantation* (2009) 87(7):956–65. doi:10.1097/TP.0b013e31819c83b5
98. Kheirabadi BS, Valdez-Delgado KK, Terrazas IB, Miranda N, Dubick MA. Is limited prehospital resuscitation with plasma more beneficial than using a synthetic colloid? An experimental study in rabbits with parenchymal bleeding. *J Trauma Acute Care Surg* (2015) 78(4):752–9. doi:10.1097/TA.0000000000000591
99. Zazzeron L, Gattinoni L, Caironi P. Role of albumin, starches and gelatins versus crystalloids in volume resuscitation of critically ill patients. *Curr Opin Crit Care* (2016) 22(5):428–36. doi:10.1097/MCC.0000000000000341
100. Pati S, Potter DR, Baimukanova G, Farrel DH, Holcomb JB, Schreiber MA. Modulating the endotheliopathy of trauma: factor concentrate versus fresh frozen plasma. *J Trauma Acute Care Surg* (2016) 80(4):576–84. doi:10.1097/TA.0000000000000961
101. McQuilten ZK, Bailey M, Cameron PA, Stanworth SJ, Venardos K, Wood EM, et al. Fibrinogen concentration and use of fibrinogen supplementation with cryoprecipitate in patients with critical bleeding receiving massive transfusion: a bi-national cohort study. *Br J Haematol* (2017) 179(1):131–41. doi:10.1111/bjh.14804
102. Yakovlev S, Mikhailenko I, Cao C, Zhang L, Strickland DK, Medved L. Identification of VLDLR as a novel endothelial cell receptor for fibrin that modulates fibrin-dependent transendothelial migration of leukocytes. *Blood* (2012) 119(2):637–44. doi:10.1182/blood-2011-09-382580
103. Deng X, Cao Y, Huby MP, Duan C, Baer L, Peng Z, et al. Adiponectin in fresh frozen plasma contributes to restoration of vascular barrier function after hemorrhagic shock. *Shock* (2016) 45(1):50–4. doi:10.1097/SHK.0000000000000458
104. Bluher M, Mantzoros CS. From leptin to other adipokines in health and disease: facts and expectations at the beginning of the 21st century. *Metabolism* (2015) 64(1):131–45. doi:10.1016/j.metabol.2014.10.016
105. van Meurs M, Castro P, Shapiro NI, Lu S, Yano M, Maeda N, et al. Adiponectin diminishes organ-specific microvascular endothelial cell activation associated with sepsis. *Shock* (2012) 37(4):392–8. doi:10.1097/SHK.0b013e318248225e
106. Xu SQ, Mahadev K, Wu X, Fuchsel L, Donnelly S, Scalia RG, et al. Adiponectin protects against angiotensin II or tumor necrosis factor alpha-induced endothelial cell monolayer hyperpermeability: role of cAMP/PKA signaling. *Arterioscler Thromb Vasc Biol* (2008) 28(5):899–905. doi:10.1161/ATVBAHA.108.163634
107. Straat M, Muller MC, Meijers JC, Arbous MS, Spoelstra-de Man AM, Beurskens CJ, et al. Effect of transfusion of fresh frozen plasma on parameters of endothelial condition and inflammatory status in non-bleeding critically ill patients: a prospective substudy of a randomized trial. *Crit Care* (2015) 19:163. doi:10.1186/s13054-015-0828-6
108. Moore EE, Chin TL, Chapman MC, Gonzalez E, Moore HB, Silliman CC, et al. Plasma first in the field for postinjury hemorrhagic shock. *Shock* (2014) 41(Suppl 1):35–8. doi:10.1097/SHK.0000000000000110

5

Fluorescence Exclusion: A Simple Method to Assess Projected Surface, Volume and Morphology of Red Blood Cells Stored in Blood Bank

Camille Roussel[1,2,3,4,5†], *Sylvain Monnier*[6†], *Michael Dussiot*[3,5], *Elisabeth Farcy*[4], *Olivier Hermine*[3,4,5,7], *Caroline Le Van Kim*[1,2,3], *Yves Colin*[1,2,3], *Matthieu Piel*[6,8], *Pascal Amireault*[1,2,3,5*†] *and Pierre A. Buffet*[1,2,3,4,7†]

[1] Biologie Intégrée du Globule Rouge UMR_S1134, Institut National de la Santé et de la Recherche Médicale, Université Paris Diderot, Sorbonne Paris Cité, Université de La Réunion, Université des Antilles, Paris, France, [2] Institut National de la Transfusion Sanguine, Paris, France, [3] Laboratoire d'Excellence GR-Ex, Paris, France, [4] Université Paris Descartes, Paris, France, [5] Laboratory of Cellular and Molecular Mechanisms of Hematological Disorders and Therapeutic Implications U1163, Centre National de la Recherche Scientifique ERL 8254, Institut National de la Santé et de la Recherche Médicale, Université Paris Descartes, Sorbonne Paris Cité, Paris, France, [6] Institut Curie, Centre National de la Recherche Scientifique, UMR 144, PSL Research University, Paris, France, [7] Assistance Publique des Hôpitaux de Paris, Paris, France, [8] Institut Pierre-Gilles de Gennes, PSL Research University, Paris, France

***Correspondence:**
Pascal Amireault
pamireault@ints.fr

† These authors have contributed equally to this work.

Red blood cells (RBC) ability to circulate is closely related to their surface area-to-volume ratio. A decrease in this ratio induces a decrease in RBC deformability that can lead to their retention and elimination in the spleen. We recently showed that a subpopulation of "small RBC" with reduced projected surface area accumulated upon storage in blood bank concentrates, but data on the volume of these altered RBC are lacking. So far, single cell measurement of RBC volume has remained a challenging task achieved by a few sophisticated methods some being subject to potential artifacts. We aimed to develop a reproducible and ergonomic method to assess simultaneously RBC volume and morphology at the single cell level. We adapted the fluorescence exclusion measurement of volume in nucleated cells to the measurement of RBC volume. This method requires no pre-treatment of the cell and can be performed in physiological or experimental buffer. In addition to RBC volume assessment, brightfield images enabling a precise definition of the morphology and the measurement of projected surface area can be generated simultaneously. We first verified that fluorescence exclusion is precise, reproducible and can quantify volume modifications following morphological changes induced by heating or incubation in non-physiological medium. We then used the method to characterize RBC stored for 42 days in SAG-M in blood bank conditions. Simultaneous determination of the volume, projected surface area and morphology allowed to evaluate the surface area-to-volume ratio of individual RBC upon storage. We observed a similar surface area-to-volume ratio in discocytes (D) and echinocytes I (EI), which decreased in EII (7%) and EIII (24%), sphero-echinocytes (SE; 41%) and spherocytes (S; 47%). If RBC dimensions determine indeed the ability of RBC to cross the spleen, these modifications are expected to induce the rapid splenic entrapment of the most morphologically altered RBC (EIII, SE, and S) and further support the hypothesis of a rapid clearance of the "small RBC" subpopulation by the spleen following transfusion.

Keywords: red blood cell volume, red blood cells, transfusion, red blood cell storage, fluorescence exclusion, red blood cell morphology

INTRODUCTION

Surface area-to-volume ratio is a major determinant of red blood cell (RBC) deformability and ability to circulate (1). Normal discocytes (8 μm in diameter) must indeed withstand stringent deformation as they navigate along 4- to 6-μm-wide microvessels and across 1- to 2-μm-wide inter-endothelial slits in the spleen. Modifications of surface area-to-volume ratio have consequences in physiology (removal of senescent RBC) (2, 3) and pathology (anemia in hereditary spherocytosis and other RBC hemoglobin and membrane disorders) (4–6). Furthermore, RBC display a tight relationship between morphology and deformability, and these parameters may impact transfusion yield. Previous studies have shown that RBC stored in blood bank exhibit morphological alterations that become significant after 3 or 4 weeks of storage depending on the technique and the cell classification (7–10). It has been also suggested that these alterations are associated with surface and volume modifications (11). A decrease in surface area-to-volume ratio induces a decrease in RBC deformability that can lead to their retention and elimination in the spleen (12–14). We recently showed that alterations in the morphology of stored RBC was accompanied by a decrease in the projected surface area that only impacts a subpopulation of RBC (10). The proportion of this subpopulation increases upon storage but is highly variable between donors. Determination of the projected surface area of these stored RBC was conducted using imaging flow cytometry, a high throughput tool allowing a detailed and objective quantification of cell morphology and dimensions (15). Imaging flow cytometry however cannot determine cell volume hence misses the key pathophysiological feature of RBC: surface area-to-volume ratio.

So far, single cell measurement of RBC volume has remained a challenging task achieved by a few sophisticated methods, such as micropipette aspiration (16, 17), quantitative phase microscopy (18) including digital holographic microscopy (19), some of these methods are flawed by potential artifacts due to labeling (confocal laser scanning microscopy) (20) or sphering (optical scattering methods) (21). A reproducible and ergonomic method enabling the assessment of the volume and morphology of RBC at the single cell level would be a useful tool to study the storage lesion and more generally RBC physiology and pathology.

The method developed here is based on the dye exclusion principle first proposed by Gray et al. (22) and adapted recently to mammalian cells (23–25). RBC were suspended in a medium supplemented with a fluorescent dye coupled to a dextran molecule and inserted in a microfluidic chamber of fixed height. Dextran is a biocompatible polysaccharide that does not cross cell membranes; fluorescence is thus excluded from the cells which allows volume calculation as the drop in fluorescence intensity is directly related to the thickness of the object (22). RBC volume is obtained by integrating the fluorescence signal over its projected area (see Material and Methods).

This technique also generates brightfield images enabling a simultaneous precise determination of their morphology.

MATERIALS AND METHODS

Chamber Design and Fabrication

Molds were fabricated using classic soft lithography methods or micromachining (Minimill3, Minitech Machinery) (24). Pillars were evenly positioned (interpillar distance 200 μm) in the observation chamber to set a very stable height in the chamber. Their value of fluorescence provides a stable signal useful for calibration (see Volume and projected area calculation in Material and Methods). Chips were made using a mixture 1:10 of PDMS (polydimethylsiloxane) and its cross linker (Sylgard 184, Dow Corning) cured at 66°C for 2 h. Inlets and outlets were created with 2 or 3 mm punchers before bonding. Chambers were bond on glass-bottomed petri dishes (Fluorodish) using air (Harrick) plasma cleaner or corona SB (Elveflow). Chamber surface was passivated with Poly(L-lysine) grafted poly(ethylene glycol) (PLL-g-PEG, Surface Solutions) for 30 min to 1 h after bonding. This pre-treatment induces the formation of a polymeric brush that prevents RBC from adhering to the surface. Chambers can be used immediately or stored at 4°C in PBS solution for a few days before use. Prior to RBC injection, PBS was changed to Krebs-Albumin 0.5% solution (Krebs-Henseleit Buffer modified with 2 g glucose, 2.1 g sodium bicarbonate, 0.175 g calcium chloride dehydrate and 5 g AlbuMAX II Lipid-Rich BSA for 1 L sterile water, pH 7.4) supplemented with FITC-dextran. According to its composition, Krebs-Albumin medium should have a refractive index similar to classical cell culture medium and thus be estimated at 1.337 (26).

Sample Preparations

Leukoreduced RBC in Saline-Adenine-Glucose-Mannitol (SAG-M) from healthy donors were supplied by the Etablissement Français du Sang (French Blood Service) 3 days after blood collection. All units were stored in optimal blood bank conditions between 2 and 6°C and for 42 days, according to regulations. Samples were aseptically collected

---

Abbreviations: D, Discocyte; E, Echinocytes; SE, spheroechinocytes; S, spherocytes; RBC, red blood cell; MCV, Mean Corpuscular Volume; SAG-M, Saline-Adenine-Glucose-Mannitol; CPDA, Citrate-Phosphate-Dextrose-Adenine; RPMI, Roswell Park Memorial Institute medium.

to perform experiments. Just before analyses, RBC were diluted (1/50) in a Krebs-Albumin 0.5% solution. pH-related morphological alterations were induced by suspension of RBC in a Krebs-Albumin 0.5% solution after adding either HCl or NaOH up to the desired pH. Heated-RBC (HRBC) were produced by incubation of a RBC suspension at 1% hematocrit in RPMI at 50°C in a glass tube for 20 min. We used HRBC and RBC exposed to low and high pH as well-known examples of clear-cut volume and surface modifications RBC. In addition, HRBC have been repeatedly used to measure the biomechanical retention of stiff RBC *in vivo*, including in human subject (27, 28).

Fluorescence Exclusion Sample Preparation

RBC were suspended in the medium supplemented with 1 mg/mL FITC-Dextran (10 kDa) from Sigma-Aldrich. The hydrodynamic radius of the FITC-Dextran used in this study has been determined previously to be 1.86 nm (29) and thus far exceeded the maximum pore radius of the erythrocytes membrane (0.4 nm) (22, 30). RBC concentration was adjusted by modifying the dilution from 1:30 to 1:50 in order to obtain an optimal number of RBC in the chamber and avoid superimposition of RBC or contacts between them that would hamper measurements.

Imaging

Imaging was performed with an automated Nikon Eclipse-Ti microscope equipped with a 20x objective NA.0.75, or a Zeiss AxioObserver microscope equipped with a 20x objective NA.0.8. Compatibility and precision of such objectives have already been shown (25). Fluorescence and brightfield images were acquired sequentially within <0.5 s according to the microscopes manufacturers.

Volume and Projected Area Calculation

Volume calculation was performed as described (24). Briefly, image analysis was performed using homemade MatLab program (The Math Works Inc., Natick, MA, USA). Calibration of the relationship between fluorescence intensity and height was performed for each field using values of fluorescence around each RBC and over the pillars as described (25). Briefly, α is extracted using a robust fit from $I_B = \alpha \cdot h + I_0$, where I_B and I_0 are the background and pillar fluorescence respectively and h the height of the chamber. To correct for the inhomogeneity of the fluorescent lamp, background is locally subtracted and the volume is then calculated by integrating over an area S larger than cell ($V_{Cell} = \iint_S \frac{I_B(x,y) - I(x,y)}{\alpha} dS$). This procedure also integrates the dye deposition on the chamber walls that can occur after several hours. After background removal, the fluorescence value around the RBC is close to zero, the area of integration does not play a crucial role and thus limits errors that could be introduced by a precise segmentation of the cell area. Projected area was extracted from brightfield images after background removal by a basic thresholding and filling procedure using built-in MatLab functions. Briefly, a square region of interest (ROI) was defined around the cell, then a binary gradient image was obtained using the edge function, the outlines of the binary image were dilated (imdilate) and the open area were filled (imfill). Eventually, objects too small or on the edge of the ROI were discarded (imclearborder, imerode). Parameters used during this procedure were adapted by user accordingly to images quality and exposure properties.

Morphological Analysis of RBC

After acquisition, brightfield images where anonymized and randomized for blind evaluation and RBC were classified in 6 morphological categories according to Bessis et al. (31). adapted for DIC microscopy (10). namely discocytes, echinocytes (I, II and III), sphero-echinocytes and spherocytes. Small RBC were defined as previously described (10) as a morphologically altered RBC population that exhibited a decrease in projected surface area and included 3 subpopulations, namely echinocytes III, sphero-echinocytes and spherocytes.

RESULTS

Determination of RBC Volume by Fluorescence Exclusion Is Simple and Requires Limited Specific Instruments

RBC were injected in a microfluidic chamber higher than the maximum size of the cells to prevent mechanical stress (chamber height = 6.8 μm). Its height was however limited to enable the capture of images with excellent contrast. The microfluidic chamber was designed to determine the volume of large numbers of RBC within a single chamber (typically from 500 up to 1,500 RBC depending on the working concentration). Regularly spaced pillars (interpillar distance 200 μm) ensure a constant height across the whole chamber and enable the calibration of the relationship between height and fluorescence (see Material and Methods). The inlet and the outlet were in immediate proximity and a fluid bridge was established between them to easily stop the flow. This prevented any fluid flow circulation in the chamber thereby enabling measurements on still RBC (**Figure 1A**).

Brightfield (**Figure 1B**) and fluorescence (**Figure 1C**) images were acquired using a 20x objective and each acquired fluorescence image enabled the volume determination of 10 to 50 RBC, depending on the concentration. Determination of RBC morphology can be evaluated simultaneously by acquiring and analyzing the corresponding brightfield image and was achieved according to Bessis et al. (see Methods).

Training to prepare chips required a few hours to a few days. The air plasma cleaner was replaced by a cheaper corona SB (Elveflow) that efficiently activated the surfaces before bonding (see Methods). Manufacturing steps are shown in **Figure 2**.

The RBC Volume Quantification by Fluorescence Exclusion Is Precise and Reproducible

To explore the reproducibility of the chip preparation and technique, the RBC volume from a RBC concentrate at day 10 of storage was assessed, on the same day, in two chips (namely A and B), manufactured from the same mold. Volume measurement showed a normal gaussian distribution (**Figure 3A**). Comparison

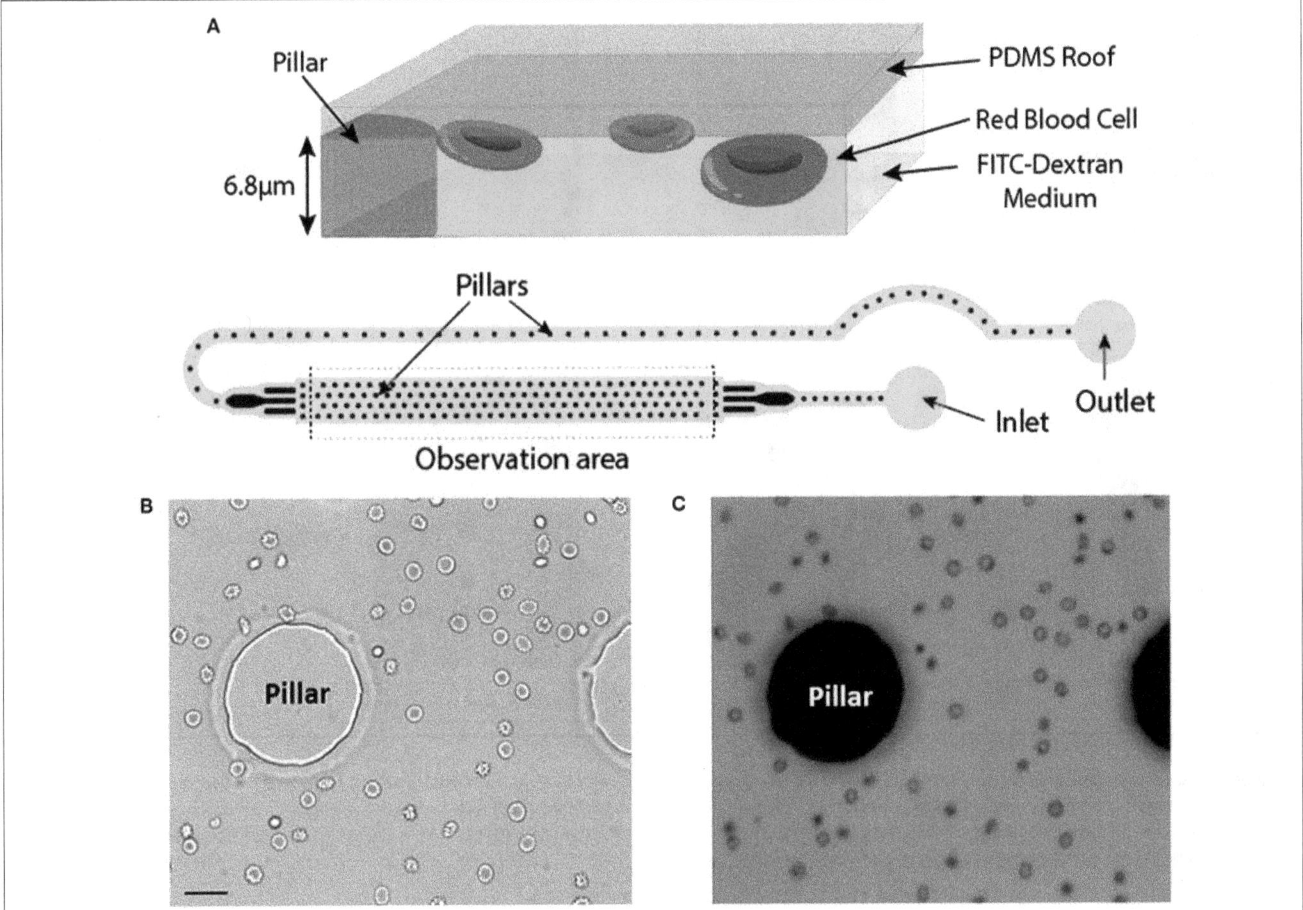

FIGURE 1 | (A) Top: Principle of the fluorescence exclusion method, bottom: design of the microfluidic chamber. **(B,C)** Brightfield and fluorescence images of the same field (x20) showing RBC stored for 42 days in SAG-M (healthy donor) scale bar = 20 µm.

of RBC volume between the two chips revealed a difference in the median volume of 3% (97 μm^3 in chip A vs 100 μm^3 in chip B) and a similar distribution (**Figure 3B**). The repetition of this experiment showed a variation of the median volume of 1.6% (97.4 vs. 99 μm^3) (data not shown). This difference is very likely due to variations in chip height that originate from the master mold itself (one mold contains several chip designs for multiplexing the PDMS chip fabrication) as the error on the height is also 3%. Other sources of error would include, the chip bonding to glass, local variations from height variation within one chip. The background cleaning step during the image processing would also contribute, but only to width distribution and not to the inter chip variations.

Precision of the technique was next assessed using samples containing an increasing concentration of RBC of reduced volume (**Figure 3C**). HRBC were used since they are known to display a loss of volume. Normalized frequency histogram of RBC volume distribution showed a progressive shift to the left when the proportion of heated RBC increased in the sample (0, 25, 50, and 100%) (**Figure 3D**). Mean volume (± SEM) of each sample was 98.4 (±0.54) μm^3, 95.0 (±0.44) μm^3, 92.4 (±0.54) μm^3, and 84.4 (±0.48) μm^3 respectively (**Figure 3E**).

Fluorescence Exclusion Measures Volume While Defining RBC Morphology

We next incubated RBC in media of acidic or basic pH to assess the RBC volume modifications associated with the pH-induced morphological modifications (**Figure 4**). Acidic pH (4.2) generated stomatocytes and sphero-stomatocytes (**Figure 4B**) which exhibited a mean 3% volume loss compared to physiological conditions (pH 7.4) (**Figure 4C**) while basic pH (9.4) generated echinocytes III, sphero-echinocytes and spherocytes (**Figure 4D**) that had lost a mean 11.4% of their volume. Differences in RBC volume were significantly different when measured either at low or normal pH ($p < 0.01$, ** Mann Whitney non-parametric test) and between high and low pH (****$p < 0.0001$).

Fluorescence Exclusion Shows a Decrease in Surface Area-to-Volume Ratio in Red Blood Cell Stored in Blood Bank Conditions

We determined the volume and the projected surface area of RBC stored for 42 days in 3 blood bank concentrates from healthy donors and correlated this measure with their

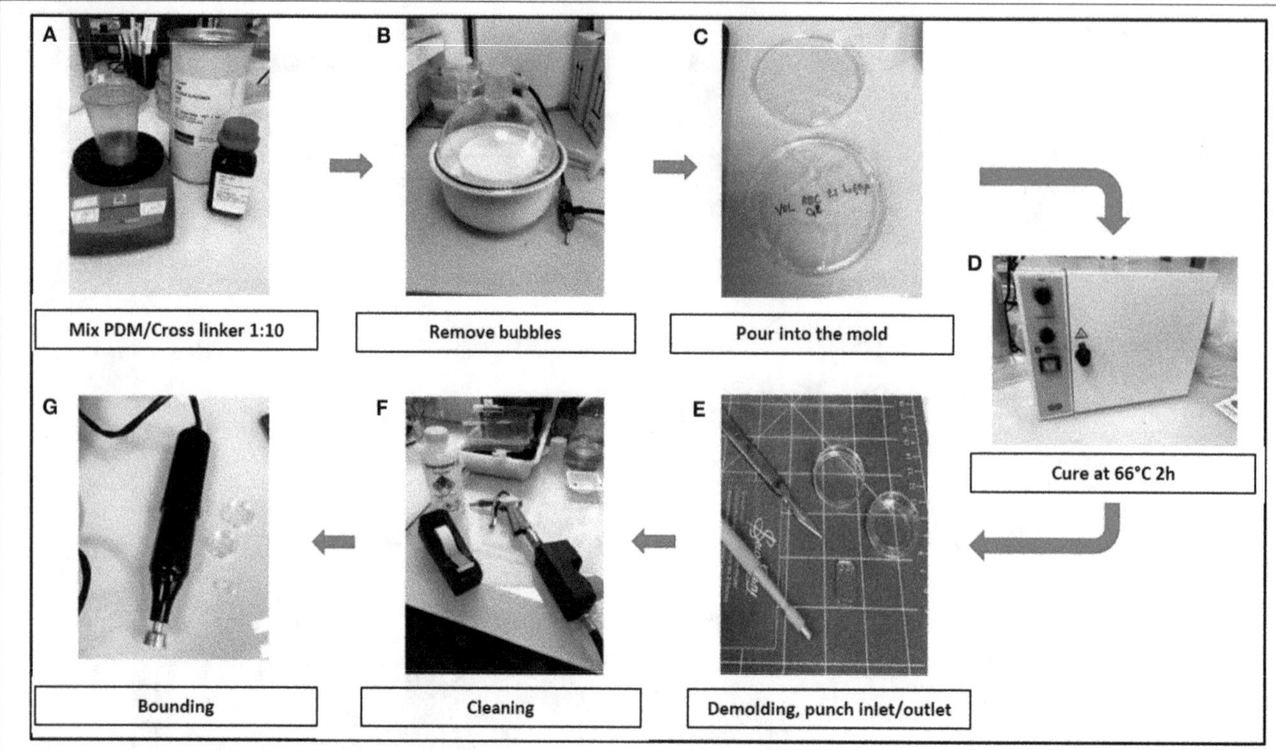

FIGURE 2 | Stepwise preparation of chips: **(A)** Chips were made using a mixture 1:10 of PDMS (polydimethylsiloxane) and its cross linker (Sylgard 184) **(B)** The mixture was degased to remove air bubbles, **(C)** poured into the mold and **(D)** cured at 66°C for 2 h. **(E)** After demolding, inlets and outlets were created with 2 or 3 mm punchers and **(F)** the surface was cleaned using isopropanol, air gun and tape before bonding. **(G)** Chambers were bond on glass-bottomed petri dishes (Fluorodish) using air plasma cleaner (Harrick) or a corona SB (Elveflow).

storage-induced morphological alterations (**Figure 5A**). For the 3 donors, surface distribution on normalized frequency plots was bimodal and confirmed the existence of a subpopulation of "small RBC" with a reduced mean projected surface area (<58 μm^2) (**Figure 5B**). Mean volume (±SD) was 86.0 ± 14.4 μm^3 for donor 1, 85.2 ±14.1 μm^3 for donor 2 and 93.9 ± 13.2 μm^3 for donor 3 (**Figure 5C**). We then determined the projected surface area, volume and surface area-to-volume ratio of RBC for each morphological category (**Figures 5D–F**).

We observed a projected surface area loss of altered RBC when compared to discocytes (D): Echinocytes (E) I, II and III exhibited a mean projected surface area loss of 2, 14, and 32% respectively while the most intensely altered RBC, namely spheroechinocytes (SE) and spherocytes (S) had lost 49 and 51% of their projected surface area, respectively. Altered RBC exhibited also a decrease in their volume although to a lesser extent. When compared to D, the mean volume loss of storage-damaged RBC was 2% (EI), 6% (EII), 10% (EIII), 14% (SE) and 6% (S). This resulted in a surface area-to-volume ratio not modified for EI and decreased of 7 and 24% for EII and EIII respectively, and of 41 and 47% for SE and S. Small RBC (EIII, SE and S) exhibited a mean decrease in surface area and volume of 40 and 11% respectively resulting in a decrease of surface area-to-volume ratio of 32%.

DISCUSSION

We adapted the fluorescence exclusion method to determine RBC volume. This method is reproducible and sensitive and allows the simultaneous measurement of volume and projected surface area together with a detailed determination of RBC morphology at a single cell level.

Several methods such as automated complete blood count and impedance-based Coulter-Counter have been described to measure cell volume, but while of major clinical impact, they have disadvantages regarding mechanistic exploration of RBC. These high-throughput methods indeed provide reproducible data but volume can only be measured on global populations of RBC and not at a single cell level (32). Light scattering in flow cytometry is also a high-throughput method which is frequently used because of the wide availability of flow cytometers. It measures individual RBC volume together with hemoglobin concentration but requires pre-treatment of the cell (sphering). Furthermore, flow cytometry does not enable fine morphological observation of RBC (32–34). Morphology, volume and surface of single RBC can be accurately assessed by micropipette aspiration (16, 17) which also provides biomechanical information such as membrane viscosity and multiple elastic moduli. Micropipette measures are however of low throughput, technically challenging, and mastered by a very few specialized teams. Moreover, mechanical constraints on the RBC during micropipette aspiration may

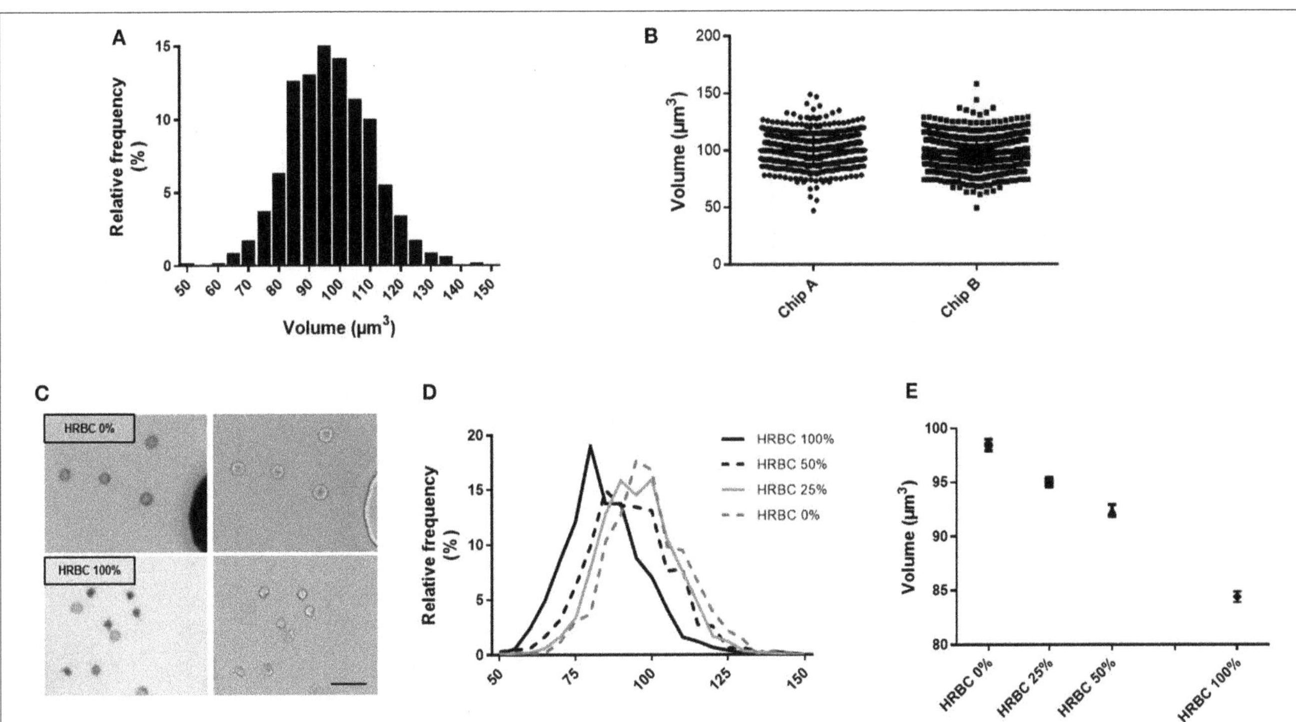

FIGURE 3 | Fluorescence exclusion to measure RBC volume: a precise and reproducible method. **(A)** Normalized frequency histogram of RBC volume distribution from a healthy donor at day 10 of storage in SAG-M. **(B)** Individual volume of RBC from a healthy donor measured using 2 differents chips manufactured from the same mold (chip A and chip B). **(C)** Fluorescence (left) and brightfield (right) images (20x) of control RBC (top) or 100% heated RBC (bottom) scale bar = 20 µm; **(D)** Normalized frequency histogram of RBC volume distribution, and (E) Mean volume (+/−SEM) of samples containing increasing concentrations of heated-RBC.

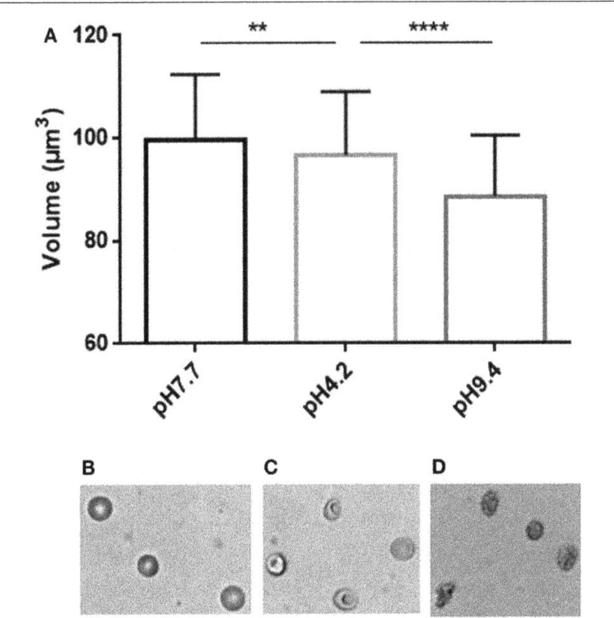

FIGURE 4 | Simultaneous determination of RBC volume and morphology using fluorescence exclusion and microscopy. **(A)** Mean (standard deviation) volume of RBC samples exposed to physiological (left), low (center) and high (right) pH. Stars represent the significance level of the Mann-Whitney statistic test, ** when $p < 0.01$, **** when $p < 0.0001$ **(B–D)** Representative brightfield images of RBC in the same samples.

generate artifactual changes in morphology or volume. Lately, new techniques to obtain RBC volume have been proposed, based on sophisticated microscopical methods and microfluidics. Guo et al. have generated a microfluidic device to measure RBC volume based on electric current modification as cells pass through a gate (MOFSET-based detection) (35). Confocal microscopy can also be used but, in addition to requiring a specific instrumentation, this technique requires membrane labeling that can modify RBC morphology (19). Quantitative phase imaging, including digital holographic microscopy can provide RBC volume and RBC refractive index, but these two parameters are measured separately in isotonic liquids of different refractive indexes and thus requires RBC adhesion to the surface or complex microfluidic setup in order to perfuse solutions (19, 36). Scanning electron microscopy has also been proposed, but its usefulness is limited by a very low throughput and the limited availability of the instrument. Not least cell fixation is required and known to induce both morphological and volume changes.

The principle of dye exclusion has been recently adapted to RBC by Schonbrun et al. (26). RBC are suspended in an index-matching absorbing solution and volume can be measured from the modification in light absorbance between the cells and the background (37). Measures with this technique are independent from cell refractive index and provide microscopic spatial resolution of single cells as well as medium throughput, but microfluidic controllers are needed.

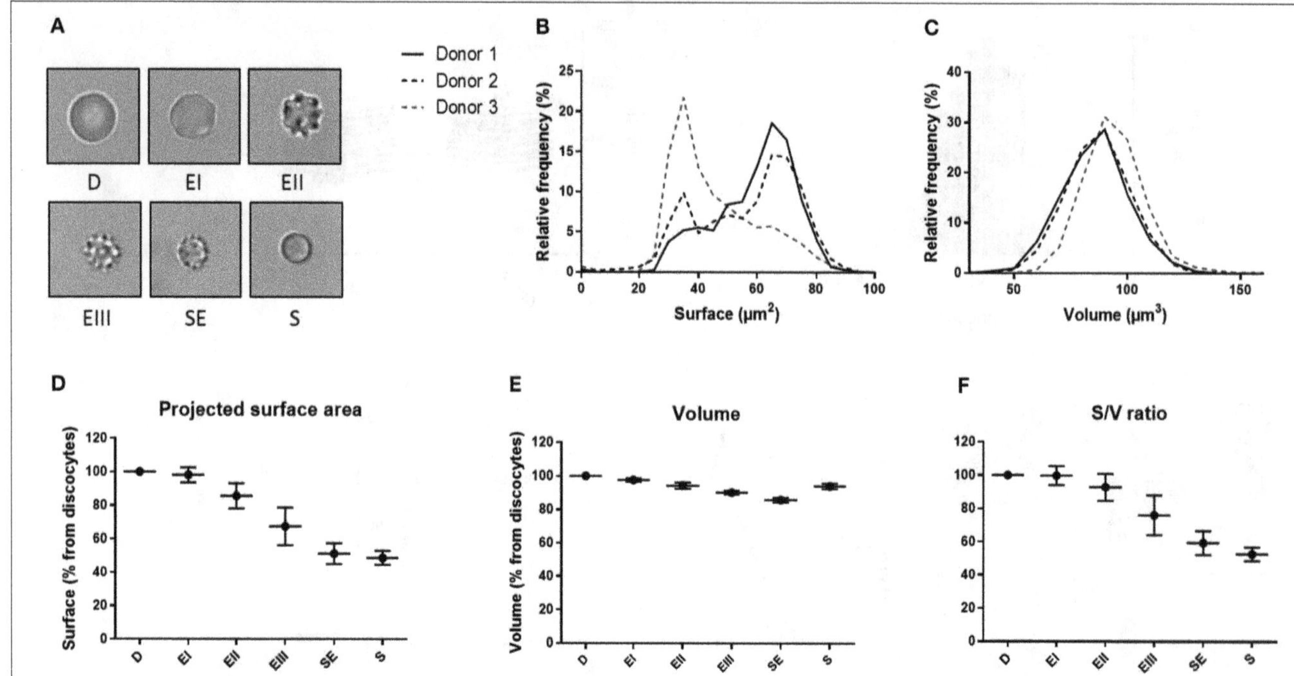

FIGURE 5 | Fluorescence exclusion shows a decrease in surface to volume ratio during storage of red blood cell concentrates. **(A)** Morphological categories of RBC as defined in the Material and Methods section, namely discocytes (D), echinocytes I (EI), echinocytes II (EII), echinocytes III (EIII), spheroechinocytes (SE) and spherocytes (S). **(B–C)** Normalized frequency of RBC projected surface area (μm^2) and RBC volume (μm^3) of RBC concentrates after 42 days of storage in SAG-M ($n = 3$). **(D–F)** Mean (SD) projected surface area, volume and projected surface area-to-volume ratio normalized to the value of discocytes (D).

Unlike most aforementioned methods, the fluorescence exclusion technique described here does not require any pre-treatment of RBC and can be performed in physiological buffer. and could then be used for long term experiments with multiple cell types [see Cadart et al. (25)]. These 2 experimental features are real assets when studying RBC. Morphology and dimensions of RBC (especially those of altered RBC) are indeed exquisitely labile and sensitive to any fluctuation in the pH of the medium, its composition and most labeling procedures. Also, the chips are loaded without requiring pressure control or any specific infusion device. RBC adherence to the surface is not warranted since the immobility of the RBC is obtained by creating a bridge of fluid between the inlet and the outlet. Not least, measuring fluorescence exclusion only requires a fluorescence microscope.

We showed that fluorescence exclusion can detects variations of volume of a RBC population as small as 3%. Mean volume of RBC populations containing increasing proportions of small heated RBC were very close to theoretical predictions. RBC heated at 50°C during 20 min exhibited a 14% volume loss. Samples containing 25 and 50% heated-RBC should have exhibited 3.5 and 7% volume loss while measured values were 3.5 and 6.1%, respectively. Reproducibility was robust when measuring the mean RBC volume in the same samples using 2 different chips. The method still has weaknesses however. In its current version it displays a relatively low throughput. Improvement is envisioned by combining the analysis program to an algorithm for automated classification of RBC morphology, as described by Piety et al. (38). Also, like imaging flow cytometry, our method measures the projected surface area of RBC, a proxy for the total RBC surface generally considered accurate but that may be suboptimal for echinocytes that exhibit membrane spicules.

Using this new method, we confirmed and expanded recent findings. We measured the projected surface area, volume and surface area-to-volume ratio of RBC stored 42 days in blood bank conditions.

Measures of the volume of the subpopulation of "small RBC" (EIII, SE and S) by fluorescence exclusion provided direct confirmation that this subpopulation exhibits an overall volume loss of 11%. Because surface loss was proportionally greater than volume loss, the result was a reduced surface area-to-volume ratio of 32%. Previous observations had shown that a reduction in surface area-to-volume ratio was correlated to splenic retention of RBC. A reduction> 21% had led to a rapid entrapment of 79% of RBC in normal human spleens perfused *ex-vivo* (14). If RBC dimensions determines indeed the ability of RBC to cross the spleen, EIII, SE and S induced by storage (i.e small RBC), that exhibit a decrease in surface area-to-volume ratio of 24, 41, and 47% respectively (resulting in an overall decrease of 32%), are expected to undergo splenic retention. Not least, the marked difference in projected surface area-to-volume ratio observed between EII and EIII, as well as between EIII and SE is consistent with the similarly marked difference in the capacity of these RBC subsets to circulate in a microfluidic device (39). These data further support the hypothesis of a rapid clearance of "small RBC" by the spleen following transfusion. Recent publications showed that approaches consisting in reducing the appearance (anaerobic storage) or selectively remove this sub-population (washing in hypotonic solution) improved the ability of stored RBC to perfuse in an artificial microvascular network (40, 41).

Little is known about volume modification of stored RBC at the single cell level. Several studies showed an increase in RBC mean corpuscular volume (MCV) upon storage (42, 43) but a recent studies using quantitative phase imaging observed no significant volume modification after 6 weeks of storage (36, 44). We observed that the volume of RBC stored in SAG-M for 42 days was smaller in EI, EII, EIII, and SE than in D (with an almost linear decrease from EI to SE). The volume of S, although reduced, was greater than that of EIII and SE. In the context of transfusion, we found no previous direct observation on the volume of the different morphological subpopulations of RBC. We are thus currently unable to address the external consistency of this somewhat unexpected observation. In physiology, RBC with irregular shape in pre-term and term neonates show a similar decline in volume from D to SE but the volume of S is lower than that of SE, when assessed by micropipette aspiration (26). The higher-than-expected volume of S that we observed using fluorescence extinction may be artefactual or correspond to alterations of transmembrane flow of ions and water, as S are the most altered RBC subpopulation in red blood cell concentrates. This may have escaped observations with micropipettes because mechanical constraints linked to the aspiration may artificially modify RBC volume. When submitted to mechanical forces, RBC can indeed undergo dehydration via the activation of the mechanosensitive cation channel, Piezo 1 (45). By contrast, our method does not require manipulation of RBC and the height of the chips (6.8 μm) protects RBC from stringent mechanical forces. These hypotheses require experimental testing. Which method is the most accurate to quantify the volume of S will be determined by future work, for example by direct comparisons using all available methods with an array of altered RBC.

The method described here has the potential to bring important insight into the ability of RBC to circulate, in the context of RBC transfusion but also in RBC membrane or volume disorders.

AUTHOR CONTRIBUTIONS

CR, SM, OH, CL, YC, MP, PA, and PB: designed the research; CR, SM, MD, and EF: performed the experiments; CR, SM, MD, and EF: analyzed the data; SM, CR, PA, and PB: wrote the paper.

ACKNOWLEDGMENTS

The authors thank Maël Leberre for the preliminary discussions on the method and EFS Nord de France for providing red cell concentrates.

REFERENCES

1. Mohandas N, Clark MR, Jacobs MS, Shohet SB. Analysis of factors regulating erythrocyte deformability. *J Clin Invest.* (1980) **66**:563–73. doi: 10.1172/JCI109888
2. Waugh RE, Narla M, Jackson CW, Mueller TJ, Suzuki T, Dale GL. Rheologic properties of senescent erythrocytes: loss of surface area and volume with red blood cell age. *Blood* (1992) **79**:1351–8.
3. Waugh RE, Sarelius IH. Effects of lost surface area on red blood cells and red blood cell survival in mice. *Am J Physiol.* (1996) **271**(6 Pt 1):C1847–1852. doi: 10.1152/ajpcell.1996.271.6.C1847
4. Perrotta S, Gallagher PG, Mohandas N. Hereditary spherocytosis. *Lancet Lond Engl.* (2008) **372**:1411–26. doi: 10.1016/S0140-6736(08)61588-3
5. Gallagher PG. Disorders of red cell volume regulation. *Curr Opin Hematol.* (2013) **20**:201–7. doi: 10.1097/MOH.0b013e32835f6870
6. Kviatkovsky I, Zeidan A, Yeheskely-Hayon D, Shabad EL, Dann EJ, Yelin D. Measuring sickle cell morphology during blood flow. *Biomed Opt Express.* (2017) **8**:1996–2003. doi: 10.1364/BOE.8.001996
7. Blasi B, D'Alessandro A, Ramundo N, Zolla L. Red blood cell storage and cell morphology. *Transfus Med Oxf Engl.* (2012) **22**:90–6. doi: 10.1111/j.1365-3148.2012.01139.x
8. Kozlova E, Chernysh A, Moroz V, Sergunova V, Gudkova O, Manchenko E. Morphology, membrane nanostructure and stiffness for quality assessment of packed red blood cells. *Sci Rep.* (2017) **7**:7846. doi: 10.1038/s41598-017-08255-9
9. Bardyn M, Rappaz B, Jaferzadeh K, Crettaz D, Tissot J-D, Moon I, et al. Red blood cells ageing markers: a multi-parametric analysis. *Blood Transfus.* (2017) **15**:239–48. doi: 10.2450/2017.0318-16
10. Roussel C, Dussiot M, Marin M, Morel A, Ndour PA, Duez J, et al. Spherocytic shift of red blood cells during storage provides a quantitative whole cell-based marker of the storage lesion. *Transfusion* (2017) **57**:1007–18. doi: 10.1111/trf.14015
11. D'Alessandro A, D'Amici GM, Vaglio S, Zolla L. Time-course investigation of SAGM-stored leukocyte-filtered red bood cell concentrates: from metabolism to proteomics. *Haematologica* (2012) **97**:107–15. doi: 10.3324/haematol.2011.051789
12. Hess JR. Red cell changes during storage. *Transfus Apher Sci.* (2010) **43**:51–9. doi: 10.1016/j.transci.2010.05.009
13. D'Alessandro A, Kriebardis AG, Rinalducci S, Antonelou MH, Hansen KC, Papassideri IS, et al. An update on red blood cell storage lesions, as gleaned through biochemistry and omics technologies. *Transfusion* (2015) **55**:205–19. doi: 10.1111/trf.12804
14. Safeukui I, Buffet PA, Perrot S, Sauvanet A, Aussilhou B, Dokmak S, et al. Surface area loss and increased sphericity account for the splenic entrapment of subpopulations of *Plasmodium falciparum* ring-infected erythrocytes. *PLoS ONE* (2013) **8**:e60150. doi: 10.1371/journal.pone.0060150
15. Samsel L, McCoy JP. Imaging flow cytometry for the study of erythroid cell biology and pathology. *J Immunol Methods* (2015) **423**:52–9. doi: 10.1016/j.jim.2015.03.019
16. Ruef P, Linderkamp O. Deformability and geometry of neonatal erythrocytes with irregular shapes. *Pediatr Res.* (1999) **45**:114–9. doi: 10.1203/00006450-199901000-00019
17. Linderkamp O, Wu PY, Meiselman HJ. Geometry of neonatal and adult red blood cells. *Pediatr Res.* (1983) **17**:250–3. doi: 10.1203/00006450-198304000-00003
18. Curl CL, Bellair CJ, Harris PJ, Allman BE, Roberts A, Nugent KA, et al. Single cell volume measurement by quantitative phase microscopy (QPM): a case

study of erythrocyte morphology. *Cell Physiol Biochem Int J Exp Cell Physiol Biochem Pharmacol.* (2006) **17**:193–200. doi: 10.1159/000094124
19. Rappaz B, Barbul A, Emery Y, Korenstein R, Depeursinge C, Magistretti PJ, et al. Comparative study of human erythrocytes by digital holographic microscopy, confocal microscopy, and impedance volume analyzer. *Cytom J Int Soc Anal Cytol.* (2008) **73**:895–903. doi: 10.1002/cyto.a.20605
20. Khairy K, Foo J, Howard J. Shapes of red blood cells: comparison of 3D confocal images with the bilayer-couple model. *Cell Mol Bioeng.* (2010) **1**:173–81. doi: 10.1007/s12195-008-0019-5
21. Mohandas N, Kim YR, Tycko DH, Orlik J, Wyatt J, Groner W. Accurate and independent measurement of volume and hemoglobin concentration of individual red cells by laser light scattering. *Blood* (1986) **68**:506–13.
22. Gray ML, Hoffman RA, Hansen WP. A new method for cell volume measurement based on volume exclusion of a fluorescent dye. *Cytometry* (1983) **3**:428–34. doi: 10.1002/cyto.990030607
23. Bottier C, Gabella C, Vianay B, Buscemi L, Sbalzarini IF, Meister J-J, et al. Dynamic measurement of the height and volume of migrating cells by a novel fluorescence microscopy technique. *Lab Chip.* (2011) **11**:3855–63. doi: 10.1039/c1lc20807a
24. Zlotek-Zlotkiewicz E, Monnier S, Cappello G, Le Berre M, Piel M. Optical volume and mass measurements show that mammalian cells swell during mitosis. *J Cell Biol.* (2015) **211**:765–74. doi: 10.1083/jcb.201505056
25. Cadart C, Zlotek-Zlotkiewicz E, Venkova L, Thouvenin O, Racine V. Le Berre M, et al. Fluorescence eXclusion Measurement of volume in live cells. *Methods Cell Biol.* (2017) **139**:103–20. doi: 10.1016/bs.mcb.2016.11.009
26. Schonbrun E, Caprio G Di, Schaak D. Dye exclusion microfluidic microscopy. (2013) **21**:8793–8. doi: 10.1364/OE.21.008793
27. Looareesuwan S, Ho M, Wattanagoon Y, White NJ, Warrell DA, Bunnag D, et al. Dynamic alteration in splenic function during acute falciparum malaria. *N Engl J Med.* (1987) **317**:675–9. doi: 10.1056/NEJM198709103171105
28. Theurl I, Hilgendorf I, Nairz M, Tymoszuk P, Haschka D, Asshoff M, et al. On-demand erythrocyte disposal and iron recycling requires transient macrophages in the liver. *Nat Med.* (2016) **22**:945–51. doi: 10.1038/nm.4146
29. Armstrong JK, Wenby RB, Meiselman HJ, Fisher TC. The hydrodynamic radii of macromolecules and their effect on red blood cell aggregation. *Biophys J.* (2004) **87**:4259–70. doi: 10.1529/biophysj.104.047746
30. Lucy JA. Ultrastructure of membranes: micellar organization. *Br Med Bull.* (1968) **24**:127–9. doi: 10.1093/oxfordjournals.bmb.a070613
31. Bessis M. Red cell shapes. An illustrated classification and its rationale. *Nouv Rev Fr Hématologie.* (1972) **12**:721–45.
32. Model MA. Methods for cell volume measurement. (2017) *Cytometry A* **93**:281–96. doi: 10.1002/cyto.a.23152
33. Tycko DH, Metz MH, Epstein EA, Grinbaum A. Flow-cytometric light scattering measurement of red blood cell volume and hemoglobin concentration. *Appl Opt.* (1985) **24**:1355. doi: 10.1364/AO.24.001355
34. Tzur A, Moore JK, Jorgensen P, Shapiro HM, Kirschner MW. Optimizing optical flow cytometry for cell volume-based sorting and analysis. *PLoS ONE* (2011) **6**:e16053. doi: 10.1371/journal.pone.0016053
35. Guo J, Ai Y, Cheng Y, Li CM, Kang Y, Wang Z. Volumetric measurement of human red blood cells by MOSFET-based microfluidic gate. *Electrophoresis* (2015) **36**:1862–5. doi: 10.1002/elps.201400365
36. Park H, Lee S, Ji M, Kim K, Son Y, Jang S, et al. Measuring cell surface area and deformability of individual human red blood cells over blood storage using quantitative phase imaging. *Sci Rep.* (2016) **6**:34257. doi: 10.1038/srep34257
37. Schonbrun E, Malka R, Di Caprio G, Schaak D, Higgins JM. Quantitative absorption cytometry for measuring red blood cell hemoglobin mass and volume. *Cytometry A* (2014) **85**:332–8. doi: 10.1002/cyto.a.22450
38. Piety NZ, Gifford SC, Yang X, Shevkoplyas SS. Quantifying morphological heterogeneity: a study of more than 1,000,000 individual stored red blood cells. *Vox Sang.* (2015) **109**:221–30. doi: 10.1111/vox.12277
39. Piety N, Reinhart WH, Pourreau PH, Abidi R, Shevkoplyas SS. Shape matters: the effect of red blood cell shape on perfusion of an artificial microvascular network. *Transfusion* (2015) **56**:844–51. doi: 10.1111/trf.13449
40. Burns JM, Yoshida T, Dumont LJ, Yang X, Piety NZ, Shevkoplyas SS. Deterioration of red blood cell mechanical properties is reduced in anaerobic storage. *Blood Transfus Trasfus Sangue.* (2016) **14**:80–8. doi: 10.2450/2015.0241-15
41. Xia H, Khanal G, Strachan BC, Vörös E, Piety NZ, Gifford SC, et al. Washing in hypotonic saline reduces the fraction of irreversibly-damaged cells in stored blood: a proof-of-concept study. *Blood Transfus.* (2017) **15**:463–71. doi: 10.2450/2017.0013-17
42. Arduini A, Minetti G, Ciana A, Seppi C, Brovelli A, Profumo A, et al. Cellular properties of human erythrocytes preserved in saline–adenine–glucose–mannitol in the presence of L-carnitine. *Am J Hematol.* (2007) **82**:31–40. doi: 10.1002/ajh.20753
43. Antonelou MH, Tzounakas VL, Velentzas AD, Stamoulis KE, Kriebardis AG, Papassideri IS. Effects of pre-storage leukoreduction on stored red blood cells signaling: a time-course evaluation from shape to proteome. *J Proteomics.* (2012) **76** Spec No.:220–38. doi: 10.1016/j.jprot.2012.06.032
44. Moon I, Yi F, Lee YH, Javidi B, Boss D, Marquet P. Automated quantitative analysis of 3D morphology and mean corpuscular hemoglobin in human red blood cells stored in different periods. *Opt Express.* (2013) **21**:30947–57. doi: 10.1364/OE.21.030947
45. Cahalan SM, Lukacs V, Ranade SS, Chien S, Bandell M, Patapoutian A. Piezo1 links mechanical forces to red blood cell volume. *eLife* (2015) **4**:1–12. doi: 10.7554/eLife.07370

The Non-Hemostatic Aspects of Transfused Platelets

*Caroline Sut[1,2], Sofiane Tariket[1,2], Cécile Aubron[3], Chaker Aloui[1], Hind Hamzeh-Cognasse[1], Philippe Berthelot[1], Sandrine Laradi[1,2], Andreas Greinacher[4], Olivier Garraud[1,5] and Fabrice Cognasse[1,2]**

[1] GIMAP-EA3064, Université de Lyon, Saint-Étienne, France, [2] Etablissement Français du Sang, Auvergne-Rhône-Alpes, Saint-Etienne, France, [3] Médecine Intensive Réanimation, Centre Hospitalier Régionale et Universitaire de Brest, Université de Bretagne Occidentale, Brest, France, [4] Institute for Immunology and Transfusion Medicine, University of Greifswald, Greifswald, Germany, [5] Institut National de Transfusion Sanguine (INTS), Paris, France

***Correspondence:**
Fabrice Cognasse
fabrice.cognasse@efs.sante.fr

Platelets transfusion is a safe process, but during or after the process, the recipient may experience an adverse reaction and occasionally a serious adverse reaction (SAR). In this review, we focus on the inflammatory potential of platelet components (PCs) and their involvement in SARs. Recent evidence has highlighted a central role for platelets in the host inflammatory and immune responses. Blood platelets are involved in inflammation and various other aspects of innate immunity through the release of a plethora of immunomodulatory cytokines, chemokines, and associated molecules, collectively termed biological response modifiers that behave like ligands for endothelial and leukocyte receptors and for platelets themselves. The involvement of PCs in SARs—particularly on a critically ill patient's context—could be related, at least in part, to the inflammatory functions of platelets, acquired during storage lesions. Moreover, we focus on causal link between platelet activation and immune-mediated disorders (transfusion-associated immunomodulation, platelets, polyanions, and bacterial defense and alloimmunization). This is linked to the platelets' propensity to be activated even in the absence of deliberate stimuli and to the occurrence of time-dependent storage lesions.

Keywords: platelets, transfusion, CD40L, serious adverse reaction, inflammation, innate immunity

INTRODUCTION

Blood platelets are small anucleate cells essentially originating from megakaryocyte (MK) fragmentation. These cells have a dense cytoskeleton that maintains their discoid shape in normal state and changes the platelets to a spherical form after their activation (1). Platelets play a key role in vascular repair and maintenance of homeostasis, particularly in primary hemostasis. The platelet membrane glycoproteins can interact with the elements of the injured endothelium, mediating their adhesion, followed by activation and finally aggregation, resulting in the formation of a thrombus formed by aggregation of interconnected platelets by fibrinogen to close the vascular gap (1, 2). Platelets also play an important role in innate and adaptive immunity by interacting directly or indirectly with other immune cells to trigger or maintain the inflammatory response (1–3). Several factors are involved in the platelet inflammatory process, in particular, by membrane expression of several immune receptors, such as cytokines (CKs), chemokines (CHs), and a large number of soluble factors contained in their granules (in α-granules, this includes CKs/CHs, immunomodulatory factors, and growth factors, etc.) (4, 5) (**Figure 1**). Moreover, platelets also release other factors: (i) growth

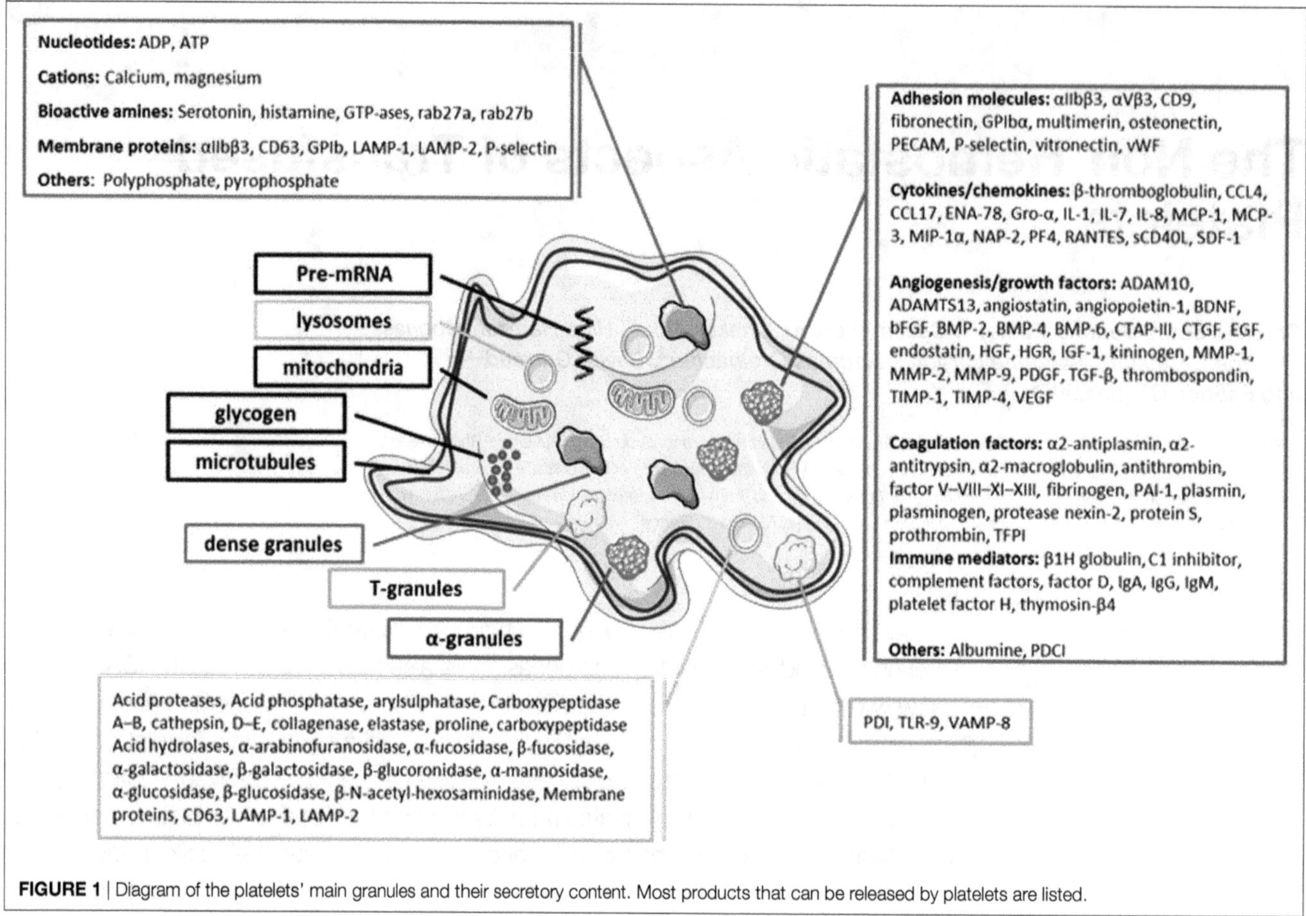

FIGURE 1 | Diagram of the platelets' main granules and their secretory content. Most products that can be released by platelets are listed.

factors promoting angiogenesis, which are also required to repair damage to inflammatory sites (6–8), (ii) clotting factors required for platelet hemostatic functions (9, 10), (iii) antibacterial peptides (1, 11), (iv) adhesion factors (12), and (v) inflammatory mediators, such as serotonin and histamine (13–15).

Platelet-derived soluble CD40L (sCD40L) is a key mediator of the immune system (16–19). Platelet receptor and signaling is important and drive the stimulated platelet granule secretion in these differential profiles—a completely new concept with regard to an anucleate cell—also appear to be strictly regulated by intraplatelet signaling pathways, depending on the stimuli (20–23). This review summarizes current information surrounding the association between inflammation and transfused platelets.

A BRIEF OVERVIEW OF PLATELET FUNCTIONS

Blood platelets are important reservoirs of soluble, preformed mediators (CKs/CHs, hemostatic factors, and immunomodulators) that are present in secretory granules, in particular, α-granules, δ-granules, and lysosomes, which are released upon their activation (1, 15, 24–28). Platelets contain a large variety of CKs/CHs, which are mainly synthesized in the MK and stored in α-granules in most cases (**Figure 1**). CKs/CHs may directly interact with cells of the innate and adaptive immune system or indirectly through immune or non-immune relay cells, such as endothelial cells. CK/CH platelets help regulate the surrounding cells, including their proliferation, differentiation, and activation (1). Interestingly, platelets also express receptors for several CKs/CHs that they secrete, showing their potential to establish autocrine and paracrine bidirectional loops. Platelet immunomodulatory factors include growth factors and CKs/CHs, but also molecules sharing the main characteristics of CHs and CKs, such as sCD40L/CD40L, soluble P-selectin/CD62P, platelet-derived growth factor AB (PDGF-AB), transforming growth factor β, interleukine 1β, regulated on activation normal T cell expressed and secreted (RANTES), and platelet factor 4 (PF4 ou CXCL4).

Although platelets have generally not been considered central to innate immunity and inflammation, this paper provides evidence that platelets may play a key role. Recent data report evidence that platelets can also recycle a number of CKs/CHs and regulatory products called biological response modifiers (BRMs) for which they also express the pairing ligand, which is the case for sCD40L (platelets are the major purveyors of this molecule in the circulation) (17, 29). Platelets also express membrane CD40 and, unlike CD40L, CD40 is detectable on the surface of resting as well as activated platelets (1).

Cytokines and other platelet products can be readily detectable at the onset of acute inflammation (8). In this regard, transfusion is an excellent model of the pathological process, as here, the mediators of inflammation are transfused with consecutively rare, but then, severe serious adverse reaction (SARs). It is currently and widely admitted that sCD40L is the master platelet-associated CKs (17, 30). When it was first described in 2001 in association with platelets, this was in the context of platelet component (PC) transfusion hazards. Subsequently, platelet-sCD40L and the CD40/CD40L pair have been described in many pathologies. The conclusion that, e.g., febrile non hemolytic transfusion reaction (FNHTRs), where sCD40L appears to be chiefly responsible for pathological symptoms, was indeed inflammatory. This conclusion seems similar to their role in diabetes, cardiovascular disease, atheromatous plaques, and inflammatory bowel disease, where CD40/CD40L have now been acknowledged as being influential (1, 31).

PLATELET INTERACTIONS WITH OTHER BLOOD CELL ELEMENTS

Interactions of sCD40L with its CD40 receptor (expressed on immune cells or other cells, such as endothelial cells) can modulate the responses of each of the different cell partners (5, 32). Indeed, platelet sCD40L, interacting with CD40 on endothelial cells, induces inflammatory responses characterized by the expression of adhesion receptors (E-selectin, P-selectin, intercellular adhesion molecule 1, vascular cell adhesion molecule 1) for the release of proinflammatory CKs/CHs (CCL2, IL-6, IL-8) and the recruitment of leukocytes to the inflammatory sites (16). The *in vitro* engagement of neutrophil CD40 by sCD40L induces the generation of reactive oxygen species (ROS) and the destruction of lung endothelial cells suggesting this factor's role in transfusion-related acute lung injury (TRALI) (33). Moreover, platelet sCD40L creates a link between innate and adaptive immunity in promoting maturation (19, 34), activation (35), secretion (36), and presentation of antigen by dendritic cells (DCs), which are cells capable of activating naive T cells to induce an adaptive immune response (5). Elzey et al. have demonstrated that platelet sCD40L can, both *in vitro* and *in vivo*, amplify the activity of pathogen-specific CD8+ T lymphocytes (Lyt), which results in the production and function of IFNγ, and in the enhancement of their lytic function (37). Iannacone has further shown that the number of cytotoxic Lyt during infection with lymphocytic choriomeningitis virus was dramatically reduced in the absence of platelets, involving CD40/CD40L: thrombocytopenia is estimated to result almost exclusively from the antiplatelet antibodies (38). CD40/CD40L also plays a major role in the interaction of $CD4^+$ T lymphocytes (and CD8+) and B lymphocytes, which supports proliferation, differentiation, and production of immunoglobulin by plasma cells. Platelet or MK-derived sCD40L, which is continuously released into the circulation in large quantities (37, 39, 40), is a key molecule regulating the immune system and increased release of sCD40L plays a major role in the pathogenesis of the immune-mediated disease.

Platelets are also essential for the formation of neutrophil extracellular traps (NETs) by neutrophils, The NET formation is an apoptotic process, most important to release of neutrophil DNA, which entraps bacteria resulting in bacterial clearance and concentrating antibacterial factors but in enhancing thrombosis. Toll-like receptor 4-activated platelets bind to neutrophils and initiate NET formation. Platelets facilitate NETosis *via* several protein interaction as CD62P-PSGL-1, involving of platelet GPIbα or neutrophil lymphocyte-function-associated-antigen-1. Moreover, platelet release several soluble factor initiate NET formation and increase bacterial clearance [CXCL4, von Willebrand factor, high-mobility group box 1 protein, thromboxane A2, and β-defensin (41)]. Platelet–leukocyte interactions has focused on platelet interactions with monocytes and neutrophils, as described above, but platelets present a role in T cell responses. Chapman et al. show elegantly that platelets express T cell costimulatory molecules, process, and present Ag in MHC class I and directly activate naive T cells in a platelet MHC class I-dependent manner. The group of Craig N. Morrell define new concept that platelets not only support and promote acquired immune responses but platelets may also directly participate in the initiation of acquired immune responses (42). While for the role in primary hemostasis, platelets primarily interact with endothelial cells, they also interact directly or indirectly *via* their released CK/CH with many of cell types, hereby, strongly influence their function. Platelets can, indeed, activate (and be mutually activated by) almost all types of leukocytes (monocytes, T-lymphocytes, B-lymphocytes, and neutrophils) and DCs (1, 30, 43). When allogeneic (donor) platelets are transfused to patients, the recipients' circulating cells make foreign encounters [e.g., by human leukocyte antigen (HLA) class I molecule expressed on platelets] and can potentially be activated by those encounters, and vice versa. This led to a recent re-examination of the concept of pathogens defense mechanisms, extending it to non-infectious "dangers" such as foreign (transfused) cells (15, 26, 27, 44, 45). PCs are stored for a maximum of 5 days (most countries) before being issued to a patient in need; prior to that, during their shelf life, platelets "spontaneously," i.e., with no acknowledged exogeneous stimulus, release a number of CKs, particularly sCD40L (17, 30) in high enough quantities to exert functional activities on target cells possessing the *ad hoc* receptors. sCD40L was found to be consistently and significantly elevated in PCs that had led to SARs comprising various syndromes, including (antibody independent) TRALI (although this is disputed in such particular case) (30, 33).

A BRIEF OVERVIEW OF PC TRANSFUSION BENEFITS AND COMPLICATIONS

Platelet component transfusions have two main indications, aimed at being either curative or prophylactic (46). Curative transfusions are given to patients presenting with active bleeding and low to very low platelet counts (in exceptional circumstances, the platelet count can be normal, but platelets are non-functional), or massive blood loss. Curative transfusions are not under debate, unlike the protocols and timing of other blood component transfusions [red blood cell concentrates (RBCCs) and fresh plasma] and/or blood derivatives, such as prothrombin complex concentrate or fibrinogen. There is no consensus on prophylactic transfusions, however, although many practitioners still recommend not exposing at-risk patients to bleed. Thresholds for transfusion and quantities of transfused platelets vary consistently in different countries and with different systems. In short, PC transfusion provides a benefit to patients and prevents bleeding and deterioration of otherwise serious clinical conditions. PC transfusion is supportive in many chemotherapy protocols and stem cell transplantation.

Platelet component transfusions can lead to adverse inflammatory reactions. The majority of adverse inflammatory reactions in patients receiving blood (recipients) appear either FNHTRs or allergy, both being clearly inflammatory conditions. FNHTR is characterized and associated with fever (≥38°C or ≥1°C above baseline, if baseline ≥37°C), or chills and rigors, but not directly with hemolysis, caused by cytokines that accumulate in the product during storage. FNHTR is also initiated by the presence of recipient antibodies reacting to donor HLA or other antigens. Allergic reactions (e.g., urticaria) occur within minutes after the start of the transfusion. Allergic reactions may be associated with mild upper respiratory symptoms, nausea, vomiting, abdominal cramps, or diarrhea. Allergic reactions could be severe (e.g., anaphylaxis). Patients can present a severe hypotension, cough, bronchospasm (respiratory distress and wheezing), laryngospasm, angioedema, urticaria, nausea, abdominal cramps, vomiting, diarrhea, shock, and/or loss of consciousness. This may be a fatal reaction. Severe allergic reactions could be dependent of (i) IgA-deficient patients who have anti-IgA antibodies, (ii) patient antibodies to plasma proteins (such as IgG, albumin, haptoglobin, transferrin, C3, C4, or cytokines), (iii) transfusing an allergen to a sensitized patient (for example, penicillin or nuts consumed by a donor), or (iv) rarely the transfusion of IgE antibodies (to drugs, food, etc.) from a donor to an allergen present in the recipient (47).

On rare occasions, PC transfusion can lead to immediate to short-delayed inflammatory adverse reactions (grades 1–3: 0.24%); however, in some cases (0.006%), grade 3 reactions can be life-threatening (48). The rationale for the relatively high number of SARs with PC transfusion [from 1/4 to 1/2 of all reported SARs, while PCs represent only about 10% of transfused blood components (BCs)] may be deduced from their propensity to secrete copious amounts of pro-inflammatory BRMs as outlined in the previous section. In addition, PC transfusion can be associated with volume overload, as PCs frequently come into large volumes and elevated levels of proteins and lipids exerting a surfactant effect (49). The latter can be prevented by close patient monitoring and by replacing 2/3 of plasma with platelet additive solutions (50). The case of TRALI and the responsibility of platelets have been presented elsewhere (45). Finally, PC transfusion carries a greater risk of bacterial contamination, which can be life threatening especially in severely immuno-compromised patients (51). The introduction of Pathogen Reduction Technologies has abrogated much of the adverse effects associated with pathogen contamination of platelet products (52, 53). Pre-storage leukoreduction proved to significantly reduce inflammatory reactions as well as viral infections (54). In brief, PC transfusions can induce unwanted effects, e.g., volume, plasma, inflammatory reactions, pathogen transmission, etc., in addition to their therapeutically intended effect, i.e., improving hemostasis. However, since PC-transfused patients are particularly fragile patients, close monitoring and careful dosing can prevent many complications such as volume overload.

PLATELET STORAGE AND OUTCOMES OF CRITICALLY ILL PATIENTS

Over the platelet storage period, certain biochemical and functional changes occur in the platelets and their storage medium. These changes, called storage lesions (**Figure 2**), include acidification of the storage medium secondary to anaerobic platelet metabolism, platelet activation (55), and an increase in CKs and lipids level in PCs (56, 57). Several authors applied a metabolomics approach to the issue of donor variability in poststorage platelet viability. Metabolomic analysis of the stored platelets identified multiple specific metabolites that correlated with either PLT recoveries or survivals after transfusion (Lipid metabolism components, caffeine, and its metabolites) (58). Interestingly, platelet storage lesion is not associated with a linear decay of metabolism, but rather with successive metabolic shifts (59). Prudent et al. review the key findings of the proteomic analyses of platelet concentrates (PCs) treated by the Mirasol Pathogen Reduction Technology, the Intercept Blood System, and the Theraflex UV-C system, respectively, and discuss the potential impact on the biological functions of platelets. The impact of the Pathogen inactivation treatment on the proteome appears to be different among the Pathogen inactivation systems (53, 60).

These storage lesions may compromise the platelets' viability and functionality, and, therefore, the transfusion's efficacy (61). They may also lead to adverse reactions in the recipients.

Critically ill patients are the second largest patient group to receive platelet products after oncology–hematology patients. Around 15% of critically ill patients require a platelet transfusion during their intensive care unit stay for treatment or prophylaxis of bleeding (62). Critically ill patients are characterized by a coexisting inflammatory state, making them theoretically more susceptible to blood product adverse reactions. A "two-hit" hypothesis has largely been used to explain the pathophysiology of transfusion adverse events including TRALI, the first hit being a pro-inflammatory condition and the second hit being the administration of antibodies or BRMs through blood component transfusion (63). Results of *in vitro* and animal studies suggest platelets storage lesions have a key effect on the occurrence of non-antibody mediated TRALI (33, 63). Khan et al. have observed an increase in sCD40L level over the PC storage period, and higher levels of sCD40L in platelet products implicated in TRALI, suggesting that the accumulation of sCD40L during platelet storage induces TRALI (33). Consistent with these findings, Vlaar et al. have found that stored platelet supernatant compared with fresh platelet supernatant led to an increase in systemic and pulmonary coagulopathy in lipopolysaccharide pretreated rats (63).

CD40/CD40L complex could be a major target in a TRALI prevention strategy. Improving the conditions in which the PCs are prepared and stored would contribute to controlling partly the risks of non-immune TRALI.

Prolonged platelet storage has been associated with a decrease in posttransfusion platelet increment and a shorter

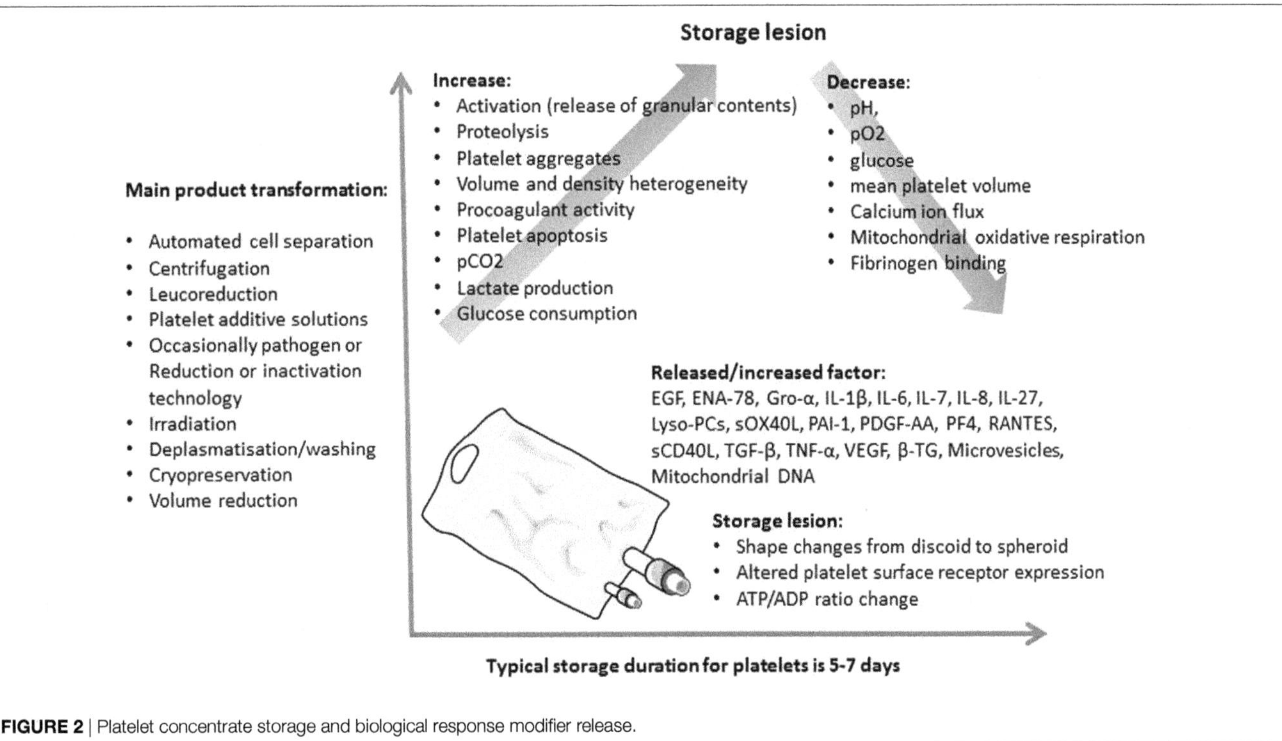

FIGURE 2 | Platelet concentrate storage and biological response modifier release.

time to next platelet transfusion in oncology–hematology patients (64–66), but the clinical consequences of the platelets storage lesions remain uncertain (66–68). To our knowledge, no study has investigated the association between transfusion efficacy and platelet storage duration in critically ill patients. Five observational studies have investigated the association between PC storage duration and critically ill patient outcomes; one included post-cardiac surgery patients only, two studies included trauma patients only, and two all critically ill patients (69–73). There was no association between mortality and storage duration in the three studies evaluating this outcome (69, 70, 73). In a study of 381 trauma patients, those receiving platelets stored for 5 days developed more complications, including sepsis, than patients transfused with platelets stored for less than 5 days (5.5% sepsis in patients receiving platelets stored for 3 days or less, versus 16.7% in patients receiving platelets stored for 5 days, $p = 0.03$) (70). After adjustment for confounders, patients receiving PCs stored for 5 days had a 2.4-fold higher risk of developing complications, including acute renal failure, acute respiratory distress syndrome, and sepsis, than patients transfused with fresher platelets (70). All these studies are retrospective and have numerous limitations in their methods making it impossible to draw any definitive conclusion on the impact of platelet storage duration on clinical-centered outcomes. Prospective research is warranted to determine whether prolonged platelet storage has an impact on the prognosis of critically ill patients. In the meantime, better understanding of platelet transfusion-related immunomodulation may help us to understand the reported association between platelet transfusion and an increased risk of hospital-acquired infections (74, 75).

TRANSFUSION-ASSOCIATED IMMUNOMODULATION

Transfusion-related immunomodulation or TRIM is a complex event with dual effects that are potentially beneficial, but in general, mostly considered harmful (76). The long-term effect of transfusions is suspected to modulate (dampen) immune responses and consequently favor the emergence of secondary malignancies and infections. It is, however, extremely difficult to decipher the respective roles of causal pathologies in severely sick intensive care patients or patients receiving chemotherapy and immunosuppressants, monoclonals and biosimilars, and BCs. TRIM induced by PCs would be best understood in patients having received PCs only, but it is almost impossible to delineate the immunosuppressive role of platelets relative to red blood cells as only very few patients receive PCs and no RBCCs. Furthermore, in case of plasma-rich BCs, plasma polyreactive immunoglobulins (Igs) may counterbalance certain immunosuppressive effects. In short, whether PC transfusions may be immunomodulatory remains elusive and difficult to assess, though it would be of interest to investigate this in order to provide patients with optimized care.

PLATELETS, POLYANIONS, AND BACTERIAL DEFENSE

While the above-described mechanisms clearly indicate that platelets interfere with the immune system, only a few studies clearly show a causal link between platelet activation and immune-mediated disorders. One well-investigated example of the role of platelets in mediating immune reactions is the interaction of platelets with heparin.

The adverse drug effect of heparin-induced thrombocytopenia (HIT) will, therefore, be used to exemplify the interaction of platelets and the immune system. HIT is a prothrombotic adverse drug reaction caused by the transient production of IgG-class platelet-activating antibodies that recognize multimolecular complexes of the positively charged PF4 and the polyanion drug heparin. These antibodies activate platelets and also monocytes *via* their FcγRIIa receptors. This causes transformation of an immune reaction into a prothrombotic reaction, resulting in massive thrombin generation and paradox thrombotic complications. If unrecognized, the risk for new thrombosis in affected patients is 5% per day and the risk of mortality is 25–30% (77). There is no doubt that with HIT, platelets mediate an extremely powerful reaction, which results from concomitant activation of the immune system and the coagulation system.

The reason for this massive response is that HIT is likely a misdirected bacterial host defense (78). PF4 binds charge-related to Gram-negative and Gram-positive bacteria. On Gram-negative bacteria, lipid-A is the binding site for PF4 (79). The binding site of PF4 on Gram-positive bacteria has not yet been identified. The question raised is how and why PF4 induces such a potentially dangerous immune response.

The following section summarizes our recently proposed working model (80, 81). All bacteria expose strong negative charges on their surface. This negative charge is likely a mechanism by which bacteria are kept apart from each other, and by which bacteria are protected from phagocytosis. The zeta potential-mediated repulsive forces generated by the negative charges push bacteria apart from each other and away from their "predators" (the reader is invited to watch the following YouTube video demonstrating this principle https://www.youtube.com/watch?v=Kb-m1uDoWfU). Eukaryotic cells, however, must not have this strong negative charge as the repulsive forces would be incompatible with a complex multicellular organism. In view of this consideration, we propose that a strong negative charge is a fundamental feature of prokaryotes. In line with this concept, basic mechanisms of the innate immune system, like the alternative and classic complement pathway, the intrinsic clotting system with factor XII and factor XI, as well as the kininogen–bradykinin pathway are strongly activated by negative charges (82). However, the adaptive immune system (T cell receptors, B cell receptors, antibodies) do not recognize charge, they recognize structures. The platelet-derived CH PF4 has the role of translating charge into structure. After binding to negative charges, PF4 undergoes complex structural changes [for review, see Ref. (83, 84)]. These structural changes expose a neoepitope, which is recognized by anti-PF4/polyanion antibodies, the same antibodies that induce HIT. After binding of anti-PF4/P antibodies to PF4-labeled bacteria, these opsonized bacteria mediate very efficient phagocytosis by granulocytes (78). The evolutionary advantage of using such a mechanism is that it enables an early IgG response toward bacteria the organism has not seen before. The newly encountered bacteria also bind PF4; PF4 undergoes its conformational change due to the negative charge on the bacteria surface and is then recognized by the preformed anti-PF4/P antibodies. In line with this concept, most likely a secondary immune reaction, natural anti-PF4/P antibodies are found in the general population where their presence is highly correlated with the presence of chronic infections like chronic periodontal disease (85). On the basis of this concept, these antibodies must be very common. Indeed, the adverse drug reaction HIT has helped to prove this. In HIT, anti-PF4/P IgG are formed in high titer between day 5 and day 10 (86). As B cells cannot produce IgG antibodies during a primary immune response within 5–10 days, HIT is always a secondary immune reaction, even in patients who have never received heparin before. As 65% of patients develop these antibodies after cardiac surgery, a plausible explanation for such frequent primary immunization is the above-outlined concept of bacterial infection-related priming of the immune system.

However, the above-outlined concept of the role of PF4 and platelets as mediators between innate and specific immunity places platelets in a very special position, bridging two major parts of our immune defense system. Platelets secrete or expose many molecules with a specific role in immunity. Little information exists on how platelet storage modifies the structure of these molecules or their spatial presentation within platelet compartments or on the platelet surface. As exemplified by the structural changes of CH PF4 induced by polyanions like heparin, conformational changes in these proteins may transmit a danger signal to the transfusion recipient's immune system, which erroneously triggers potent pathogen defense mechanisms, resulting in adverse transfusion reactions. Although this has not been shown yet, it is conceivable that other platelet-derived mediators such as sCD40L intensify and probably orchestrate the interaction of platelets and other immune cells with pathogens. If misdirected, this can cause SARs. The adverse drug reaction of HIT provides one of the most prominent examples of the potentially deleterious consequences for patients.

The risk that our immune system develops autoimmune-like reactions toward platelet proteins when they are modified during storage is probably quite low, although such autoimmune reactions may occur. Again, this has been demonstrated for the immune reaction toward conformationally changed PF4. In the past decade, it has become recognized that certain patients present with clinical symptoms and laboratory features of HIT despite not having previously received heparin either in the recent past or at all. Sera from these patients contain antibodies that strongly activate platelets even in the absence of heparin. To date, ≈20 cases of spontaneous HIT syndrome have been reported (87–96). In the plasma of these patients, antibodies are found, which bind to PF4 with such high avidity that they cluster two PF4 molecules, thereby inducing the same conformational change as polyanions. These clusters of conformationally changed PF4 attach to platelets and endothelial cells, giving the immune system a false signal of the presence of strong negative charges, which prompts the above-described bacterial defense mechanism.

As the negative charge is a danger signal for the human defense system, bacteria have naturally developed counteracting methods to hide this danger signal. One of which is long lipopolysaccharide (LPS) chains covering and "hiding" the negative charges or the Fc-part of the anti-PF4/P antibodies bound to conformational-changed PF4 on the bacteria surface. Lipid A is the basis of LPS.

PF4 has a diameter of 5 nm; when an IgG molecule (which is about 10 nm long) binds to conformationally changed PF4 bound to lipid A, the entire complex has a height of about 15–18 nm. The LPS chain, however, can reach lengths of up to 25 nm. This covers the Fc part of the antibody and thereby recognition of opsonized bacteria by the immune system's Fc receptors. However, platelets, in addition to PF4, secrete polyphosphates from their δ-granules. Polyphosphates are also negatively charged and bind to the PF4 molecule on the bacteria surface, attracting other PF4 molecules and finally forming large multimolecular PF4/polyphosphate complexes, which extend well out of the bacteria's LPS shield (97). This has two effects: conformationally changed PF4 is now exposed for antibody recognition, and consequently several anti-PF4/P antibodies can bind to these complexes on the bacterial surface, forming immune complexes, which are then readily recognized by the Fc receptors of human defense cells.

Platelets also found a new way in which platelets defend against bacteria. When platelets are incubated with *Escherchia coli* in the presence of PF4 and anti-PF4/P antibodies, platelets kill up to 75% of *E. coli* by direct platelet bacteria interaction. Upon investigating this mechanism in more detail, we found a new way in which platelets defend bacteria. It is well established that platelets can internalize IgG-coated targets (98–100); however, it is debated whether phagocytosis of bacteria (i.e., *Staphylococcus aureus*) (101) is really a major mechanism for bacterial host defense (102, 103). Although platelets store bactericidal substances in their α-granules (12), α-granules are designed to be released and it is unlikely that phagocytosed bacteria are transported within the platelet into the α-granule. Such a mechanism would be incompatible with platelet shape change during activation where platelets are spread thinly over a large area with the α-granules concentrated within the immediate granulomere zone (104). We propose an alternative mechanism, where platelets cover bacteria by widely extending their membranes and then actively contracting them, thereby centralizing bacteria until they are very close to the granulomere of the platelets, where the substances with antibacterial potency are stored (105). When a threshold concentration of platelet-activating signals is reached due to platelet interaction with the opsonized bacteria, the activated platelets release their α-granules preferentially at the site of the bacteria, thereby locally reaching high concentrations of antibacterial substances. This phenomenon is similar to the pore-forming perforin released from the granules at the immunological synapse potentiated by cytotoxic T lymphocytes (106).

The above-outlined mechanisms are not the only ways in which platelets interfere with bacteria and other pathogens (107–110). Through complex mechanisms involving the platelet Fc-receptor FcγRIIA (111–113), glycoprotein αIIbβ3, GPIbα, complement receptors (e.g., gC1q-R), and toll-like receptors (e.g., TLR-2 and TLR-4), platelets interact with bacteria and become activated by bacteria (27, 114). Upon activation, platelets release antimicrobial substances such as ROS, antimicrobial peptides, defensins, kinocidins, and proteases (11, 115–117). Taken together, there is ample evidence that platelets play an important role in the defense against pathogens.

Recognition of pathogens by platelets is at least partly mediated by conformationally changed endogenous, platelet-derived proteins. The challenge for transfusion medicine and immunohematology is to identify whether platelet proteins with an important role in danger signaling are also conformationally changed during platelet processing and storage, thereby presenting a danger signal with an increased risk of triggering misdirected host defense mechanisms.

PLATELETS, POLYMORPHISMS, AND ALLOIMMUNIZATION

Platelet component transfusions are extremely difficult to match for surface antigens between donors and recipients, apart from the ABO groups (A and/or B antigens can be variably expressed on platelets) (118). Moreover, platelets exhibit numerous copies of highly polymorphic HLA class I antigens. The functions associated with HLA class I molecules on platelets are currently under debate, as platelets are not consensually considered capable of presenting antigens. HLA transfer to other cells has recently been evidenced experimentally in mice, opening up novel avenues on the subject. HLA immunization of patients is not uncommon, but pre-storage leukoreduction has proven to be tremendously efficacious in limiting it, since leukocytes—10-times more loaded with HLA moieties than platelets—seem to potentiate immunization against platelet antigens, HLA, and human platelet antigens (HPA) (119). HPA are actually polymorphic variants of platelet glycoproteins, representing "platelet-specific blood groups." Almost 20 such molecules are recognized as being immunogenic, with less than five being implicated in the most frequent immunization, while the others stand for rare antigens. Those HPA antigens usually come in two antithetical moieties termed "a" and "b," "a" being the frequent allele and "b" the rarest. In certain circumstances, HLA or HPA testing and matching is the only option available to efficiently transfuse refractory patients; indeed, patients presenting with allogeneous anti-HLA and/or HPA Abs may destroy transfused platelets especially if Abs are directed at frequent Ags, leading to refractory states and imposing cross-matching of donor PCs against recipients' plasma whenever possible (outside emergency situations) (120); rarely, transfer of allogenous Ags onto recipient's platelets may create aggravated thrombocytopenic states with posttransfusion purpura (121). Transfusion of pooled platelets may be an option to saturate allo-Abs and give a chance to increase the patient's platelet count during the critical phase (at the expense of creating further immunization, however). Regarding female patients having been alloimmunized during pregnancies, it is preferable to transfuse them using either HPA (HLA) typed, or cross-matched, PCs, to avoid the rebound of allo-Abs and refractoriness (122). It should be noted that as residual red blood cells exist even in very small numbers in PCs, patients transfused with PCs can be immunized against red blood cell antigens, especially when these are highly immunogenic such as Rhesus-D; this occurrence is nevertheless infrequent. Whereas it is strongly advised not to transfuse a Rhesus D negative female recipient in child-bearing age with platelets obtained from a Rhesus D positive donor unless prophylaxis is available if needed; Rhesus D negative men and females with no longer child-bearing potential are assumed to be safely transfused by Rh D positive donor's PCs (especially pooled PCs according to recently published studies) (123); the case of Rhesus negative men (such as HSC transplanted) undergoing repeated PC transfusion is debated but should be discussed for Rh-D prophylaxis (124). Finally, it has recently been hypothesized that ABO mismatched platelets favor alloimmunization (125), although this hypothesis has yet to be ascertained with respect to its clinical impact.

CONCLUSION

In conclusion, transfusion of platelets is generally safe and largely beneficial to patients. On rare occasions, SARs (which cannot be prevented by current measures), occur with clinical presentation of acute inflammation. In all cases investigated to date, either based on clinical observations or tested experimentally, BRMs (comprising chiefly of CKs and CHs and related molecules such as sCD40L) are found to be in close association. Potentially, these SARs are misdirected physiological defense mechanisms. This we have exemplified by the complex pathogenesis of HIT, which, however, involves just one of the many immunomodulatory CHs released by platelets. Additional safety measures to prevent those SARs would be beneficial to patients; however, it is likely they would be extremely difficult to establish and would not be cost effective. Again, transfusion-linked inflammation is likely the result of a combination of factors related to the donor, the BC, and the recipient. The only factor that can be targeted at present is the BC and measures to improve BC quality are being implemented when identified within the industry, in partnership with blood establishments. The identification of parameters that may be related to patients (recipients) would be desirable to identify at-risk patients and apply measures to prevent the severity of the hazards. If parameters are linked to donors, the situation becomes much more difficult, because further medical investigations in donors would scarcely be acceptable, and would have the potential to jeopardize BC stocks. How can one explain to a generous blood donor that he or she is perfectly safe and healthy, but "at risk" of inflicting harm on "certain" recipients? This problem is medically, ethically, and psychologically difficult to address. Alternatively, transfusion medicine may become one of the first medical specialties where personalized medicine comes into effect: "How can a given patient be given the BC most suited to his or her condition"?

AUTHOR CONTRIBUTIONS

CS, CA, HH-C, AG, OG, and FC: wrote the paper. CS, ST, CA, ChA, HH-C, PB, SL, AG, OG, and FC: participated in all steps of the process and reviewed the manuscript.

ACKNOWLEDGMENTS

The authors are grateful to the technical and medical staff and personnel of the Etablissement Français du Sang (EFS), Auvergne-Rhône-Alpes, Saint-Etienne, France for collecting and contributing data to this study. They would also like to thank the blood donors. This work was supported by grants from the Etablissement Français du Sang (Grant APR), France, the Agence Nationale de la Sécurité et du Médicament et des Produits de Santé (ANSM-AAP-2012-011, Reference 2012S055), the Agence Nationale de la Recherche (ANR-12-JSV1-0012-01), and the association Les Amis de Rémi, Savigneux, France.

REFERENCES

1. Semple JW, Italiano JE Jr, Freedman J. Platelets and the immune continuum. *Nat Rev Immunol* (2011) 11(4):264–74. doi:10.1038/nri2956
2. Boilard E, Blanco P, Nigrovic PA. Platelets: active players in the pathogenesis of arthritis and SLE. *Nat Rev Rheumatol* (2012) 8(9):534–42. doi:10.1038/nrrheum.2012.118
3. Mantovani A, Garlanda C. Platelet-macrophage partnership in innate immunity and inflammation. *Nat Immunol* (2013) 14(8):768–70. doi:10.1038/ni.2666
4. Garraud O, Hamzeh-Cognasse H, Cognasse F. Platelets and cytokines: how and why? *Transfus Clin Biol* (2012) 19(3):104–8. doi:10.1016/j.tracli.2012.02.004
5. Garraud O, Hamzeh-Cognasse H, Pozzetto B, Cavaillon JM, Cognasse F. Bench-to-bedside review: platelets and active immune functions – new clues for immunopathology? *Crit Care* (2013) 17(4):236. doi:10.1186/cc12716
6. Whiteheart SW. Platelet granules: surprise packages. *Blood* (2011) 118(5):1190–1. doi:10.1182/blood-2011-06-359836
7. Peterson JE, Zurakowski D, Italiano JE Jr, Michel LV, Fox L, Klement GL, et al. Normal ranges of angiogenesis regulatory proteins in human platelets. *Am J Hematol* (2010) 85(7):487–93. doi:10.1002/ajh.21732
8. Jenne CN, Urrutia R, Kubes P. Platelets: bridging hemostasis, inflammation, and immunity. *Int J Lab Hematol* (2013) 35(3):254–61. doi:10.1111/ijlh.12084
9. Gremmel T, Frelinger AL III, Michelson AD. Platelet physiology. *Semin Thromb Hemost* (2016) 42(3):191–204. doi:10.1055/s-0035-1564835
10. Kieffer N, Guichard J, Farcet JP, Vainchenker W, Breton-Gorius J. Biosynthesis of major platelet proteins in human blood platelets. *Eur J Biochem* (1987) 164(1):189–95. doi:10.1111/j.1432-1033.1987.tb11010.x
11. Yeaman MR. Platelets: at the nexus of antimicrobial defence. *Nat Rev Microbiol* (2014) 12(6):426–37. doi:10.1038/nrmicro3269
12. Blair P, Flaumenhaft R. Platelet alpha-granules: basic biology and clinical correlates. *Blood Rev* (2009) 23(4):177–89. doi:10.1016/j.blre.2009.04.001
13. Thon JN, Italiano JE. Platelets: production, morphology and ultrastructure. *Handb Exp Pharmacol* (2012) 210:3–22. doi:10.1007/978-3-642-29423-5_1
14. McNicol A, Israels SJ. Platelet dense granules: structure, function and implications for haemostasis. *Thromb Res* (1999) 95(1):1–18. doi:10.1016/S0049-3848(99)00015-8
15. Garraud O, Tariket S, Sut C, Haddad A, Aloui C, Chakroun T, et al. Transfusion as an inflammation hit: knowns and unknowns. *Front Immunol* (2016) 7:534. doi:10.3389/fimmu.2016.00534
16. Henn V, Slupsky JR, Grafe M, Anagnostopoulos I, Forster R, Muller-Berghaus G, et al. CD40 ligand on activated platelets triggers an inflammatory reaction of endothelial cells. *Nature* (1998) 391(6667):591–4. doi:10.1038/35393
17. Phipps RP, Kaufman J, Blumberg N. Platelet derived CD154 (CD40 ligand) and febrile responses to transfusion. *Lancet* (2001) 357(9273):2023–4. doi:10.1016/S0140-6736(00)05108-4
18. Freedman JE. CD40-CD40L and platelet function: beyond hemostasis. *Circ Res* (2003) 92(9):944–6. doi:10.1161/01.RES.0000074030.98009.FF
19. Blumberg N, Spinelli SL, Francis CW, Taubman MB, Phipps RP. The platelet as an immune cell-CD40 ligand and transfusion immunomodulation. *Immunol Res* (2009) 45(2–3):251–60. doi:10.1007/s12026-009-8106-9
20. Damien P, Cognasse F, Lucht F, Suy F, Pozzetto B, Garraud O, et al. Highly active antiretroviral therapy alters inflammation linked to platelet cytokines in HIV-1-infected patients. *J Infect Dis* (2013) 208(5):868–70. doi:10.1093/infdis/jit260
21. Berthet J, Damien P, Hamzeh-Cognasse H, Arthaud CA, Eyraud MA, Zeni F, et al. Human platelets can discriminate between various bacterial LPS isoforms via TLR4 signaling and differential cytokine secretion. *Clin Immunol* (2012) 145(3):189–200. doi:10.1016/j.clim.2012.09.004

22. McNicol A, Agpalza A, Jackson EC, Hamzeh-Cognasse H, Garraud O, Cognasse F. *Streptococcus sanguinis*-induced cytokine release from platelets. *J Thromb Haemost* (2011) 9(10):2038–49. doi:10.1111/j.1538-7836.2011.04462.x
23. Cognasse F, Hamzeh-Cognasse H, Berthet J, Damien P, Lucht F, Pozzetto B, et al. Altered release of regulated upon activation, normal T-cell expressed and secreted protein from human, normal platelets: contribution of distinct HIV-1MN gp41 peptides. *AIDS* (2009) 23(15):2057–9. doi:10.1097/QAD.0b013e328330da65
24. Kapur R, Zufferey A, Boilard E, Semple JW. Nouvelle cuisine: platelets served with inflammation. *J Immunol* (2015) 194(12):5579–87. doi:10.4049/jimmunol.1500259
25. Elzey BD, Sprague DL, Ratliff TL. The emerging role of platelets in adaptive immunity. *Cell Immunol* (2005) 238(1):1–9. doi:10.1016/j.cellimm.2005.12.005
26. Cognasse F, Garraud O, Pozzetto B, Laradi S, Hamzeh-Cognasse H. How can non-nucleated platelets be so smart? *J Thromb Haemost* (2016) 14(4):794–6. doi:10.1111/jth.13262
27. Garraud O, Cognasse F. Are platelets cells? And if yes, are they immune cells? *Front Immunol* (2015) 6:70. doi:10.3389/fimmu.2015.00070
28. Heijnen H, van der Sluijs P. Platelet secretory behaviour: as diverse as the granules … or not? *J Thromb Haemost* (2015) 13(12):2141–51. doi:10.1111/jth.13147
29. Andre P, Nannizzi-Alaimo L, Prasad SK, Phillips DR. Platelet-derived CD40L: the switch-hitting player of cardiovascular disease. *Circulation* (2002) 106(8):896–9. doi:10.1161/01.CIR.0000028962.04520.01
30. Cognasse F, Payrat JM, Corash L, Osselaer JC, Garraud O. Platelet components associated with acute transfusion reactions: the role of platelet-derived soluble CD40 ligand. *Blood* (2008) 112(12):4779–80. doi:10.1182/blood-2008-05-157578
31. Boilard E, Nigrovic PA, Larabee K, Watts GF, Coblyn JS, Weinblatt ME, et al. Platelets amplify inflammation in arthritis via collagen-dependent microparticle production. *Science* (2010) 327(5965):580–3. doi:10.1126/science.1181928
32. Henn V, Steinbach S, Buchner K, Presek P, Kroczek RA. The inflammatory action of CD40 ligand (CD154) expressed on activated human platelets is temporally limited by coexpressed CD40. *Blood* (2001) 98(4):1047–54. doi:10.1182/blood.V98.4.1047
33. Khan SY, Kelher MR, Heal JM, Blumberg N, Boshkov LK, Phipps R, et al. Soluble CD40 ligand accumulates in stored blood components, primes neutrophils through CD40, and is a potential cofactor in the development of transfusion-related acute lung injury. *Blood* (2006) 108(7):2455–62. doi:10.1182/blood-2006-04-017251
34. Perros AJ, Christensen AM, Flower RL, Dean MM. Soluble mediators in platelet concentrates modulate dendritic cell inflammatory responses in an experimental model of transfusion. *J Interferon Cytokine Res* (2015) 35(10):821–30. doi:10.1089/jir.2015.0029
35. Martinson J, Bae J, Klingemann HG, Tam Y. Activated platelets rapidly up-regulate CD40L expression and can effectively mature and activate autologous ex vivo differentiated DC. *Cytotherapy* (2004) 6(5):487–97. doi:10.1080/14653240410005249
36. Ma DY, Clark EA. The role of CD40 and CD154/CD40L in dendritic cells. *Semin Immunol* (2009) 21(5):265–72. doi:10.1016/j.smim.2009.05.010
37. Elzey BD, Ratliff TL, Sowa JM, Crist SA. Platelet CD40L at the interface of adaptive immunity. *Thromb Res* (2011) 127(3):180–3. doi:10.1016/j.thromres.2010.10.011
38. Iannacone M. Platelet-mediated modulation of adaptive immunity. *Semin Immunol* (2016) 28(6):555–60. doi:10.1016/j.smim.2016.10.008
39. Aloui C, Prigent A, Sut C, Tariket S, Hamzeh-Cognasse H, Pozzetto B, et al. The signaling role of CD40 ligand in platelet biology and in platelet component transfusion. *Int J Mol Sci* (2014) 15(12):22342–64. doi:10.3390/ijms151222342
40. Ferroni P, Basili S, Davi G. Platelet activation, inflammatory mediators and hypercholesterolemia. *Curr Vasc Pharmacol* (2003) 1(2):157–69. doi:10.2174/1570161033476772
41. Kral JB, Schrottmaier WC, Salzmann M, Assinger A. Platelet interaction with innate immune cells. *Transfus Med Hemother* (2016) 43(2):78–88. doi:10.1159/000444807
42. Chapman LM, Aggrey AA, Field DJ, Srivastava K, Ture S, Yui K, et al. Platelets present antigen in the context of MHC class I. *J Immunol* (2012) 189(2):916–23. doi:10.4049/jimmunol.1200580
43. Elzey BD, Tian J, Jensen RJ, Swanson AK, Lees JR, Lentz SR, et al. Platelet-mediated modulation of adaptive immunity. A communication link between innate and adaptive immune compartments. *Immunity* (2003) 19(1):9–19. doi:10.1016/S1074-7613(03)00177-8
44. Garraud O, Chabert A, Hamzeh-Cognasse H, Laradi S, Cognasse F. Platelets and immunity: from physiology to pathology. *Transfus Clin Biol* (2017) 24(2):83–6. doi:10.1016/j.tracli.2017.04.004
45. Tariket S, Sut C, Hamzeh-Cognasse H, Laradi S, Pozzetto B, Garraud O, et al. Transfusion-related acute lung injury: transfusion, platelets and biological response modifiers. *Expert Rev Hematol* (2016) 9(5):497–508. doi:10.1586/17474086.2016.1152177
46. Connell NT. Transfusion medicine. *Prim Care* (2016) 43(4):651–9. doi:10.1016/j.pop.2016.07.004
47. Funk M (ed). Chapter 27: non-infectious complications of blood transfusion. 18th ed. *AABB Technical Manual*. Bethesda: AABB (2014).
48. ANSM. *Rapport d'activité hémovigilance 2015*. (2016). Available from: http://ansm.sante.fr/var/ansm_site/storage/original/application/27ce3d0739821882c0cd87041b8050a7.pdf
49. Sharma S, Sharma P, Tyler LN. Transfusion of blood and blood products: indications and complications. *Am Fam Physician* (2011) 83(6):719–24.
50. Wagner T, Vetter A, Dimovic N, Guber SE, Helmberg W, Kroll W, et al. Ultrastructural changes and activation differences in platelet concentrates stored in plasma and additive solution. *Transfusion* (2002) 42(6):719–27. doi:10.1046/j.1537-2995.2002.00125.x
51. Osterman JL, Arora S. Blood product transfusions and reactions. *Emerg Med Clin North Am* (2014) 32(3):727–38. doi:10.1016/j.emc.2014.04.012
52. Hechler B, Ravanat C, Gachet C. Amotosalen/UVA pathogen inactivation technology reduces platelet activability, induces apoptosis and accelerates clearance. *Haematologica* (2017) 102:e502–3. doi:10.3324/haematol.2017.180539
53. Tissot JD, Bardyn M, Sonego G, Abonnenc M, Prudent M. The storage lesions: from past to future. *Transfus Clin Biol* (2017) 24(3):277–84. doi:10.1016/j.tracli.2017.05.012
54. Wadhwa M, Krailadsiri P, Dilger P, Gaines Das R, Seghatchian MJ, Thorpe R. Cytokine levels as performance indicators for white blood cell reduction of platelet concentrates. *Vox Sang* (2002) 83(2):125–36. doi:10.1046/j.1423-0410.2002.00203.x
55. Cognasse F, Hamzeh-Cognasse H, Lafarge S, Acquart S, Chavarin P, Courbil R, et al. Donor platelets stored for at least 3 days can elicit activation marker expression by the recipient's blood mononuclear cells: an in vitro study. *Transfusion* (2009) 49(1):91–8. doi:10.1111/j.1537-2995.2008.01931.x
56. Silliman CC, Dickey WO, Paterson AJ, Thurman GW, Clay KL, Johnson CA, et al. Analysis of the priming activity of lipids generated during routine storage of platelet concentrates. *Transfusion* (1996) 36(2):133–9. doi:10.1046/j.1537-2995.1996.36296181925.x
57. Cardigan R, Sutherland J, Wadhwa M, Dilger P, Thorpe R. The influence of platelet additive solutions on cytokine levels and complement activation in platelet concentrates during storage. *Vox Sang* (2003) 84(1):28–35. doi:10.1046/j.1423-0410.2003.00257.x
58. Zimring JC, Slichter S, Odem-Davis K, Felcyn JR, Kapp LM, Bell LN, et al. Metabolites in stored platelets associated with platelet recoveries and survivals. *Transfusion* (2016) 56(8):1974–83. doi:10.1111/trf.13631
59. Paglia G, Sigurjonsson OE, Rolfsson O, Valgeirsdottir S, Hansen MB, Brynjolfsson S, et al. Comprehensive metabolomic study of platelets reveals the expression of discrete metabolic phenotypes during storage. *Transfusion* (2014) 54(11):2911–23. doi:10.1111/trf.12710
60. Prudent M, D'Alessandro A, Cazenave JP, Devine DV, Gachet C, Greinacher A, et al. Proteome changes in platelets after pathogen inactivation – an inter-laboratory consensus. *Transfus Med Rev* (2014) 28(2):72–83. doi:10.1016/j.tmrv.2014.02.002
61. Rosenfeld BA, Herfel B, Faraday N, Fuller A, Braine H. Effects of storage time on quantitative and qualitative platelet function after transfusion. *Anesthesiology* (1995) 83(6):1167–72. doi:10.1097/00000542-199512000-00006
62. Lieberman L, Bercovitz RS, Sholapur NS, Heddle NM, Stanworth SJ, Arnold DM. Platelet transfusions for critically ill patients with thrombocytopenia. *Blood* (2014) 123(8):1146–51; quiz 280. doi:10.1182/blood-2013-02-435693
63. Vlaar AP, Hofstra JJ, Kulik W, van Lenthe H, Nieuwland R, Schultz MJ, et al. Supernatant of stored platelets causes lung inflammation and coagulopathy in a novel in vivo transfusion model. *Blood* (2010) 116(8):1360–8. doi:10.1182/blood-2009-10-248732
64. Slichter SJ, Davis K, Enright H, Braine H, Gernsheimer T, Kao KJ, et al. Factors affecting posttransfusion platelet increments, platelet refractoriness,

and platelet transfusion intervals in thrombocytopenic patients. *Blood* (2005) 105(10):4106–14. doi:10.1182/blood-2003-08-2724

65. Heim D, Passweg J, Gregor M, Buser A, Theocharides A, Arber C, et al. Patient and product factors affecting platelet transfusion results. *Transfusion* (2008) 48(4):681–7. doi:10.1111/j.1537-2995.2007.01613.x
66. Triulzi DJ, Assmann SF, Strauss RG, Ness PM, Hess JR, Kaufman RM, et al. The impact of platelet transfusion characteristics on posttransfusion platelet increments and clinical bleeding in patients with hypoproliferative thrombocytopenia. *Blood* (2012) 119(23):5553–62. doi:10.1182/blood-2011-11-393165
67. MacLennan S, Harding K, Llewelyn C, Choo L, Bakrania L, Massey E, et al. A randomized noninferiority crossover trial of corrected count increments and bleeding in thrombocytopenic hematology patients receiving 2- to 5- versus 6- or 7-day-stored platelets. *Transfusion* (2015) 55(8):1856–65; quiz 5. doi:10.1111/trf.13038
68. Kreuger AL, Caram-Deelder C, Jacobse J, Kerkhoffs JL, van der Bom JG, Middelburg RA. Effect of storage time of platelet products on clinical outcomes after transfusion: a systematic review and meta-analyses. *Vox Sang* (2017) 112(4):291–300. doi:10.1111/vox.12494
69. Welsby IJ, Lockhart E, Phillips-Bute B, Campbell ML, Mathew JP, Newman MF, et al. Storage age of transfused platelets and outcomes after cardiac surgery. *Transfusion* (2010) 50(11):2311–7. doi:10.1111/j.1537-2995.2010.02747.x
70. Inaba K, Branco BC, Rhee P, Blackbourne LH, Holcomb JB, Spinella PC, et al. Impact of the duration of platelet storage in critically ill trauma patients. *J Trauma* (2011) 71(6):1766–73; discussion 73–4. doi:10.1097/TA.0b013e31823bdbf9
71. Juffermans NP, Vlaar AP, Prins DJ, Goslings JC, Binnekade JM. The age of red blood cells is associated with bacterial infections in critically ill trauma patients. *Blood Transfus* (2012) 10(3):290–5. doi:10.2450/2012.0068-11
72. Juffermans NP, Prins DJ, Vlaar AP, Nieuwland R, Binnekade JM. Transfusion-related risk of secondary bacterial infections in sepsis patients: a retrospective cohort study. *Shock* (2011) 35(4):355–9. doi:10.1097/SHK.0b013e3182086094
73. Flint A, Aubron C, Bailey M, Bellomo R, Pilcher D, Cheng AC, et al. Duration of platelet storage and outcomes of critically ill patients. *Transfusion* (2017) 57(3):599–605. doi:10.1111/trf.14056
74. Aubron C, Flint AW, Bailey M, Pilcher D, Cheng AC, Hegarty C, et al. Is platelet transfusion associated with hospital-acquired infections in critically ill patients? *Crit Care* (2017) 21(1):2. doi:10.1186/s13054-016-1593-x
75. Engele LJ, Straat M, van Rooijen IHM, de Vooght KMK, Cremer OL, Schultz MJ, et al. Transfusion of platelets, but not of red blood cells, is independently associated with nosocomial infections in the critically ill. *Ann Intensive Care* (2016) 6(1):67. doi:10.1186/s13613-016-0173-1
76. Frazier SK, Higgins J, Bugajski A, Jones AR, Brown MR. Adverse reactions to transfusion of blood products and best practices for prevention. *Crit Care Nurs Clin North Am* (2017) 29(3):271–90. doi:10.1016/j.cnc.2017.04.002
77. Greinacher A. Clinical practice. Heparin-induced thrombocytopenia. *N Engl J Med* (2015) 373(3):252–61. doi:10.1056/NEJMcp1411910
78. Krauel K, Potschke C, Weber C, Kessler W, Furll B, Ittermann T, et al. Platelet factor 4 binds to bacteria, [corrected] inducing antibodies cross-reacting with the major antigen in heparin-induced thrombocytopenia. *Blood* (2011) 117(4):1370–8. doi:10.1182/blood-2010-08-301424
79. Krauel K, Weber C, Brandt S, Zahringer U, Mamat U, Greinacher A, et al. Platelet factor 4 binding to lipid A of Gram-negative bacteria exposes PF4/heparin-like epitopes. *Blood* (2012) 120(16):3345–52. doi:10.1182/blood-2012-06-434985
80. Greinacher A, Selleng K, Warkentin TE. Autoimmune heparin-induced thrombocytopenia. *J Thromb Haemost* (2017) 15(11):2099–114. doi:10.1111/jth.13813
81. Nguyen TH, Medvedev N, Delcea M, Greinacher A. Anti-platelet factor 4/polyanion antibodies mediate a new mechanism of autoimmunity. *Nat Commun* (2017) 8:14945. doi:10.1038/ncomms14945
82. Oikonomopoulou K, Ricklin D, Ward PA, Lambris JD. Interactions between coagulation and complement – their role in inflammation. *Semin Immunopathol* (2012) 34(1):151–65. doi:10.1007/s00281-011-0280-x
83. Delcea M, Greinacher A. Biophysical tools to assess the interaction of PF4 with polyanions. *Thromb Haemost* (2016) 116(5):783–91. doi:10.1160/TH16-04-0258
84. Cai Z, Yarovoi SV, Zhu Z, Rauova L, Hayes V, Lebedeva T, et al. Atomic description of the immune complex involved in heparin-induced thrombocytopenia. *Nat Commun* (2015) 6:8277. doi:10.1038/ncomms9277
85. Greinacher A, Holtfreter B, Krauel K, Gatke D, Weber C, Ittermann T, et al. Association of natural anti-platelet factor 4/heparin antibodies with periodontal disease. *Blood* (2011) 118(5):1395–401. doi:10.1182/blood-2011-03-342857
86. Warkentin TE, Kelton JG. Temporal aspects of heparin-induced thrombocytopenia. *N Engl J Med* (2001) 344(17):1286–92. doi:10.1056/NEJM200104263441704
87. Warkentin TE, Makris M, Jay RM, Kelton JG. A spontaneous prothrombotic disorder resembling heparin-induced thrombocytopenia. *Am J Med* (2008) 121(7):632–6. doi:10.1016/j.amjmed.2008.03.012
88. Jay RM, Warkentin TE. Fatal heparin-induced thrombocytopenia (HIT) during warfarin thromboprophylaxis following orthopedic surgery: another example of 'spontaneous' HIT? *J Thromb Haemost* (2008) 6(9):1598–600. doi:10.1111/j.1538-7836.2008.03040.x
89. Pruthi RK, Daniels PR, Nambudiri GS, Warkentin TE. Heparin-induced thrombocytopenia (HIT) during postoperative warfarin thromboprophylaxis: a second example of postorthopedic surgery 'spontaneous' HIT. *J Thromb Haemost* (2009) 7(3):499–501. doi:10.1111/j.1538-7836.2008.03263.x
90. Warkentin TE, Basciano PA, Knopman J, Bernstein RA. Spontaneous heparin-induced thrombocytopenia syndrome: 2 new cases and a proposal for defining this disorder. *Blood* (2014) 123(23):3651–4. doi:10.1182/blood-2014-01-549741
91. Greinacher A. Me or not me? The danger of spontaneity. *Blood* (2014) 123(23):3536–8. doi:10.1182/blood-2014-04-566836
92. Perrin J, Barraud D, Toussaint-Hacquard M, Bollaert PE, Lecompte T. Rapid onset heparin-induced thrombocytopenia (HIT) without history of heparin exposure: a new case of so-called 'spontaneous' HIT. *Thromb Haemost* (2012) 107(4):795–7. doi:10.1160/TH11-12-0825
93. Okata T, Miyata S, Miyashita F, Maeda T, Toyoda K. Spontaneous heparin-induced thrombocytopenia syndrome without any proximate heparin exposure, infection, or inflammatory condition: atypical clinical features with heparin-dependent platelet activating antibodies. *Platelets* (2015) 26(6):602–7. doi:10.3109/09537104.2014.979338
94. Mallik A, Carlson KB, DeSancho MT. A patient with 'spontaneous' heparin-induced thrombocytopenia and thrombosis after undergoing knee replacement. *Blood Coagul Fibrinolysis* (2011) 22(1):73–5. doi:10.1097/MBC.0b013e328340ff11
95. Ketha S, Smithedajkul P, Vella A, Pruthi R, Wysokinski W, McBane R. Adrenal haemorrhage due to heparin-induced thrombocytopenia. *Thromb Haemost* (2013) 109(4):669–75. doi:10.1160/TH12-11-0865
96. Warkentin TE, Safyan EL, Linkins LA. Heparin-induced thrombocytopenia presenting as bilateral adrenal hemorrhages. *N Engl J Med* (2015) 372(5):492–4. doi:10.1056/NEJMc1414161
97. Brandt S, Krauel K, Jaax M, Renne T, Helm CA, Hammerschmidt S, et al. Polyphosphates form antigenic complexes with platelet factor 4 (PF4) and enhance PF4-binding to bacteria. *Thromb Haemost* (2015) 114(6):1189–98. doi:10.1160/TH15-01-0062
98. Antczak AJ, Vieth JA, Singh N, Worth RG. Internalization of IgG-coated targets results in activation and secretion of soluble CD40 ligand and RANTES by human platelets. *Clin Vaccine Immunol* (2011) 18(2):210–6. doi:10.1128/CVI.00296-10
99. Worth RG, Chien CD, Chien P, Reilly MP, McKenzie SE, Schreiber AD. Platelet FcgammaRIIA binds and internalizes IgG-containing complexes. *Exp Hematol* (2006) 34(11):1490–5. doi:10.1016/j.exphem.2006.06.015
100. Riaz AH, Tasma BE, Woodman ME, Wooten RM, Worth RG. Human platelets efficiently kill IgG-opsonized *E. coli*. *FEMS Immunol Med Microbiol* (2012) 65(1):78–83. doi:10.1111/j.1574-695X.2012.00945.x
101. Youssefian T, Drouin A, Masse JM, Guichard J, Cramer EM. Host defense role of platelets: engulfment of HIV and *Staphylococcus aureus* occurs in a specific subcellular compartment and is enhanced by platelet activation. *Blood* (2002) 99(11):4021–9. doi:10.1182/blood-2001-12-0191
102. White JG. Why human platelets fail to kill bacteria. *Platelets* (2006) 17(3):191–200. doi:10.1080/09537100500441234
103. White JG. Platelets are covercytes, not phagocytes: uptake of bacteria involves channels of the open canalicular system. *Platelets* (2005) 16(2):121–31. doi:10.1080/09537100400007390

104. Peters CG, Michelson AD, Flaumenhaft R. Granule exocytosis is required for platelet spreading: differential sorting of alpha-granules expressing VAMP-7. *Blood* (2012) 120(1):199–206. doi:10.1182/blood-2011-10-389247
105. Palankar R, Kohler TP, Krauel K, Wesche J, Hammerschmidt S, Greinacher A. Platelets kill bacteria by bridging innate and adaptive immunity via PF4 and FcgammaRIIA. *J Thromb Haemost* (2018). doi:10.1111/jth.13955
106. Basu R, Whitlock BM, Husson J, Le Floc'h A, Jin W, Oyler-Yaniv A, et al. Cytotoxic T cells use mechanical force to potentiate target cell killing. *Cell* (2016) 165(1):100–10. doi:10.1016/j.cell.2016.01.021
107. Assinger A. Platelets and infection – an emerging role of platelets in viral infection. *Front Immunol* (2014) 5:649. doi:10.3389/fimmu.2014.00649
108. Hamzeh-Cognasse H, Damien P, Chabert A, Pozzetto B, Cognasse F, Garraud O. Platelets and infections – complex interactions with bacteria. *Front Immunol* (2015) 6:82. doi:10.3389/fimmu.2015.00082
109. Speth C, Rambach G, Lass-Florl C. Platelet immunology in fungal infections. *Thromb Haemost* (2014) 112(4):632–9. doi:10.1160/TH14-01-0074
110. McMorran BJ, Wieczorski L, Drysdale KE, Chan JA, Huang HM, Smith C, et al. Platelet factor 4 and Duffy antigen required for platelet killing of *Plasmodium falciparum*. *Science* (2012) 338(6112):1348–51. doi:10.1126/science.1228892
111. Arman M, Krauel K, Tilley DO, Weber C, Cox D, Greinacher A, et al. Amplification of bacteria-induced platelet activation is triggered by FcgammaRIIA, integrin alphaIIbbeta3, and platelet factor 4. *Blood* (2014) 123(20):3166–74. doi:10.1182/blood-2013-11-540526
112. Moriarty RD, Cox A, McCall M, Smith SGJ, Cox D. *Escherichia coli* induces platelet aggregation in an FcγRIIa-dependent manner. *J Thromb Haemost* (2016) 14(4):797–806. doi:10.1111/jth.13226
113. Watson CN, Kerrigan SW, Cox D, Henderson IR, Watson SP, Arman M. Human platelet activation by *Escherichia coli*: roles for FcgammaRIIA and integrin alphaIIbbeta3. *Platelets* (2016) 27(6):535–40. doi:10.3109/09537104.2016.1148129
114. Kerrigan SW, Cox D. Platelet-bacterial interactions. *Cell Mol Life Sci* (2010) 67(4):513–23. doi:10.1007/s00018-009-0207-z
115. Tang YQ, Yeaman MR, Selsted ME. Antimicrobial peptides from human platelets. *Infect Immun* (2002) 70(12):6524–33. doi:10.1128/IAI.70.12.6524-6533.2002
116. Trier DA, Gank KD, Kupferwasser D, Yount NY, French WJ, Michelson AD, et al. Platelet antistaphylococcal responses occur through P2X1 and P2Y12 receptor-induced activation and kinocidin release. *Infect Immun* (2008) 76(12):5706–13. doi:10.1128/IAI.00935-08
117. Kraemer BF, Campbell RA, Schwertz H, Cody MJ, Franks Z, Tolley ND, et al. Novel anti-bacterial activities of beta-defensin 1 in human platelets: suppression of pathogen growth and signaling of neutrophil extracellular trap formation. *PLoS Pathog* (2011) 7(11):e1002355. doi:10.1371/journal.ppat.1002355
118. Dasararaju R, Marques MB. Adverse effects of transfusion. *Cancer Control* (2015) 22(1):16–25. doi:10.1177/107327481502200104
119. Sahu S, Hemlata, Verma A. Adverse events related to blood transfusion. *Indian J Anaesth* (2014) 58(5):543–51. doi:10.4103/0019-5049.144650
120. Stanworth SJ, Navarrete C, Estcourt L, Marsh J. Platelet refractoriness – practical approaches and ongoing dilemmas in patient management. *Br J Haematol* (2015) 171(3):297–305. doi:10.1111/bjh.13597
121. Lubenow N, Eichler P, Albrecht D, Carlsson LE, Kothmann J, Rossocha WR, et al. Very low platelet counts in post-transfusion purpura falsely diagnosed as heparin-induced thrombocytopenia. Report of four cases and review of literature. *Thromb Res* (2000) 100(3):115–25. doi:10.1016/S0049-3848(00)00311-X
122. Zeller M, Canadian Blood Services. Chapter18: platelet transfusion – alloimmunization and management of platelet refractorisness. *Clinical Guide to Transfusion*. (2016). Available from: https://professionaleducation.blood.ca/en/transfusion/clinical-guide/platelet-transfusion-alloimmunization-and-management-platelet.
123. Cid J, Carbasse G, Pereira A, Sanz C, Mazzara R, Escolar G, et al. Platelet transfusions from D+ donors to D- patients: a 10-year follow-up study of 1014 patients. *Transfusion* (2011) 51(6):1163–9. doi:10.1111/j.1537-2995.2010.02953.x
124. Chambost H. [Platelet transfusion and immunization anti-Rh1: implication for immunoprophylaxis]. *Transfus Clin Biol* (2014) 21(4–5):210–5. doi:10.1016/j.tracli.2014.08.137
125. Valsami S, Dimitroulis D, Gialeraki A, Chimonidou M, Politou M. Current trends in platelet transfusions practice: the role of ABO-RhD and human leukocyte antigen incompatibility. *Asian J Transfus Sci* (2015) 9(2):117–23. doi:10.4103/0973-6247.162684

Measuring Post-transfusion Recovery and Survival of Red Blood Cells: Strengths and Weaknesses of Chromium-51 Labeling and Alternative Methods

Camille Roussel[1,2,3,4,5], Pierre A. Buffet[1,2,3,5,6] and Pascal Amireault[1,2,3,4*]

[1] Biologie Intégrée du Globule Rouge UMR_S1134, INSERM, Univ. Paris Diderot, Sorbonne Paris Cité, Univ. de la Réunion, Univ. des Antilles, Paris, France, [2] Institut National de la Transfusion Sanguine, Paris, France, [3] Laboratoire d'Excellence GR-Ex, Paris, France, [4] Laboratory of Cellular and Molecular Mechanisms of Hematological Disorders and Therapeutic Implications U1163/CNRS ERL 8254, INSERM, CNRS, Univ Paris Descartes, Sorbonne Paris Cité, Paris, France, [5] Université Paris Descartes, Paris, France, [6] Assistance publique des hôpitaux de Paris, Paris, France

***Correspondence:**
Pascal Amireault
pamireault@ints.fr

The proportion of transfused red blood cells (RBCs) that remain in circulation is an important surrogate marker of transfusion efficacy and contributes to predict the potential benefit of a transfusion process. Over the last 50 years, most of the transfusion recovery data were generated by chromium-51 (^{51}Cr)-labeling studies and were predominantly performed to validate new storage systems and new processes to prepare RBC concentrates. As a consequence, our understanding of transfusion efficacy is strongly dependent on the strengths and weaknesses of ^{51}Cr labeling in particular. Other methods such as antigen mismatch or biotin-based labeling can bring relevant information, for example, on the long-term survival of transfused RBC. These radioactivity-free methods can be used in patients including from vulnerable groups. We provide an overview of the methods used to measure transfusion recovery in humans, compare their strengths and weaknesses, and discuss their potential limitations. Also, based on our understanding of the spleen-specific filtration of damaged RBC and historical transfusion recovery data, we propose that RBC deformability and morphology are storage lesion markers that could become useful predictors of transfusion recovery. Transfusion recovery can and should be accurately explored by more than one method. Technical optimization and clarification of concepts is still needed in this important field of transfusion and physiology.

Keywords: transfusion recovery, red blood cell, spleen, red blood cell morphology, red blood cell deformability, storage lesion

INTRODUCTION

Each year, more than 85 million red blood cells (RBCs) units are transfused worldwide. This demanding human and organizational task is conducted by national or local organizations. Collection, transformation, storage (for a maximum of 35–49 days), and distribution of blood products are tightly quality controlled, most commonly at the national level. In industrialized countries, most of the transfused RBCs are stored as red cell concentrates (RCC), from which plasma, platelets, and leukocytes have been almost entirely removed, usually using centrifugation and/or leukoreduction filters.

The objective of an RCC transfusion is to increase the oxygenation capacity of the recipient by increasing the number of functional RBC in circulation. Improvement in tissue oxygenation following transfusion is arguably the most relevant marker of transfusion efficacy but measuring it is technically and logistically challenging in patients and impossible in healthy volunteers in whom tissue oxygenation is not altered. Measuring the proportion of RBCs that remain in circulation after transfusion thus appears as a suitable surrogate marker to evaluate the efficacy of a transfusion. That a reasonable proportion of transfused RBC stays in circulation for long enough to operate the expected correction is indeed a prerequisite for transfusion efficacy.

Early studies have identified that, after storage, a variable proportion of transfused RBC is removed from the circulation in the first 24 h following transfusion (1). Then, the remaining transfused RBCs have a normal survival. Although the long-term survival of RBC is an important parameter to evaluate transfusion efficacy, most studies have focused on the measure of the 24 h transfusion recovery.

Several techniques have been developed and used in the last 100 years to measure transfusion recovery. Transfusion recovery using chromium-51 (^{51}Cr) labeling is now a regulation criterion to license new storage systems or RCC preparation processes by the Food and Drug Administration (FDA). The FDA threshold to approve a preparation and storage process of RBC is a maximum 1% *in vitro* hemolysis and a 24 h *in vivo* recovery of at least 75% after reinfusion of autologous ^{51}Cr-labeled RBC in healthy volunteers, at the limit of storage (2). The ^{51}Cr-labeling technique was first used in the early 1950s and became the gold standard in the 1970s when the International Committee for Standardization in Hematology (3) proposed it as the reference technique. The use of a standardized protocol is essential to compare studies distant in space or time. Over the last 50 years, most of the transfusion recovery data were generated by ^{51}Cr-labeling studies, mostly to validate new storage systems and RCC preparation processes. As a consequence, our understanding of transfusion efficacy strongly depends on the strengths and weaknesses of ^{51}Cr labeling. However, other methods have been developed and validated, the advantages and limitations of which deserve careful analysis.

We will provide a brief overview of the methods used to measure transfusion recovery in humans. We will compare their strengths and weaknesses and critically analyze their potential limitations. Also, based on our understanding of the spleen-specific filtration of damaged RBC, we will discuss the relevance of storage lesion markers to predict transfusion recovery. We will finally discuss the current state of knowledge in the RBC transfusion field and propose future directions. Animal studies published in the recent years on this topic are beyond the scope of this analysis.

METHODS USED FOR TRANSFUSION RECOVERY STUDIES

Differential Agglutination (DA)

Differential agglutination was the first method used to measure transfusion recovery of a complete RCC (1, 4). In the 24 h post-transfusion blood sample, RBCs from the donor or the recipient are agglutinated with an appropriate antiserum, and the remaining RBCs are counted (5, 6). Similarly, an automated DA technique was developed where agglutinates are removed automatically and the remaining hemoglobin is quantified colorimetrically (7–13). The "100%" initial point is calculated from the prediction of the recipient's normal blood volume (using its height and weight). Alternatively, the initial point can be obtained from an estimation of the recipient's red cell volume using radioactive labeling of "fresh" RBC.

Radioactive Labeling Methods With ^{51}Cr and Other Isotopes

Here, 15–30 ml of RBCs from a donor is labeled with ^{51}Cr (14) and injected to the recipient (most of the time the donor himself) (15–31). RBC recovery is quantified after transfusion by taking a blood sample at early time points (5, 7.5, 10, 12.5, and 15 min) and 24 h after injection. In each sample, a radioactivity count number is acquired, and the initial point is extrapolated by linear regression. Alternatively, transfusion recovery can be evaluated using the technetium-99 (^{99m}Tc)/^{51}Cr double-labeling technique (32–43). In this method, the recipient's RBC volume is first evaluated using a known amount of "fresh" RBC labeled with ^{99m}Tc (^{32}P and ^{52}Cr were also used in older studies) (44–46), which is then used to calculate transfusion recovery. Similarly, ^{51}Cr labeling can be associated with ^{125}I-labeled albumin to evaluate the recipient's plasma volume, which is then used in the calculation of transfusion recovery (35, 46–48). A reduced transfusion recovery was observed in some studies (34, 46, 48) that compared the double labeling with the single-labeling method. This is probably due to an undervaluation of the very short-term component of survival when using the single-label method (since some RBCs are rapidly removed from the circulation in the very first minutes following injection) and suggests that the double-label method is worth the extra complexity.

Biotinylation

Red blood cells from a donor (5–30 ml) are labeled with biotin and injected to the recipient. RBC recovery is usually quantified after transfusion by taking a blood sample at an early time point (10 min) and 24 h after injection (49, 50). Fluorescent labeling of biotinylated RBC and flow cytometry detection quantify the proportion of transfused RBC. By labeling RBC with different densities of biotin, it is possible to evaluate the recovery of up to three RBC populations in the same recipient. Care must be taken to avoid too high concentrations of biotin since it has been correlated with increase of transfused RBC clearance and anti-biotin antibodies in the recipient (51). A GMP grade biotin is now available and could be used in countries where radioactive labeling procedures are not authorized (52). This method theoretically allows the determination of transfused RBC characteristics.

Minor Antigen Mismatch

In the minor antigen mismatch method, an antibody directed against a minor antigen (e.g., Fy), which differs between the donor and the recipient, is used to determine, by flow cytometry, the proportion of transfused RBC in the 24 h post-transfusion sample (53, 54). No manipulation of the transfused RBC is necessary, and recovery is evaluated after the transfusion of a complete RCC, but the measure is dependent on the prediction of the recipient blood volume (from its height and weight). Theoretically, the characteristics of transfused RBC can be observed after transfusion.

Increase in Blood Counts

A simple method to evaluate transfusion recovery is to measure the increase in blood count (hemoglobin level or hematocrit) between a pretransfusion sample and post-transfusion samples (55–58). Limitations from such a method include the limited accuracy of the blood count measure and the unknown recipient's blood volume (and its variable response to transfusion) that both contribute to the inaccuracy of the measure.

LIMITATIONS OF EXISTING RECOVERY STUDIES

Strengths and weaknesses of the different methods are summarized in **Table 1**. One of the potential bias of the chromium or biotinylation techniques stems from the labeling protocol necessary to perform these studies. In the normal transfusion setup, RBCs are transfused to the recipient directly from the bag while in these two methods, RBCs are manipulated, centrifuged, and incubated in PBS or saline solution. It is conceivable that these steps modify labeled RBC in a way that affects their ability to stay in circulation, although a recent study showed that some RBC properties are only slightly modified by the biotinylation protocol (59). The situation is different with DA and minor antigen mismatch, as these techniques do not require any RBC manipulation before transfusion, thereby eliminating this potential source of artifact.

Another potential limitation of the accuracy of the ^{51}Cr or biotinylation techniques is the infusion of a relatively small volume (5–30 ml) of RBC rather than a complete RCC. Transfusion recovery may indeed be influenced by the volume of transfused RBC. To explore this possibility and mimic more closely a complete RCC transfusion, ^{51}Cr-labeled or biotinylated RBC could be co-transfused with the rest of the RCC. One study (60) reported a lower transfusion recovery of an entire unit (using automated DA) when compared with a 10–30 ml transfusion volume (using ^{51}Cr labeling). However, it is not possible to ascertain that the "volume of transfusion" was responsible for this difference since other potential factors related to the method used to quantify transfusion recovery method (automated DA vs ^{51}Cr) may have impacted the observation. The exact clearance mechanism(s) of potentially damaged RBC stored for many weeks are not well known. To what extent transfusion recovery data using a small amount of RBC accurately predict the outcome of a complete—or massive—RCC transfusion remains therefore an open question.

To reduce the risk of adverse events including transmission of infectious diseases, most of the transfusion recovery studies are conducted using autologous transfusion of stored RBC to healthy volunteers. In this setup, conditions of transfusion are probably appropriate to evaluate storage and donor effects. However, they do not take into consideration the possible complex interaction between damaged-stored RBC and potential recipient specificities related to its physiopathological condition. Along this line, it has been shown that survival of transfused RBC is abnormally low in some thalassemia patients with splenomegaly (61). Normal survival was restored following splenectomy suggesting that the spleen is where most RBCs that were no longer present in the circulation 24 h after transfusion had been retained. This is an example of how the medical condition of the recipient can impact transfusion recovery.

STORAGE LESION, TRANSFUSION RECOVERY, AND SPLEEN FILTRATION

Storage Lesion and Transfusion Recovery

Recently, a number of prospective clinical studies have been conducted to evaluate the potential benefit of transfusing RCC stored for a short period (61–66). These studies have shown that transfusion of RCC stored for a short period does not reduce in-hospital morbidity or mortality in adult and children transfused for acute anemia. The "standard of care" collection and storage processes thus appear to be currently adequate when (accurately) assessed on clinical endpoints. However, these complex prospective clinical studies assessing predominantly safety may be difficult to conduct in some cohorts, such as chronically transfused patients, where the long-term impact of transfusions may be even more relevant. In addition, clinical studies of safety did not specifically examine the effect of transfusing RCC stored for a long period (more than 35 days) and did not directly address the efficacy of the procedure. This evaluation could be important in light of the well-documented RBC alterations that accumulate during hypothermic storage (67). The clinical relevance of this storage "lesion" to predict the efficacy and safety of the transfusion for the recipient is still a matter of controversy but suggests that RBC quality does not remain stable during storage.

It has been assumed that the decrease in transfusion recovery related to storage is due to RBC damages that accumulate after several weeks of storage. Studies performed more than 50 years ago have shown indeed that the extent of the storage lesion increases with storage duration while transfusion recovery decreases accordingly (5, 8, 10, 45). Few studies have directly explored the correlation between *in vitro* markers of storage lesion and *in vivo* recovery. In these studies, three markers (intracellular ATP, deformability, and morphology) have been shown to correlate with transfusion recovery (**Box 1**). The proportion of RBC removed from circulation (calculated from transfusion recovery) could correspond to the proportion of RBC, damaged during the storage process, which are over a recipient "clearance threshold." If this assumption is correct, an optimal marker of storage lesion should identify and quantify the subpopulation of RBC that undergoes early premature clearance.

The spleen has a specific filtering function that operates the clearance of damaged or senescent RBC from the circulation. Knowledge on the spleen filtration process is therefore relevant to understand transfusion recovery.

TABLE 1 | Strengths and weaknesses of the different methods to measure transfusion recovery.

Method	Principle	Strengths	Weaknesses
Differential agglutination (DA)	Red blood cells (RBCs) from the donor or recipient are agglutinated, and the remaining RBCs are counted	• Transfusion recovery of a normal transfusion volume can be determined • One or more RBC populations can be quantified in parallel • The persistence of transfused RBC in circulation may be followed for several weeks • The method can be used in patients, in infants, pregnant women, and any vulnerable group • RBCs from the donor or the recipient are not manipulated before transfusion	• Quantification is inaccurate when/if agglutination is incomplete • Only allogeneic RBC transfusion can be studied with this method • The method is dependent on the prediction of the recipient's blood volume (from its height and weight) or the calculation of the recipient RBC volume using radioactivity
Automated DA	RBCs from the donor or recipient are agglutinated and the remaining hemoglobin is quantified	• Variability is reduced when an automated procedure is used	
Chromium-51 (^{51}Cr)	Donor RBCs are labeled with ^{51}Cr and then injected to the recipient Recovery is quantified in serial samples	• This is a reference Food and Drug Administration-approved method to test new devices/procedures for transfusion/storage • The procedure is standardized which allows comparison between different studies • Autologous RBC transfusion can be studied with this method	• Only relatively small volumes (15–30 ml) of labeled RBC can be transfused • Elution of ^{51}Cr from RBC limits the evaluation of long-term persistence in circulation (less than 30 days) • There are regulatory, logistical, and technical constraints related to the use of radioactivity • Protected populations cannot be studied because recipients are exposed to radioactivity • RBCs from the donor are manipulated before transfusion
Technetium-99 (^{99m}Tc) /^{51}Cr	Blood volume in the recipient is first evaluated using a known amount of tracer "fresh" RBC labeled with ^{99m}Tc	• Quantification is expected to be more robust because recipient's RBC volume is measured with ^{99m}Tc-labeled RBC	
Biotin	One or more donor RBC populations are labeled with different concentrations of biotin then quantified in serial samples by flow cytometry	• The persistence of transfused RBC in circulation may be followed for several weeks • Up to 3 RBC populations can be quantified in parallel • Autologous RBC transfusion can be studied with this method • The method can be used in patients, in infants, pregnant women, and any vulnerable group • The characteristics of transfused RBC can be observed after transfusion	• Only relatively small volumes (15–30 ml) of labeled RBC can be transfused • The recipient is at risk of developing anti-biotin antibodies • RBCs from the donor are manipulated before transfusion
Antigen mismatch	Following transfusion of compatible RBC, minor antigen differences (e.g., Fy) are used to quantify RBC from the donor by flow cytometry	• Transfusion recovery of a normal transfusion volume can be determined • The persistence of transfused RBC in circulation may be followed for several weeks • One or more RBC populations can be quantified in parallel • The characteristics of transfused RBC can be observed after transfusion • The method can be used in patients, in infants, pregnant women, and any vulnerable group • RBCs from the donor or the recipient are not manipulated before transfusion	• Only compatible transfusions with at least 1 minor antigen difference can be studied with this method • The method is dependent on the prediction of the recipient's blood volume (from its height and weight)
Increase in blood counts	Blood hemoglobin levels (or hematocrit) are measured before and after transfusion	• Transfusion recovery of a normal transfusion volume can be determined • The method can be used in patients, in infants, pregnant women, and any vulnerable group • RBCs from the donor or the recipient are not manipulated before transfusion	• The quantification is inaccurate when the blood volume of the recipient is abnormal • Processes or interventions other than transfusion can impact on hemoglobin blood level (or hematocrit)

Spleen Filtration Capacity

In the splenic circulation, RBCs engage into two parallel pathways, the fast or slow microcirculations (71). In the fast and "closed" microcirculation, RBCs remain in endothelialized pathways and transit from arterioles to the venous sinus lumen through pathways in the perifollicular zone (72). In the slow and "open" microcirculation, RBCs navigate in tortuous microcirculatory beds of the red pulp, devoid of endothelium, before returning to the venous circulation by squeezing through 1- to 2-µm-wide slits between endothelial cells in the wall of sinuses (71, 73). Macrophages account for approximately half the volume of the cords, and their abundance facilitates direct RBC–macrophage interactions (71). The spleen likely contributes through one or more of these mechanisms to the clearance of transfused RBC.

BOX 1 | Connecting storage lesion with transfusion recovery.

Intracellular ATP

An inverse correlation between the intracellular content in ATP in the RCC and transfusion recovery has been reported in a number of studies (1, 7, 9, 44). ATP content declines during long-term hypothermic incubation in a non-physiological solution. This is probably at the root of most RBC alterations that accumulate during storage. Intracellular ATP quantification remains, however, difficult to standardize and allows evaluation of the RCC quality at a cell population rather than a single-cell level.

Morphology

At least two studies using the ^{51}Cr technique have shown that morphological modifications of RBC in a RCC do correlate with transfusion recovery. In the first study, the proportion of RBC with a discoid shape was positively correlated with transfusion recovery (16), while in the second, the morphology index after rejuvenation correlated with recovery (20). An evaluation of RBC morphology thus seems a good potential predictor of transfusion recovery provided that individual RBC shape can be categorized reliably. However, morphology analyses are low-throughput and operator-dependent making them difficult to standardize and implement. New technologies such as imaging flow cytometry may help circumvent this problem. We have recently identified a subpopulation of small spherocytic RBC that appears and expands during storage with wide variations between donors (68). This spherocytic shift could be a relevant marker as it readily identifies a subpopulation of RBC expected to be cleared rapidly after transfusion. However, direct evidence is lacking that small spherocytic RBC are prematurely cleared following transfusion, hence account for all or part of a suboptimal recovery.

Deformability

A recent study in patients with thalassemia showed that the increase in hemoglobin following transfusion was inversely correlated to the proportion of "less deformable" RBC in the RCC (57). In this study, a cell flow analyzer (69) was used to measure the elongation index of individual RBC that adheres to a polystyrene slide. Deformability can also be evaluated by measuring an RBC elongation index using ektacytometry (70). Both technologies have shown a decrease in RBC deformability during storage but the cell flow analyzer, although not commercially available has the advantage of measuring individual RBC elongation. In principle, the automated rheoscope and cell analyzer would provide interesting individual cell data on the evolution of RBC during storage.

Intensity and kinetics of this clearance depend on the proportion of altered RBC in an RCC and on the intensity of the alterations. In physiologic conditions, the spleen can process at least 20 ml of RBC per day. It is conceivable that its filtration capacity might be overwhelmed by the amount of damaged RBC transfused, potentially leaving in circulation RBC that should normally be removed.

Spleen Filtration Threshold

The spleen-specific filtration process can trigger the clearance of senescent or altered RBC based on the sensing of surface modifications, mechanical alterations, or a combination of both. Inter-endothelial slits in the spleen exert a stringent challenge on RBC and retain least deformable ones (74, 75). Macrophages sense the shape and altered deformability of RBC and phagocytize them (76). In hereditary spherocytosis, morphology and deformability of RBC are linked (77), surface area-to-volume ratio being the main major determinant of RBC ability to cross narrow inter-endothelial slits in the spleen (74, 78). *Ex vivo* experiments with human spleens have confirmed the correlation between RBC retention in the spleen and the loss in projected surface area (79). Retention was almost complete when more than 17.5% of surface area had been lost. There is therefore a "splenic clearance threshold" that senses biomechanical and morphological changes of RBC which has also been determined by modeling *in silico* (75). Deformability and morphology of transfused RBC are expected to be very important determinants of transfusion recovery.

CONCLUSION

Recovery of autologous RBC in healthy non-anemic recipients using ^{51}Cr labeling, 24 h after transfusion, is the method usually performed to determine the validity of the RCC preparation/storage processes. When examining transfusion recovery studies, we identified three parameters, namely transfusion volume, labeling protocol and the recipient pathophysiological state that have been under-evaluated and may impact the determination of transfusion recovery. For example, monocytes and macrophages, that possess a limited clearance capacity (80), could be saturated and leave in circulation damaged RBC when a large volume of RBC is transfused. Such an assumption is supported by data showing that transfusion of more than five RCC leads to a decreased deformability of circulating RBC (81). In the case of the labeling protocol, it has been shown that RBC stored for a long period are "primed" and more sensitive to an incubation in medium at 37°C (82) and may react differently when incubated in non-physiological solutions used in certain labeling protocol. Also, the observation that transfusion recovery is reduced in recipients with a splenomegaly (4, 61, 83) strongly suggests that individual characteristics or a pathological condition in the recipient impacts the recovery and survival of transfused RBC, even in absence of alloantibodies. These technical differences between transfusion recovery studies in healthy volunteers and transfusion of an anemic patient in a medical context suggest that available transfusion recovery data may not reflect transfusion efficacy in anemic recipients in some physiopathological conditions. A better understanding of RBC clearance mechanisms is warranted and could be explored by conducting transfusion recovery studies. In doing so, an appropriate experimental design, considering the strengths, weaknesses of the available methods, should be selected. As such, antigen mismatch method appears to offer a number of theoretical advantages over the other methods but would ideally be coupled with a non-radioactive labeling method to evaluate the RBC volume in the recipient.

That some storage lesion markers correlate with transfusion recovery reinforces the potential relevance of these *in vitro* studies which may deliver clinically relevant information. However, in the current conditions of blood collection and processing, this correlation between transfusion recovery and storage lesion remains poorly explored. Identification of a marker that could predict transfusion recovery would be a valuable tool for transfusion medicine and help to bridge the gap between storage lesion and the morbi-mortality studies. Future studies that evaluate transfusion recovery should be designed to include selected storage lesion markers to verify potential correlations. Deformability and morphology, preferably at the individual RBC level, appear as key potential markers since both spleen physiology and historical transfusion recovery data identify them as potentially predictive of transfusion recovery.

In vitro studies have shown that marked RBC alterations appear and worsen during storage, but a paradox remains since clinical studies have not found correlations between using RCC stored for a short time (generally less than 7–10 days) and improved clinical outcome. This apparent discrepancy is a source of interrogation in the transfusion community. Clinical studies were appropriately designed to guide transfusion policy. The current conclusion is that there would be no benefit at keeping "fresh blood" for specific situations. The impact of studying storage "lesion" has been questioned as well as the medical relevance of cellular alterations that do not translate into any negative outcome. Is storage "lesion" merely a misnomer, to be replaced advantageously by storage "changes"? This is not so sure yet. Many have argued that clinical studies did not assess the effect of transfusing RCC stored for more than 28 days, while storage lesion studies indicate that the extent of damage rapidly increases after 4 weeks of storage (84). Furthermore, clinical studies were not designed to assess transfusion efficacy and particularly the influence of storage duration on transfusion recovery. On the other hand, *in vitro* studies of the storage lesion are not often correlated with *in vivo* recovery. *In vitro* studies of the storage lesion and clinical studies deliver complementary information while addressing different questions. Studies that explore both dimensions of knowledge are difficult to implement since their designs differ. Large safety studies collect simple data from many patients while transfusion recovery collects complex repetitive samples, which are analyzed using relatively sophisticated methods. The way forward is probably to set-up ancillary recovery studies in the context of large safety trials.

AUTHOR CONTRIBUTIONS

All the authors listed have made a contribution to the work and approved it for publication.

REFERENCES

1. Ashby W. The determination of the length of life of transfused blood corpuscles in man. *J Exp Med* (1919) 29(3):267–81. doi:10.1084/jem.29.3.267
2. Hess JR. Biomedical Excellence for Safer Transfusion (BEST) Collaborative. Scientific problems in the regulation of red blood cell products. *Transfusion* (2012) 52(8):1827–35. doi:10.1111/j.1537-2995.2011.03511.x
3. Recommended methods for radioisotope red cell survival studies. *Blood* (1971) 38(3):378–86.
4. Klein HG, Anstee DJ. *Mollison's Blood Transfusion in Clinical Medicine.* 11th ed. Chichester: Wiley-Blackwell (2008). 912 p.
5. Mollison PL, Young IM. Failure of in vitro tests as a guide to the value of stored blood. *Br Med J* (1941) 2(4222):797–800. doi:10.1136/bmj.2.4222.797
6. Mollison PL, Sloviter HA, Chaplin H. Survival of transfused red cells previously stored for long periods in the frozen state. *Lancet* (1952) 2(6733):501–5. doi:10.1016/S0140-6736(52)90290-0
7. Szymanski IO, Valeri CR, McCallum LE, Emerson CP, Rosenfield RE. Automated differential agglutination technic to measure red cell survival. I. Methodology. *Transfusion* (1968) 8(2):65–73. doi:10.1111/j.1537-2995.1968.tb02397.x
8. Szymanski IO, Valeri CR. Automated differential agglutination technic to measure red cell survival. II. Survival in vivo of preserved red cells. *Transfusion* (1968) 8(2):74–83. doi:10.1111/j.1537-2995.1968.tb02398.x
9. Valeri CR, Landrock RD, Pivacek LE, Gray AD, Fink JG, Szymanski IO. Quantitative differential agglutination method using the Coulter Counter to measure survival of compatible but identifiable red blood cells. *Vox Sang* (1985) 49(3):195–205. doi:10.1111/j.1423-0410.1985.tb00793.x
10. Szymanski IO, Dean HM, Valeri CR, Bougas JA, Desforges JF. Measurement of erythrocyte survival during open-heart surgery. *Transfusion* (1970) 10(4):163–70. doi:10.1111/j.1537-2995.1970.tb00726.x
11. Szymanski IO, Valeri CR. Lifespan of preserved red cells. *Vox Sang* (1971) 21(2):97–108. doi:10.1111/j.1423-0410.1971.tb00566.x
12. Szymanski IO, Valeri CR. Evaluation of double 51Cr technique. *Vox Sang* (1968) 15(4):287–92. doi:10.1159/000467074
13. Valeri CR. Factors influencing the 24-hour posttransfusion survival and the oxygen transport function of previously frozen red cells preserved with 40 per cent W-V glycerol and frozen at -80°C. *Transfusion* (1974) 14(1):1–15. doi:10.1111/j.1537-2995.1974.tb04478.x
14. Moroff G, Sohmer PR, Button LN. Proposed standardization of methods for determining the 24-hour survival of stored red cells. *Transfusion* (1984) 24(2):109–14. doi:10.1046/j.1537-2995.1984.24284173339.x
15. Deverdier CH, Garby L, Hjelm M, Hoegman C. Adenine in blood preservation: posttransfusion viability and biochemical changes. *Transfusion* (1964) 4:331–8. doi:10.1111/j.1537-2995.1964.tb02883.x
16. Haradin AR, Weed RI, Reed CF. Changes in physical properties of stored erythrocytes relationship to survival in vivo. *Transfusion* (1969) 9(5):229–37. doi:10.1111/j.1537-2995.1969.tb04929.x
17. Herve P, Lamy B, Peters A, Toubin M, Bidet AC. Preservation of human erythrocytes in the liquid state: biological results with a new medium. *Vox Sang* (1980) 39(4):195–204. doi:10.1111/j.1423-0410.1980.tb01857.x
18. Beutler E, Kuhl W, West C. The osmotic fragility of erythrocytes after prolonged liquid storage and after reinfusion. *Blood* (1982) 59(6):1141–7.
19. Högman CF, Hedlund K. Storage of red cells in a CPD/SAGM system using Teruflex PVC. *Vox Sang* (1985) 49(3):177–80. doi:10.1111/j.1423-0410.1985.tb00790.x
20. Högman CF, de Verdier CH, Ericson A, Hedlund K, Sandhagen B. Studies on the mechanism of human red cell loss of viability during storage at +4 degrees C in vitro. I. Cell shape and total adenylate concentration as determinant factors for posttransfusion survival. *Vox Sang* (1985) 48(5):257–68. doi:10.1111/j.1423-0410.1985.tb00181.x
21. AuBuchon JP, Estep TN, Davey RJ. The effect of the plasticizer di-2-ethylhexyl phthalate on the survival of stored RBCs. *Blood* (1988) 71(2):448–52.
22. Davey RJ, Carmen RA, Simon TL, Nelson EJ, Leng BS, Chong C, et al. Preparation of white cell-depleted red cells for 42-day storage using an integral in-line filter. *Transfusion* (1989) 29(6):496–9. doi:10.1046/j.1537-2995.1989.29689318446.x
23. Moore GL, Hess JR, Ledford ME. In vivo viability studies of two additive solutions in the postthaw preservation of red cells held for 3 weeks at 4 degrees C. *Transfusion* (1993) 33(9):709–12. doi:10.1046/j.1537-2995.1993.33994025017.x
24. Greenwalt TJ, Dumaswala UJ, Rugg N. Studies in red blood cell preservation 10. 51Cr recovery of red cells after liquid storage in a glycerol-containing additive solution. *Vox Sang* (1996) 70(1):6–10. doi:10.1111/j.1423-0410.1996.tb00988.x
25. Hess JR, Rugg N, Knapp AD, Gormas JF, Silberstein EB, Greenwalt TJ. Successful storage of RBCs for 9 weeks in a new additive solution. *Transfusion* (2000) 40(8):1007–11. doi:10.1046/j.1537-2995.2000.40081007.x

26. Hess JR, Rugg N, Gormas JK, Knapp AD, Hill HR, Oliver CK, et al. RBC storage for 11 weeks. *Transfusion* (2001) 41(12):1586–90. doi:10.1046/j.1537-2995.2001.41121586.x
27. Valeri CR, Ragno G, Pivacek L, O'Neill EM. In vivo survival of apheresis RBCs, frozen with 40-percent (wt/vol) glycerol, deglycerolized in the ACP 215, and stored at 4 degrees C in AS-3 for up to 21 days. *Transfusion* (2001) 41(7):928–32. doi:10.1046/j.1537-2995.2001.41070928.x
28. Hess JR, Rugg N, Joines AD, Gormas JF, Pratt PG, Silberstein EB, et al. Buffering and dilution in red blood cell storage. *Transfusion* (2006) 46(1):50–4. doi:10.1111/j.1537-2995.2005.00672.x
29. Dumont LJ, AuBuchon JP. Evaluation of proposed FDA criteria for the evaluation of radiolabeled red cell recovery trials. *Transfusion* (2008) 48(6):1053–60. doi:10.1111/j.1537-2995.2008.01642.x
30. Cancelas JA, Dumont LJ, Maes LA, Rugg N, Herschel L, Whitley PH, et al. Additive solution-7 reduces the red blood cell cold storage lesion. *Transfusion* (2015) 55(3):491–8. doi:10.1111/trf.12867
31. Rapido F, Brittenham GM, Bandyopadhyay S, La Carpia F, L'Acqua C, McMahon DJ, et al. Prolonged red cell storage before transfusion increases extravascular hemolysis. *J Clin Invest* (2017) 127(1):375–82. doi:10.1172/JCI90837
32. Mishler JM, Darley JH, Haworth C, Mollison PL. Viability of red cells stored in diminished concentration of citrate. *Br J Haematol* (1979) 43(1):63–7. doi:10.1111/j.1365-2141.1979.tb03720.x
33. Card RT, Mohandas N, Mollison PL. Relationship of post-transfusion viability to deformability of stored red cells. *Br J Haematol* (1983) 53(2):237–40. doi:10.1111/j.1365-2141.1983.tb02016.x
34. Heaton WA, Keegan T, Holme S, Momoda G. Evaluation of 99mtechnetium/51chromium post-transfusion recovery of red cells stored in saline, adenine, glucose, mannitol for 42 days. *Vox Sang* (1989) 57(1):37–42. doi:10.1159/000460998
35. Moroff G, Holme S, Heaton WA, Kevy S, Jacobson M, Popovsky M. Effect of an 8-hour holding period on in vivo and in vitro properties of red cells and factor VIII content of plasma after collection in a red cell additive system. *Transfusion* (1990) 30(9):828–32. doi:10.1046/j.1537-2995.1990.30991048790.x
36. Heaton WA, Holme S, Smith K, Brecher ME, Pineda A, AuBuchon JP, et al. Effects of 3–5 log10 pre-storage leucocyte depletion on red cell storage and metabolism. *Br J Haematol* (1994) 87(2):363–8. doi:10.1111/j.1365-2141.1994.tb04923.x
37. Reid TJ, Babcock JG, Derse-Anthony CP, Hill HR, Lippert LE, Hess JR. The viability of autologous human red cells stored in additive solution 5 and exposed to 25 degrees C for 24 hours. *Transfusion* (1999) 39(9):991–7. doi:10.1046/j.1537-2995.1999.39090991.x
38. Hess JR, Rugg N, Knapp AD, Gormas JF, Silberstein EB, Greenwalt TJ. Successful storage of RBCs for 10 weeks in a new additive solution. *Transfusion* (2000) 40(8):1012–6. doi:10.1046/j.1537-2995.2000.40081012.x
39. Hess JR, Hill HR, Oliver CK, Lippert LE, Rugg N, Joines AD, et al. Twelve-week RBC storage. *Transfusion* (2003) 43(7):867–72. doi:10.1046/j.1537-2995.2003.00442.x
40. Yoshida T, AuBuchon JP, Tryzelaar L, Foster KY, Bitensky MW. Extended storage of red blood cells under anaerobic conditions. *Vox Sang* (2007) 92(1):22–31. doi:10.1111/j.1423-0410.2006.00860.x
41. Yoshida T, AuBuchon JP, Dumont LJ, Gorham JD, Gifford SC, Foster KY, et al. The effects of additive solution pH and metabolic rejuvenation on anaerobic storage of red cells. *Transfusion* (2008) 48(10):2096–105. doi:10.1111/j.1537-2995.2008.01812.x
42. Cancelas JA, Slichter SJ, Rugg N, Pratt PG, Nestheide S, Corson J, et al. Red blood cells derived from whole blood treated with riboflavin and ultraviolet light maintain adequate survival in vivo after 21 days of storage. *Transfusion* (2017) 57(5):1218–25. doi:10.1111/trf.14084
43. Cancelas JA, Gottschall JL, Rugg N, Graminske S, Schott MA, North A, et al. Red blood cell concentrates treated with the amustaline (S-303) pathogen reduction system and stored for 35 days retain post-transfusion viability: results of a two-centre study. *Vox Sang* (2017) 112(3):210–8. doi:10.1111/vox.12500
44. Gabrio BW, Donohue DM, Finch CA. Erythrocyte preservation. V. Relationship between chemical changes and viability of stored blood treated with adenosine. *J Clin Invest* (1955) 34(10):1509–12. doi:10.1172/JCI103202
45. Shields CE. Effect of adenine on stored erythrocytes evaluated by autologous and homologous transfusions. *Transfusion* (1969) 9(3):115–9. doi:10.1111/j.1537-2995.1969.tb05528.x
46. Heaton WA, Keegan T, Hanbury CM, Holme S, Pleban P. Studies with nonradioisotopic sodium chromate. II. Single- and double-label 52Cr/51Cr posttransfusion recovery estimations. *Transfusion* (1989) 29(8):703–7. doi:10.1046/j.1537-2995.1989.29890020444.x
47. Simon TL, Marcus CS, Myhre BA, Nelson EJ. Effects of AS-3 nutrient-additive solution on 42 and 49 days of storage of red cells. *Transfusion* (1987) 27(2):178–82. doi:10.1046/j.1537-2995.1987.27287150195.x
48. Valeri CR, Pivacek LE, Palter M, Dennis RC, Yeston N, Emerson CP, et al. A clinical experience with ADSOL preserved erythrocytes. *Surg Gynecol Obstet* (1988) 166(1):33–46.
49. Strauss RG, Mock DM, Widness JA, Johnson K, Cress G, Schmidt RL. Posttransfusion 24-hour recovery and subsequent survival of allogeneic red blood cells in the bloodstream of newborn infants. *Transfusion* (2004) 44(6):871–6. doi:10.1111/j.1537-2995.2004.03393.x
50. Peters AL, Beuger B, Mock DM, Widness JA, de Korte D, Juffermans NP, et al. Clearance of stored red blood cells is not increased compared with fresh red blood cells in a human endotoxemia model. *Transfusion* (2016) 56(6):1362–9. doi:10.1111/trf.13595
51. Mock DM, Widness JA, Veng-Pedersen P, Strauss RG, Cancelas JA, Cohen RM, et al. Measurement of posttransfusion red cell survival with the biotin label. *Transfus Med Rev* (2014) 28(3):114–25. doi:10.1016/j.tmrv.2014.03.003
52. Ohlmann P, Kemperman G, Basten J, Viaud-Massuard M, Ravanat C. Synthesis of the first GMP grade biotin-3-sulfo hydroxysuccinimide is now available to label blood cells intended for human transfusion studies. In: Devine DA, editor. *Vox Sanguinis. Proceedings of the 28th Regional Congress of the ISBT; 2017 Nov 25–28; Guangzhou, China*. Copenhagen: Wiley-Blackwell (2017). p. 5–191.
53. Zeiler T, Müller JT, Kretschmer V. Flow-cytometric determination of survival time and 24-hour recovery of transfused red blood cells. *Transfus Med Hemother* (2003) 30(1):14–9. doi:10.1159/000069340
54. Luten M, Roerdinkholder-Stoelwinder B, Schaap NPM, de Grip WJ, Bos HJ, Bosman GJ. Survival of red blood cells after transfusion: a comparison between red cells concentrates of different storage periods. *Transfusion* (2008) 48(7):1478–85. doi:10.1111/j.1537-2995.2008.01734.x
55. Dhabangi A, Ainomugisha B, Cserti-Gazdewich C, Ddungu H, Kyeyune D, Musisi E, et al. Effect of transfusion of red blood cells with longer vs shorter storage duration on elevated blood lactate levels in children with severe anemia: the TOTAL Randomized Clinical Trial. *JAMA* (2015) 314(23):2514–23. doi:10.1001/jama.2015.13977
56. Pilania RK, Saini SS, Dutta S, Das R, Marwaha N, Kumar P. Factors affecting efficacy of packed red blood cell transfusion in neonates. *Eur J Pediatr* (2017) 176(1):67–74. doi:10.1007/s00431-016-2806-7
57. Barshtein G, Goldschmidt N, Pries AR, Zelig O, Arbell D, Yedgar S. Deformability of transfused red blood cells is a potent effector of transfusion-induced hemoglobin increment: a study with β-thalassemia major patients. *Am J Hematol* (2017) 92(9):E559–60. doi:10.1002/ajh.24821
58. Barshtein G, Pries AR, Goldschmidt N, Zukerman A, Orbach A, Zelig O, et al. Deformability of transfused red blood cells is a potent determinant of transfusion-induced change in recipient's blood flow. *Microcirculation* (2016) 23(7):479–86. doi:10.1111/micc.12296
59. de Back DZ, Vlaar R, Beuger B, Daal B, Lagerberg J, Vlaar APJ, et al. A method for red blood cell biotinylation in a closed system. *Transfusion* (2018) 58(4):896–904. doi:10.1111/trf.14535
60. Valeri CR, Zaroulis CG. Rejuvenation and freezing of outdated stored human red cells. *N Engl J Med* (1972) 287(26):1307–13. doi:10.1056/NEJM197212282872601
61. Smith CH, Schulman I, Ando RE, Stern G. Studies in Mediterranean (Cooley's) anemia. I. Clinical and hematologic aspects of splenectomy, with special reference to fetal hemoglobin synthesis. *Blood* (1955) 10(6):582–99.
62. Cooper DJ, McQuilten ZK, Nichol A, Ady B, Aubron C, Bailey M, et al. Age of red cells for transfusion and outcomes in critically ill adults. *N Engl J Med* (2017) 377(19):1858–67. doi:10.1056/NEJMoa1707572
63. Heddle NM, Cook RJ, Arnold DM, Liu Y, Barty R, Crowther MA, et al. Effect of short-term vs. long-term blood storage on mortality after transfusion. *N Engl J Med* (2016) 375(20):1937–45. doi:10.1056/NEJMoa1609014
64. Lacroix J, Hébert PC, Fergusson DA, Tinmouth A, Cook DJ, Marshall JC, et al. Age of transfused blood in critically ill adults. *N Engl J Med* (2015) 372(15):1410–8. doi:10.1056/NEJMoa1500704

65. Steiner ME, Ness PM, Assmann SF, Triulzi DJ, Sloan SR, Delaney M, et al. Effects of red-cell storage duration on patients undergoing cardiac surgery. *N Engl J Med* (2015) 372(15):1419–29. doi:10.1056/NEJMoa1414219
66. Cook RJ, Heddle NM, Lee KA, Arnold DM, Crowther MA, Devereaux PJ, et al. Red blood cell storage and in-hospital mortality: a secondary analysis of the INFORM randomised controlled trial. *Lancet Haematol* (2017) 4(11):e544–52. doi:10.1016/S2352-3026(17)30169-2
67. Fergusson DA, Hébert P, Hogan DL, LeBel L, Rouvinez-Bouali N, Smyth JA, et al. Effect of fresh red blood cell transfusions on clinical outcomes in premature, very low-birth-weight infants: the ARIPI randomized trial. *JAMA* (2012) 308(14):1443–51. doi:10.1001/2012.jama.11953
68. Roussel C, Dussiot M, Marin M, Morel A, Ndour PA, Duez J, et al. Spherocytic shift of red blood cells during storage provides a quantitative whole cell-based marker of the storage lesion. *Transfusion* (2017) 57(4):1007–18. doi:10.1111/trf.14015
69. Relevy H, Koshkaryev A, Manny N, Yedgar S, Barshtein G. Blood banking-induced alteration of red blood cell flow properties. *Transfusion* (2008) 48(1):136–46. doi:10.1111/j.1537-2995.2007.01491.x
70. Mohandas N, Clark MR, Jacobs MS, Shohet SB. Analysis of factors regulating erythrocyte deformability. *J Clin Invest* (1980) 66(3):563–73. doi:10.1172/JCI109888
71. Groom AC, Schmidt EE, MacDonald IC. Microcirculatory pathways and blood flow in spleen: new insights from washout kinetics, corrosion casts, and quantitative intravital videomicroscopy. *Scanning Microsc* (1991) 5(1):159–173; discussion 173–174.
72. Buffet PA, Safeukui I, Deplaine G, Brousse V, Prendki V, Thellier M, et al. The pathogenesis of *Plasmodium falciparum* malaria in humans: insights from splenic physiology. *Blood* (2011) 117(2):381–92. doi:10.1182/blood-2010-04-202911
73. Buffet PA, Milon G, Brousse V, Correas J-M, Dousset B, Couvelard A, et al. Ex vivo perfusion of human spleens maintains clearing and processing functions. *Blood* (2006) 107(9):3745–52. doi:10.1182/blood-2005-10-4094
74. Mohandas N, Gallagher PG. Red cell membrane: past, present, and future. *Blood* (2008) 112(10):3939–48. doi:10.1182/blood-2008-07-161166
75. Pivkin IV, Peng Z, Karniadakis GE, Buffet PA, Dao M, Suresh S. Biomechanics of red blood cells in human spleen and consequences for physiology and disease. *Proc Natl Acad Sci U S A* (2016) 113(28):7804–9. doi:10.1073/pnas.1606751113
76. SosaleNG, RouhiparkouhiT, BradshawAM, DimovaR, LipowskyR, DischerDE. Cell rigidity and shape override CD47's "self"-signaling in phagocytosis by hyperactivating myosin-II. *Blood* (2015) 125(3):542–52. doi:10.1182/blood-2014-06-585299
77. Perrotta S, Gallagher PG, Mohandas N. Hereditary spherocytosis. *Lancet* (2008) 372(9647):1411–26. doi:10.1016/S0140-6736(08)61588-3
78. Waugh RE, Narla M, Jackson CW, Mueller TJ, Suzuki T, Dale GL. Rheologic properties of senescent erythrocytes: loss of surface area and volume with red blood cell age. *Blood* (1992) 79(5):1351–8.
79. Safeukui I, Buffet PA, Deplaine G, Perrot S, Brousse V, Ndour A, et al. Quantitative assessment of sensing and sequestration of spherocytic erythrocytes by the human spleen. *Blood* (2012) 120(2):424–30. doi:10.1182/blood-2012-01-404103
80. Noyes WD, Bothwell TH, Finch CA. The role of the reticulo-endothelial cell in iron metabolism. *Br J Haematol* (1960) 6:43–55. doi:10.1111/j.1365-2141.1960.tb06216.x
81. Frank SM, Abazyan B, Ono M, Hogue CW, Cohen DB, Berkowitz DE, et al. Decreased erythrocyte deformability after transfusion and the effects of erythrocyte storage duration. *Anesth Analg* (2013) 116(5):975–81. doi:10.1213/ANE.0b013e31828843e6
82. Burger P, Kostova E, Bloem E, Hilarius-Stokman P, Meijer AB, van den Berg TK, et al. Potassium leakage primes stored erythrocytes for phosphatidylserine exposure and shedding of pro-coagulant vesicles. *Br J Haematol* (2013) 160(3):377–86. doi:10.1111/bjh.12133
83. Greenberg MS, Jandl JH. The selective destruction of transfused compatible normal red cells in two patients with splenomegaly. *J Lab Clin Med* (1957) 49(2):233–45.
84. Prudent M, Tissot J-D, Lion N. In vitro assays and clinical trials in red blood cell aging: lost in translation. *Transfus Apher Sci* (2015) 52(3):270–6. doi:10.1016/j.transci.2015.04.006

A Conceptual Framework for Optimizing Blood Matching Strategies: Balancing Patient Complications Against Total Costs Incurred

Joost H. J. van Sambeeck [1,2]*, Puck D. de Wit* [3]*, Jessie Luken* [4]*, Barbera Veldhuisen* [4,5]*, Katja van den Hurk* [3]*, Anne van Dongen* [3]*, Maria M. W. Koopman* [6]*, Marian G. J. van Kraaij* [6,7,8]*, C. Ellen van der Schoot* [5]*, Henk Schonewille* [5]*, Wim L. A. M. de Kort* [3,9] *and Mart P. Janssen* [1*]

[1] Department of Transfusion Technology Assessment, Sanquin Research, Amsterdam, Netherlands, [2] Center for Healthcare Operations Improvement and Research, University of Twente, Enschede, Netherlands, [3] Department of Donor Studies, Sanquin Research, Amsterdam, Netherlands, [4] Sanquin Diagnostic Services, Amsterdam, Netherlands, [5] Sanquin Research and Landsteiner Laboratory, Department of Experimental Immunohematology, Academic Medical Center, University of Amsterdam, Amsterdam, Netherlands, [6] Department of Transfusion Medicine, Sanquin Blood Bank, Amsterdam, Netherlands, [7] Department of Donor Affairs, Sanquin Blood Bank, Amsterdam, Netherlands, [8] Department of Clinical Transfusion Research, Sanquin Research, Amsterdam, Netherlands, [9] Department of Social Medicine, Academic Medical Center, Amsterdam, Netherlands

***Correspondence:**
Mart P. Janssen
m.janssen@sanquin.nl*

Alloimmunization is currently the most frequent adverse blood transfusion event. Whilst completely matched donor blood would nullify the alloimmunization risk, this is practically infeasible. Current matching strategies therefore aim at matching a limited number of blood groups only, and have evolved over time by systematically including matching strategies for those blood groups for which (serious) alloimmunization complications most frequently occurred. An optimal matching strategy for controlling the risk of alloimmunization however, would balance alloimmunization complications and costs within the entire blood supply chain, whilst fulfilling all practical requirements and limitations. In this article the outline of an integrated blood management model is described and various potential challenges and prospects foreseen with the development of such a model are discussed.

Keywords: blood supply chain, alloimmunization, cost-effectiveness, optimization, modeling

1. INTRODUCTION

In a utopian world every blood transfusion would be handled like an organ transplant, which means that one would try to find a perfect match between donor and recipient. The reality however is that completely matched donor blood is impossible in practice due to the abundance of blood group antigens, costs associated with blood typing, and complications the logistics for such a scheme would impose. As a consequence only a handful of blood group antigens are matched, posing transfusion recipients at risk for alloimmunization and associated transfusion complications. An ideal matching strategy would be one that minimizes the risk of alloimmunization, is cost-effective, and fits within the practical limitations of the blood supply chain. In the past, matching strategies have been guided by the frequency of alloimmunization incidents, without systematically considering all consequences such strategies impose on the blood supply. Since a selected matching strategy will either directly or indirectly affect the entire blood supply chain (**Figure 1**), an integrated approach is required. Such an approach would, for any particular blood matching strategy, allow balancing the costs of donor recruitment, donor typing, inventory management, blood product logistics, patient blood typing, and alloimmunization complications in transfusion recipients. Besides costs also the effects of transfusion complications on patients health should be taken into account. This article describes the outline of a generic integrated blood management model, its components, their interaction and potential complicating factors and limitations currently foreseen for such a model.

We will first provide a description of all elements within the blood transfusion chain that are relevant to such a blood management model. Next we will describe how various elements are combined into an integrated model. Finally, we will discuss which challenges are foreseen with the implementation of the model and potential prospects. Challenges will concern knowledge required for shaping the modeling structure and the availability of data for various model parameters. Not only will the model guide the search for a rational choice of an optimal matching strategy, it will create transparency for the decision arena: the balance between costs and patient outcomes will become explicit for whatever optimal decision is selected. Secondly, by developing an integrated model, any blind spots in knowledge regarding any of the elements of the decision model will become visible and will have to be filled in.

The elements identified for the integrated blood management model are: the patient population, transfusion practice, predisposition of transfusion complications, typing and matching strategies, and the donor population. Note that as the patient is the primary concern, it is the patient that should be the starting point of the analysis. From there we will work our way back through the blood transfusion chain toward the donor population.

2. TRANSFUSED PATIENTS, EXPOSURE AND TRANSFUSION COMPLICATIONS

Blood transfusion is one of the most common medical procedures performed in hospitals. Despite its benefits, patients exposed to red blood cell (RBC) alloantigens may produce antibodies, which can cause acute or delayed hemolytic transfusion reactions (HTR). In addition, upon pregnancy in alloimmunized women, hemolytic disease of the fetus and newborn (HDFN) may occur. Not all patients form antibodies after RBC transfusion. According to current views, most are so-called non-responders and will never form antibodies despite numerous transfusions. Others seem to have an increased immunization risk and develop multiple antibodies after a few antigenic exposures, these are referred to as the (hyper)responders (1). It is currently not possible to prospectively identify patients that will form antibodies. In the absence of phenotypic matching, RBC alloimmunization risks vary between patient groups; it occurs in less than 5% of all transfusion recipients, increases to about 10–30% in patients with thalassemia, auto-immune hemolytic anemia or myelodysplastic syndromes, and can be

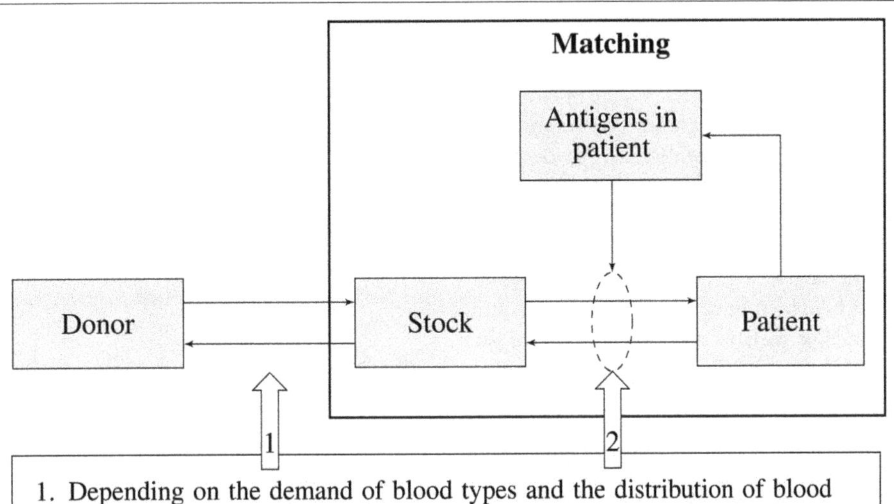
Matching
Antigens in patient
Donor
Stock
Patient
1
2
1. Depending on the demand of blood types and the distribution of blood products currently available in stock, donors with particular blood types are needed.
2. The requirement of particular blood types directly affects the availability of blood products in stock. This is therefore directly affected by the patient's characteristics (blood type and blood use) in combination with the matching strategy applied.

FIGURE 1 | Schematic overview of blood type matching and its impact on the blood supply chain.

more than 50% in sickle cell anemia patients (2, 3). In addition, patients with antibodies are at increased risk for additional antibody development upon subsequent transfusions (4, 5). During pregnancy, maternal RBC antibodies against paternal inherited antigens can pose the child at risk for HDFN. Besides anti-D, anti-E, anti-K, and anti-c are the most frequently encountered antibodies with the potential to seriously complicate pregnancy if the fetus carries the cognate antigen. The risk for severe HDFN in these fetuses, requiring intra-uterine or postnatal (exchange) transfusion, is estimated to be 12% for anti-K, 8.5% for anti-c and about 1% for anti-E. While for anti-D, administration of anti-D immunoglobulin (besides preventive D-matching) has reduced the risk of D immunization from 15% to 0.3%, such measures are not available or not always applied for other antigens, which are in the majority of cases elicited by previous transfusions (6).

The impact of transfusion reactions may vary widely, ranging from serologic observations or mild symptomatic anemia only, to life-threatening complications and death. It is obvious that with increasing severity, costs of treatment will also increase, although studies reporting on such associations and associated costs are currently limited or completely lacking (7). Maximum benefits of alloimmunization prevention can be obtained by administering extended antigen matched blood to patients who have an a priori high risk for alloimmunization. Therefore, unraveling genetic and environmental conditions enhancing RBC immunization would support preventive strategies. Although most studies on this subject have been performed in sickle cell disease (SCD) patients, factors such as age, sex, inflammatory status, MHC class-II genotype, polymorphisms associated with immune modulation and altered immune (regulatory) cells and disease or therapy associated immunosuppression seem to influence the immune response toward transfusion exposed alloantigens (1, 8–13). Due to logistic constraints, elaborate preventive matching based on a responder-profile is expected to be only feasible for a small proportion of patients. Targeting patients with (chronic) elective transfusions is likely to be feasible. Also, two recent prospective studies showed that less than 50% of surgery patients, who according to the local hospital pre-operative blood-ordering schedule had a high transfusion risk, were actually transfused. Extensive preventive matching as a routine policy is therefore expected to require a substantial amount of additional work and costs. Moreover, about 25% of patients required more than the anticipated number of RBC units during surgery and extended matched units were not readily available (14, 15).

As the blood management model is aiming to optimize strategies for preventing HTRs, the risk of alloimmunization in patients, its associated cost and health impact needs to be explicated. The ongoing Dutch R-fact study in which the predisposition for formation of antibodies is studied will allow modeling the likelihood of antibody formation. This information, combined with data on blood use for various patient groups, which will be obtained from the Dutch PROTON study (in which detailed transfusion data from a large number of hospitals are combined in a Dutch Transfusion Datawarehouse), will provide the information required to model the likelihood of HTRs in various patient groups. Research on the cost and health impact associated with HTRs will also be required to complete the model for patient and health outcome of transfusion complications.

3. CURRENT MATCHING STRATEGIES IN THE NETHERLANDS

In the Netherlands all RBC transfusions are compatible for ABO and D antigens. Since 2011 the guideline for selection of RBC units prescribes preventive matching for specific blood group antigens for different patient subgroups. Since 2004 it has been policy to select K-negative RBCs for women aged under 45, which in 2011 was extended with matching for c and E. These measures aim to prevent HDFN. In the updated guideline four patients groups with a putative increased risk of alloimmunization were defined, on grounds of either underlying disease, transfusion frequency, or potential (hyper-)respondership. The four patient groups concern (1) patients with autoimmune hemolytic disease; (2) patients with myelodysplastic syndrome and (3) patients with an immediate early antibody (IEA) against a clinically relevant RBC antigen. For these three patient subgroups Rh phenotype (CcDEe) and K compatible RBCs are selected. Finally, the fourth group consists of patients with hemoglobinopathies (SCD or thalassemia) for whom Rh phenotype, K and Fy(a) compatible RBCs are selected, and whenever available, Jk(b), S or s compatible RBCs. The recommended matching strategies formulated in Dutch transfusion guidelines are summarized in **Table 1** (16).

Apart from these specific patient groups, patients in the Netherlands are routinely tested for the presence of IEAs prior to RBC transfusions. When IEAs are detected, both their specificity and clinical importance are investigated. In case of a clinical important IEAs it is essential to select donor erythrocytes that are negative for corresponding antigens to prevent HTRs. Furthermore, dependent on the matching strategy, it may be required that donor erythrocytes are compatible with other antigens of the patient (extended matched), to prevent the formation of additional IEAs. Because antibodies may lose detectability over time, accurate recording and accessibility of patient antibody formation is of the utmost importance (17–19). Besides in-hospital records, a national database is available in the Netherlands (TRIX, Transfusion Register Irregular antibodies and X(cross)-matching), in which hospitals register patients with RBC antibodies and cross-match problems (20). This system is accessed for the evanesced antibodies in all patients

TABLE 1 | Matching strategies for various patient groups as recommended in the 2011 Dutch Transfusion guideline.

Patient group	Matching strategy
Sickle cell anemia and thalassemia	Rh phenotype, K and Fy(a) (and if available, Jk(b), S and s)
Autoimmune hemolytic anemia	Rh phenotype and K
Myelodysplastic syndrome	Rh phenotype and K
Alloimmunized with clinical important antibodies	Rh phenotype and K
Woman of childbearing age	c, E and K

with a transfusion request to prevent re-exposure to the cognate antigen. However, these registrations will not prevent re-exposure due to an inadequate antibody follow-up after transfusion.

The blood management model will have to accommodate matching strategies currently implemented as well as various extended matching strategies. The model should incorporate all costs involved for various matching strategies considered (e.g., costs of personnel and materials used).

4. TYPING THE DONOR POPULATION

Different matching strategies will pose different requirements on the availability of typed blood products. The required number of typed blood products, the variation in its demand, and the required service level (the probability of not being able to deliver a requested typed blood product) will determine the number of typed blood products that will have to be available in stock at any time, and hence the level of typed donors. A large typed donor population has the advantage that in most cases donor erythrocytes can be selected directly from inventory, even when blood products need to be typed negative for combinations of antigens. However, there will always be a balance between the additional efforts required to fulfill requirements for typed blood products and extending the pool of elaborately typed donors.

5. DONOR RECRUITMENT

Transfusing matched blood is only feasible if there are enough donors that are typed negative for specific (combinations of) blood group antigens. For instance, many Blood Services in Western countries have a structural shortage of Fy(a)-neg, Fy(b)-neg, e-neg donors. This blood type is most common in populations from Sub-Saharan Africa, of which relatively few individuals are enrolled as blood donors (21). In addition, in many countries a broad variety of ethnic minority populations exist. Shifting immigration patterns and mixing of these populations will increase the demand for rare blood type combinations. A valuable side effect of recruiting among minority groups is a potentially increase of donors for HLA-matched substances of human origin, such as stem cells. Blood Services therefore need to identify which specific ethnic minority populations to focus on in terms of rare blood type prevalence.

6. INTEGRATION

In the previous sections various elements of the blood transfusion chain and their interdependencies were discussed (see **Figure 1**). Each of these elements and their interactions need to be modeled in order to allow evaluation of the impact of a particular matching strategy on the transfusion risk of patients (i.e., acute and delayed HTRs) and on other parts of the blood supply chain (e.g., the availability of matched blood products, costs of type and screen, storage, outdating, and targeted donor recruitment). The main elements of the blood supply chain and the associated sub-models describing various interactions required for an integrated blood management model is depicted in **Figure 2**.

The starting point for any evaluation is the blood matching strategy, as this, in combination with the patient mix, will determine the demand for particular blood products. Depending on the matching strategy and patient mix (patient subgroups) there will be a risk of antibody formation and subsequent risk for adverse transfusion complications. Moreover, the combination of patient mix and associated matching strategy will determine the demand for typed blood products in the inventory. The availability of typed blood products in the inventory is dependent on the availability of typed blood donors, which again is dependent on the efforts and requirements of targeted donor recruitment.

The assessment of the transfusion complication risk requires estimates of the likelihood of antibody formation and subsequent transfusion reactions in patients given a particular matching strategy. Such estimates should incorporate the transfusion pattern and the ethnic (blood type) composition of various patient sub-groups. Also, antigen specific estimates for the likelihood of developing antibodies as well as for transfusion complications are required. The likelihood of transfusion complications in combination with cost and the health impact

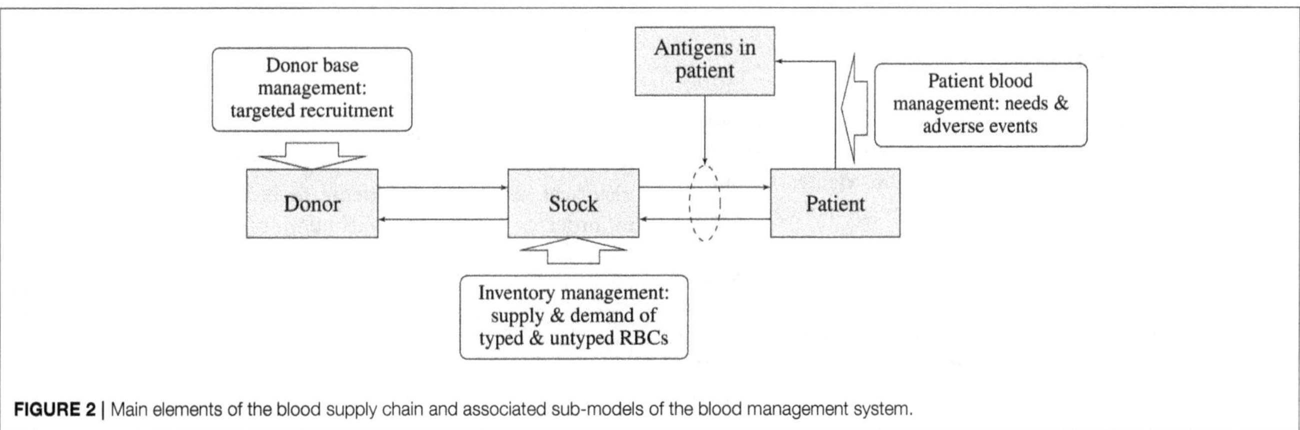

FIGURE 2 | Main elements of the blood supply chain and associated sub-models of the blood management system.

will allow estimation and subsequent balancing of the costs and benefits from the matching strategy applied.

To enable matching blood for transfusion recipients antigen and antibody profiles of patient subgroups have to be determined. Next, compatible RBC units have to be selected from inventory. Detailed information on blood use and the antigen profiles per patient group allows assessment of the blood inventory required to meet patient needs. This will be a description of the required inventory both in terms of amount and composition of RBCs in various stocks along the blood transfusion chain. Blood product demand will show a stochastic behavior and a realistic blood management model will therefore have to be able to accommodate such random variations. Given the patient mix, matching strategy and associated transfusion characteristics, for any pre-specified acceptability rate for the unavailability of (matched) blood products and inventory management strategy, the required blood inventory size and composition can be determined. The resulting costs and effects for the complete blood transfusion chain (outdating, size of the inventory, logistics, and material handling costs) can now be estimated. Note that the unavailability of matched blood products will impact the likelihood of transfusion complications in patients. Therefore, optimization of the overall blood transfusion chain will require a separate sub-optimization for the inventory management strategy.

The availability of compatible RBC units required in the inventory is directly linked to the availability of typed donors and hence guides the typing strategy and targeted donor recruitment efforts. The typing strategy will be aiming at fulfilling the requirements for maintaining sufficient inventory levels, but this will be dependent on the availability of specific antigen profiles in the (typed) donor population. Whenever these are insufficient, targeted donor recruitment efforts will have to ensure adequacy of the desired antigen profiles in the un-typed donor population, and ultimately those in the typed donor population. Estimates for the costs of recruiting specific donor subgroups in order to ensure a sufficient level of typed blood groups in the donor population are required to estimate the costs for maintaining the required inventory levels. Other than in the inventory management, which is an in-line process, it is presumed that the required levels of typed donors will be met by increasing donor recruitment efforts.

7. DISCUSSION

In this article we discussed a conceptual framework for a blood management model which allows optimization of blood matching strategies. The model links various elements from the blood transfusion chain to allow an assessment of the full impact of any particular matching strategy. The approach is unique in the sense that in the past matching strategies were guided by the prevention of transfusions complications observed with the administration of blood products, without consideration its impact on the underlying blood supply process. In theory this new approach seems sensible, however, in practice there will be a number of complicating factors.

First of all, except for some specific patient subgroups there is only limited evidence available on the effectiveness of matching strategies for the prevention of transfusion complications. Despite the fact that transfusion complications are accurately analyzed, patient exposure is far more difficult to ascertain. More evidence however has been gained for the risks of alloimmunization in various patient cohorts in the Netherlands in the ongoing Risk-Factors for alloimmunization after red blood Cell Transfusion (R-FACT) study (22). This concerted collaboration of several large hospitals will provide the information required to model risk factors for some patient subgroups. Also, looking back at the reduction of transfusion complications after implementation of altered matching strategies may support inference on its effectiveness. However, this effect may also be confounded by transfusion practice.

Another complicating factor is the impact of transfusion complications on patients, as this may vary from serologic observations or mild symptomatic anemia to life-threatening complications and death. Not only are predictors for predisposing factors lacking, but the impact of various levels of transfusion complications on patient health (apart from death) are not readily available, and neither are the associated costs. Assessing costs of complications is complex as it requires separation of the costs of patient treatment from costs of complications which are confounded by definition. Similar complications occur when estimating the impact on patient health. Nonetheless, an increasing number of publications on the impact of transfusion complications are becoming available (23–25).

In most settings detailed information on transfusion practice (number of transfused blood products for specific patient subgroups and the variation herein) is lacking. In the PROTON II study for a large number of Dutch hospitals detailed information on blood transfusions administered to patients is collected in one central datawarehouse (26). These data consist not only of transfused products, but also patient diagnosis and lab results. These data are indispensable when modeling the logistics of the blood supply in general, and for specific patient groups. Optimized inventory and dispatching strategies can be developed for both hospital and regional distribution centers and may be tailored to specified matching strategies. Note that with data on blood use the requirements and constraints for such models are available.

For the assessment of the risk of transfusion reactions (depending on the matching strategy) information on historical exposure of patients to blood products is required in order to assess the likelihood of antibody development. Such data is at present only available at a large scale for Denmark and Sweden where long term follow-up data on transfused patients is recorded in the SCANDAT database (27, 28). Such information may be used to estimate an approximate risk of exposure to red blood cells in other settings.

The development of an integrated blood management model will increase transparency in costs and effects of selected matching strategies and is therefore -if applied- expected to contribute to an improved efficiency in blood transfusion practice.

AUTHOR CONTRIBUTIONS

JvS, PdW, JL, BV, KvdH, AvD, MK, MvK, CvdS, HS, WdK, and MJ design of the framework. JvS, PdW, BV, KvdH, AvD, HS, and MJ initial draft of the paper. All authors review and update of the final paper.

REFERENCES

1. Gehrie EA, Tormey CA. The influence of clinical and biological factors on transfusion-associated non-ABO antigen alloimmunization: responders, hyper-responders, and non-responders. *Transfus Med Hemother.* (2014) 41:420–9. doi: 10.1159/000369109
2. Verduin EP, Brand A, Schonewille H. Is female sex a risk factor for red blood cell alloimmunization after transfusion? A systematic review. *Transfus Med Rev.* (2012) 26:342–53. doi: 10.1016/j.tmrv.2011.12.001
3. Verduin EP, Brand A, Middelburg RA, Schonewille H. Female sex of older patients is an independent risk factor for red blood cell alloimmunization after transfusion. *Transfusion* (2015) 55(6 pt 2):1478–85. doi: 10.1111/trf.13111
4. Schonewille H, Van De Watering LM, Brand A. Additional red blood cell alloantibodies after blood transfusions in a nonhematologic alloimmunized patient cohort: is it time to take precautionary measures? *Transfusion* (2006) 46:630–5. doi: 10.1111/j.1537-2995.2006.00764.x
5. Higgins JM, Sloan SR. Stochastic modeling of human RBC alloimmunization: evidence for a distinct population of immunologic responders. *Blood* (2008) 112:2546–53. doi: 10.1182/blood-2008-03-146415
6. Koelewijn JM, De Haas M, Vrijkotte TG, Bonsel GJ, Der Schoot V, Ellen C. One single dose of 200 μg of antenatal RhIG halves the risk of anti-D immunization and hemolytic disease of the fetus and newborn in the next pregnancy. *Transfusion* (2008) 48:1721–9. doi: 10.1111/j.1537-2995.2008.01742.x
7. Janssen M, van Tilborgh A, de Vooght K, Bokhorst A, Wiersum-Osselton J. Direct costs of transfusion reactions–an expert judgement approach. *Vox Sanguinis* (2018) 113:143–51. doi: 10.1111/vox.12614
8. Bauer MP, Wiersum-Osselton J, Schipperus M, Vandenbroucke JP, Briët E. Clinical predictors of alloimmunization after red blood cell transfusion. *Transfusion* (2007) 47:2066–71. doi: 10.1111/j.1537-2995.2007.01433.x
9. Körmöczi GF, Mayr WR. Responder individuality in red blood cell alloimmunization. *Transfus Med Hemother.* (2014) 41:446–51. doi: 10.1159/000369179
10. Zalpuri S, Evers D, Zwaginga JJ, Schonewille H, Vooght KM, Cessie S, et al. Immunosuppressants and alloimmunization against red blood cell transfusions. *Transfusion* (2014) 54:1981–7. doi: 10.1111/trf.12639
11. Yazdanbakhsh K. Mechanisms of sickle cell alloimmunization. *Transfus Clin Biol.* (2015) 22:178–81. doi: 10.1016/j.tracli.2015.05.005
12. Tatari-Calderone Z, Gordish-Dressman H, Fasano R, Riggs M, Fortier C, Campbell AD, et al. Protective effect of HLA-DQB1 alleles against alloimmunization in patients with sickle cell disease. *Hum Immunol.* (2016) 77:35–40. doi: 10.1016/j.humimm.2015.10.010
13. Meinderts SM, Sins JW, Fijnvandraat K, Nagelkerke SQ, Geissler J, Tanck MW, et al. Nonclassical FCGR2C haplotype is associated with protection from red blood cell alloimmunization in sickle cell disease. *Blood* (2017) 130:2121–30. doi: 10.1182/blood-2017-05-784876
14. Elebute MO, Choo L, Mora A, MacRury C, Llewelyn C, Purohit S, et al. Transfusion of prion-filtered red cells does not increase the rate of alloimmunization or transfusion reactions in patients: results of the UK trial of prion-filtered versus standard red cells in surgical patients (PRISM A). *Brit J Haematol.* (2013) 160:701–8. doi: 10.1111/bjh.12188
15. Schonewille H, Honohan Á, Van Der Watering LM, Hudig F, Te Boekhorst PA, Koopman-van Gemert AW, et al. Incidence of alloantibody formation after ABO-D or extended matched red blood cell transfusions: a randomized trial (MATCH study). *Transfusion* (2016) 56:311–20. doi: 10.1111/trf.13347
16. CBO. *CBO Blood Transfusion Guideline.* (2011). Available online at: http://www.isbtweb.org/fileadmin/user_upload/blood-transfusion-guideline.pdf
17. Ramsey G, Smietana S. Long-term follow-up testing of red cell alloantibodies. *Transfusion* (1994) 34:122–4. doi: 10.1046/j.1537-2995.1994.34294143938.x
18. Schonewille H, Haak HL, Van Zijl AM. RBC antibody persistence. *Transfusion* (2000) 40:1127–31. doi: 10.1046/j.1537-2995.2000.40091127.x
19. Reverberi R. The persistence of red cell alloantibodies. *Blood Transfus.* (2008) 6:225. doi: 10.2450/2008.0021-08
20. TRIX Register. Dutch Transfusion Register for Irregular Antibodies (2017). Available online at: https://www.sanquin.nl/producten-diensten/trix/
21. van Dongen A, Mews M, de Kort W, Wagenmans E. Missing Minorities: a survey based description of the current state of minority blood donor recruitment across 23 countries. *Divers Equal Health Care* (2016) 13:138–45. doi: 10.21767/2049-5471.100042
22. Zalpuri S, Zwaginga JJ, Van der Bom J. Risk factors for alloimmunisation after red blood cell transfusions (R-FACT): a case cohort study. *BMJ Open* (2012) 2:e001150. doi: 10.1136/bmjopen-2012-001150
23. Nickel RS, Hendrickson JE, Fasano RM, Meyer EK, Winkler AM, Yee MM, et al. Impact of red blood cell alloimmunization on sickle cell disease mortality: a case series. *Transfusion* (2016) 56:107–14. doi: 10.1111/trf.13379
24. Santos B, Portugal R, Nogueira C, Loureiro M. Hyperhemolysis syndrome in patients with sickle cell anemia: report of three cases. *Transfusion* (2015) 55(6 pt 2):1394–8. doi: 10.1111/trf.12993
25. Gehrie EA, Ness PM, Bloch EM, Kacker S, Tobian AA. Medical and economic implications of strategies to prevent alloimmunization in sickle cell disease. *Transfusion* (2017) 57:2267–76. doi: 10.1111/trf.14212
26. van Hoeven LR, Hooftman BH, Janssen MP, de Bruijne MC, de Vooght KM, Kemper P, et al. Protocol for a national blood transfusion data warehouse from donor to recipient. *BMJ Open* (2016) 6:e010962. doi: 10.1136/bmjopen-2015-010962
27. Edgren G, Hjalgrim H, Tran TN, Rostgaard K, Shanwell A, Titlestad K, et al. A population-based binational register for monitoring long-term outcome and possible disease concordance among blood donors and recipients. *Vox Sanguinis* (2006) 91:316–23. doi: 10.1111/j.1423-0410.2006.00827.x
28. Edgren G, Rostgaard K, Vasan SK, Wikman A, Norda R, Pedersen OB, et al. The new Scandinavian Donations and Transfusions database (SCANDAT2): a blood safety resource with added versatility. *Transfusion* (2015) 55:1600–6. doi: 10.1111/trf.12986

9

Emerging Infectious Agents and Blood Safety in Latin America

*José Eduardo Levi**

Hospital Israelita Albert Einstein, São Paulo, Brazil

***Correspondence:**
José Eduardo Levi
jose.levi@einstein.br

Historically, emerging infectious agents have been an important driving force toward the enhancement of blood safety, illustrated by the sharp reduction in the transmission of infectious agents by blood transfusion after human immunodeficiency virus (HIV) epidemics. In general, Latin American (LATAM) countries have introduced screening for microorganisms with proven blood transmission with some delay in comparison to developed countries, but, nowadays, all LATAM countries comply with a minimum standard of screening which includes Hepatitis B, C, HIV, *Treponema pallidum*, and *Trypanosoma cruzi*. Noticeably, all those agents, in addition to HTLV, cause chronic infections. By contrast, in the last decade, the region has witnessed explosive outbreaks of arboviral diseases, representing a new challenge to the blood system, threatening not only blood safety but also availability. So far, the clinical impact of transfusion-transmitted Dengue, Chikungunya, or Zika has not been evident, precluding immediate reaction from the authorities. A number of other arboviruses are endemic in the region and may, unpredictably, originate new epidemics. Several measures must be taken in preparedness for the potential emergence of another arbodisease.

Keywords: blood transfusion, arboviruses, Latin America, Zika, Dengue, Chikungunya

INTRODUCTION

The first agent verified to be transmitted by blood transfusion was the malaria protozoa (1) followed by Syphilis, the latter leading to the introduction of predonation testing in the first decades of the previous century (2). During the next 70 years, the safety of blood transfusions was gradually increased, covering a growing range of agents, more importantly the hepatitis viruses and human immunodeficiency virus (HIV). In common, all these pathologies have a short symptomatic acute phase and a variable rate of progression to a chronic asymptomatic period that may last through life. Blood units collected from unaware infected donors are averted from being transfused by detecting specific antibodies against those agents. With the exception of the hepatitis B virus (HBV) surface antigen (HBsAg) detection, the hallmark of prevention by laboratorial analysis has been the development and implementation of imunoassays, including, in some countries, the anti-hepatitis B core antigen (anti-HBc), that detects occult B carriers lacking, by definition, detectable HBsAg.

By the beginning of the millennia, the evolution of nucleic acid testing (NAT) allowed their incorporation to the blood screening routine, in order to interdict window-period donations, pursuing for an unattainable zero risk. A better selection of candidate donors with more stringent epidemiological and behavioral restrictions, summed to the arsenal of screening tests, have dropped the risk of transfusion transmission of infectious agents to a very low level, being nowadays a rare event (3).

Latin American (LATAM) countries are in general still struggling to motivate the population to donate blood voluntarily and regularly. Donations in the region are commonly insufficient for sustaining the transfusion demand, thereby resulting in a permanent blood shortage. In many countries, most of the donations come from replacement, often familiar donors (4) and emphasis is given to transform those into altruistic regular donors. Surprisingly, it has been observed that in some centers, repeat donors pose a risk that is similar or even higher than first-time donors concerning HIV transmission (5). This observation is justified by a fraction of repeat donors being indeed composed of HIV test seekers (6).

With some delay in comparison to developed countries, the four most important screening targets, HBV, HCV, HIV, and Syphillis, in addition to *Trypanosoma cruzi*, of local uttermost importance, were fully implemented in the 1990s (4). Seroprevalence of these agents were and are still much higher when compared to those verified in blood donors from Europe, Japan, Canada, and the US (3, 4, 7).

In this scenario, the explosive outbreaks of arboviruses with a high rate of asymptomatic subjects with a short-term viremia is new to the LATAM blood transfusion community; thus, there is a lot of uncertainty in how to deal with it. There are several proposed measures to mitigate this situation: averting blood collection in affected regions, applying pathogen reduction methods for plasma and platelet concentrates, adopting NAT and quarantine while waiting for post-donation information of donor's health. Some countries may implement all them and others one or none. Certainly, this variability is not only due to scientific gaps in our knowledge but also to the resources available and political determination in each country or region. **Table 1** summarizes selected features of the arboviruses representing today potential threats to the blood supply in LATAM.

EMERGING VIRUSES

Dengue

Viruses transmitted by arthropods (arboviruses) have always been of concern to human health but never much in the radar of blood banks. Dengue was the first arbovirus to cause epidemics in a global scale in the twenty-first century, globally affecting millions, from the Far East to the Americas. In LATAM, Brazil has been the country with the largest number of cases, experiencing yearly outbreaks from moderate to high intensity. Moreover, all four serotypes are now endemic, but there is still a large number of subjects naïve to at least one of the four serotypes, meaning that outbreaks will continue to occur.

TABLE 1 | Selected features of emerging viruses representing a potential threat to the blood supply in Latin America, 2018.

	Arbovirus		
	Chikungunya	**Dengue**	**Zika**
Family/genus	Togaviridae/ alphavirus	Flaviviridae/ flavivirus	Flaviviridae/ flavivirus
Enveloped	Yes	Yes	Yes
Viremic blood donors	Yes	Yes	Yes
Proven TT	No	Yes	Yes
NAT screening commercially available	No	No	Yes
Inactivated by PIT[a]	Yes	Yes	Yes
Vaccine available	No	Yes	No

[a]*Pathogen reduction/inactivation technologies.*

The main impact of dengue outbreaks to the blood system is the fall in the number of candidate donors, thus shortening the supply of blood products, aggravated by the universal practice of transfusing dengue patients with low platelet counts (8). As most dengue infections are asymptomatic, it is likely that such infected subjects are be able to donate and thus eventually transmit the dengue virus to recipients. This possibility was demonstrated by several studies detecting viremic donors in Brazil (9–11), Honduras (9), Mexico (12), and Puerto Rico (13) among others.

However, there is an obvious discrepancy in between the dengue incidence and rates of viremia verified among blood donors during outbreaks and the paucity of reports of dengue cases by the transfusional route (TT-DENV). The most comprehensive study on TT-DENV showed that recipients have an approximately 36% risk to get the virus from a viremic donor, but was unable to depict dengue-specific symptoms on those infected (11). Several reasons have been presented to explain this (un)finding, discussed in detail elsewhere (14), but may be summarized as follows: it seems that dengue viruses are well adapted to the mosquito to human cycle, and, passage through the invertebrate host and inoculation by its bite are required to cause disease on us. So, although TT-DENV is a recognized risk in many endemic countries in LATAM, preventive measures were never taken, since it did not convince clinicians and authorities of its morbidity for recipients. However, it is necessary to emphasize that, in rare instances, severe dengue-associated symptoms were observed on recipients of viremic donations (13, 15), thereby leading to the implementation of laboratorial screening in Puerto Rico, first by using NS1 antigen testing further replaced by NAT (16) but in nowhere else in LATAM.

West Nile Virus (WNV)

The diverse outcome of the different Flaviviruses causing human diseases requires that each viral species to be studied in depth, making analogies and generic Flavivirus models of little practical utility. This was well illustrated when the WNV arrived to the US by the end of the previous century. It took about 2 years to get enough evidence of its aggressiveness when acquired by blood transfusion or organ transplantation (17), since there was no previous recognition of any arbovirus transmission by these modes. When this link was unquestionably proven, it triggered a fast response from the transfusion medicine community, culminating in the introduction of screening by NAT (18). As WNV moved so fast from East to West US, it seemed inevitable that it would spread further South to LATAM, since susceptible vectors are abundant in the region and there is a huge migration of bird species that may harbor high titer viremias, from US and Canada to South America. Contrary to expectations, WNV was never able to cause human outbreaks in LATAM (19).

Zika

The trajectory of Zika virus (ZKV) from an obscure agent to a global health emergence has been comprehensively described (20). The well-studied outbreak in French Polynesia revealed the important association of ZKV to Guillain-Barré syndrome (21), while Brazil was the country to raise and prove the hypothesis of a shocking causal association of this Flavivirus to microcephaly and other fetal neural abnormalities (22). Concerns about blood safety were raised by Musso and co-workers in French Polynesia where NAT, pathogen inactivation and quarantine were deployed to protect the blood supply (23). So far, there are only two published clusters of TT-ZKV, both from Brazil (24, 25). Similar to TT-DENV, on those reports it was shown that ZKV was indeed transmitted to transfusion recipients but they did not develop any symptom associated with Zika disease. In French Polynesia, look-back of 12 recipients transfused with red blood cells from ZKV-RNA$^+$ donors has not also identified any post-transfusion symptoms (23). Even though solid evidence for a severe clinical outcome of TT-ZKV is still missing, the precautionary principle led Fundação Pró-Sangue/Hemocentro de São Paulo, Brazil, to develop a validated in-house NAT (26) and adopt it, from February 2016 on, to provide Zika-RNA-free blood units to approximately 20 pregnant women per month. In Martinique, Guadaloupe, and the French Guyana, pregnant women received blood collected in mainland France (Xavier de Lamballerie, personal communication) while donations were screened by individual NAT in Marseille, France (27). This policy of prioritizing groups at higher risk such as pregnant and highly transfused fertile women, and fetuses was further advocated by experts and organizations in the field (28) and WHO (29). In the US, in observation of FDA recommendations, blood collection was halted in Puerto Rico in between March and April 2016, resumed when NAT screening was introduced in late April. Approximately 0.5% of the donors were found viremic, peaking to 1.8% in July 2016 (30). Mosquito-borne and travel-associated cases in the continental US led the FDA to extend the recommendation of NAT screening to the whole country, being implemented by September/October 2016 and indeed depicting some infected donors, the majority with a recent travel history to an endemic area (31, 32). No country in LATAM so far followed this policy. The sharp decline in Zika incidence in LATAM in 2017 reduced the pressure and debate over this issue. High seroprevalence rates are observed today in the most affected areas of Brazil, what may prevent new large outbreaks in the near future (22, 33).

Chikungunya

Chikungunya (CHKV), in common with Zika and Dengue, is also transmitted by mosquitos from the *Aedes* genus, causing similar symptoms, making difficult to perform a diagnosis relying solely on clinical manifestations. Noticeably, arthralgia is much more pronounced and may last for months in some patients.

Its transmission by blood transfusion remains theoretical since no single case of TT-CHKV has ever been published. CHKV was introduced to LATAM in 2013, hitting first the Saint Martin Island in the Caribbean, brought probably from the South Pacific. The implicated CHKV Asian strain rapidly spread over the Caribbean and to South, Central, and North America (34). In the French West Indies, concerns about blood safety led to early implementation of a lab-developed NAT, in addition to pathogen reduction and quarantine (35). They were able to detect four viremic donors, two of them developed fever after donation and the other two remained asymptomatic. A large outbreak occurred a few months later in Puerto Rico with up to 2.1% of donors testing CHKV-RNA$^+$ (36). In contrast to the fast adoption of NAT for WNV, upon solid evidence of the clinical impact of TT-WNV, and for Zika, even lacking such parallel data, NAT for CHKV was never implemented in Puerto Rico.

From the Caribbean, the Asian strain spread first to the Northern countries of South America; Colombia, Venezuela, Suriname, Guyana, and the French overseas territory of French Guyana (37). The Brazilian Amazon state of Amapá, contiguous to the French Guyana, was the first to report autochthonous cases in September 2014. Curiously, at about the same time, an infected individual brought the East–South–Central Africa (ECSA) strain to the Northeastern state of Bahia, resulting in hundreds of cases and the establishment of this lineage as endemic in the region (38). In the following years, growing number of presumed CHKV cases were verified in Brazil, 38,499 in 2015, 271,824 in 2016, and approximately 200,000 in 2017, with dozens of deaths (39, 40). It is suspected that another arbovirus, Mayaro (MAYV), belonging to the same Alphavirus genus from the *Togaviridae* family, may be hidden among cases attributed to CHKV (41) and DENV (42).

There is a fear in LATAM in general, that huge outbreaks of CHKV will take place in the next years, since the majority of the population is still naïve to this virus. Strategies to mitigate the risk of TT-CHKV are not being actively discussed, since the risk of getting infected by mosquitoes is much higher and the associated clinical picture absolutely clear. In LATAM countries, with several social and health demands, it is debatable whether the resources to prevent a few TT-CHKV should not be invested in vector control, in order to benefit a larger number of inhabitants, including blood recipients that are off course also susceptible to mosquitoes' bites in daily life outside blood transfusion settings. However, availability of, in development, arboviral multiplex NATs allowing for simultaneous detection of Dengue, Chikungunya, and Zika and/ or pathogen reduction technologies acting on whole blood (43) or components, necessarily including red cells (44) may perhaps result in cost-effective measures to be implemented in endemic areas, home to the majority of the LATAM population.

AUTHOR CONTRIBUTIONS

The author confirms being the sole contributor of this work and approved it for publication.

REFERENCES

1. Bruce-Chwatt LJ. Transfusion malaria. *Bull WHO* (1974) 50:337–46.
2. Stansbury LG, Hess JR. Blood transfusion in World War I: the roles of Lawrence Bruce Robertson and Oswald Hope Robertson in the "most important medical advance of the war". *Transfus Med Rev* (2009) 23:232–6. doi:10.1016/j.tmrv.2009.03.007
3. Perkins HA, Busch MP. Transfusion-associated infections: 50 years of relentless challenges and remarkable progress. *Transfusion* (2010) 50:2080–99. doi:10.1111/j.1537-2995.2010.02851.x
4. WHO/PAHO. *Supply of Blood for Transfusion in Latin American and Caribbean Countries 2012 and 2013*. Washington, DC: OPS (2015). Available from: http://www.who.int
5. de Almeida-Neto C, Goncalez TT, Birch RJ, de Carvalho SM, Capuani L, Leão SC, et al. Risk factors for human immunodeficiency virus infection among Brazilian blood donors: a multicentre case-control study using audio computer-assisted structured interviews. *Vox Sang* (2013) 105(2):91–9. doi:10.1111/vox.12028
6. Levi JE, Lira SM, Bub CB, Polite MB, Terzian CC, Kutner JM. Contrasting HCV and HIV seroepidemiology in 11 years of blood donors screening in Brazil. *Transfus Med* (2017) 27(4):286–91. doi:10.1111/tme.12427
7. Schmunis GA, Zicker F, Cruz JR, Cuchi P. Safety of blood supply for infectious diseases in Latin American countries, 1994–1997. *Am J Trop Med Hyg* (2001) 65(6):924–30. doi:10.4269/ajtmh.2001.65.924
8. Lye DC, Archuleta S, Syed-Omar SF, Low JG, Oh HM, Wei Y, et al. Prophylactic platelet transfusion plus supportive care versus supportive care alone in adults with dengue and thrombocytopenia: a multicentre, open-label, randomised, superiority trial. *Lancet* (2017) 389(10079):1611–8. doi:10.1016/S0140-6736(17)30269-6
9. Linnen JM, Vinelli E, Sabino EC, Tobler LH, Hyland C, Lee TH, et al. Dengue viremia in blood donors from Honduras, Brazil, and Australia. *Transfusion* (2008) 48:1355–62. doi:10.1111/j.1537-2995.2008.01772.x
10. Dias LL, Amarilla AA, Poloni TR, Covas DT, Aquino VH, Figueiredo LT. Detection of dengue virus in sera of Brazilian blood donors. *Transfusion* (2012) 52:1667–71. doi:10.1111/j.1537-2995.2012.03729.x
11. Sabino EC, Loureiro P, Lopes ME, Capuani L, McClure C, Chowdhury D, et al. Transfusion based transmission of dengue virus and associated clinical symptoms during the 2012 epidemic in Brazil. *J Infect Dis* (2016) 213:694–702. doi:10.1093/infdis/jiv326
12. Arellanos-Soto D, B-d Cruz V, Mendoza-Tavera N, Ramos-Jiménez J, Cázares-Taméz R, Ortega-Soto A, et al. Constant risk of dengue virus infection by blood transfusion in an endemic area in Mexico. *Transfus Med* (2015) 25(2):122–4. doi:10.1111/tme.12198
13. Stramer SL, Linnen JM, Carrick JM, Foster GA, Krysztof DE, Zou S, et al. Dengue viremia in blood donors identified by RNA and detection of dengue transfusion transmission during the 2007 dengue outbreak in Puerto Rico. *Transfusion* (2012) 52:1657–66. doi:10.1111/j.1537-2995.2012.03566.x
14. Levi JE. Dengue virus and blood transfusion. *J Infect Dis* (2016) 213:689–90. doi:10.1093/infdis/jiv322
15. Levi JE, Nishiya A, Félix AC, Salles NA, Sampaio LR, Hangai F, et al. Real-time symptomatic case of transfusion-transmitted dengue. *Transfusion* (2015) 55:961–4. doi:10.1111/trf.12944
16. Matos D, Tomashek KM, Perez-Padilla J, Muñoz-Jordán J, Hunsperger E, Horiuchi K, et al. Probable and possible transfusion-transmitted dengue associated with NS1 antigen-negative but RNA confirmed-positive red blood cells. *Transfusion* (2016) 56(1):215–22. doi:10.1111/trf.13288
17. Pealer LN, Marfin AA, Petersen LR, Lanciotti RS, Page PL, Stramer SL, et al. Transmission of West Nile virus through blood transfusion in the United States in 2002. West Nile Virus Transmission Investigation Team. *N Engl J Med* (2003) 349:1236–45. doi:10.1056/NEJMoa030969
18. Dodd RY, Foster GA, Stramer SL. Keeping blood transfusion safe from West Nile virus: American Red Cross experience, 2003 to 2012. *Transfus Med Rev* (2015) 29:153–61. doi:10.1016/j.tmrv.2015.03.001
19. Elizondo-Quiroga D, Elizondo-Quiroga A. West Nile virus and its theories, a big puzzle in Mexico and Latin America. *J Glob Infect Dis* (2013) 5(4):168–75. doi:10.4103/0974-777X.122014
20. Hills SL, Fischer M, Petersen LR. Epidemiology of Zika virus Infection. *J Infect Dis* (2017) 216(Suppl_10):S868–74. doi:10.1093/infdis/jix434
21. Musso D, Bossin H, Mallet HP, Besnard M, Broult J, Baudouin L, et al. Zika virus in French Polynesia 2013–14: anatomy of a completed outbreak. *Lancet Infect Dis* (2017). doi:10.1016/S1473-3099(17)30446-2
22. de Araújo TVB, Rodrigues LC, de Alencar Ximenes RA, de Barros Miranda-Filho D, Montarroyos UR, de Melo APL, et al. Association between Zika virus infection and microcephaly in Brazil, January to May, 2016: preliminary report of a case-control study. *Lancet Infect Dis* (2016) 16:1356–63. doi:10.1016/S1473-3099(16)30318-8
23. Bierlaire D, Mauguin S, Broult J, Musso D. Zika virus and blood transfusion: the experience of French Polynesia. *Transfusion* (2017) 57:729–33. doi:10.1111/trf.14028
24. Barjas-Castro ML, Angerami RN, Cunha MS, Suzuki A, Nogueira JS, Rocco IM, et al. Probable transfusion-transmitted Zika virus in Brazil. *Transfusion* (2016) 56:1684–8. doi:10.1111/trf.13681
25. Motta IJ, Spencer BR, Cordeiro da Silva SG, Arruda MB, Dobbin JA, Gonzaga YBM, et al. Evidence for transmission of Zika virus by platelet transfusion. *N Engl J Med* (2016) 375:1101–3. doi:10.1056/NEJMc1607262
26. Stone M, Lanteri MC, Bakkour S, Deng X, Galel SA, Linnen JM, et al. Relative analytical sensitivity of donor nucleic acid amplification technology screening and diagnostic real-time polymerase chain reaction assays for detection of Zika virus RNA. *Transfusion* (2017) 57:734–47. doi:10.1111/trf.14031
27. Gallian P, Cabié A, Richard P, Paturel L, Charrel RN, Pastorino B, et al. Zika virus in asymptomatic blood donors in Martinique. *Blood* (2017) 129(2):263–6. doi:10.1182/blood-2016-09-737981
28. Musso D, Stramer SL; AABB Transfusion-Transmitted Diseases Committee, Busch MP; International Society of Blood Transfusion Working Party on Transfusion-Transmitted Infectious Diseases. Zika virus: a new challenge for blood transfusion. *Lancet* (2016) 387(10032):1993–4. doi:10.1016/S0140-6736(16)30428-7
29. WHO. *Interim Guidance. Maintaining a Safe and Adequate Blood Supply during Zika Virus Outbreaks*. (2016). WHO/ZIKV/HS/16.1. Available from: http://www.who.int
30. Adams L, Bello-Pagan M, Lozier M, Ryff KR, Espinet C, Torres J, et al. Update: ongoing Zika virus transmission—Puerto Rico, November 1, 2015-July 7, 2016. *MMWR Morb Mortal Wkly Rep* (2016) 65:774–9.
31. Williamson PC, Linnen JM, Kessler DA, Shaz BH, Kamel H, Vassallo RR, et al. First cases of Zika virus-infected US blood donors outside states with areas of active transmission. *Transfusion* (2017) 57:770–8. doi:10.1111/trf.14041
32. Galel SA, Williamson PC, Busch MP, Stanek D, Bakkour S, Stone M, et al. First Zika-positive donations in the continental United States. *Transfusion* (2017) 57:762–9. doi:10.1111/trf.14029
33. Netto EM, Moreira-Soto A, Pedroso C, Höser C, Funk S, Kucharski AJ, et al. High Zika virus seroprevalence in Salvador, northeastern Brazil limits the potential for further outbreaks. *MBio* (2017) 8:e1390–1317. doi:10.1128/mBio.01390-17
34. Chen R, Puri V, Fedorova N, Lin D, Hari KL, Jain R, et al. Comprehensive genome scale phylogenetic study provides new insights on the global expansion of chikungunya virus. *J Virol* (2016) 90(23):10600–11. doi:10.1128/JVI.01166-16
35. Gallian P, de Lamballerie X, Salez N, Piorkowski G, Richard P, Paturel L, et al. Prospective detection of chikungunya virus in blood donors, Caribbean 2014. *Blood* (2014) 123:3679–81. doi:10.1182/blood-2014-03-564880
36. Simmons G, Brès V, Lu K, Liss NM, Brambilla DJ, Ryff KR, et al. High incidence of chikungunya virus and frequency of viremic blood donations during epidemic, Puerto Rico, USA, 2014. *Emerg Infect Dis* (2016) 22(7):1221–8. doi:10.3201/eid2207.160116
37. Bajak A. US assesses virus of the Caribbean. *Nature* (2014) 152:124–5. doi:10.1038/512124a
38. Nunes MR, Faria NR, de Vasconcelos JM, Golding N, Kraemer MU, de Oliveira LF, et al. Emergence and potential for spread of chikungunya virus in Brazil. *BMC Med* (2015) 13:102. doi:10.1186/s12916-015-0348-x
39. BRAZIL. *Boletim Epidemiológico: Monitoramento dos casos de dengue, febre de chikungunya e febre pelo vírus Zika até a Semana Epidemiológica*. (2017). Available from: http://portalsaude.saude.gov.br

40. Brito CA. Alert: severe cases and deaths associated with chikungunya in Brazil. *Rev Soc Bras Med Trop* (2017) 50(5):585–9. doi:10.1590/0037-8682-0479-2016
41. Esposito DLA, Fonseca BALD. Will Mayaro virus be responsible for the next outbreak of an arthropod-borne virus in Brazil? *Braz J Infect Dis* (2017) 21(5):540–4. doi:10.1016/j.bjid.2017.06.002
42. Zuchi N, Heinen LB, Santos MA, Pereira FC, Slhessarenko RD. Molecular detection of Mayaro virus during a dengue outbreak in the state of Mato Grosso, Central-West Brazil. *Mem Inst Oswaldo Cruz* (2014) 109:820–3. doi:10.1590/0074-0276140108
43. Allain JP, Goodrich R. Pathogen reduction of whole blood: utility and feasibility. *Transfus Med* (2017) 27(Suppl 5):320–6. doi:10.1111/tme.12456
44. Aubry M, Laughhunn A, Santa Maria F, Lanteri MC, Stassinopoulos A, Musso D. Amustaline (S-303) treatment inactivates high levels of chikungunya virus in red-blood-cell components. *Vox Sang* (2018). doi:10.1111/vox.12626

10

How Can Eastern/Southern Mediterranean Countries Resolve Quality and Safety Issues in Transfusion Medicine?

Antoine Haddad[1,2], Tarek Bou Assi[3,4] and Olivier Garraud[2,5]*

[1] Department of Clinical Pathology and Blood Banking, Sacré-Coeur Hospital, Lebanese University, Beirut, Lebanon, [2] EA3064, Faculty of Medicine of Saint-Etienne, University of Lyon, Saint-Etienne, France, [3] Department of Laboratory Medicine, Psychiatric Hospital of the Cross, Jal El Dib, Lebanon, [4] Department of Laboratory Medicine and Blood Banking, Saint Joseph Hospital, Dora, Lebanon, [5] Institut National de la Transfusion Sanguine, Paris, France

***Correspondence:**
Antoine Haddad
anthadd@gmail.com

Unlike their Western counterparts, some of the Eastern/Southern Mediterranean countries lack centralized coordinated blood transfusion services leading to an unequal blood safety level. This was recently highlighted by a recent World Health Organization (WHO) regional committee report in which WHO urges these countries to establish and implement a national blood system with well-coordinated blood transfusion activities and to make attempts to reach 100% voluntary non-remunerated blood donation. The objective is thus to meet the same levels or standards as Western countries in term of self-sufficiency and blood safety. This raises the question whether these countries can either comply with Western countries' guidelines and experiences or develop their own safety scheme based on proper sociopolitical and economic features. Another option is to identify efficient and cost-effective strategies setup successfully in neighbor countries sharing cultural and economic features. To address this issue—and make an attempt to achieve this goal—we designed a number of surveys specifically addressed to Mediterranean countries, which were sent out to the national authorities; so far, five surveys aim at covering all aspects in blood collection, processing, testing, inventory and distribution, as well as patient immune-hematological testing and follow-up (including surveillance and vigilances). It is anticipated that such practice can help identifying and then sharing the more successful and cost-effective experiences, and be really focused on Mediterranean areas while not necessarily copying and pasting experiences designed for Western/Northern areas with significantly distinct situations.

Keywords: transfusion, Southern Mediterranean, Eastern Mediterranean, quality, safety, VNRD, blood supply

INTRODUCTION

Despite having lower to upper middle-income economies, Eastern/Southern Mediterranean countries, compared with high-income countries (often referred to as either Western or Northern countries), provide similar transfusion therapies for a wide range of diseases and conditions. This comprises, among others, care for thalassemia major, and to a lesser extent, sickle cell disease patients, and assistance to transplantation programs, including stem cells (1, 2). However, unlike their Western counterparts, some of these countries lack centralized or coordinated blood transfusion services resulting in different levels of blood safety in terms of quantity and quality: insufficient blood supply, unequal availability of blood components (BCs) and nationwide health-care coverage, inadequate financial and human resources, etc. (3, 4). All of which were regularly highlighted by World Health Organization (WHO) reports, urging these countries to establish and implement a national blood system with well-coordinated blood transfusion activities. In parallel to its recommendation on blood use and surveillance, WHO also advised all countries to achieve a 100% voluntary non-remunerated blood donation (VNRBD) objective by the year 2020 (recently postponed to 2025 for Eastern Mediterranean countries) (5, 6). In stating this, WHO considers that the fundamental strategy to ensure timely access to safe and sufficient supplies of blood and blood products is the development of a nationally coordinated blood transfusion service based on VNRBDs without any other alternative (7).

CURRENT QUESTIONS ADDRESSED BY DEVELOPING COUNTRIES REGARDING THEIR BLOOD COLLECTION AND TRANSFUSION PROGRAMS

Almost all countries in the process of implementing or strengthening their own national blood transfusion program must address seven key questions:

- (ai) How can we meet the clinical demand and become self-sufficient in procuring BCs?
- (aii) How can we guarantee donors' safety during blood collection?
- (aiii) How can we ensure BCs are issued at the safest level (at least regarding transfusion-transmitted infections and immunohematological compatibility)?
- (aiv) How can we ensure a quality management-driven organization?
- (av) How can we set up a surveillance system to follow-up donors, the BC chain process and recipients?
- (avi) How can we guarantee optimal clinical use of blood and ensure Patient Blood Management (PBM) while avoiding inadequate transfusions and/or loss of expired blood products?
- (avii) How can we educate all staff categories (and/or other stakeholders)?

It is evident that not all countries are at the same level of progress toward these goals. In fact, the majority face a number of obstacles such as (8):

- (bi) Available financial and human resources (including educational level).
- (bii) Cultural habits, traditions, and experiences (including perception of blood donation or infusion and quality management).
- (biii) Unfavorable epidemiological conditions (active circulation of vectors, viruses, and other pathogens that may be transmitted by blood).
- (biv) Multiethnic population with antigenic diversity that makes immunohematological matching difficult to achieve for some patients.

These goals cannot be achieved without a strong commitment from the public authorities and the backing of the Ministry of Health in the country concerned.

Bearing in mind that quality, safety, education, surveillance, and vigilance program apply to all three aspects, the blood transfusion process can commonly be reported as a three-legged stool, i.e., the "A, B, C" of the process:

A. Donors, donations, and/or blood collection.
B. BCs (i.e., blood outside the donor and not yet transfused to the recipient).
C. Recipients.

THE "A, B, C" OF THE BLOOD COLLECTION AND TRANSFUSION PROCESS WITH SPECIAL REFERENCE TO DEVELOPING COUNTRIES

Donors/Donations/Blood Collection

It would be tempting to start with the "A" leg of the stool; however, it must be borne in mind that blood donation and/or collection only exist because there is a demand. There are three major approaches for analyzing this demand: (i) a passive analysis, which is the easiest and consists in retrospectively reviewing all BCs issued over a defined period of time for predefined clinical situations (obstetrical bleeding, trauma, malaria, etc.); (ii) an active or prospective analysis, more difficult to address, which consists in predicting the needs in a given population to fulfill certain clinical indications such as cancer therapy, transplantation, and internal medicine; (iii) a combined (active and passive) analysis, which simultaneously reviews historical data and prospects the needs based on the development of the patient recruitment processes. Therefore, it is instrumental to stratify the actual needs and anticipate any increase in blood demand based on the available hospital strategies to recruit patients and on the consensuses regarding transfusion strategies for every patient category. All of the above is aimed at defining whether a system is self-sufficient or not. Indeed, can anyone consider a system self-sufficient when it only ensures BCs on a daily basis (emergency or/and bleeding situations) as regularly seen in developing countries? Consequently, it can be deduced that self-sufficiency is difficult to define and should be driven by audits assessing both short (or daily basis) and long-term needs.

Once the demand is defined, blood collection programs can be launched to build up inventories. Here again, there are essentially two main pathways: the first applies to small Hospital Blood Banks (HBBs) and consists in fulfilling the arbitrary need on a daily basis. The second—usually seen in larger settings—is based on a program, adjusted according to the statistical consumption of blood. The latter is more suitable with the VNRD-based blood supply system where mobile drives in partnership with non-governmental organizations (NGOs) such as the Red Cross/Red Crescent, can eventually be planned in advance.

The respective values of VNRD and replacement donation can now be discussed.

Replacement donation consists in donating blood voluntarily in case a relative is in need, therefore contributing to blood bank replenishment. This donation mode is predominant in almost all Mediterranean countries. In fact, a recent Greek study found that donors seem to be more sensitized by the need in BCs rather than altruism, contrary to what is seen in VNRD systems (9). The donation is addressed specifically to the bank and not to the patient, since the donor and recipient are not required to have an identical blood group. The recipient will be transfused with already processed BCs, bearing in mind that the anonymity process is always guaranteed. No direct benefits are provided by the patient, donor or blood bank. However, indirect benefits cannot be ruled out for each party. Based on the literature, replacement donation should not be abandoned since it is more efficient in small facilities where the collection of blood and inventory replenishment occurs at all times simultaneously with the BC delivery activity (10).

However, both systems have their own advantages and disadvantages (11). The VNRD system clearly favors intergroup solidarity (region and nation), while the replacement system favors intragroup solidarity (village or neighborhood, family, and work station). Complying with WHO recommendations and abandoning replacement donation should, if adopted, be scheduled progressively and strongly encouraged and supported by the national authorities.

The following two examples appear to illustrate this statement: (a) the first is the Lebanese experience (12). In this country, blood banking does indeed largely depend on replacement donors for several reasons: decentralized system, predominance of the private health-care sector over the public (i.e., a fragmented system) and the cultural habits of its inhabitants who are used to react in emergency situations (13). Recently, NGOs started taking initiatives to promote national solidarity and VNRD and have made considerable progress (14). However, this should be further encouraged by the national authorities who lack complete involvement (12) due to political issues. Meanwhile, should Lebanon encourage family replacement donors who meet all the classical criteria of VNRD to donate regularly? In fact, some authors consider these donors legitimate and indispensable (10, 15). (b) The second experience is the Moroccan one where VNRD is highly valued and where national authorities are fully involved under the blessing of the Royal Family. In fact, the Royal Family has been photographed while donating blood and their pictures are displayed in blood centers clearly to motivate donors and promote voluntary blood donation. Despite cultural similarities with Lebanon, Morocco, which is a centralized state, seems to be on the right track toward achieving 100% VNRD (the WHO target).

VNRD is recognized as the universal goal for all countries since it fully respects the ethical issues of donation; however, replacement donation might be regarded as ethically valuable and efficient in some cultures. In addition, some authors estimate that replacement donors are as safe as VNRD and less costly to health-care systems (16, 17).

In our opinion, an interesting but highly debatable strategy that can significantly alleviate the burden of transfusion-transmitted infections in endemic areas (i.e., Africa) is to establish financial contracts with "safe" donors (committed to safe behavior). However, such compensation would fall into the for-profit category according to the Nuffield Council on Bioethics (18), which raises two points: (a) The first is that this strategy is beneficial to patients in terms of supply and safety, as these donors ought to be at least as safe as or most probably safer than ordinary donors. (b) The second is related to ethical issues: are ethical values so inflexible, universal, and really independent from culture? This is perhaps debatable.

Emerging transfusion systems should also consider donor hemovigilance—set up over a decade after patient hemovigilance—especially when populations' iron stores are threatened by many local reasons such as ethnicity, nutritional aspects, and digestive parasitosis. Furthermore, the frequency of donations also has a strong impact on donor safety and the depletion of iron stores. Finally, the ethics of donation or collection is now regarded as a strong pillar of safety (19).

Thus, it would be an interesting option for each country to consider the establishment of a Blood Supply Committee to discuss the organization and ethical issues of blood supply according to local characteristics and constraints. This committee should comprise not only of professionals and authorities but also representatives from various branches of human and social sciences (economy, ethics, sociology, etc.), and other stakeholders.

BC Processing and Quality Management

The "B" leg of the transfusion stool encompasses the BCs and the quality management system. Nowadays, blood is collected, anticoagulated—which is a manipulation—and processed. Any BCs that are made available need to be defined (whole blood, red blood cell concentrates, plasma for therapeutic use, platelet components, etc.), along with their characteristics (volumes, active compounds with their minimum therapeutic levels, quality indicators, etc.). Furthermore, BCs can be either leukoreduced or not, and, if so, certain indicators must be defined such as date and time, pre- or post-storage (at bedside) leukoreduction and its efficacy, storage conditions (temperature), storage period, and expiry date. BC modifications such as irradiation, pathogen inactivation where available, volume reduction, washing, and splitting or pooling must be considered to define what is accepted by the system and what is not, and in which conditions. Quality indicators at all stages may be set up to monitor each part of the entire process (20).

Finally, testing of either the donor or the donated blood product is mandatory and not optional, but its extent and the decision tree upon biological findings may vary between systems. Indeed, no transfusion system can consider not testing donors for HIV, but not all HIV tests are equal nor are they confirmatory. Furthermore, some systems now retest previously donated BCs (using frozen plasma samples) in the event of positivity on the current donation.

However, not all systems allow the retrieval of historical samples. All of this depends on the organization, policy, and resources allocated to blood testing. An issue which is likely addressed in well-established systems is the definition of acceptance or rejection criteria for a given product (volume, quality, infectious safety level, extended blood grouping/phenotype, and residual leukocyte count to control or reduce inflammation). In fact, defining the infectious safety of a given BC (e.g., for a given virus) is a very difficult task. For example, is the residual risk of HIV-1 infection defined by less than 1 in 10^6 donations, considered within the acceptable range? This may be unacceptable in countries that control HIV transmission well (i.e., in Europe or the USA), but unachievable in countries with a high prevalence of HIV in their population such as Middle Africa (21). It is clearly not the responsibility of HBB or Blood Establishment (BE) professionals to define such criteria, but rather the national public health authorities.

Recipients (the Beneficiaries of BC Transfusions)

The "C" leg of the transfusion stool represents the recipients. Once the BC is qualified for issuing (and subsequently labeled), which is the main responsibility of the BE alongside the procurement of BCs that meet the demand, there remain a large number of tasks that the HBBs still have to perform, as they have to match the immunogenic and immunophenotypic characteristics of donor and recipient bloods. This is never a simple process in high-income countries and can be extremely difficult in low-income countries due to scarce resources: BCs in the inventory, resources to type and match bloods, etc. The financial burden of transfusions in high-income countries, where BC access was not restricted, has been extensive for decades with probable over-transfusion (22, 23). Those countries have now started to reduce unnecessary transfusions, implementing recommendations on Optimal Blood Use (OBU) and operating the so-called PBM programs (24, 25). Should low-income countries, where over-transfusion does not likely exist, start implementing PBM programs? And should they also apply OBU programs? We would be tempted to answer yes to both questions. In fact, both programs are aimed at improving the quality of medical services delivered to patients in need and reducing complications. Issuing recommendations that follow the general (universal) standards and are adapted to the actual situation of the country/system would be beneficial to both patients and the transfusion systems.

The major issue that developing countries face is the scarcity of surveillance and hemovigilance programs, with limited resources to recognize and report adverse reactions to implement improvement programs based on quality management. Another obstacle is the lack of evaluation of applicable or newly developed practices. Finally, hospital transfusion committees should be encouraged since they have proved to support transfusion safety in many places (26).

CONCLUDING REMARKS

All of the foregoing raises the question of whether Eastern/Southern Mediterranean countries can either comply with Western countries' guidelines and experiences or develop their own safety scheme based on proper sociopolitical and economic features. Another option (which does not necessarily contradict the previous ones) is to identify efficient and cost-effective strategies in neighboring countries that have had successful experiences and share similar cultural and economic features. To address this issue, and attempt to achieve this goal, we designed a number of surveys addressed specifically to Southern/Eastern Mediterranean countries that were sent out to national authorities when they existed, or to pre-identified blood banking specialists. So far, five surveys (comprising of 45 pages in total) have been produced and disseminated aimed at covering all aspects of blood activities [1—organization of the national transfusion service related to donors and staff; 2—prevention of infectious risks and prevalence of infectious diseases; 3—type, quantity, and specifications of produced blood products; 4—quality management system and the specifications of the environment of transfusion practices (education, vigilance, and invoicing); and 5—conditions of release and the use of blood and blood products] to collect and analyze data and standards. The surveys include series of questions tracking carefully all transfusion procedures that can be answered with a YES or NO and sometimes a box exists for some questions to place comments. All Southern/Eastern Mediterranean countries were targeted but only eight (Southern: Egypt, Morocco, Tunisia, Mauritania, and Algeria; Eastern: Lebanon, Jordan, and Palestine) responded to these surveys, which are currently being analyzed and validated before their communication. The preliminary results indicate that the organization of blood service in these countries is heterogeneous, as some countries have national systems and some others a decentralized organization; all countries nevertheless face similar challenges; to cite some: the blood supply relies mainly on replacement male donors; there is no clear strategy to secure the infectious safety of blood (and for instance no nuclear acid testing); there is not always an adequate quality management system; there is an evident lack of proper education; hemovigilance, when existing, is stammering, alongside all vigilances and surveillance processes. Some interesting experiences (e.g., universal leukoreduction in Lebanon, production of derived plasma products in Morocco, etc.) deserve to be highlighted and discussed regarding their outcomes and cost-effectiveness. It is anticipated that such a practice can help identify and then share the more successful and cost-effective experiences, and really focus on Mediterranean areas while not necessarily copying and pasting experiences designed for Western/Northern areas with significantly distinct situations in terms of donors, recipients, politics, economics, and even ethical and philosophical baseline.

AUTHOR CONTRIBUTIONS

AH and OG designed and wrote the paper. TA assisted with the writing and critical revision of the paper.

ACKNOWLEDGMENTS

AH is completing a PhD program at the University of Saint-Etienne and he wishes to acknowledge Association Recherche et Transfusion (Paris, France) for its support in the PETM/s (Program "Epidémiologie Transfusionnelle Méditerranéenne"/Sud) project, presented in part in this paper, and the association Les Amis de Rémi (Savigneux, France), together with the University of Lyon, Saint-Etienne.

REFERENCES

1. Saffi M, Howard N. Exploring the effectiveness of mandatory premarital screening and genetic counseling programmes for β-thalassaemia in the Middle East: a scoping review. *Public Health Genomics* (2015) 18:193–203. doi:10.1159/000430837
2. Amato A, Grisanti P, Mastropietro F, Lerone M, Cappabianca MP, Ponzini D, et al. Epidemiology and screening of sickle cell anemia in the Mediterranean area and in developing countries. *Ig Sanita Pubbl* (2014) 70:41–52.
3. Darbandi A, Mashati P, Yami A, Gharehbaghian A, Namini MT, Gharehbaghian A. Status of blood transfusion in World Health Organization-Eastern Mediterranean Region (WHO-EMR): successes and challenges. *Transfus Apher Sci* (2017) 56:448–53. doi:10.1016/j.transci.2017.04.003
4. Cheraghali AM. Blood safety concerns in the Eastern Mediterranean region. *Hepat Mon* (2011) 11:422–6.
5. World Health Organisation. *The Melbourne Declaration on 100% Voluntary Non-Remunerated Donation of Blood and Blood Components*. (2009). Available from:http://www.who.int/worldblooddonorday/MelbourneDeclarationWBDD09.pdf
6. World Health Organization, Regional Office for the Eastern Mediterranean. *Strategic Framework for Blood Safety and Availability 2016–2025*. (2016). Available from: http://www.who.int/iris/handle/10665/250402
7. World Health Organization. *Global Status Report on Blood Safety and Availability*. (2016). Available from: http://apps.who.int/iris/bitstream/10665/254987/1/9789241565431-eng.pdf
8. Roberts DJ, Field S, Delaney M, Bates I. Problems and approaches for blood transfusion in the developing countries. *Hematol Oncol Clin North Am* (2016) 30:477–95. doi:10.1016/j.hoc.2015.11.011
9. Kalargirou AA, Beloukas AI, Kosma AG, Nanou CI, Saridi MI, Kriebardis AG. Attitudes and behaviours of Greeks concerning blood donation: recruitment and retention campaigns should be focused on need rather than altruism. *Blood Transfus* (2014) 12:320–9. doi:10.2450/2014.0203-13
10. Allain JP, Sibinga CT. Family donors are critical and legitimate in developing countries. *Asian J Transfus Sci* (2016) 10:5–11. doi:10.4103/0973-6247.164270
11. Asenso-Mensah K, Achina G, Appiah R, Owusu-Ofori S, Allain JP. Can family or replacement blood donors become regular volunteer donors? *Transfusion* (2014) 54:797–804. doi:10.1111/trf.12216
12. Haddad A, Bou Assi T, Garraud O. Can a decentralized blood system ensure self-sufficiency and blood safety? The Lebanese experience. *J Public Health Policy* (2017) 38:359–65. doi:10.1057/s41271-017-0076-x
13. Samaha H, Irani-Hakimeh N, Hajj I. Disaster-preparedness plan at Saint George Hospital University Medical Center during the summer 2006 war and blockade on Lebanon. *Paper Presented at the XVII Regional Congress of the International Society of Blood Transfusion, 23 June 2007*. Madrid, Spain (2007).
14. Ceccaldi J, Thibert JB, Haddad A, Bouësseau MC, Pottier R, Danic B, et al. [Not-for-profit: a report from the fourth annual symposium of ethics held by the national institute for blood transfusion (France)]. *Transfus Clin Biol* (2017) 24:76–82. doi:10.1016/j.tracli.2017.04.003
15. Allain JP. Moving on from voluntary non-remunerated donors: who is the best blood donor? *Br J Haematol* (2011) 154:763–9. doi:10.1111/j.1365-2141.2011.08708.x
16. Allain JP, Sarkodie F, Asenso-Mensah K, Owusu-Ofori S. Relative safety of first-time volunteer and replacement donors in West Africa. *Transfusion* (2010) 50:340–3. doi:10.1111/j.1537-2995.2009.02444.x
17. Bates I, Manyasi G, Medina Lara A. Reducing replacement donors in Sub-Saharan Africa: challenges and affordability. *Transfus Med* (2007) 17:434–42. doi:10.1111/j.1365-3148.2007.00798.x
18. Nuffield Council on Bioethics. *Human Bodies: Donation for Medicine and Research*. (2011). Available from: http://nuffieldbioethics.org/wp-content/uploads/2014/07/Donation_full_report.pdf
19. Tissot JD, Garraud O. Ethics and blood donation: a marriage of convenience. *Presse Med* (2016) 45:e247–52. doi:10.1016/j.lpm.2016.06.016
20. The Council of Europe (EDQM). *Guide to the Preparation, Use and Quality Assurance of Blood Components*. (2017). Available from: https://www.edqm.eu/en/publications-transfusion-and-transplantation
21. Garraud O, Filho LA, Laperche S, Tayou-Tagny C, Pozzetto B. The infectious risks in blood transfusion as of today – a no black and white situation. *Presse Med* (2016) 45:e303–11. doi:10.1016/j.lpm.2016.06.022
22. Goodnough LT, Maggio P, Hadhazy E, Shieh L, Hernandez-Boussard T, Khari P, et al. Restrictive blood transfusion practices are associated with improved patient outcomes. *Transfusion* (2014) 54:2753–9. doi:10.1111/trf.12723
23. Politsmakher A, Doddapaneni V, Seeratan R, Dosik H. Effective reduction of blood product use in a community teaching hospital: when less is more. *Am J Med* (2013) 126:894–902. doi:10.1016/j.amjmed.2013.06.013
24. Spahn DR, Vamvakas EC. Is best transfusion practice alone best clinical practice? *Blood Transfus* (2013) 11:172–4. doi:10.2450/2012.0283-12
25. Schmidt AE, Refaai MA, Blumberg N. Past, present and forecast of transfusion medicine: what has changed and what is expected to change? *Presse Med* (2016) 45:e253–72. doi:10.1016/j.lpm.2016.06.017
26. Politis C, Wiersum JC, Richardson C, Robillard P, Jorgensen J, Renaudier P, et al. The international haemovigilance network database for the surveillance of adverse reactions and events in donors and recipients of blood components: technical issues and results. *Vox Sang* (2016) 111:409–17. doi:10.1111/vox.12447

11

Parvovirus B19: What Is the Relevance in Transfusion Medicine?

David Juhl* and Holger Hennig

Institute of Transfusion Medicine, University Hospital of Schleswig-Holstein, Lübeck, Germany

****Correspondence:***
David Juhl
david.juhl@uksh.de

Parvovirus B19 (B19V) has been discovered in 1975. The association with a disease was unclear in the first time after the discovery of B19V, but meanwhile, the usually droplet transmitted B19V is known as the infectious agent of the "fifth disease," a rather harmless children's illness. But B19V infects erythrocyte progenitor cells and thus, acute B19V infection in patients with a high erythrocyte turnover may lead to a life-threatening aplastic crisis, and acutely infected pregnant women can transmit B19V to their unborn child, resulting in a hydrops fetalis and fetal death. However, in many adults, B19V infection goes unnoticed and thus many blood donors donate blood despite the infection. The B19V infection does not impair the blood cell counts in healthy blood donors, but after the acute infection with extremely high DNA concentrations exceeding 10^{10} IU B19V DNA/ml plasma is resolved, B19V DNA persists in the plasma of blood donors at low levels for several years. That way, many consecutive donations that contain B19V DNA can be taken from a single donor, but the majority of blood products from donors with detectable B19V DNA seem not to be infectious for the recipients from several reasons: first, many recipients had undergone a B19V infection in the past and have formed protective antibodies. Second, B19V DNA concentration in the blood product is often too low to infect the recipient. Third, after the acute infection, the presence of B19V DNA in the donor is accompanied by presumably neutralizing antibodies which are protective also for the recipient of his blood products. Thus, transfusion-transmitted (TT-) B19V infections are very rarely reported. Moreover, in most blood donors, B19V DNA concentration is below 1,000 IU/ml plasma, and no TT-B19V infections have been found by such low-viremic donations. Cutoff for an assay for B19V DNA blood donor screening should, therefore, be approximately 1,000 IU/ml plasma, if a general screening of blood donors for single donation blood components is considered at all: for the overwhelming majority of transfusion recipients, B19V infection is not relevant as well as for the blood donors. B19V DNA screening of vulnerable patients after transfusion seems to be a more reasonable approach than general blood donor screening.

Keywords: parvovirus B19 infection, B19V, blood donors, transfusion-transmitted infection, blood donor screening

INTRODUCTION

Parvovirus B19 (B19V) has been described first in 1975: Cossard and colleagues (1) found "parvovirus-like particles" in the sera of nine blood donors and two patients. Meanwhile, these "parvovirus-like particles" are known to be B19V, a small, single-stranded DNA virus of approximately 5,500 nucleotides of which three different genotypes worldwide are existent. Genotype 1 is predominant worldwide, while genotype 2 is found only sporadically in Europe and the Americas. Genotype 3 seems to be widespread predominantly in north- and west-Africa (2). The diameter of B19V is between 19 and 25 nm, and it is a "bare" virus without any envelope. The icosahedral capsid consists of two structure proteins: VP1 and the smaller VP2 one. VP2 is the main protein in the capsid with a percentage of approximately 95% of the capsid while 5% of the capsid consists of VP1 (2, 3). The genome also encodes, besides for VP1 and VP2, for the non-structure protein NS1 which is essential for the replication of the viral DNA and responsible for the host cell apoptosis (4).

The tropism of B19V is very specific: B19V infects only cells with the blood group antigen P (globosid) on their surface (5). The antigen P is expressed on erythrocyte precursor cells and megakaryocytes as well as on endothelia cells, placental cells, and fetal myocardium.

Crucial for virus entry into the host cell is besides the P-antigen on the cell surface a distinct part of VP1, the unique amino-terminal region VP1u (6). The role of antibodies against epitopes on VP1 in the protection of erythrocyte progenitor cell and in the termination of the acute B19V infection underlines the importance of VP1 for the establishment of the infection by host cell entry (7, 8). Although B19V enters all cells with the antigen P, a productive infection with virus replication and the formation of progeny viruses happens only in erythrocyte progenitor cells, leading to the apoptosis of the infected cell.

However, many infections with B19V are asymptomatic or manifests only with mild of unspecific symptoms, flu-like symptoms, or arthralgia. The association of B19V with a disease was initially unclear (1) but only several years later, B19V could be linked to an exanthematous children's disease, the erythema infectiosum or fifth disease (9).

The ability to enter P-antigen expressing tissues, may explain the distinct clinical picture of B19V infection in some patient at risk for a more severe course of the infection: acute infection causes an affection of a large number of erythrocyte precursors with consecutive apoptosis. Mass apoptosis of these cells may lead to a short-time arrest of hematopoiesis and slight drop of the hemoglobin value (10) or the hematocrit, respectively, but due to the life span of red cells of approximately 140 days, severe anemia due B19V infection in patients without high erythrocyte turnover are rare and only single cases have been reported (11–13). However, in patients with increased red blood cell destruction resulting in high erythrocyte turnover and a shorter half-life of red cells from other reasons, e.g., hemolytic anemia or hemoglobinopathies, already the short-time hematopoetic arrest due to B19V infection can cause a life-threatening aplastic crisis (4).

Penetration of other cells with the P-antigen on their surface can induce some other clinical pictures of B19V infection: the typical rash during the erythema infectiosum may be a sign of the B19V infection of cutaneous endothelial cells, although a deposit of immune complexes, formed by antigen-bound antibodies is also a possible explanation.

In non-immune, antibody-negative pregnant women, B19V-infection can be transmitted *via* the placenta to the unborn child. In first-trimester pregnancies, transplacental infection of the fetus can lead to miscarriage, in the second or third trimester, infection of fetal erythrocyte precursor cells in the liver, which is the site of fetal haematopoesis, and infection of myocardial cells causes a severe fetal illness with anemia and myocardial failure, a clinical picture that is called hydrops fetalis.

After the experimental infection of otherwise healthy volunteer subjects, the course of the B19V infection was characterized in detail first in 1985 (14): B19V is naturally droplet transmitted by aerosol *via* the upper respiratory tract, and the infection of the volunteers in this study was thus performed by intranasal inoculation with B19V. Already few days after infection, B19V was detectable in the plasma of the infected volunteers, and virus levels reached a peak 6–10 days after infection was induced. In this acute stage of infection, viral DNA at a concentration of more than 10^{10} IU/ml (15) plasma is detectable, followed by IgM antibody formation which precedes the appearance of IgG antibodies about some days (14, 16). Individuals, in whom IgG antibodies against B19V are present, are considered to be immune against a new infection with any B19V genotype.

Due to the infection path *via* droplet transmission, many infections occur during childhood: while in infants at an age of below 5 years, in only 2% antibodies against B19V are detectable as a marker of a past infection, the percentage of antibody-positive infants increases with the age: between an age of 5 and 9, in 21% of infants antibodies against B19V are detectable and 36% in adolescents between 10 and 19 years. In 49% of adults, between an age of 20 and 39 years, antibodies against B19V were detectable in this study (17). In Germany, in 66.9% of the adolescents at an age of 18–19 years, antibodies against B19V are detectable, also indicating that many infections occur already during childhood. Overall 72.1% of the adults between 18 and 79 years in Germany tested positive for anti-B19V-IgG as a marker for an infection anytime in the past (18).

B19V INFECTION IN BLOOD DONORS

Seroprevalence of B19V in Blood Donors

As shown by Anderson et al. (14) and known for other viral infections, also infection with B19V is accompanied by the formation of B19V-specific IgG antibodies, which are detectable for many years or even lifelong. The rate of B19V IgG-positive blood donors, the seroprevalence, thus serves for the assessment of the rate of donors who have had a B19V infection at any time in the past. Data about the prevalence of antibodies against B19V are available from several countries (**Table 1**). The seroprevalence differed between 9.78 and 79.1% in the different countries, but not only geographical differences might led to the differing seroprevalence rates but also differences in the numbers of investigated donors as well as different sensitivities in the antibody tests that were used.

Data about the seroprevalence of B19V in German blood donors are lacking. However, the seroprevalence of B19V in blood donors is likely similar to that in the general adult population and can probably be transformed to the blood donor population: the seroprevalence of B19V in adults from the age of 18 years in Germany has been assessed to 72.1% and these individuals can be considered as probably immune against a B19V infection (18).

TABLE 1 | Seroprevalence, measured by anti-parvovirus B19 IgG determination, in blood donors.

Country	Seroprevalence (%)	No of investigated donors	Reference
Spain	9.78	92	(19)
India	27.96	1,633	(20)
Russia	29.70	1,000	(21)
Chile	55	400	(22)
Brazil	55.30	47	(23)
China	55.43	184	(24)
Brazil	60	100	(25)
Spain	64.70	136	(26)
Tunisia	65	378	(27)
Belgium	74	441	(27)
Italy	79.10	446	(28)

TABLE 2 | Prevalence of parvovirus B19 (B19V) DNA in blood donations.

Country	Prevalence of B19V DNA (%)	No of investigated donations	Pool size	Reference
UK	0.03	20,000	500	(31)
Japan	0.6	1,000	10	(32)
USA	0.1	9,568	50	(33)
Belgium	0.16	16,859	480	(34)
Portugal	0.12	5,025	10	(35)
Germany/Austria	0.013[a] and 0.26[a]	2.8 million	96	(36)
USA	0.88	5,020	Single donation	(37)
The Netherlands	0.006	6.5 million	480	(38)
Korea	0.1	10,032	24	(39)
China	0.58	3,957	Single donation	(40)
Brazil	1	100	Single donation	(25)
Germany	0.61	53,789	96	(41)
China	0.06[b]	5,040	96	(42)
	0.079[b]	5,030	96	
Brazil	1	91	Single donation	(43)

[a]*Prevalence of B19V DNA was assessed for high (>10⁶ IU B19V DNA/ml plasma) and low (<10⁶ IU B19V DNA/ml plasma) viremic donations.*

[b]*Prevalence data were assessed for source plasma and for whole blood donors separately.*

Prevalence of B19V DNA in Blood Donors

Provided that 72% (or slightly less) of all blood donors are immune against B19V due to the presence of antibodies formed by a B19V infection in the past, the remaining blood donors without detectable antibodies are susceptible for a B19V infection. As the acute infection is often asymptomatic, especially in adults, affected blood donors are often not apparently ill and hence are allowed to donate blood. That way, viremic donations can be taken and B19V DNA can be detected in the plasma by nucleic acid testing (NAT). In the last years, with the availability of international standards (29, 30), it became common, to express the viral load of a blood sample by the quantity of B19V DNA in "International Units per milliliter (IU/ml)" rather than genome equivalents with one international unit being approximately equivalent to 0.6–0.8 genome equivalents (29).

Several reports about the prevalence of B19V DNA in blood donors or blood donations, respectively, have been published in the past 15 years. Investigation of blood donations for B19V DNA showed that detection of B19V DNA in blood donations is not a rare event: Already in studies performed in the 1990s, in 0.03–0.6% of all blood donations, detection of B19V DNA was reported (31–33). An overview about the prevalence of B19V DNA in blood donations as well as the number of investigated donations and the pool size is provided in **Table 2**.

The early prevalence data from the 1990s could be confirmed by more recently published reports: B19V DNA was present in one out of 625 (or 0.16%) donations in Belgium between 1999 and 2000 (34). As in many studies dealing with the issue of B19V DNA in blood donations, the screening for B19V DNA in this study was performed by minipool-testing: That means, not each single donation is tested for B19V DNA, but several donations are brought and tested together by NAT.

In another study from the USA, 5,020 archived samples collected in the years 2000 and 2003, were investigated for B19V DNA. The prevalence was 0.88% (37) and considerably higher compared to a further study that was performed in the Netherlands (38) between 2003 and 2009: 6.5 million blood donations have been tested for B19V DNA. However, donations with a concentration of B19V DNA below 1×10^6 IU/ml plasma were not considered in the study. With the limitation that only donations with a high DNA concentration were considered, 411 out of the 6.5 million donations (or 0.006%) tested positive for B19V DNA.

In a Chinese study (40), 3,957 donor samples were screened for B19V DNA, 23 of those samples (0.58%) tested positive. In this study as well as in the study from the USA, only samples with lower DNA concentration had been detected (2.48×10^2–6.38×10^4 IU/ml and <20–1,869 IU/ml plasma), in contrast to the Dutch study. Acute B19V infections with high DNA concentrations seemed to be only shortly detectable, and thus, a large number of blood donations have to be screened for B19V DNA in order to detect a high viremic donation.

In another study from Austria and Germany (36), 2.8 million donations were screened for B19V DNA by minipools within 4 years. Minipools with a B19V DNA concentration $>10^5$ IU/ml were resolved to identify the high viremic donation and the positive donation was discarded, but minipools with a lower B19V DNA concentration were not resolved. That way, 12.7 positive donations per 100,000 donations (0.13%) with a high viral load ($>10^5$ IU/ml) were found and, presumably, 261.5 positive donations per 100,000 (0.26%) donations with a low ($<10^5$ IU/ml) viral load.

In a recent study (41) concerning the issue of B19V DNA in blood donations was performed also in Germany: 53,789 donations from overall 23,889 donors (first time and repeat blood donors) were screened for B19V DNA within 1 year. In 326 donations (0.61%), B19V DNA was detectable, in most cases at a low concentration. Only in eight donations, more than 10^5 IU B19V DNA/ml plasma were detectable.

Also the incidence as well as the prevalence of B19V DNA in blood donors were assessed in this study: 77/17,231 repeat blood donors were B19V DNA positive when tested first time during the study period and from 34/17,231 repeat blood donors, at least one negative sample were drawn, before they became infected during the study period. By these data, the prevalence of B19V DNA was calculated to be 0.45% and the annual incidence to be 0.20%.

The results of these studies are compatible with each other although a comparison of these studies is difficult due to differences in the size of the study population, the pool size [e.g., 480 donations in the Belgium study (34) vs 96 in the German/Austrian study (36) or vs single donation testing in the US study (37)] and use of different tests with a different analytical sensitivity for B19V DNA screening. Moreover, it is known that the occurrence of acute B19V infections follows a seasonal pattern, with many infections in spring and less or no infections in autumn (38). The point in time when a study was performed might, therefore, influence the prevalence of B19V DNA, especially if the study did not comprise the period of an entire year. It is also known, that in some years B19V epidemics occur, with a higher number of acute B19V infections in 1 year, while in other years only few B19V infections happen (38, 44).

COURSE OF THE B19V INFECTION IN BLOOD DONORS

Clinical Course

At present, there are no studies available which investigated systematically the clinical picture of the B19V infection in blood donors. However, in many otherwise healthy individuals like blood donors, the infection often goes unnoticed or presents with only mild or unspecific symptoms. One can assume that B19V infections in blood donors demonstrate a likewise course and from that reason, many B19V-infected blood donors appear to donate and are allowed to donate in the absence of any signs of disease.

Hematological Course

As B19V affects erythrocyte precursor cells and megakaryocytes, a change in the hematological parameter (hemoglobin and platelets) could be expected in blood donors and was already described after the experimental infection of a low number of otherwise healthy individuals (14). The relation between B19V infection and blood count in blood donors has been investigated in one study in Germany (41): blood counts of 345 samples with detectable B19V DNA were compared to 100 B19V DNA-negative controls. While no differences in the quantity of leukocytes, erythrocytes, and platelets were observed, the mean hemoglobin value, the hematocrit, the mean corpuscular volume, the mean cellular hemoglobin value, and the mean hemoglobine concentration of the 345 B19V DNA-positive samples were statistical significant lower than the 100 controls. However, although statistical significant, the differences were only moderate and without any clinical relevance. Also, in the context of acute B19V infection with high DNA concentration, no major differences in the blood count could be observed in comparison to controls or to the B19V DNA-negative samples of the same donors which were drawn before the B19V infection.

Course of the Viremia

The course of the viremia during B19V infection in blood donors is well investigated. The results of the first study, which investigated the course of the viremia after the infection, led to the conclusion that viremia is rapidly cleared in acutely infected, not immune compromised individuals (14). However, the method used to detect B19V DNA (dot-plot hybridization) was less sensitive compared to the methods that are currently used in the blood donor screening, but such a sensitive method was not available at that time. Especially in recent studies, the concentration of B19V DNA, measured in the plasma by NAT, serves as parameter for the level of the viremia of blood donors. And despite the use of more sensitive methods for the detection of B19V DNA, until the beginning of the last decade, the viremia in the acute B19V infection was considered as a rather short phenomenon, lasting only for several weeks (45, 46). The duration of viremia in blood donors has been estimated to be 17.5 days (95% CI 11.0–53.0) (47). The persistence of the virus or chronic infections were considered as extremely rare (48) and a longlasting viremia as a phenomenon that is limited to more severely ill and immunocompromised individuals rather than blood donors, although the data of Jordan and colleagues (33) already suggested that a longer period of viremia might be possible: at least one of the 11 B19V DNA-positive donors in this study was tested positive again during a follow-up investigation performed over 5 months later.

Compatible with this observation were the results of a longitudinal study from France (49): 76 patients who suffered from hemoglobinopathies, and were thus, like blood donors, not immunocompromised, have been followed up for several years. In six of these patients, persistence of B19V DNA at low levels (10–100 IU B19V DNA/ml plasma) for several years (up to 60 months) was determined. Also in a Japanese study, 20 B19V DNA-positive blood donors were followed up for several years and investigated for B19V DNA biannual. A decline of the B19V DNA concentration was found to be below 10^4 IU B19V DNA/ml plasma after 1 year and 10^3 IU/ml plasma after 2 years, subsequently, B19V DNA concentration persisted between 10^3 and 10^1 IU B19V DNA/ml plasma in the third and fourth year (50). In a German-Austrian Study (36), a rapid decline in the median B19V DNA concentration from 4.85×10^7 to 4.6×10^2 IU/ml within approximately 12 weeks was observed. Another study (51) investigated the duration of B19 viremia in 75 blood donors, in whom several consecutive samples could be investigated during 5.5 years. In this period, only in a minority of blood donors, the entire duration of viremia could be assessed, as the last B19V DNA-negative sample before infection *and* a B19V DNA-negative sample after the infection became available, indicating a long duration of viremia. However, the mean interval between drawing the first positive sample and the last positive samples in the study period was 21.5 months (range: 2.3–52.4 months; 95% CI: 19.1–23.9 months). Compatible with the rapid decline of B19V DNA concentration in the former studies (36, 41), a rapid decline of the B19V DNA concentration from a mean value of 2.23×10^8 IU B19V DNA/ml plasma (95% CI: 0–6.48×10^8 IU/ml plasma) to a mean value of 1,598 IU B19V DNA/ml plasma (95% CI: 1,157–2,039 IU/ml plasma) was assessed between the first B19V DNA-positive sample and the second sample, which has been taken after a mean time of 135.8 days later. B19V DNA then persisted in the donors who could be investigated for a longer period, for several years at low (10^2–10^3 IU/ml plasma) or very low levels (<10^2 IU/ml plasma).

Persistence of B19V DNA has been proven (52–54) in several tissues (e.g., liver, heart, tonsils, synovia) and it has been suggested that, after acute infection, possibly bare B19V DNA, and *not* mature virions, are released from these tissues into the plasma (53, 55). A recent study provided evidence that the positive detection of B19V DNA in the plasma of blood donors approximately 6 months after acute infection is based on bare DNA strands and not on mature, infectious virions. These DNA strands may persist for years after the acute infection (56). Based on this assumption, most of the B19V DNA-positive donations, namely those with low DNA concentrations, might not be infectious for the recipients and the persistence of B19V DNA in blood donors after the decrease of the peak B19V DNA concentration might be irrelevant.

Humoral Immune Response in B19V-Infected Donors

The humoral immune response in the B19V infection in blood donors has already been studied thoroughly and might influence the assessment of the importance in Transfusion Medicine. Already Anderson and colleagues (14) observed the typical antibody response in experimentally infected individuals with formation of anti-B19V IgM in the second week after infection, followed by the formation of anti-B19V IgG few days later. However, the epitope specificity (anti-NS1, anti-VP1, anti-VP2) of these antibodies was not reported.

Early studies on blood donors reported the prevalence of IgG and IgM antibodies in B19V DNA-positive blood donors: in the Netherlands (38), a subgroup of 67 out 411 B19V DNA-positive blood donors was investigated for antibodies of both classes. In 47 (70%) of the B19V DNA-positive donors, no antibodies against B19V were detected, neither of the IgM nor of the IgG class. 16 (24%) donors tested positive for anti-B19 IgM, and 4 (6%) tested positive for IgG *and* IgM. A further characterization of these antibodies was not performed and the findings of this study (no antibodies or predominant IgM detectable) are compatible with acute B19V infections in the investigated blood donors and not with longlasting infections. A German-Austrian study (36) was the first, which investigated the course of the humoral immune response in relation to the B19V DNA concentration by investigation of follow-up samples from 50 B19V-infected donors. IgG antibodies against epitopes on the viral capsids (VP1, VP2) were detectable in approximately one-third of the donors in the first sample, which has been taken during the acute infection. Already in the first follow-up sample, taken 12 weeks thereafter, in all of the donors, IgG antibodies against epitopes on the viral capsid, were detectable. These antibodies were also detectable in a second follow-up sample. As these IgG antibodies were directed against epitopes on the virus surface (VP1 and VP2), it can be hypothesized that these antibodies are able to neutralize the virions by hindering their binding to the cellular receptor on the target cells for B19V. This assumption was corroborated by another experiment in this study: samples with high B19V DNA concentrations and with low B19V DNA concentrations were filtered through a protein G column. Afterward, the DNA concentration was assessed again, and the reduction of B19V DNA after protein G filtration was significantly higher in samples with low DNA concentration compared to those samples with high DNA concentration. This finding indicated the presence of strong binding, high avide IgG antibodies on the surface of B19V, leading to clearance of B19V in the sample by adsorption of IgG-binded virions to the protein G *via* the Fc-fragment of the IgG.

In another study from Germany (51), the humoral immune response in 75 B19V-infected blood donors was investigated, 29 of them had an acute B19V infection during the study period, in the remaining donors, the infection occurred before the study period. Overall 410 samples with detectable B19V DNA have been provided by these donors within 5.5 years and could be considered in the study. That way, the course of B19V infection in blood donors could be studied over a longer period. Besides B19V DNA, samples were investigated for anti-B19V IgM, quantitative for anti-B19V IgG, and the avidity of anti-B19V IgG antibodies was determined. In only six samples with high B19V DNA concentrations, no anti-B19V IgG was detectable. The decrease of B19V DNA concentration was accompanied by an increase of the anti-B19V IgG titer, compatible with the findings of another study (41). Out of 29 donors with an acute, recently acquired B19V infection, in 24 (82.8%) already IgG antibodies, directed against epitopes on VP1 and VP2 with high avidity, were detectable. In five donors, no IgG antibodies against B19V were detectable in the first B19V DNA-positive donation, but at the point in time, when the next follow-up samples was drawn from these donors, also anti-B19V IgG with high avidity, directed against viral capsid proteins, were detectable. The study could also demonstrate that detection of anti-B19V IgM is not a suitable marker for the acute B19V infection as B19V IgM could not be detected in many donors during the acute infection.

TRANSFUSION-TRANSMITTED (TT-) B19V INFECTION BY BLOOD PRODUCTS, IN PARTICULAR BY SINGLE DONATION BLOOD PRODUCTS

Data suggesting a B19V transmission by plasma derivates are available since the 1990s (57, 58). Due to its physicochemical properties, B19V is hard to inactivate or to remove by processes used for other viruses during the manufacturing process of plasma derivatives. In addition, because of the prevalence of B19V DNA among blood donors, the entering of a donation with high DNA concentration in a plasma pool for fractionation is not a rare event, leading to the contamination of the plasma pool from several thousand donations. Thus, it is not astonishing that in a large number of plasma pools for fractionation, B19V DNA is detectable, when untested donations are entering in a pool (59) and that many TT-B19V infections by plasma derivatives have been reported in the past (57). To avoid further manufacturing of such plasma pools, B19V DNA testing of plasma pools or plasma units for fractionation is recommended by the Food and

Drug Administration. The B19V DNA concentration should not exceed 10^4 IU B19V DNA/ml plasma,[1] a level that is considered as the maximum acceptable in plasma pools for fractionation. Nevertheless, there is further evidence for a B19V transmission by plasma derivatives despite the exclusion of plasma donations or plasma pools with high B19V DNA concentration for fractionation (60).

Measures to avoid potential B19V transmission by single donation blood products have not been established so far in many countries, although the first cases of TT-B19V infection were reported also in 1990s (61, 62). Despite the frequent detection of B19V DNA in blood donors, suspected TT-B19V infections are rarely reported in Germany, a country in which several millions of transfusions are carried out annually.[2] If a case of viral transmission by transfusions is suspected in Germany, the German authority has to be informed according to the German transfusion act. However, the publications of this authority in which suspected cases of TT infection were reported during the period from 1997 to 2012, included no cases of suspected TT-B19V infection.[3,4] In 2013, seven B19 infections in a donor and two in 2014 were reported, but infection of these donors never led to a transmission to the recipients of their blood components and no suspected cases of a TT-B19V infection due to an overt infection in a recipient of single-donor blood components was reported to the German authority by a treating physician.[5] TT-B19V infections hence seem to be either a rare event or with a low clinical relevance, so that many infections are overlooked by the treating physicians. Also data reported to the Serious Hazard Of Transfusion (SHOT-) registry in the UK support this assumption: only one case of major morbidity due to a TT-B19V infection has been reported to SHOT between 1996 and 2016 (63).

Initially, only blood products provided from donors with high B19V DNA concentrations seemed to be infectious for their recipients. In a study from the USA, a fourfold increase in the IgG antibody titer in an already anti-IgG antibody-positive recipient of a red blood cell concentrate from a donor with 2.9×10^{10} IU B19V DNA/ml plasma was detected. The authors interpreted their finding as an anamnestic immune response, triggered by a TT-B19V infection through the red blood cell concentrate (15), but they detected no TT-B19V infection through blood products with a B19V DNA concentration of less than 10^6 IU/ml plasma and concluded, that transmission with blood components from donors with a lower B19V DNA concentration do either not occur or are at least a rare event. Shortly later, a TT-B19V infection in a susceptible, antibody-negative recipient by a red blood cell concentrate from an antibody-negative donor with an acute B19V infection was reported. The B19V DNA concentration in the donor's plasma was 5×10^9 IU/ml, the genome of the B19V of the donor and the recipient shared 100% of their sequences, making the red blood cell concentrate as the origin of infection very probable (64).

However, the threshold DNA concentration in blood donors that was considered as being infectious for the recipients of their single donation blood products decreased more and more in the following years. Already in the year 2011, it could be demonstrated that red blood cell concentrates from B19V-infected donors with DNA concentration of 10^5 IU/ml plasma are probably able to transmit B19V by their donation: after transfusion of red blood cell concentrates from nine out of 18 donors with a DNA concentration of 10^5 IU B19V DNA/ml plasma or more, an infection in the recipients occurred, but no TT-B19V infection was observed after transfusion of red blood cell concentrates from donors with less than 10^5 IU B19V DNA/ml plasma. In this study, phylogenetic analysis of B19V in the donors and the infected recipients yielded the blood products as the probable origin of infection (65). In donors with lower B19V DNA concentration ($<10^5$ IU/ml plasma) without transmission of B19V infections to the recipients, a higher proportion of probably neutralizing antibodies was detectable. Besides the lower DNA concentration, the presence of such antibodies might also be protective for the recipients of the blood products. But already in the same years, transmissions of B19V infections through blood donations from donors with still lower DNA concentrations were reported: In a Japanese study (66), a TT-B19V infection through a red blood cell concentrate provided by a donor with a B19V DNA concentration of 5.1×10^3 IU B19V DNA/ml plasma and proved by genome sequence analysis, occurred. Also IgG and IgM antibodies were detectable in the donor's plasma, demonstrating that antibodies in the donor are not always protective for the recipient of his blood products. Although a further probable TT-B19V infection after transfusion of a red blood cell concentrate from a donor with low ($10^{3.2}$ IU B19V DNA/ml plasma) DNA concentration and *with* detectable B19V IgG antibodies was reported (67), single donation blood products with such a low B19V DNA concentration, seem not to be infective in either case: no TT-B19V infections have been observed after transfusion of 15 single donation blood products (eight red blood cell concentrates, four pooled platelet concentrates, and three fresh frozen plasma) from donors with a B19V DNA concentration between 10^3 and 10^4 IU B19V DNA/ml plasma (68).

In the latest report of a TT-B19V infection, a red blood cell concentrate taken from a donor with a B19V DNA concentration of 1.1×10^4 B19V DNA/ml plasma was the probable source of the infection. The B19V infection of the recipient has been accompanied by an immune thrombocytopenia (69).

It is noteworthy that, in only three of the recent studies, the symptomatology of the transfusion recipient finally led to the investigation of the donor: in one Japanese study (66), the infections in the recipients became evident due to more or less serious, miscellaneous symptoms like reticulocytopenia, delayed recovery of red blood cells after chemotherapy or pure red cell aplasia, and also rash or febrile disease. In France (67), a recipient suffered from erythroblastopenia after transfusion of a red blood

[1] https://www.fda.gov/downloads/BiologicsBloodVaccines/GuidanceCompliance RegulatoryInformation/Guidances/Blood/ucm078510.pdf.

[2] http://www.pei.de/DE/infos/meldepflichtige/meldung-blutprodukte-21-transfusionsgesetz/berichte/berichte-21tfg-node.html.

[3] http://www.pei.de/SharedDocs/Downloads/vigilanz/haemovigilanz/publikationen/haemovigillanz-bericht-1997-2008.pdf;jsessionid=734FDB0D86C7B79C8E95E0E9AE86EF2F.1_cid329?__blob=publicationFile&v=1.

[4] http://www.pei.de/SharedDocs/Downloads/vigilanz/haemovigilanz/publikationen/haemovigilanz-bericht-2011.pdf?__blob=publicationFile&v=6.

[5] http://www.pei.de/SharedDocs/Downloads/vigilanz/haemovigilanz/publikationen/haemovigilanz-bericht-2013-2014.pdf?__blob=publicationFile&v=4.

cell concentrate due to sickle cell disease, and in Japan again, fever and thrombocytopenia led to the diagnosis of B19V infection (69). In the other studies (15, 64, 65, 68), positive screening of blood donors for B19V DNA induced the retrospective investigation of the recipients of their blood products, in whom no B19V infection had been suspected so far. Retrospective analysis of the red blood cell counts in one study (68) revealed a slight drop of the hemoglobin values in the two infected recipients after transfusion of red blood cell concentrate. However, the slight decrease of the hemoglobin level might also be attributed to other reasons like allogeneic blood stem cell transplantation, or iatrogen due to excessive blood sample withdrawal. No specific symptoms were specified later by the affected recipients in another study (66) and no symptoms in the recipients have been reported in two further studies (64, 65).

CONCLUSION: WHAT IS THE RELEVANCE OF B19V IN TRANSFUSION MEDICINE AND WHAT CAN BE DONE?

Approximately 30% of the potential blood donors starting at an age of 18 years have no antibodies against B19V and are thus susceptible for new B19V infections. And as B19V infection often go unnoticed especially in adults, B19V-infected donors cannot be recognized by clinical symptoms or evident aberrances in the blood count and are, therefore, allowed to donate. From that reasons, detection of B19V DNA in blood donations is not a rare finding, at least in comparison to other transfusion-transmissible viral agents like HIV, HCV, and HBV. Unlike suggested in the past, B19 viremia after the acute infection is not a short phenomenon limited to several days or weeks, but persistence of B19V DNA for months to years, also in otherwise healthy blood donors, seems to be the norm rather than the exception and that way, multiple consecutive B19V DNA-positive donations can be taken even from a single donor. However, high DNA concentrations indicates peak viremia in the acute infection, but shortly after the acute infection DNA concentration decreases rapidly, accompanied by formation of potentially neutralizing IgG antibodies.

That TT-B19V infections are seldom reported by treating physicians may serve as an indication of the minor relevance of B19V for the transfusion of single donation blood components, either because they do not occur at all or because of their missing clinical consequences. In many reports, dealing with the issue of TT-B19V infection, only the detection of B19V DNA in the donor induced the investigation of the usually asymptomatic recipient of the blood products, and it was not a symptomatic transfusion recipient who was the cause for the investigation of a donor for a B19V infection. This could indicate that the overwhelming majority of TT-B19V infections (if they occur at all) are overlooked by the treating physicians either due to missing or only mild and unspecific symptoms and only single cases of TT-B19V infections with severe consequences were reported (66, 67, 69).

To avoid TT-B19V infections, several measures have been proposed: In Japan, screening for B19V is performed by hemagglutination assay to avoid donations with high viral load entering a plasma pool for fractionation (66, 70). However, the method is less sensitive, detects only donations with a very high viral load and, therefore, more suitable to detect plasma donation that should not enter a plasma pool for fractionation due to their high B19 viral load. As many single donations with lower viral loads and thus the potential to transmit B19V to recipient are overlooked by this assay, the performance in blood donor screening for single donation blood products is not reasonable.

The most efficient method to avoid TT-B19V infections is a general blood donor screening for B19V DNA by NAT. This can be also done by minipools, in which multiple donations are brought together for NAT screening. Screening assays nowadays have a sufficient sensitivity (36, 71, 72) to reliably detect donations even with minimal amounts of B19V DNA. On the basis of the current knowledge, maximal security in terms of avoiding a TT-B19V infection is provided, if the sensitivity of the assay is sufficient to detect a single donation with a B19V DNA concentration of 10^3 IU B19V DNA/ml plasma.

In contrast to NAT screening of blood donations, anti-B19V IgM screening is not suitable to detect blood donations at risk for the transmission of a B19V infection: although IgM is generally regarded as formed during the acute B19V infection, IgM antibodies are not always detectable during the peak viremia in the acute infection stage (51). Reasons might be a pre-seroconversion acute infection when B19V DNA precedes the antibody formation or the disappearance of IgM antibodies during the Ig-class switch.

Another, antibody testing-based strategy for providing "B19V safe" single donation blood components has been proposed in the Netherlands (73): single-donor blood components can be considered as "B19V safe" if they are donated from donors, in whom anti-B19V IgG has been detected in two separate samples, taken after an interval of at least 6 months. And although B19V DNA is usually detectable over a longer period than 6 months after seroconversion (unlike believed at that time), the measured concentration is low, the detection of B19V DNA is probably based on bare DNA strands and, moreover, B19V DNA accompanied by the presence of protective antibodies in at least all donors with ongoing B19V infection. This approach warrants more protection against TT-B19V infection by single-donor blood products. However, anti-B19V IgG testing, preferably fully automated, is required just as an efficient algorithm, which warrants anti-B19V IgG testing after 6 months and then the declaration of single donation blood products as "B19V safe."

Besides donor screening for B19V DNA, inactivation or removal by the virions is applied during the manufacturing process for plasma derivates. Measures like pasteurization or treatment with low pH were effective in the elimination of B19V (74) as well as nanofiltration (75) and an additional gain of security concerning the transmission B19V by plasma derivatives can be expected.

Some data are currently available concerning the effectiveness of pathogen reduction technologies like the amotosalen/UVA treatment or the riboflavin/UV-light treatment of cellular blood products in the inactivation of B19V. By such treatment, a considerably reduction of human or porcine B19V has been reported (76). However, a possible transmission of B19V by an amotosalen/UVA treated pooled platelet concentrate has been also reported recently (77), making a final conclusion about the effectiveness of pathogen inactivation of B19V in cellular blood products currently difficult.

Whether a general screening for B19V DNA or implementation of other measures for providing "B19V safe" single donation blood components is meaningful should be debated thoroughly. According to current knowledge, B19V seems to be of minor relevance in the administration of single-donor blood components. Symptomatic TT-B19V infection are very rarely reported by clinicians. This may be because they rarely occur for donor reasons: the viral load, if mature virions are present at all in the donor, is too low and/or circulating virions are neutralized by coexisting anti-B19V IgG antibodies with specificity for VP1, protecting the recipient against the infection. Also patient reasons are possible: the seroprevalence in the patient population is comparable to that of the general population. This means that approximately 70% of the transfusion recipients have antibodies against B19V and are probably immune. Another explanation is that TT-B19V infections occur, but are overlooked by the treating physician because they do not have any clinical relevance.

Unlike other transfusion-transmissible viruses (e.g., HBV, HCV, HIV), B19V infections can be well treated, e.g., by transfusion of further red blood cells or by administration of i.v. IgG, and thereby major consequences of TT-B19V infections can be prevented. Moreover, HBV, HCV, and HIV pose a threat for a majority or almost all transfusion recipients and cannot or hardly be community acquired, in contrast to B19V, which is droplet-transmissible but against which already 70% of transfusion recipients are immune.

Hence, another approach than a general blood donor screening to protect recipients for TT-B19V infection is to generate awareness in clinicians for the possibility of TT-B19V infections. Distinct susceptible patient groups for a more severe course of a potential B19V infection (e.g., pregnant women, immunosupressed patients, patients with high erythrocyte turnover) should be investigated thoroughly for symptoms of a B19V infection after transfusion and also performance of a B19V NAT screening in the patient can be considered. In this way, not only rarely occurring TT-B19V infections but also the presumably more frequently occurring community-acquired B19V infections can be detected.

AUTHOR CONTRIBUTIONS

DJ and HH reviewed the literature and wrote the manuscript.

REFERENCES

1. Cossart YE, Field AM, Cant B, Widdows D. Parvovirus-like particles in human sera. *Lancet* (1975) 1(7898):72–3. doi:10.1016/S0140-6736(75)91074-0
2. Blümel J, Burger R, Drosten C, Gröner A, Gürtler L, Heiden M, et al. Parvovirus B19 – revised. *Transfus Med Hemother* (2010) 37(6):339–50. doi:10.1159/000322190
3. Servant-Delmas A, Lefrère JJ, Morinet F, Pillet S. Advances in human B19 erythrovirus biology. *J Virol* (2010) 84(19):9658–65. doi:10.1128/JVI.00684-10
4. Young NS, Brown KE. Parvovirus B19. *N Engl J Med* (2004) 350(6):586–97. doi:10.1056/NEJMra030840
5. Brown KE, Anderson SM, Young NS. Erythrocyte P antigen: cellular receptor for B19 parvovirus. *Science* (1993) 262(5130):114–7. doi:10.1126/science.8211117
6. Zádori Z, Szelei J, Lacoste MC, Li Y, Gariépy S, Raymond P, et al. A viral phospholipase A2 is required for parvovirus infectivity. *Dev Cell* (2001) 1(2):291–302. doi:10.1016/S1534-5807(01)00031-4
7. Bansal GP, Hatfield JA, Dunn FE, Kramer AA, Brady F, Riggin CH, et al. Candidate recombinant vaccine for human B19 parvovirus. *J Infect Dis* (1993) 167(5):1034–44. doi:10.1093/infdis/167.5.1034
8. Saikawa T, Anderson S, Momoeda M, Kajigaya S, Young NS. Neutralizing linear epitopes of B19 parvovirus cluster in the VP1 unique and VP1-VP2 junction regions. *J Virol* (1993) 67(6):3004–9.
9. Anderson MJ, Jones SE, Fisher-Hoch SP, Lewis E, Hall SM, Bartlett CL, et al. Human parvovirus, the cause of erythema infectiosum (fifth disease)? *Lancet* (1983) 1(8338):1378. doi:10.1016/S0140-6736(83)92152-9
10. Potter CG, Potter AC, Hatton CS, Chapel HM, Anderson MJ, Pattison JR, et al. Variation of erythroid and myeloid precursors in the marrow and peripheral blood of volunteer subjects infected with human parvovirus (B19). *J Clin Invest* (1987) 79(5):1486–92. doi:10.1172/JCI112978
11. Osaki M, Matsubara K, Iwasaki T, Kurata T, Nigami H, Harigaya H, et al. Severe aplastic anemia associated with human parvovirus B19 infection in a patient without underlying disease. *Ann Hematol* (1999) 78(2):83–6. doi:10.1007/s002770050477
12. Qian XH, Zhang GC, Jiao XY, Zheng YJ, Cao YH, Xu DL, et al. Aplastic anaemia associated with parvovirus B19 infection. *Arch Dis Child* (2002) 87(5):436–7. doi:10.1136/adc.87.5.436
13. Ideguchi H, Ohno S, Ishigatsubo Y. A case of pure red cell aplasia and systemic lupus erythematosus caused by human parvovirus B19 infection. *Rheumatol Int* (2007) 27(4):411–4. doi:10.1007/s00296-006-0227-z
14. Anderson MJ, Higgins PG, Davis LR, Willman JS, Jones SE, Kidd IM, et al. Experimental parvoviral infection in humans. *J Infect Dis* (1985) 152(2): 257–65. doi:10.1093/infdis/152.2.257
15. Kleinman SH, Glynn SA, Lee TH, Tobler LH, Schlumpf KS, Todd DS, et al. A linked donor-recipient study to evaluate parvovirus B19 transmission by blood component transfusion. *Blood* (2009) 114(17):3677–83. doi:10.1182/blood-2009-06-225706
16. Klein HG. Transfused B19V: B-nign, B-ware, B-gone? *Blood* (2009) 114(17):3509–11. doi:10.1182/blood-2009-09-239939
17. Anderson LJ, Tsou C, Parker RA, Chorba TL, Wulff H, Tattersall P, et al. Detection of antibodies and antigens of human parvovirus B19 by enzyme-linked immunosorbent assay. *J Clin Microbiol* (1986) 24(4): 522–6.
18. Röhrer C, Gärtner B, Sauerbrei A, Böhm S, Hottenträger B, Raab U, et al. Seroprevalence of parvovirus B19 in the German population. *Epidemiol Infect* (2008) 136(11):1564–75. doi:10.1017/S0950268807009958
19. Mata Rebón M, Bartolomé Husson C, Bernárdez Hermida I. Seroprevalence of anti-human parvovirus B19 antibodies in a sample of blood donors in Galicia. *Enferm Infecc Microbiol Clin* (1998) 16(1):25–7.
20. Kumar S, Gupta RM, Sen S, Sarkar RS, Philip J, Kotwal A, et al. Seroprevalence of human parvovirus B19 in healthy blood donors. *Med J Armed Forces India* (2013) 69(3):268–72. doi:10.1016/j.mjafi.2012.11.009
21. Filatova EV, Zubkova NV, Novikova NA, Golitsina LN, Kuznetsov KV. Detection of parvovirus B19 markers in blood samples of donors. *Zh Mikrobiol Epidemiol Immunobiol* (2010) 5:67–70.
22. Gaggero A, Rivera J, Calquín E, Larrañaga CE, León O, Díaz P, et al. Seroprevalence of IgG antibodies against parvovirus B19 among blood donors from Santiago, Chile. *Rev Med Chil* (2007) 135(4):443–8.
23. Slavov SN, Kashima S, Silva-Pinto AC, Covas DT. Genotyping of human parvovirus B19 among Brazilian patients with hemoglobinopathies. *Can J Microbiol* (2012) 58(2):200–5. doi:10.1139/w11-119
24. Wei Q, Li Y, Wang JW, Wang H, Qu JG, Hung T. Prevalence of anti-human parvovirus B19 IgG antibody among blood donors in Jilin province. *Zhonghua Shi Yan He Lin Chuang Bing Du Xue Za Zhi* (2006) 20(2):60–2.

25. Slavov SN, Haddad SK, Silva-Pinto AC, Amarilla AA, Alfonso HL, Aquino VH, et al. Molecular and phylogenetic analyses of human parvovirus B19 isolated from Brazilian patients with sickle cell disease and β-thalassemia major and healthy blood donors. *J Med Virol* (2012) 84(10):1652–65. doi:10.1002/jmv.23358
26. Muñoz S, Alonso MA, Fernández MJ, Muñoz JL, García-Rodríguez JA. Seroprevalence versus parvovirus B19 in blood donors. *Enferm Infecc Microbiol Clin* (1998) 16(4):161–2.
27. Letaïef M, Vanham G, Boukef K, Yacoub S, Muylle L, Mertens G. Higher prevalence of parvovirus B19 in Belgian as compared to Tunisian blood donors: differential implications for prevention of transfusional transmission. *Transfus Sci* (1997) 18(4):523–30. doi:10.1016/S0955-3886(97)00049-0
28. Manaresi E, Gallinella G, Morselli Labate AM, Zucchelli P, Zaccarelli D, Ambretti S, et al. Seroprevalence of IgG against conformational and linear capsid antigens of parvovirus B19 in Italian blood donors. *Epidemiol Infect* (2004) 132(5):857–62. doi:10.1017/S0950268804002389
29. Saldanha J, Lelie N, Yu MW, Heath A; B19 Collaborative Study Group. Establishment of the first World Health Organization International Standard for human parvovirus B19 DNA nucleic acid amplification techniques. *Vox Sang* (2002) 82(1):24–31. doi:10.1046/j.1423-0410.2002.00132.x
30. Baylis SA, Chudy M, Blümel J, Pisani G, Candotti D, José M, et al. Collaborative study to establish a replacement World Health Organization International Standard for parvovirus B19 DNA nucleic acid amplification technology (NAT)-based assays. *Vox Sang* (2010) 98(3):441–6. doi:10.1111/j.1423-0410.2009.01288.x
31. McOmish F, Yap PL, Jordan A, Hart H, Cohen BJ, Simmonds P. Detection of parvovirus B19 in donated blood: a model system for screening by polymerase chain reaction. *J Clin Microbiol* (1993) 31(2):323–8.
32. Yoto Y, Kudoh T, Haseyama K, Suzuki N, Oda T, Katoh T, et al. Incidence of human parvovirus B19 DNA detection in blood donors. *Br J Haematol* (1995) 91(4):1017–8. doi:10.1111/j.1365-2141.1995.tb05427.x
33. Jordan J, Tiangco B, Kiss J, Koch W. Human parvovirus B19: prevalence of viral DNA in volunteer blood donors and clinical outcomes of transfusion recipients. *Vox Sang* (1998) 75(2):97–102. doi:10.1046/j.1423-0410.1998.7520097.x
34. Thomas I, Di Giambattista M, Gérard C, Mathys E, Hougardy V, Latour B, et al. Prevalence of human erythrovirus B19 DNA in healthy Belgian blood donors and correlation with specific antibodies against structural and non-structural viral proteins. *Vox Sang* (2003) 84(4):300–7. doi:10.1046/j.1423-0410.2003.00299.x
35. Henriques I, Monteiro F, Meireles E, Cruz A, Tavares G, Ferreira M, et al. Prevalence of parvovirus B19 and hepatitis A virus in Portuguese blood donors. *Transfus Apher Sci* (2005) 33(3):305–9. doi:10.1016/j.transci.2005.06.002
36. Schmidt M, Themann A, Drexler C, Bayer M, Lanzer G, Menichetti E, et al. Blood donor screening for parvovirus B19 in Germany and Austria. *Transfusion* (2007) 47(10):1775–82. doi:10.1111/j.1537-2995.2007.01443.x
37. Kleinman SH, Glynn SA, Lee TH, Tobler L, Montalvo L, Todd D, et al. Prevalence and quantitation of parvovirus B19 DNA levels in blood donors with a sensitive polymerase chain reaction screening assay. *Transfusion* (2007) 47(10):1756–64. doi:10.1111/j.1537-2995.2007.01341.x
38. Kooistra K, Mesman HJ, de Waal M, Koppelman MH, Zaaijer HL. Epidemiology of high-level parvovirus B19 viraemia among Dutch blood donors, 2003–2009. *Vox Sang* (2011) 100(3):261–6. doi:10.1111/j.1423-0410.2010.01423.x
39. Oh DJ, Lee YL, Kang JW, Kwon SY, Cho NS. Investigation of the prevalence of human parvovirus B19 DNA in Korean plasmapheresis donors. *Korean J Lab Med* (2010) 30(1):58–64. doi:10.3343/kjlm.2010.30.1.58
40. Ke L, He M, Li C, Liu Y, Gao L, Yao F, et al. The prevalence of human parvovirus B19 DNA and antibodies in blood donors from four Chinese blood centers. *Transfusion* (2011) 51(9):1909–18. doi:10.1111/j.1537-2995.2011.03067.x
41. Juhl D, Steppat D, Görg S, Hennig H. Parvovirus b19 infections and blood counts in blood donors. *Transfus Med Hemother* (2014) 41(1):52–9. doi:10.1159/000357650
42. Han T, Li C, Zhang Y, Wang Y, Wu B, Ke L, et al. The prevalence of hepatitis A virus and parvovirus B19 in source-plasma donors and whole blood donors in China. *Transfus Med* (2015) 25(6):406–10. doi:10.1111/tme.12259
43. Slavov SN, Otaguiri KK, Covas DT, Kashima S. Prevalence and viral load of human parvovirus B19 (B19V) among blood donors in South-East Brazil. *Indian J Hematol Blood Transfus* (2016) 32:323–5. doi:10.1007/s12288-015-0607-1
44. Juhl D, Thiessen U, Glessing P, Görg S, Hennig H. Experiences with the NAT testing for parvovirus B19 (B19V) and hepatitis A virus (HAV) in a five years period. Abstract. *Transfus Med Hemother* (2017) 44(Suppl 1):47. doi:10.1159/000481444
45. Schleuning M. Parvovirus-B19-Infektionen: Sind es nur harmlose Ringelröteln? *Dtsch Arztebl* (1996) 93(43):A–2781/B–2362/C–2098.
46. Modrow S. Parvovirus B19: Ein Infektionserreger mit vielen Erkrankungsbildern. *Dtsch Arztebl* (2001) 98(24):A–1620/B–1390/C–1293.
47. Zaaijer HL, Koppelman MH, Farrington CP. Parvovirus B19 viraemia in Dutch blood donors. *Epidemiol Infect* (2004) 132(6):1161–6. doi:10.1017/S0950268804002730
48. Brown KE, Young NS, Alving BM, Barbosa LH. Parvovirus B19: implications for transfusion medicine. Summary of a workshop. *Transfusion* (2001) 41(1):130–5. doi:10.1046/j.1537-2995.2001.41010130.x
49. Lefrère JJ, Servant-Delmas A, Candotti D, Mariotti M, Thomas I, Brossard Y, et al. Persistent B19 infection in immunocompetent individuals: implications for transfusion safety. *Blood* (2005) 106(8):2890–5. doi:10.1182/blood-2005-03-1053
50. Matsukura H, Shibata S, Tani Y, Shibata H, Furuta RA. Persistent infection by human parvovirus B19 in qualified blood donors. *Transfusion* (2008) 48(5):1036–7. doi:10.1111/j.1537-2995.2008.01704.x
51. Juhl D, Görg S, Hennig H. Persistence of parvovirus B19 (B19V) DNA and humoral immune response in B19V-infected blood donors. *Vox Sang* (2014) 107(3):226–32. doi:10.1111/vox.12162
52. Eis-Hübinger AM, Reber U, Abdul-Nour T, Glatzel U, Lauschke H, Pütz U. Evidence for persistence of parvovirus B19 DNA in livers of adults. *J Med Virol* (2001) 65(2):395–401. doi:10.1002/jmv.2047
53. Norja P, Hokynar K, Aaltonen LM, Chen R, Ranki A, Partio EK, et al. Bioportfolio: lifelong persistence of variant and prototypic erythrovirus DNA genomes in human tissue. *Proc Natl Acad Sci U S A* (2006) 103(19):7450–3. doi:10.1073/pnas.0602259103
54. Kuethe F, Lindner J, Matschke K, Wenzel JJ, Norja P, Ploetze K, et al. Prevalence of parvovirus B19 and human bocavirus DNA in the heart of patients with no evidence of dilated cardiomyopathy or myocarditis. *Clin Infect Dis* (2009) 49(11):1660–6. doi:10.1086/648074
55. Plentz A, Würdinger M, Kudlich M, Modrow S. Low-level DNAemia of parvovirus B19 (genotypes 1–3) in adult transplant recipients is not associated with anaemia. *J Clin Virol* (2013) 58(2):443–8. doi:10.1016/j.jcv.2013.07.007
56. Molenaar-de Backer MW, Russcher A, Kroes AC, Koppelman MH, Lanfermeijer M, Zaaijer HL. Detection of parvovirus B19 DNA in blood: viruses or DNA remnants? *J Clin Virol* (2016) 84:19–23. doi:10.1016/j.jcv.2016.09.004
57. Parsyan A, Candotti D. Human erythrovirus B19 and blood transfusion – an update. *Transfus Med* (2007) 17(4):263–78. doi:10.1111/j.1365-3148.2007.00765.x
58. Marano G, Vaglio S, Pupella S, Facco G, Calizzani G, Candura F, et al. Human parvovirus B19 and blood product safety: a tale of twenty years of improvements. *Blood Transfus* (2015) 13(2):184–96. doi:10.2450/2014.0174.14
59. Jia J, Ma Y, Zhao X, Guo Y, Huangfu C, Fang C, et al. Prevalence of human parvovirus B19 in Chinese plasma pools for manufacturing plasma derivatives. *Virol J* (2015) 12:162. doi:10.1186/s12985-015-0396-z
60. Soucie JM, De Staercke C, Monahan PE, Recht M, Chitlur MB, Gruppo R, et al. Evidence for the transmission of parvovirus B19 in patients with bleeding disorders treated with plasma-derived factor concentrates in the era of nucleic acid test screening. *Transfusion* (2013) 53(6):1217–25. doi:10.1111/j.1537-2995.2012.03907.x
61. Zanella A, Rossi F, Cesana C, Foresti A, Nador F, Binda AS, et al. Transfusion-transmitted human parvovirus B19 infection in a thalassemic patient. *Transfusion* (1995) 35(9):769–72. doi:10.1046/j.1537-2995.1995.35996029163.x
62. Cohen BJ, Beard S, Knowles WA, Ellis JS, Joske D, Goldman JM, et al. Chronic anemia due to parvovirus B19 infection in a bone marrow transplant patient after platelet transfusion. *Transfusion* (1997) 37(9):947–52. doi:10.1046/j.1537-2995.1997.37997454023.x
63. *SHOT-Report.* (2016). Available from: https://www.shotuk.org/wp-content/uploads/SHOT-Report-2016_web_11th-July.pdf
64. Yu MY, Alter HJ, Virata-Theimer ML, Geng Y, Ma L, Schechterly CA, et al. Parvovirus B19 infection transmitted by transfusion of red blood cells

confirmed by molecular analysis of linked donor and recipient samples. *Transfusion* (2010) 50(8):1712–21. doi:10.1111/j.1537-2995.2010.02591.x
65. Hourfar MK, Mayr-Wohlfart U, Themann A, Sireis W, Seifried E, Schrezenmeier H, et al. Recipients potentially infected with parvovirus B19 by red blood cell products. *Transfusion* (2011) 51(1):129–36. doi:10.1111/j.1537-2995.2010.02780.x
66. Satake M, Hoshi Y, Taira R, Momose SY, Hino S, Tadokoro K. Symptomatic parvovirus B19 infection caused by blood component transfusion. *Transfusion* (2011) 51(9):1887–95. doi:10.1111/j.1537-2995.2010.03047.x
67. Servant-Delmas A, Laperche S, Mercier M, Michel Y, Garbarg-Chenon A, Boyeldieu D, et al. Limits of sequencing and phylogenetic analysis to assess B19V transmission by single-donor blood component. *Vox Sang* (2011) 100(2):254–5. doi:10.1111/j.1423-0410.2010.01390.x
68. Juhl D, Özdemir M, Dreier J, Görg S, Hennig H. Look-back study on recipients of parvovirus B19 (B19V) DNA-positive blood components. *Vox Sang* (2015) 109(4):305–11. doi:10.1111/vox.12295
69. Nagaharu K, Sugimoto Y, Hoshi Y, Yamaguchi T, Ito R, Matsubayashi K, et al. Persistent symptomatic parvovirus B19 infection with severe thrombocytopenia transmitted by red blood cell transfusion containing low parvovirus B19 DNA levels. *Transfusion* (2017) 57(6):1414–8. doi:10.1111/trf.14088
70. Sato H, Takakura F, Kojima E, Fukada K, Okochi K, Maeda Y. Screening of blood donors for human parvovirus B19. *Lancet* (1995) 346(8984):1237–8. doi:10.1016/S0140-6736(95)92950-9
71. Koppelman MH, Cuijpers HT, Wessberg S, Valkeajärvi A, Pichl L, Schottstedt V, et al. Multicenter evaluation of a commercial multiplex polymerase chain reaction test for screening plasma donations for parvovirus B19 DNA and hepatitis A virus RNA. *Transfusion* (2012) 52(7):1498–508. doi:10.1111/j.1537-2995.2012.03705.x
72. Molenaar-de Backer MW, de Waal M, Sjerps MC, Koppelman MH. Validation of new real-time polymerase chain reaction assays for detection of hepatitis A virus RNA and parvovirus B19 DNA. *Transfusion* (2016) 56(2):440–8. doi:10.1111/trf.13334
73. Groeneveld K, van der Noordaa J. Blood products and parvovirus B19. *Neth J Med* (2003) 61(5):154–6.
74. Blümel J, Rinckel LA, Lee DC, Roth NJ, Baylis SA. Inactivation and neutralization of parvovirus B19 genotype 3. *Transfusion* (2012) 52(7):1490–7. doi:10.1111/j.1537-2995.2012.03573.x
75. Menconi MC, Maggi F, Zakrzewska K, Salotti V, Giovacchini P, Farina C, et al. Effectiveness of nanofiltration in removing small non-enveloped viruses from three different plasma-derived products. *Transfus Med* (2009) 19(4):213–7. doi:10.1111/j.1365-3148.2009.00931.x
76. Schlenke P. Pathogen inactivation technologies for cellular blood components: an update. *Transfus Med Hemother* (2014) 41(4):309–25. doi:10.1159/000365646
77. Gowland P, Fontana S, Stolz M, Andina N, Niederhauser C. Parvovirus B19 passive transmission by transfusion of Intercept® blood system-treated platelet concentrate. *Transfus Med Hemother* (2016) 43(3):198–202. doi:10.1159/000445195

12

Reflections on Dry Eye Syndrome Treatment: Therapeutic Role of Blood Products

*Victor J. Drew[1,2], Ching-Li Tseng[1,2], Jerard Seghatchian[3] and Thierry Burnouf[1,2]**

[1] International PhD Program of Biomedical Engineering, College of Biomedical Engineering, Taipei Medical University, Taipei, Taiwan, [2] College of Biomedical Engineering, Graduate Institute of Biomedical Materials and Tissue Engineering, Taipei Medical University, Taipei, Taiwan, [3] Independent Researcher, London, United Kingdom

Correspondence:
Thierry Burnouf
thburnouf@gmail.com

Dry eye syndrome (DES) is a multifactorial, frequent, pathology characterized by deficient tear production or increased evaporation of tears and associated with ocular surface alteration and inflammation. It mostly affects, but not exclusively, older individuals and leads to varying degrees of discomfort and decreased quality of life. Although the typical treatments of DES rely on using artificial tears, polyunsaturated fatty acids, integrin antagonists, anti-inflammatory agents, or on performing punctal occlusion, recently, standardized blood-derived serum eye drops (SED) are generating much interest as a new physiological treatment option. The scientific rationale in using SED for treating or releasing the symptoms of DES is thought to lie in its composition in multiple factors that resembles that of tears and contributes to the healing and protection of the ocular surface. This manuscript seeks to provide relevant background information on the management of DES, and on the increasing role that various types of SED or platelet lysates, from autologous or allogeneic origins, are playing in the improved therapeutic management of this pathology. The increasing role played by blood establishments in producing better-standardized SED is also addressed.

Keywords: dry eye syndrome, keratoconjunctivitis, artificial tears, serum eye drop, platelet lysate, blood

DRY EYE SYNDROME (DES): EPIDEMIOLOGY, PATHOLOGY, AND SOCIO-ECONOMIC IMPACTS

Epidemiology

Dry eye syndrome, also known as dry eye disease or keratoconjunctivitis sicca (KCS), is among the most common ocular complaints that older patients seek eye care for (1). Often under-recognized, DES is a multifactorial disease associated with varying degrees of discomfort and decreased quality of life (2). Awareness of DES varies much among populations, largely influenced by criteria used for self-diagnosis. For instance, in a survey conducted in Japan, 33% of participants estimated to be affected by DES (3). DES prevalence increases with age. One study found that there are no significant differences in DES prevalence in men of differing races or regions in the United States (1). Females of all age groups have a greater likelihood of developing DES than males, with DES prevalence increasing with age (4). Schaumberg et al. estimate that, in the United States, 1.68 million men over the age of 50 years experience DES and this number is expected to grow to 2.79 million by 2030 as life expectancy increases (1), whereas a previous health study found that over 3.23 million women are currently suffering from DES (4).

In another study, it was extrapolated that 4.3 million people over 65 years in the United States suffer from ocular irritation at least occasionally (5).

Pathology

Dry eye syndrome pathology is typically divided into two types: deficient tear production or the evaporation of tears. Deficiency in tear production can be further divided into two more categories: Sjögren's syndrome (SS), which is an autoimmune disease, or non-Sjögren's syndrome (non-SS) (2, 6–8). Evaporation of tears refers to the loss of water from the ocular surface and is often the result of a meibomian gland dysfunction leading to a lipid bilayer deficiency in the tear film. The meibomian gland loses its function with age, leading to tear film instability and evaporation of tears; the quality and function of the meibomian gland has been linked, at least in part, to androgen levels (9). As males have higher androgen levels than females, this is consistent with the higher frequency of DES in females, especially after menopause.

Deficiency of tears caused by the decrease of aqueous tear production or excessive tear evaporation could increase osmolarity, with deleterious effects on the ocular surface. DES is associated with inflammation, and tear hyperosmolarity is an important mediator of this inflammation (2). Hyperosmolarity is associated with a key pathogenic mechanism of DES with negative effects on epithelial cells, including decreased cell volume, damage to DNA repair systems, increased apoptosis, and increased oxidative stress (2). It also stimulates multiple inflammatory events involving metalloproteinase-9 (MMP-9), tumor necrosis factor-alpha (TNF-α), and mitogen-activated protein kinase (MAPK) (2). Indeed, overexpression of proinflammatory cytokines/chemokines on the ocular surface has been found to be associated with the symptoms of dry eye (10–12), including interleukin (IL)-1β, IL-6, IL-17, IL-22, interferon-γ, tumor necrosis factor α (TNF-α), chemokine (C-Cmotif) ligand 2 (CCL2), and matrix metalloproteinases (13, 14).

In addition to dryness, symptoms associated with DES include pain, burning sensations, eye fatigue, redness, blurred vision, discharge, contact lens intolerance, sensitivity to light, and the feeling of foreign bodies present in the ocular region (2). Depending on the severity of DES, some patients experience problems carrying out basic daily activities such as reading, watching television, using a computer, driving a vehicle, and working (15). The discomfort caused by DES has also been tied to depression and decreased quality of life (2, 16–18). Furthermore, one study conducted a battery of tests, including tear function and ocular surface evaluations, and questionnaires on DES patients and determined a correlation between lower DES symptoms and patient happiness, suggesting that DES may influence a patient's psychiatric well-being (19). A study of depression in DES subjects identified that these patients experience poor sleep quality (16). DES patients tend to sleep later, less, and use more sleep medications and antidepressants than non-affected subjects. However, antidepressants are being investigated as a potential contributor to DES (20), and patients with severe DES that progressively worsens over time suffer from increased anxiety and other mood disorders (2, 16).

Socio-economic Impacts

Dry eye syndrome places a substantial economic burden on society due to hospital visits, medical costs, surgeries, and drugs, in addition to indirect costs such as loss of productivity (21). In the United States, the average DES patient makes approximately 6 hospital visits annually at a total cost of nearly $800 USD, adding up to a national cost of nearly $4 billion USD. These costs have risen over the years. When taking loss of productivity into account, annual societal costs are estimated to exceed $55 billion in the United States (22). In Europe, the estimated annual cost for ophthalmologist-managed care ranged from approximately $270 USD in France to $1,100 USD in the United Kingdom (21). In Japan, DES patient annual medical costs amounted to roughly $470 USD, mostly for drugs (21). Additionally, loss of work productivity in Japan was calculated to be approximately $536 USD per patient (21, 23). Surprisingly, the economic burden of DES due to loss of productivity drastically outweighed the direct expenses from receiving care from healthcare professionals or prescription drugs (22). Although the apparent costs vary among countries, the real costs of DES in each country are likely higher than data shows when taking into account that the purchase of over-the-counter artificial tears is not always incorporated into cost calculations (24) and data are incomplete, in particular in some parts of Asia (21).

CURRENT THERAPEUTIC STRATEGIES

The past 5 years have witnessed substantial developments in DES treatment options. Current treatment strategies that are not based on blood products include artificial tears, lubricants, steroids, immunosuppressant eye drops, dietary supplements associated with eyelid cleansing, and in more extreme case, anti-inflammatory drugs or punctal occlusion, a procedure consisting of inserting a plug into the tear drainage area to maintain tears in the eyes. Generally, such treatments, which can be combined, are selected based on disease severity and medical history of the patient. For the majority of DES cases, treatments focus on alleviating symptoms rather than addressing the causes of DES (6–8). Treatment effectiveness on symptoms must be regularly assessed (25). Regular use of artificial tears, anti-inflammatory drops, or punctal plugs provides only transient release and can often induce ocular side effects.

Artificial Tears

The main functions of artificial tears are to increase moisture and provide lubrication of the ocular surface (26). There is a variety of artificial tear formulations available, differing in osmolarity, viscosity, electrolyte content, preservative content, and solute combinations (27). Artificial tears are currently formulated as osmoprotectants, with the purpose of restoring cell volume, decreasing cell stress, and reducing inflammatory reactions that occur under hyperosmotic conditions (28). One eye drop product uses propylene glycol (PG), polyethylene glycol (PEG), and hydroxypropyl guar (HP-Guar) with polyquaternium-1 preservative, which decreased ocular surface inflammation and DES symptom severity (29). Similarly, another eyedrop formulated using hyaluronic acid (HA) and trehalose stabilizes the bilipid membranes and protects labile proteins from desiccation, as well as prevents oxidative damage (30, 31).

A recent Cochrane analysis (27) could not identify whether different over-the-counter artificial tears provide "similar relief of signs and symptoms when compared with each other or placebo." However, 0.2% polyacrylic acid-based artificial tears were found to be more effective than 1.4% polyvinyl alcohol-based artificial tears. In addition, artificial tears are not free of inducing some adverse events.

One limitation of artificial tears is the lack of some of the components of natural tears such as lipids, salts, proteins, and hydrocarbons, as well as growth factors, immunoglobulins, albumin, and vitamins present in serum, as discussed later (28, 32–34). Additional possible drawbacks of artificial tears include the presence of preservatives and other potentially toxic and allergenic compounds (35). Benzalkonium chloride (BAK), the most frequently used preservative compound in eye drops, may contribute to hyperosmolarity by disrupting tear films. BAK-induced damage extends to destruction of goblet cells, the corneal epithelium barrier, and deeper ocular tissues including release of proinflammatory cytokines, oxidative stress, and apoptosis (35). These factors should be taken into consideration when prescribing DES treatments.

Polyunsaturated Fatty Acids (PUFAs)

Omega 3 and 6 fatty acids are essential fatty acids that cannot be synthesized in the human body. Their improper balance can lead to an omega 6 proinflammatory effect (8). Dietary supplementation of polyunsaturated fatty acids (PUFAs) may help manage DES (8, 36). In a randomized, double-blind study, omega-3 supplementation promoted tear film stabilization, reducing tear evaporation and DES symptoms as a result of increased goblet cell counts and improved epithelial cell morphology (8, 36). Balanced combination of omega-3 and omega-6 was recently found to attenuate contact lens-related DES (37).

Integrin Antagonist

Lymphocyte function-associated antigen-1 (LFA-1), an integrin expressed on T-cells, is upregulated in the conjunctiva of DES patients (38). The interaction between LFA-1 and intercellular adhesion molecule-1 (ICAM-1) is key in T-cell adhesion with endothelial cells, as well as for T-cell interaction with antigen presenting cells (38). One approach to treat DES aimed to block the interaction between LFA-1 and ICAM-1. A small LFA-1 antagonist called Lifitegrast (SAR 1118) demonstrated in phase III clinical trials to significantly and safely relieve DES symptoms (39). Lifitegrast acts as an antagonist to LFA-1, resulting in the inhibition of T-cell activation, migration, and proliferation (40). However, other parameters to assess ocular function, such as Schirmer's test results, tear breakup time, and inferior corneal staining, did not improve significantly (41). In July 2016, Xiidra® was the first United States Food and Drug Administration (US-FDA)-approved LFA-1 agonist for treating DES (40).

Anti-Inflammatory Therapies and Immunomodulators

Corticosteroids are one among several anti-inflammatory drugs to treat DES. In addition to reducing cellular infiltration, restoring vascular permeability and inhibiting chemotaxis, corticosteroids decrease fibroblast proliferation, reduce capillary dilation and suppress collagen deposition (40). They are considered highly effective toward the treatment of immune-mediated inflammatory diseases (40). However, their efficacy is limited to short-term usage (4 weeks or less) (41) as long term use leads to intraocular pressure and the formation of cataracts (40, 42). A combination with anti-inflammation agent (epigallocatechin gallate, EGCG) and mucoadhesive component, hyaluronic acid (HA) was used for the treatment of DES in a rabbit experimental model (43). Its therapeutic effect was evidenced via increased tear production, inflammation relief, and corneal epithelium recovery providing an alternative inflammatory inhibition agent for clinical DES treatment.

Cyclosporine is preferred over corticosteroids as a long-term treatment for DES. Cyclosporine A is a topical immunomodulator, first approved by the FDA in 2002 (Restasis®) for treating dry eye by increasing tear production (44) and by the European Union in 2015 (Ikervis®) (45). When administered topically, cyclosporine A acts as an immunomodulator, and when administered systemically, it acts as an immunosuppressant (8). This drug elicits anti-inflammatory properties by inhibiting cell-mediated reactions and preventing the release of proinflammatory cytokines, while upregulating the production of anti-inflammatory cytokines (44). Multiple studies have reported minimal side effects associated with topical application of cyclosporine A, under conditions increasing tear production and conjunctival goblet cell density (8, 45–47).

Punctal Occlusion

Lacrimal punctal occlusion by plug is the most common non-pharmacological therapy for DES (48, 49). Although many authors recommend temporary occlusion by plugs as a trial treatment, permanent occlusion can be achieved through surgical obstruction of the lacrimal punctum. It has been described as being like "blocking the drain in a tub and collecting the water dripping from the tap" (50), which in other words means preventing tear drainage toward the nasal cavity by physically blocking the lacrimal punctum/canaliculus. Punctal occlusion is typically recommended for patients suffering from DES symptoms after failed attempts of using traditional aqueous treatment options (49). Although punctal occlusion may improve DES symptoms, there is a concern that it could retain unhealthy tears on the ocular surface causing irritation (51) and does not decrease tear cytokines and MMP-9 levels (52). An international panel of dry eye specialists recommended that factors associated with inflammation be handled prior to performing punctal occlusion (53). A study comparing the effects of administering punctal occlusion alone versus a punctal plug regime in combination with cyclosporine treatment demonstrated that for the near term, punctal occlusion, alone or with cyclosporine, yielded swift improvement in moisture. However, for the long term, treatment regimes involving punctal occlusion in combination with cyclosporine produced equal or superior results to treatment regimes using occlusion plugs only (50). A recent Cochrane study has identified a "very low-certainty evidence on symptomatic improvement" of punctal occlusion, commonly associated with epiphora and inflammatory conditions (54).

BLOOD PRODUCT-BASED DES TREATMENT OPTIONS

Scientific Rationale

Human blood has been for many decades the source of a wide range of cell-based or protein-based therapeutic products. Cellular products include red blood cell (erythrocyte) concentrates, buffy coats/granulocytes concentrates, and platelet (thrombocyte) concentrates. Therapeutic proteins encompass coagulation factors, albumin, and immunoglobulins. More recently, new platelet-derived preparations, rich in growth factors, have been increasingly used for therapeutic applications in wound healing, tissue repair and regeneration (55), and *in vitro* clinical-grade cell propagation and tissue engineering (56).

There is now great interest in the application of human blood derived products as eye drops for DES. The most common blood product used as eye drops is serum, which is obtained by a physiological clotting process of blood collected without anticoagulant, as described in details below. The therapeutic benefits of blood-derived serum eye drops (SED) are probably multifactorial and may be explained by a composition that, in part, shares similarities with that of tears (32–34, 57). Like tears, SED contains carbohydrates, lipids, and various electrolytes, but 10 times more proteins including albumin, fibronectin, and transferrin (33). SED contains natural antimicrobial components, like complement component (58), and IgG, but less lysozyme than tears (32). Tears and SED provide vitamins and both share a similar osmolality (close to 300 mosm/l) as they contain comparable sodium and anion levels, and a similar pH (close to pH 7.4) (33, 59, 60). Potassium ion levels are about five times higher in tears than in SED, but calcium ions and phosphate levels are less in tears than in SED (33). However, the total protein content of tears is only about 10% that of SED (33). IgA is the major immunoglobulin in tears, playing a role in protecting against infections. Vitamin A is less in tears than in serum. Vitamin C and glutathione antioxidants are present at higher levels in tears than in serum. Most importantly, SED, like tears (61), also contain a mixture of cell growth promoting agents (62, 63), since blood clotting is associated with a degranulation of the platelets and a release of a plethora of growth factors from their alpha-granules (56, 64, 65). Growth factor composition is said to be qualitatively equivalent in tears and serum, but concentrations may be higher in serum, as is the case for transforming growth factor-beta (TGF-β) and platelet-derived growth factor (PDGF). **Table 1** presents some of the known similarities existing between tears and SED.

Serum Eye Drop

Preparation

Serum refers to the fluid portion of blood, devoid of cellular components that is obtained by letting blood collected without an anticoagulant to clot. It is typically prepared by collecting blood from patients (autologous source) or donors (allogeneic source), allowing the blood to clot for several hours prior to a centrifugation step at ca. 3,000 × *g* for approximately 10 min at 20–25°C to recover a supernatant serum. Serum may be passed through a 0.22-µm pore-sized filter for bacterial sterilization and clarification (34, 57, 66). In such a preparation, the platelets are not concentrated compared to the level found in the blood circulation, by contrast to newer SED formulation made from platelet concentrates where platelets are threefold to fivefold enriched compared to blood. When SED are made from platelet concentrates for transfusion, the content of serum plasma protein depends upon whether the platelets are suspended in 100% plasma or a mixture of plasma and platelet additive solution (PAS).

An informative survey of methods used at international levels to prepare SED has recently been conducted by the Biomedical Excellence for Safer Transfusion (BEST) Collaborative (67). A summary of the preparation methods of SED is illustrated in **Figure 1**. Briefly, this survey indicates that SED for clinical use are prepared by national or regional blood establishments (also known as blood centers), as well as by hospitals or medical centers. Although most centers are manufacturing SED of autologous origin, an increasing number is now producing SED from allogeneic blood donors (68–70). When the SED are from allogeneic origins, procedures are in place, e.g., by preparing SED from AB group donors to hold a single blood group inventory or by donation screening to match all blood groups to ensure hemato-immunological matching between donors and recipients. It is, however, still unknown whether presence of anti-B agglutinins affect corneal healing (67).

A small majority of centers (most likely the blood establishments familiar with the production of blood components for transfusion) prepare SED from blood collected into blood bags rather than into tubes and use larger volumes of 200 mL or more. While the clotting time to get serum may be less than 6 h, it can be up to 24 h and (somewhat surprisingly) up to 3 days in some places. Most often, the serum is centrifuged to clarify the supernatant. Most centers do not perform a bacterial filtration step, whereas others do, implying that they apply the standard close-system manufacturing practices familiar to blood establishments. A small majority of the centers dilute the serum twofold to fivefold in saline or phosphate-buffered saline solution, before immediate dispensing in 0.5–5 mL aliquots into vials/eye dropper bottles or tubing segments before freezing (67).

Formulation

To date, the optimal formulation and dilution factor of SED for DES treatment remains uncertain. This is not unexpected considering the biological complexity of the serum material compared to artificial tears. Sometimes, the serum is diluted to approach

TABLE 1 | Comparison of tears and serum composition (individual variations may affect the values).

	Tears	Serum	Physiological function possibly relevant in ocular defect treatment
Physico-chemical parameters (33, 57)			
Osmolality, mosm/l	302	300	Maintains physiological osmolality and pH
pH	7.2–7.4	7.2–7.4	
Proteins (33, 55, 56, 74)			
Total proteins, mg/mL	7.37	60–70	Support tear surface tension, physiological hydration of the ocular surface, and ocular homeostasis
Albumin, mg/mL	0.05	35–40	Anti-apoptotic activity, detoxification
Fibronectin, μg/mL	21	200–300	Adhesion protein supporting wound healing
IgG, mg/mL	0.032	8–12	Anti-microbial
IgA, mg/mL	0.41		Anti-microbial
IgM, mg/mL	–	0.5	Endotoxin binding
IgD, μg/mL	–	3–300	
IgE, μg/mL	–	0.25–0.7	
Alpha 2-macroglobulin		2.6	Anti-collagenase
Complement system			Anti-microbial; bacteriostatic
Lactoferrin, mg/mL	1.51	–	Anti-microbial and anti-inflammatory
Transferrin, mg/mL	–	2–3	Iron-carrier; anti-microbial
Lysozyme, mg/mL	1.4	6	Iron carrier; anti-microbial
Growth factors (33, 55–57, 61)			
TGF-β1, ng/mL	2–10	6–50	Epithelial and stromal repair processes
PDGF, ng/mL	0.09–1.7	30–100	Enhances mitosis and scarring
EGF, ng/mL	0.2–3	0.5–1	Accelerates the migration of epithelial cells; anti-apoptotic
HGF, ng/mL	0.2–0.5	0.1–1	Supports corneal epithelial cells
VEGF, ng/mL	0.019	1–5	Supports conjunctival endothelial permeability
Vitamins (33)			
A, ng/mL	16–20	800–1000	Prevents squamous metaplasia and helps maintain the normal histology in the conjunctiva
C, μg/mL	117	7–20	Antioxidant
Antioxidants (33)			
Tyrosine, μM	45	77	
Glutathione, μM	107	ND	
Electrolytes (33)			
Na+, mEq/L	145	135–146	
K+, mEq/L	24.1	3.5–5.0	
Ca^{2+}, mM	1.5	1.1	
Cl^-, mM	128	96–108	
HCO_3^- mM	26	21–29	
NO_3^- mM	0.14	0.19	
PO_4^{3-} mM	0.22	1.42	
SO_4^{2-} mM	0.39	0.53	

the composition of tears and to decrease the concentration of TGF-β, which may exert an anti-proliferative activity and impair the healing of epithelial cells (33). There is, nevertheless, no real consensus yet nor evidence-based information on the optimal formulation (71). One cannot exclude that formulation may have to be adjusted to the disease treated or its extent (dryness or epithelium defect). Lower dilution factors (50%), or even no dilution at all, have been used (57, 72), while other authors have proposed to dilute SED to 20% in a sodium hyaluronate solution in particular to improve retention time and decrease the frequency of the administration (73). Higher SED concentrations have been reported to increase the speed of epithelial healing and closure in a patient recovering from laser *in situ* keratomileusis (LASIK) eye surgery (66).

Safety Aspects

Autologous SED do not essentially present risks of extraneous virus contamination when produced under GMP restricting the risks of cross-contamination or mislabeling with SED from another patient. Release testing focusing on microbial sterility of the final batch is carried out by about half of the producers that were recently surveyed (67). Preservative solutions are not added in SED; preparation procedures should therefore be carefully controlled and monitored to prevent bacterial contaminations.

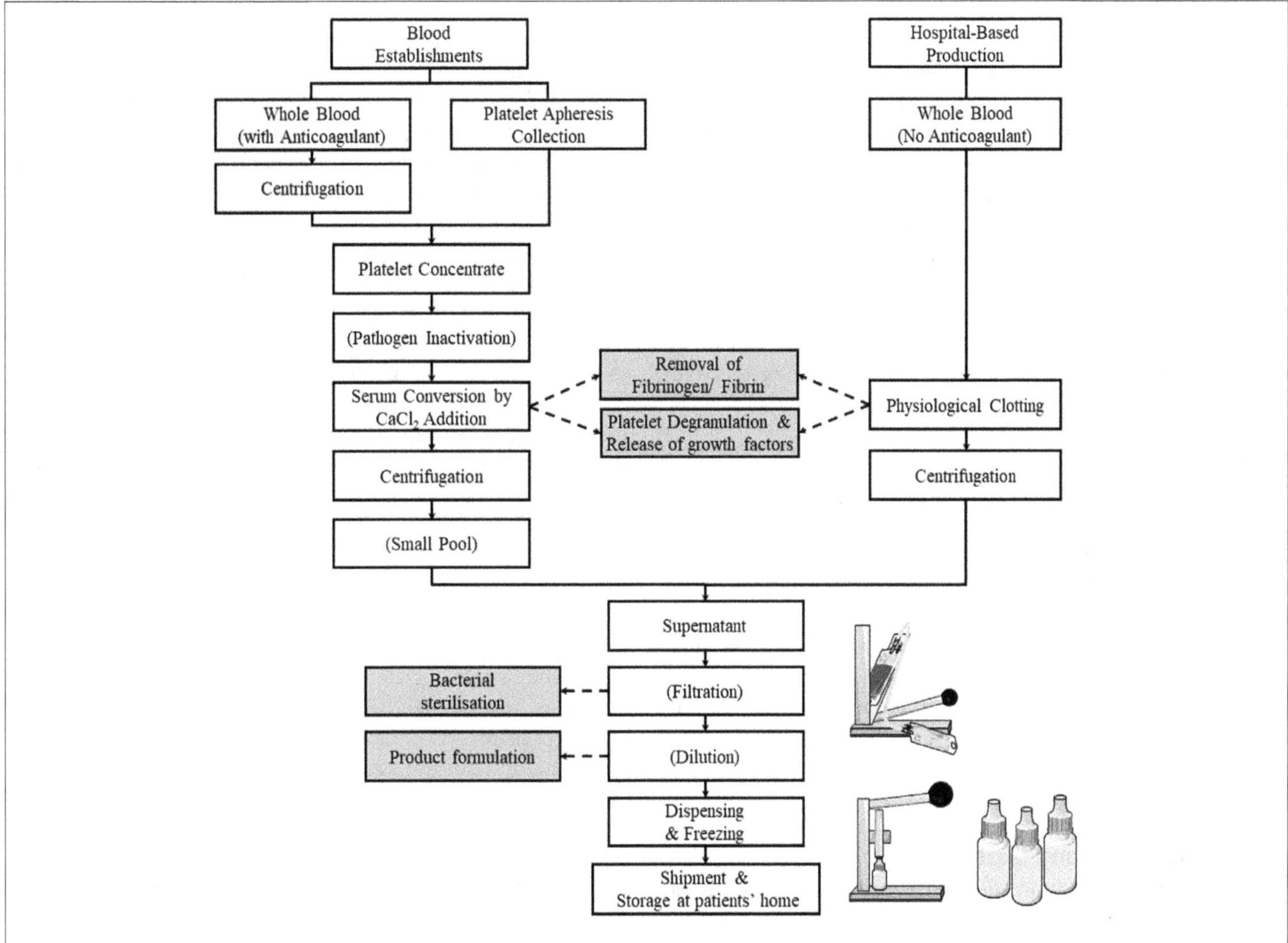

FIGURE 1 | Flowchart of the preparation methods of serum eye drop by blood establishments and hospitals. Typically, the process involves the release of the platelet growth factors by physiological or $CaCl_2$ stimulated clotting of blood (or platelet concentrates), followed by centrifugation, filtration (optional), dilution (optional), dispensing, and freezing.

Allogeneic blood donors donating blood for the production of SED should be screened for virus markers using the same standards that are applied to donations devoted to the manufacturer of transfused blood products (67, 74, 75). The main transfusion transmitted infections associated with allogeneic serum are viruses, most notably human immunodeficiency virus, and hepatitis B and C viruses (76). Emerging viruses, like West Nile virus, Dengue virus, Chikungunya virus, Ebola virus, and Zika virus, may also be a potential threat (77). However, efficient safety measures in place in blood establishments, namely donors' screening and donation testing, dramatically restrict the risks of viral transmissions in a regulated blood collection jurisdiction (78). Particular future attention may need to address the pathological consequences of risks of transmission of other blood-borne viruses, such as the Herpes simplex virus, that may lead to ocular complications and affect vision (79).

Photochemical pathogen inactivation methods are in use for transfused plasma and platelet concentrates (80, 81), but they are not a current option as no dedicated or licensed pathogen inactivation treatment has been approved for application to therapeutic serum, although experimental studies have shown applicability to serum for cell expansion (82). As therapeutic platelet concentrates can be pathogen-inactivated using licensed treatment, this may speed-up the development of allogeneic pathogen-inactivated SED for clinical use (67). The well-established solvent-detergent (S/D) treatment, already applied to a wide range of biopharmaceutical preparations and plasma products (76), was experimentally proven applicable to rabbit SED (83). This S/D-treated rabbit serum was used as allogeneic SED equivalent to treat DES-rabbits, showing promising results. The safety and efficacy of such S/D-treated SED was demonstrated through the restoration of a corneal epithelium in a DES rabbit model. This preclinical study supports the possibility of using S/D virally inactivated SED to treat DES for the application of allogeneic human SED (83).

Shipment and Storage

Most often, patients themselves collect the SED from the production site and store the bottles at home in a domestic freezer. The typical specified shelf life set by producers of SED ranges from 3 to 12 months until thawing and up to 24 h to 1 week after thawing. Currently, SED storage at patients' home is not specifically controlled and is under patients' responsibility

(33, 67). Studies have suggested that SED can be stored liquid at 4°C for up to 1 month, or frozen at −20°C or −80°C for up to 3 to 6 months, and in the dark to limit the decay in vitamin A (62, 71, 72). The stability of factors in serum, such as vitamin A, EGF, and TGF-β, was shown over up to 9 months. However, stability evaluations based on functional or biological activity (e.g., using cell cultures or animal models), rather than immunological tests (e.g., ELISA measurement of growth factors), should be conducted to determine the shelf-life. Furthermore, variations in the preparation methods of SED may impact its quality and properties (57, 72, 84) and, potentially, influence its long-term stability. Topical application of SED, which do not contain preservatives in order to prevent toxicity, requires careful handling to avoid microbial contamination.

Regulations

The regulatory status of current SED varies, but these preparations are typically regulated as blood products with variations from country to country depending upon jurisdictions (85). The increasing number of blood centers producing SED should eventually lead to the recognition and regulation of SED as a blood product, and to the establishments of international guidelines underlying their manufacture, and efforts towards implementing guidelines for standardization and product specifications. Clinical trials are expected to provide more rigorous information of clinical efficacy in various ocular pathologies and guidance for optimal products' performance and clinical outcomes (67).

Clinical Rationale and Experience

The clinical strategy behind administering autologous serum is to take a comprehensive approach to treating dry eye, rather than just serve as a lubricant. Recent studies and review papers generally confirm the benefit of SED, from autologous or allogeneic sources, providing improved tear film stability, ocular surface health, and subjective comfort in refractory DES (57, 59, 71, 86–93). According to a Cochrane review based on a limited number of randomized clinical trials, autologous SED alleviate dry eye symptoms better than artificial eye drops for the first couple of weeks, but data still remain inconclusive at determining clinical efficacy over long-term periods (72). Therefore, randomized clinical trials involving larger cohorts of various patient groups should be conducted to better delineate the short-term and long-term benefit of SED in the treatment of DES and other ocular diseases (26, 72, 87).

Cost Consideration and Reimbursement Policy

Cost is a major limitation of using autologous SED. In the United States, most health insurance providers do not cover this form of dry eye treatment, resulting in out-of-pocket costs between $175 and $250 for a 2-month supply. The cost of this treatment may therefore makes it an option to consider for patients who have already exhausted more conventional forms of dry eye treatment.

Pending Issues

Autologous versus Allogeneic Products

Currently, there is no universal consensus of criteria on suitable patient selection for autologous blood donation (72). Another disadvantage of using autologous serum is that occasionally the frequent drawing of blood can be inconvenient to patients with prolonged treatment (59). For the elderly and for newborns with serious infections, autologous serum products may be unavailable or contraindicated (94). Cultural considerations are also playing some role. Patients of many Asian cultures, especially the elderly Chinese and Taiwanese, hold the belief that frequent venipuncture causes weakness and makes them more prone to bacterial infection (94). Also some people fear phlebotomy. Additionally, some patients may be too old to donate due to poor venous access or do not possess blood suitable for conversion into autologous SED due to clinical conditions such as previous cerebrovascular accidents, cardiovascular disease, anemia, use of anticoagulant medications or coagulation factor deficiency, or presence of inflammatory mediators (59, 70, 92). Allogeneic serum consists of the same general substances as those in autologous serum, but from a different source and provides a potential alternative treatment for these patients (59). Allogeneic SED are thus being researched for their efficacy in treating a variety of eye disorders associated with DES including persistent corneal epithelial defect (PED), KCS, chronic graft-versus-host disease (cGVHD), and many more (69, 88, 94). In other words, some ocular pathologies may actually benefit from SED made from allogeneic source, rather than autologous.

The use of allogeneic SED poses some risks of its own including the transmission of blood-borne pathogens, hypersensitivity and immune reactions, and potential legal or ethical concerns (59). To overcome some of the risks associated with allogeneic serum, some researchers have limited their investigations to SED obtained from family members (69). It has been reported that these eye drops are clinically comparable to autologous serum (94), but obtaining blood from family members does not imply the absence of risks, including infectious one's. A ready-made, ABO-specific allogeneic eye drop study involving 34 patients (20 patients with KCS and 14 with PED) observed no side effects in any of the subjects and recorded objective improvement in 59% of the subjects. Of patients with KCS, relief was reported in 80% of the patients after allogeneic eye drop treatment (69). In a separate study investigating allogeneic serum in 36 PED patients, the epithelial defect of 16 subjects had healed in 2 weeks time (94). These results were confirmed with the observation of partial or full corneal changes in 16 of the 20 patients. This particular study supports the clinical potential for, and safety of, allogeneic eye drops. However, several immunological and physiological concerns still need to be given due consideration, namely ABO and HLA antibodies that may initiate inflammation (69). As such the virus safety and immune-hematological screening criteria of blood donations used to make allogeneic SED should be in line with those used for blood components for transfusion.

Due to the risk of transfusion-transmitted infections, it is highly recommended that manufacturers and documenters of allogeneic blood products implement good manufacturing practice as is recommended for the collection of blood components by blood establishments (67, 74, 75, 85).

Newer and Emerging Strategies Using Other Blood Products

Various other blood-derived preparations can be considered as therapeutic options to relieve DES symptoms and improve patients' quality of life. It was identified, using a dry eye rat model, that plasma albumin provides a therapeutic benefit that was attributed to suppression of apoptosis (95). Albumin added to an eye drop formulation also helps to relieve DES symptoms in a rabbit model (96). Recent trends in development of blood products to treat DES focus on using blood fractions enriched in platelets (therefore equivalent to therefore somewhat equivalent to what is typically known as platelet-rich-plasma or PRP) as source material as the combination of platelet growth factors is believed to provide a scientific rationale to support its healing potential of DES (69). In the above-mentioned international survey (67), four centers manufacture eye drops either from (a) platelet-rich plasma (PRP) from human cords, (b) autologous platelet rich plasma donations, or (c) plasma. There is great interest in producing SED from PRP or platelet concentrate, as this blood fraction contains a threefold to fivefold higher platelet count than does whole blood.

A product termed Eye-PRP ("E-PRP") is prepared by collecting whole blood in the presence of a 3.2% sodium citrate anticoagulant solution (97) in order to avoid serum formation. Anticoagulated whole blood is centrifuged to sediment red blood cells and to recover a platelet-enriched supernatant plasma. This PRP is then directly divided into aliquots of 3–4 mL and stored in 4°C refrigeration for 1 week or stored in −20°C freezer for extended periods (97, 98). Growth factors in E-PRP act to stimulate angiogenesis, promote cell repair, and activate macrophages (97). These essential molecules are actually commonly used in ophthalmology to promote epithelial wound healing of the cornea (98). 89% of patients using E-PRP eye drops four to six times per day reported subjective absence of DES symptoms. Benefits extended to include increased visual acuity, increased tear production, and improvements in ocular surface condition (98). A similar conclusion was reached by a study investigating the effect of this PRP on human lacrimal function (99).

An alternative to autologous serum and E-PRP is "plasma rich in growth factors" (PRGF). PRGF contains, like serum and E-PRP, a number of platelet growth factors, including platelet-derived growth factor, angiopoietin-1 (ANG-1), epidermal growth factor (EGF), VEGF, and many more (100, 101). PRGF can be prepared by collecting 30 mL of whole blood in tubes containing 3.8% sodium citrate and centrifuging the tubes, using soft spin, at 460 × *g* at room temperature for 8 min. The plasma supernatant portion is recovered, and the platelets are activated using 22.8 mM calcium chloride (102). Addition of calcium chloride induces a process of serum-conversion where a fibrin clot is generated, and growth factors are released due to platelet activation and degranulation. Afterward, the growth factor-rich supernatant serum is collected and filtered. It can be diluted with 0.9% sodium chloride down to 20%. All of these steps are performed under sterile conditions. The final product is distributed into eye drop dispensers, ready for use. For immediate usage, the eye drops could be stored in 4°C refrigeration up to 1 week, and for long-term storage, at −20°C for no longer than 3 months. Patients administer eye drop solution four times per day. Treatment cycles last approximately 3 months, but treatment can be extended several more months to include more cycles if symptoms do not improve. A study investigating the efficacy of PRGF to treat DES reported that out of 16 patients, 75% experienced moderate to substantial improvements. Use of PRGF has demonstrated an ability to reduce symptoms of squamous metaplasia in patients suffering from DES (101).

As mentioned above, the development of human platelet lysates (HPL) manufactured from platelet concentrates collected following the licensed procedures in place to prepare blood products for transfusion is very likely and opens the roadmap for the development of more standardized SED (103).

Finally, recently, a limited case study was conducted in the UK where patients applied a drop of whole blood to the affected eye(s) four times daily for 8 weeks. Significant improvements were noted in several parameters, such as visual acuity, corneal staining, tear break-up time (TBUT), and ocular comfort index (OCI), but not Schirmer's test (104).

CONCLUSION AND FUTURE PROSPECTS

Dry eye syndrome is a common eye condition with a range of causes and degrees of severity and tremendous socioeconomic implications in addition to reductions in quality of life. There is a wide variety of medical products and procedures currently available or under development for the treatment of DES, each with their own advantages and disadvantages. Emerging treatment options include products derived from whole blood, such as autologous or allogeneic SED, E-PRP, PRGF, and HPL.

Relevant questions regarding the production method, quality, efficacy and safety of blood products used to treat DES remain, as already identified in particular with regards to standardization and formulation (87, 103). Similar to most claimed applications of platelet-derived preparations used in regenerative medicine, work is needed to design and standardize SED production methods to yield formulations with optimized blood proteins and growth factors composition to best address various DES and ocular pathologies. Reliable *in vitro* tests should be identified and validated as predictor of clinical outcomes (87). Furthermore, pre-clinical studies using valid animal models (105) to delineate the respective contribution of the plasma and platelet proteomes in the benefits of blood-derived eye drops in releasing DES symptoms should be performed. As is the case in other fields of regenerative medicine (106), dedicated platelet lysates may be needed to tackle the specific micro-environment of the diseased tissues and promote optimal repair strategies. An increasing involvement of blood establishments in producing SED is expected to contribute to improve standardization, quality, and safety (67).

In summary, blood products are well known for their benefits in relieving a variety of symptoms associated with DES. Many new and emerging blood products are currently being assessed for the presence of key growth factors and their overall effects weighed against their potential risks. Ultimately, as more evidence-based knowledge is obtained on the specific growth factors and their direct impact, patients with ocular defects should be able to receive personalized treatments, better customized to their individual needs and pathology, which are becoming the buzzword of all clinical interventions.

AUTHOR CONTRIBUTIONS

VJD and TB wrote the first draft. CLT made additions. JS reviewed and modified the final draft. All authors approved the final version.

REFERENCES

1. Schaumberg DA, Dana R, Buring JE, Sullivan DA. Prevalence of dry eye disease among US men: estimates from the physicians' health studies. *Arch Ophthalmol* (2009) 127(6):763–8. doi:10.1001/archophthalmol.2009.103
2. Barabino S, Labetoulle M, Rolando M, Messmer EM. Understanding symptoms and quality of life in patients with dry eye syndrome. *Ocul Surf* (2016) 14(3):365–76. doi:10.1016/j.jtos.2016.04.005
3. Shimmura S, Shimazaki J, Tsubota K. Results of a population-based questionnaire on the symptoms and lifestyles associated with dry eye. *Cornea* (1999) 18(4):408–11. doi:10.1097/00003226-199907000-00003
4. Schaumberg DA, Sullivan DA, Buring JE, Dana MR. Prevalence of dry eye syndrome among US women. *Am J Ophthalmol* (2003) 136(2):318–26. doi:10.1016/S0002-9394(03)00218-6
5. Schein OD, MUÑO B, Tielsch JM, Bandeen-Roche K, West S. Prevalence of dry eye among the elderly. *Am J Ophthalmol* (1997) 124(6):723–8. doi:10.1016/S0002-9394(14)71688-5
6. Pflugfelder SC, Solomon A, Stern ME. The diagnosis and management of dry eye: a twenty-five-year review. *Cornea* (2000) 19(5):644–9. doi:10.1097/00003226-200009000-00009
7. Messmer EM. The pathophysiology, diagnosis, and treatment of dry eye disease. *Dtsch Arztebl Int* (2015) 112(5):71. doi:10.3238/arztebl.2015.0071
8. Nebbioso M, Fameli V, Gharbiya M, Sacchetti M, Zicari AM, Lambiase A. Investigational drugs in dry eye disease. *Expert Opin Investig Drugs* (2016) 25(12):1437–46. doi:10.1080/13543784.2016.1249564
9. Sullivan BD, Evans JE, Dana MR, Sullivan DA. Influence of aging on the polar and neutral lipid profiles in human meibomian gland secretions. *Arch Ophthalmol* (2006) 124(9):1286–92. doi:10.1001/archopht.124.9.1286
10. Yoon KC, De Paiva CS, Qi H, Chen Z, Farley WJ, Li DQ, et al. Expression of Th-1 chemokines and chemokine receptors on the ocular surface of C57BL/6 mice: effects of desiccating stress. *Invest Ophthalmol Vis Sci* (2007) 48(6):2561–9. doi:10.1167/iovs.07-0002
11. Mrugacz M, Ostrowska L, Bryl A, Szulc A, Zelazowska-Rutkowska B, Mrugacz G. Pro-inflammatory cytokines associated with clinical severity of dry eye disease of patients with depression. *Adv Med Sci* (2017) 62(2):338–44. doi:10.1016/j.advms.2017.03.003
12. Liu R, Gao C, Chen H, Li Y, Jin Y, Qi H. Analysis of Th17-associated cytokines and clinical correlations in patients with dry eye disease. *PLoS One* (2017) 12(4):e0173301. doi:10.1371/journal.pone.0173301
13. Luo L, Li DQ, Doshi A, Farley W, Corrales RM, Pflugfelder SC. Experimental dry eye stimulates production of inflammatory cytokines and MMP-9 and activates MAPK signaling pathways on the ocular surface. *Invest Ophthalmol Vis Sci* (2004) 45(12):4293–301. doi:10.1167/iovs.03-1145
14. Tan X, Sun S, Liu Y, Zhu T, Wang K, Ren T, et al. Analysis of Th17-associated cytokines in tears of patients with dry eye syndrome. *Eye (Lond)* (2014) 28(5):608–13. doi:10.1038/eye.2014.38
15. Miljanović B, Dana R, Sullivan DA, Schaumberg DA. Impact of dry eye syndrome on vision-related quality of life. *Am J Ophthalmol* (2007) 143(3):409–15.e2. doi:10.1016/j.ajo.2006.11.060
16. Ayaki M, Kawashima M, Negishi K, Kishimoto T, Mimura M, Tsubota K. Sleep and mood disorders in dry eye disease and allied irritating ocular diseases. *Sci Rep* (2016) 6:22480. doi:10.1038/srep22480
17. Zheng Y, Wu X, Lin X, Lin H. The prevalence of depression and depressive symptoms among eye disease patients: a systematic review and meta-analysis. *Sci Rep* (2017) 7:46453. doi:10.1038/srep46453
18. Wan KH, Chen LJ, Young AL. Depression and anxiety in dry eye disease: a systematic review and meta-analysis. *Eye (Lond)* (2016) 30(12):1558–67. doi:10.1038/eye.2016.186
19. Kawashima M, Uchino M, Yokoi N, Uchino Y, Dogru M, Komuro A, et al. Associations between subjective happiness and dry eye disease: a new perspective from the Osaka study. *PLoS One* (2015) 10(4):e0123299. doi:10.1371/journal.pone.0123299
20. Mrugacz M, Ostrowska L, Łazarczyk-Kirejczyk J, Bryl A, Mrugacz G, Stefańska E, et al. Dry eye disease in patients treated with antidepressants. *Klin Oczna* (2013) 115(2):111–4.
21. McDonald M, Patel DA, Keith MS, Snedecor SJ. Economic and humanistic burden of dry eye disease in Europe, North America, and Asia: a systematic literature review. *Ocul Surf* (2016) 14(2):144–67. doi:10.1016/j.jtos.2015.11.002
22. Yu J, Asche CV, Fairchild CJ. The economic burden of dry eye disease in the United States: a decision tree analysis. *Cornea* (2011) 30(4):379–87. doi:10.1097/ICO.0b013e3181f7f363
23. Mizuno Y, Yamada M, Shigeyasu C. Annual direct cost of dry eye in Japan. *Clin Ophthalmol* (2012) 6:755–60. doi:10.2147/OPTH.S30625
24. Clegg JP, Guest JF, Lehman A, Smith AF. The annual cost of dry eye syndrome in France, Germany, Italy, Spain, Sweden and the United Kingdom among patients managed by ophthalmologists. *Ophthalmic Epidemiol* (2006) 13(4):263–74. doi:10.1080/09286580600801044
25. McMonnies CW. Measurement of symptoms pre- and post-treatment of dry eye syndromes. *Optom Vis Sci* (2016) 93(11):1431–7. doi:10.1097/OPX.0000000000000965
26. Pan Q, Angelina A, Zambrano A, Marrone M, Stark WJ, Heflin T, et al. Autologous serum eye drops for dry eye. *Cochrane Database Syst Rev* (2013) 8:CD009327. doi:10.1002/14651858.CD009327.pub2
27. Pucker AD, Ng SM, Nichols JJ. Over the counter (OTC) artificial tear drops for dry eye syndrome. *Cochrane Database Syst Rev* (2016) 2:CD009729. doi:10.1002/14651858.CD009729.pub2
28. Simmons PA, Liu H, Carlisle-Wilcox C, Vehige JG. Efficacy and safety of two new formulations of artificial tears in subjects with dry eye disease: a 3-month, multicenter, active-controlled, randomized trial. *Clin Ophthalmol* (2015) 9:665–75. doi:10.2147/OPTH.S78184
29. Fernandez KB, Epstein SP, Raynor GS, Sheyman AT, Massingale ML, Dentone PG, et al. Modulation of HLA-DR in dry eye patients following 30 days of treatment with a lubricant eyedrop solution. *Clin Ophthalmol* (2015) 9:1137–45. doi:10.2147/OPTH.S81355
30. Pinto-Bonilla JC, del Olmo-Jimeno A, Llovet-Osuna F, Hernández-Galilea E. A randomized crossover study comparing trehalose/hyaluronate eyedrops and standard treatment: patient satisfaction in the treatment of dry eye syndrome. *Ther Clin Risk Manag* (2015) 11:595. doi:10.2147/TCRM.S77091
31. Chiambaretta F, Doan S, Labetoulle M, Rocher N, Fekih LE, Messaoud R, et al. A randomized, controlled study of the efficacy and safety of a new eyedrop formulation for moderate to severe dry eye syndrome. *Eur J Ophthalmol* (2017) 27(1):1–9. doi:10.5301/ejo.5000836
32. Yamada C, King KE, Ness PM. Autologous serum eyedrops: literature review and implications for transfusion medicine specialists. *Transfusion* (2008) 48(6):1245–55. doi:10.1111/j.1537-2995.2008.01665.x
33. Tsubota K, Higuchi A. Serum application for the treatment of ocular surface disorders. *Int Ophthalmol Clin* (2000) 40(4):113–22. doi:10.1097/00004397-200010000-00009
34. Lopez-Garcia JS, Garcia-Lozano I, Rivas L, Martinez-Garchitorena J. Use of autologous serum in ophthalmic practice. *Arch Soc Esp Oftalmol* (2007) 82:9–20.
35. Baudouin C, Labbé A, Liang H, Pauly A, Brignole-Baudouin F. Preservatives in eyedrops: the good, the bad and the ugly. *Prog Retin Eye Res* (2010) 29(4):312–34. doi:10.1016/j.preteyeres.2010.03.001
36. Bhargava R, Kumar P, Phogat H, Kaur A, Kumar M. Oral omega-3 fatty acids treatment in computer vision syndrome related dry eye. *Cont Lens Anterior Eye* (2015) 38(3):206–10. doi:10.1016/j.clae.2015.01.007

37. Wang L, Chen X, Hao J, Yang L. Proper balance of omega-3 and omega-6 fatty acid supplements with topical cyclosporine attenuated contact lens-related dry eye syndrome. *Inflammopharmacology* (2016) 24(6):389–96. doi:10.1007/s10787-016-0291-2
38. Perez VL, Pflugfelder SC, Zhang S, Shojaei A, Haque R. Lifitegrast, a novel integrin antagonist for treatment of dry eye disease. *Ocul Surf* (2016) 14(2):207–15. doi:10.1016/j.jtos.2016.01.001
39. Holland EJ, Luchs J, Karpecki PM, Nichols KK, Jackson MA, Sall K, et al. Lifitegrast for the treatment of dry eye disease: results of a phase III, randomized, double-masked, placebo-controlled trial (OPUS-3). *Ophthalmology* (2017) 124(1):53–60. doi:10.1016/j.ophtha.2016.09.025
40. Bielory BP, Shah SP, O'Brien TP, Perez VL, Bielory L. Emerging therapeutics for ocular surface disease. *Curr Opin Allergy Clin Immunol* (2016) 16(5):477–86. doi:10.1097/ACI.0000000000000309
41. Tauber J, Karpecki P, Latkany R, Luchs J, Martel J, Sall K, et al. Lifitegrast ophthalmic solution 5.0% versus placebo for treatment of dry eye disease: results of the randomized phase III OPUS-2 study. *Ophthalmology* (2015) 122(12):2423–31. doi:10.1016/j.ophtha.2015.08.001
42. Cutolo CA, Barabino S, Bonzano C, Traverso CE. The use of topical corticosteroids for treatment of dry eye syndrome. *Ocul Immunol Inflamm* (2017):1–10. doi:10.1080/09273948.2017.1341988
43. Tseng CL, Hung YJ, Chen ZY, Fang HW, Chen KH. Synergistic effect of artificial tears containing epigallocatechin gallate and hyaluronic acid for the treatment of rabbits with dry eye syndrome. *PLoS One* (2016) 11(6):e0157982. doi:10.1371/journal.pone.0157982
44. Wan KH, Chen LJ, Young AL. Efficacy and safety of topical 0.05% cyclosporine eye drops in the treatment of dry eye syndrome: a systematic review and meta-analysis. *Ocul Surf* (2015) 13(3):213–25. doi:10.1016/j.jtos.2014.12.006
45. Agarwal P, Rupenthal ID. Modern approaches to the ocular delivery of cyclosporine A. *Drug Discov Today* (2016) 21(6):977–88. doi:10.1016/j.drudis.2016.04.002
46. Stevenson D, Tauber J, Reis BL. Efficacy and safety of cyclosporin A ophthalmic emulsion in the treatment of moderate-to-severe dry eye disease: a dose-ranging, randomized trial. The cyclosporin A phase 2 study group. *Ophthalmology* (2000) 107(5):967–74. doi:10.1016/S0161-6420(00)00035-X
47. Wilson SE, Perry HD. Long-term resolution of chronic dry eye symptoms and signs after topical cyclosporine treatment. *Ophthalmology* (2007) 114(1):76–9. doi:10.1016/j.ophtha.2006.05.077
48. Bourkiza R, Lee V. A review of the complications of lacrimal occlusion with punctal and canalicular plugs. *Orbit* (2012) 31(2):86–93. doi:10.3109/01676830.2011.648802
49. Yazdani C, McLaughlin T, Smeeding JE, Walt J. Prevalence of treated dry eye disease in a managed care population. *Clin Ther* (2001) 23(10):1672–82. doi:10.1016/S0149-2918(01)80136-3
50. Cohen EJ. Punctal occlusion. *Arch Ophthalmol* (1999) 117(3):389–90. doi:10.1001/archopht.117.3.389
51. Roberts CW, Carniglia PE, Brazzo BG. Comparison of topical cyclosporine, punctal occlusion, and a combination for the treatment of dry eye. *Cornea* (2007) 26(7):805–9. doi:10.1097/ICO.0b013e318074e460
52. Tong L, Beuerman R, Simonyi S, Hollander DA, Stern ME. Effects of punctal occlusion on clinical signs and symptoms and on tear cytokine levels in patients with dry eye. *Ocul Surf* (2016) 14(2):233–41. doi:10.1016/j.jtos.2015.12.004
53. Liu D, Sadhan Y. Surgical punctal occlusion: a prospective study. *Br J Ophthalmol* (2002) 86(9):1031–4. doi:10.1136/bjo.86.9.1031
54. Ervin AM, Law A, Pucker AD. Punctal occlusion for dry eye syndrome. *Cochrane Database Syst Rev* (2017) 6:CD006775. doi:10.1002/14651858.CD006775.pub3
55. Burnouf T, Goubran HA, Chen TM, Ou KL, El-Ekiaby M, Radosevic M. Blood-derived biomaterials and platelet growth factors in regenerative medicine. *Blood Rev* (2013) 27(2):77–89. doi:10.1016/j.blre.2013.02.001
56. Burnouf T, Strunk D, Koh MB, Schallmoser K. Human platelet lysate: replacing fetal bovine serum as a gold standard for human cell propagation? *Biomaterials* (2016) 76:371–87. doi:10.1016/j.biomaterials.2015.10.065
57. Geerling G, Maclennan S, Hartwig D. Autologous serum eye drops for ocular surface disorders. *Br J Ophthalmol* (2004) 88(11):1467–74. doi:10.1136/bjo.2004.044347
58. Burnouf T, Chou ML, Wu YW, Su CY, Lee LW. Antimicrobial activity of platelet (PLT)-poor plasma, PLT-rich plasma, PLT gel, and solvent/detergent-treated PLT lysate biomaterials against wound bacteria. *Transfusion* (2013) 53(1):138–46. doi:10.1111/j.1537-2995.2012.03668.x
59. Hussain M, Shtein RM, Sugar A, Soong HK, Woodward MA, DeLoss K, et al. Long-term use of autologous serum 50% eye drops for the treatment of dry eye disease. *Cornea* (2014) 33(12):1245–51. doi:10.1097/ICO.0000000000000271
60. Anitua E, Muruzabal F, Tayebba A, Riestra A, Perez VL, Merayo-Lloves J, et al. Autologous serum and plasma rich in growth factors in ophthalmology: preclinical and clinical studies. *Acta Ophthalmol* (2015) 93(8):e605–14. doi:10.1111/aos.12710
61. Klenkler B, Sheardown H, Jones L. Growth factors in the tear film: role in tissue maintenance, wound healing, and ocular pathology. *Ocul Surf* (2007) 5(3):228–39. doi:10.1016/S1542-0124(12)70613-4
62. Tsubota K, Goto E, Fujita H, Ono M, Inoue H, Saito I, et al. Treatment of dry eye by autologous serum application in Sjögren's syndrome. *Br J Ophthalmol* (1999) 83(4):390–5. doi:10.1136/bjo.83.4.390
63. Setten GBV, Tervo T, Tervo K, Tarkkanen A. Epidermal growth factor (EGF) in ocular fluids: presence, origin and therapeutical considerations. *Acta Ophthalmol* (1992) 202:54–9.
64. Nurden AT. The biology of the platelet with special reference to inflammation, wound healing and immunity. *Front Biosci (Landmark Ed)* (2018) 23:726–51. doi:10.2741/4613
65. Nurden AT, Nurden P, Sanchez M, Andia I, Anitua E. Platelets and wound healing. *Front Biosci* (2008) 13:3532–48.
66. von Hofsten J, Egardt M, Zetterberg M. The use of autologous serum for the treatment of ocular surface disease at a Swedish tertiary referral center. *Int Med Case Rep J* (2016) 9:47. doi:10.2147/IMCRJ.S97297
67. Marks DC, van der Meer PF; Biomedical Excellence for Safer Transfusion (BEST) Collaborative. Serum eye drops: a survey of international production methods. *Vox Sang* (2017) 112(4):310–7. doi:10.1111/vox.12502
68. Espinosa A, Hjorth-Hansen H, Aasly K, Teigum I, Sivertsen G, Seghatchian J. Implementation of a standardised method for the production of allogeneic serum eye drops from regular blood donors in a Norwegian University Hospital: some methodological aspects and clinical considerations. *Transfus Apher Sci* (2015) 53(1):88–91. doi:10.1016/j.transci.2015.05.014
69. Harritshoj LH, Nielsen C, Ullum H, Hansen MB, Julian HO. Ready-made allogeneic ABO-specific serum eye drops: production from regular male blood donors, clinical routine, safety and efficacy. *Acta Ophthalmol* (2014) 92(8):783–6. doi:10.1111/aos.12386
70. Badami KG, McKellar M. Allogeneic serum eye drops: time these became the norm? *Br J Ophthalmol* (2012) 96(8):1151–2. doi:10.1136/bjophthalmol-2012-301668
71. Cho YK, Huang W, Kim GY, Lim BS. Comparison of autologous serum eye drops with different diluents. *Curr Eye Res* (2013) 38(1):9–17. doi:10.3109/02713683.2012.720340
72. Pan Q, Angelina A, Marrone M, Stark WJ, Akpek EK. Autologous serum eye drops for dry eye. *Cochrane Database Syst Rev* (2017) 2:CD009327. doi:10.1002/14651858.CD009327.pub3
73. Lopez-Garcia JS, Garcia-Lozano I, Rivas L, Ramirez N, Raposo R, Mendez MT. Autologous serum eye drops diluted with sodium hyaluronate: clinical and experimental comparative study. *Acta Ophthalmol* (2014) 92(1):e22–9. doi:10.1111/aos.12167
74. WHO. *Recommendations for the Production, Quality Control and Regulation of Plasma for Fractionation*. Geneva: World Health Organization (2005). Available from: http://www.who.int/biologicals/publications/ECBS%202005%20Annex%204%20Human%20Plasma%20Fractionation.pdf
75. WHO. WHO guidelines on good manufacturing practices for blood establishments. *WHO Tech Rep Ser* (2011) 961:148–214.
76. Burnouf T, Radosevich M. Reducing the risk of infection from plasma products: specific preventative strategies. *Blood Rev* (2000) 14:94–110. doi:10.1054/blre.2000.0129
77. Dodd RY. Emerging pathogens and their implications for the blood supply and transfusion transmitted infections. *Br J Haematol* (2012) 159:135–42. doi:10.1111/bjh.12031
78. Kiely P, Gambhir M, Cheng AC, McQuilten ZK, Seed CR, Wood EM. Emerging infectious diseases and blood safety: modeling the transfusion-transmission risk. *Transfus Med Rev* (2017) 31(3):154–64. doi:10.1016/j.tmrv.2017.05.002
79. Yawn BP, Wollan PC, St Sauver JL, Butterfield LC. Herpes zoster eye complications: rates and trends. *Mayo Clin Proc* (2013) 88(6):562–70. doi:10.1016/j.mayocp.2013.03.014

80. Drew VJ, Barro L, Seghatchian J, Burnouf T. Towards pathogen inactivation of red blood cells and whole blood targeting viral DNA/RNA: design, technologies, and future prospects for developing countries. *Blood Transfus* (2017) 15(6):512–21. doi:10.2450/2017.0344-16
81. Devine DV, Schubert P. Pathogen inactivation technologies: the advent of pathogen-reduced blood components to reduce blood safety risk. *Hematol Oncol Clin North Am* (2016) 30(3):609–17. doi:10.1016/j.hoc.2016.01.005
82. Stahle MU, Brandhorst D, Korsgren O, Knutson F. Pathogen inactivation of human serum facilitates its clinical use for islet cell culture and subsequent transplantation. *Cell Transplant* (2011) 20(5):775–81. doi:10.3727/0963689 10X539056
83. Tseng CL, Chen ZY, Renn TY, Hsiao SH, Burnouf T. Solvent/detergent virally inactivated serum eye drops restore healthy ocular epithelium in a rabbit model of dry-eye syndrome. *PLoS One* (2016) 11(4):e0153573. doi:10.1371/journal.pone.0153573
84. Liu L, Hartwig D, Harloff S, Herminghaus P, Wedel T, Geerling G. An optimised protocol for the production of autologous serum eyedrops. *Graefes Arch Clin Exp Ophthalmol* (2005) 243(7):706–14. doi:10.1007/s00417-004-1106-5
85. EDQM. *Good Practice Guidelines for Blood Establishments and Hospital Blood Banks Required to Comply with EU Directive 2005/62/EC – Guide to the Preparation, Use and Quality Assurance of Blood Components. Recommendation No. R (95) 15.* 18th ed. Strasbourg, France: European Directorate for the Quality of Medicines & HealthCare (2015).
86. Alio JL, Rodriguez AE, Ferreira-Oliveira R, Wrobel-Dudzinska D, Abdelghany AA. Treatment of dry eye disease with autologous platelet-rich plasma: a prospective, interventional, non-randomized study. *Ophthalmol Ther* (2017) 6(2):285–93. doi:10.1007/s40123-017-0100-z
87. van der Meer PF, Seghatchian J, Marks DC. Quality standards, safety and efficacy of blood-derived serum eye drops: a review. *Transfus Apher Sci* (2016) 54(1):164–7. doi:10.1016/j.transci.2016.01.022
88. Chiang C-C, Lin J-M, Chen W-L, Tsai Y-Y. Allogeneic serum eye drops for the treatment of severe dry eye in patients with chronic graft-versus-host disease. *Cornea* (2007) 26(7):861–3. doi:10.1097/ICO.0b013e3180645cd7
89. Noble BA, Loh RSK, MacLennan S, Pesudovs K, Reynolds A, Bridges LR, et al. Comparison of autologous serum eye drops with conventional therapy in a randomised controlled crossover trial for ocular surface disease. *Br J Ophthalmol* (2004) 88:647–52. doi:10.1136/bjo.2003.026211
90. Kojima T, Ishida R, Dogru M, Goto E, Matsumoto Y, Kaido M, et al. The effect of autologous serum eyedrops in the treatment of severe dry eye disease: a prospective randomized case-control study. *Am J Ophthalmol* (2005) 139(2):242–6. doi:10.1016/j.ajo.2004.08.040
91. Jeng BH, Dupps WJ Jr. Autologous serum 50% eyedrops in the treatment of persistent corneal epithelial defects. *Cornea* (2009) 28(10):1104–8. doi:10.1097/ICO.0b013e3181a2a7f6
92. Na KS, Kim MS. Allogeneic serum eye drops for the treatment of dry eye patients with chronic graft-versus-host disease. *J Ocul Pharmacol Ther* (2012) 28(5):479–83. doi:10.1089/jop.2012.0002
93. Celebi AR, Ulusoy C, Mirza GE. The efficacy of autologous serum eye drops for severe dry eye syndrome: a randomized double-blind crossover study. *Graefes Arch Clin Exp Ophthalmol* (2014) 252(4):619–26. doi:10.1007/s00417-014-2599-1
94. Chiang CC, Chen WL, Lin JM, Tsai YY. Allogeneic serum eye drops for the treatment of persistent corneal epithelial defect. *Eye (Lond)* (2009) 23(2):290–3. doi:10.1038/sj.eye.6703079
95. Higuchi A, Ueno R, Shimmura S, Suematsu M, Dogru M, Tsubota K. Albumin rescues ocular epithelial cells from cell death in dry eye. *Curr Eye Res* (2007) 32(2):83–8. doi:10.1080/02713680601147690
96. Shimmura S, Ueno R, Matsumoto Y, Goto E, Higuchi A, Shimazaki J, et al. Albumin as a tear supplement in the treatment of severe dry eye. *Br J Ophthalmol* (2003) 87(10):1279–83. doi:10.1136/bjo.87.10.1279
97. Alio JL, Rodriguez AE, WróbelDudzinska D. Eye platelet-rich plasma in the treatment of ocular surface disorders. *Curr Opin Ophthalmol* (2015) 26(4):325–32. doi:10.1097/ICU.0000000000000169
98. Alio JL, Arnalich-Montiel F, Rodriguez AE. The role of "eye platelet rich plasma (E-PRP)" for wound healing in ophthalmology. *Curr Pharm Biotechnol* (2012) 13(7):1257–65. doi:10.2174/138920112800624355
99. Avila MY. Restoration of human lacrimal function following platelet-rich plasma injection. *Cornea* (2014) 33(1):18–21. doi:10.1097/ICO.0000000000000016
100. Anitua E, de la Fuente M, Riestra A, Merayo-Lloves J, Muruzabal F, Orive G. Preservation of biological activity of plasma and platelet-derived eye drops after their different time and temperature conditions of storage. *Cornea* (2015) 34(9):1144–8. doi:10.1097/Ico.0000000000000489
101. Lopez-Plandolit S, Morales MC, Freire V, Grau AE, Duran JA. Efficacy of plasma rich in growth factors for the treatment of dry eye. *Cornea* (2011) 30(12):1312–7. doi:10.1097/ICO.0b013e31820d86d6
102. Anitua E. Plasma rich in growth factors: preliminary results of use in the preparation of future sites for implants. *Int J Oral Maxillofac Implants* (1999) 14(4):529–35.
103. Seghatchian J, Espinosa A, Burnouf T. Quality, safety and sustained therapeutic efficacy of blood-derived serum eye drops to treat dry eye syndrome: R&D road map for future progress. *Transfus Apher Sci* (2016) 54(1):168–9. doi:10.1016/j.transci.2016.01.023
104. Than J, Balal S, Wawrzynski J, Nesaratnam N, Saleh GM, Moore J, et al. Fingerprick autologous blood: a novel treatment for dry eye syndrome. *Eye (Lond)* (2017) 31(12):1655–63. doi:10.1038/eye.2017.118
105. Tseng CL, Seghatchian J, Burnouf T. Animal models to assess the therapeutic efficacy of human serum and serum-converted platelet lysates for dry eye syndrome: seeing is believing. *Transfus Apher Sci* (2015) 53(1):95–8. doi:10.1016/j.transci.2015.05.016
106. Chou ML, Wu JW, Gouel F, Jonneaux A, Timmerman K, Renn TY, et al. Tailor-made purified human platelet lysate concentrated in neurotrophins for treatment of Parkinson's disease. *Biomaterials* (2017) 142:77–89. doi:10.1016/j.biomaterials.2017.07.018

13

Toward the Relevance of Platelet Subpopulations for Transfusion Medicine

*Stefan Handtke[1], Leif Steil[2], Andreas Greinacher[1] and Thomas Thiele[1]**

[1]*Institut für Immunologie und Transfusionsmedizin, Greifswald, Germany,* [2]*Interfakultäres Institut für Funktionelle Genomforschung, Greifswald, Germany*

Correspondence:
Thomas Thiele
thielet@uni-greifswald.de

Circulating platelets consist of subpopulations with different age, maturation state and size. In this review, we address the association between platelet size and platelet function and summarize the current knowledge on platelet subpopulations including reticulated platelets, procoagulant platelets and platelets exposing signals to mediate their clearance. Thereby, we emphasize the impact of platelet turnover as an important condition for platelet production *in vivo*. Understanding of the features that characterize platelet subpopulations is very relevant for the methods of platelet concentrate production, which may enrich or deplete particular platelet subpopulations. Moreover, the concept of platelet size being associated with platelet function may be attractive for transfusion medicine as it holds the perspective to separate platelet subpopulations with specific functional capabilities.

Keywords: platelet subpopulation, platelet size, platelet turnover, platelet clearance, platelet maturation

INTRODUCTION

Platelets recognize vessel damage, trigger coagulation and enhance clot formation at the site of injury (1). Beyond hemostasis, platelets also act as mediators in immunity and inflammation (2–5).

Circulating platelets differ in age, maturation state, or density. An obvious physical feature of platelets is their size, which can vary substantially among platelets of one individual. It was an early concept, that large platelets represent a rather young and reactive platelet subpopulation (6). Later, this concept was abandoned when consecutive experiments demonstrated no clear correlation between platelet size and age (7, 8).

The observation that some platelets have particular procoagulant capabilities led to the concept of platelet subpopulations with different biological functions (9). Other examples for platelet subpopulations are reticulated (rather young) platelets and platelets exposing signals mediating their clearance from the circulation (rather old platelets). It is conceivable albeit unclear, whether other platelet subpopulations exist which play a more pronounced role in immunological or inflammatory processes, e.g. by expression of CD40 or release of CD40L (10, 11).

Epidemiological studies found an association between an increased platelet size and thrombotic outcomes in patients with cardiovascular disease (12) resulting in a revival of the "old" hypothesis of an association between a larger platelet size and enhanced platelet function in hemostasis.

Clarifying the hypothesis of different biological features of platelet subpopulations is potentially relevant for transfusion medicine. Enrichment of distinct platelet subpopulations in platelet concentrates (PCs) during production may modulate the biological effects of PCs.

In this review, we summarize the current knowledge on platelet subpopulations with a special emphasis on platelet size, its association with platelet function and the impact of platelet turnover on platelet production.

SIZE AS A PLATELET CHARACTERISTIC

Platelet Formation, Turnover, and their Role for Platelet Size

Platelet size is genetically determined and relatively stable over the lifetime in healthy individuals. Genome wide association studies in healthy subjects identified several genes associated with platelet size (13–18).

Under steady-state conditions, platelets are generated from megakaryocytes in the bone marrow after stimulation with thrombopoietin. The amount of circulating thrombopoietin is regulated by the mass of circulating platelets. They bind thrombopoietin, providing a negative feedback mechanism to control thrombopoiesis (19). In mice, thrombopoietin administration increases platelet size (20) whereas in humans the opposite seems to be the case (21).

In the bone marrow, preplatelet intermediates are formed as extensions of elongated megakaryocyte-pseudopodia and released into the sinusoidal blood vessels (22, 23). Glycoprotein Ib mediates transmigration of megakaryocytes into the sinusoids *via* the small GTPases Cdc42 and RhoA (24). Preplatelets convert into barbell-shaped proplatelets that form platelets (23, 25) mediated by integrin αIIbβIII signaling (26). Platelet size is established during the formation of barbell proplatelets from circular preplatelets and limited by microtubule bundling, elastic bending, and actin-myosin-spectrin cortex forces (27).

Thrombopoiesis in the bone marrow is spatially regulated (28) but platelet maturation does not end in the bone marrow. Preplatelets are also formed from proplatelets in the circulation (29) and can maturate in the lungs (30).

In vivo, the mechanisms of proplatelet formation are very dynamic and influenced by platelet turnover (31). In case of inflammation an alternative pathway of platelet production can occur. Nishimura et al. found that increased serum levels of the inflammatory cytokine IL-1α induce platelet release by the rupture of megakaryocytes as a distinct mechanism in the absence of elevated thrombopoietin (32). *Via* this mechanism, larger platelets are produced than in thrombopoietin-stimulated megakaryocytes in mice.

We have established a model of enhanced platelet production in healthy volunteers using platelet apheresis showing that platelet apheresis stimulated platelet production leads to reversible changes in the platelet proteome (33). This further indicates an impact of platelet turnover on the phenotype of circulating human platelets.

Platelet Size and Function during Steady-State Platelet Production

Most studies identified large platelets as a subpopulation with a higher prohemostatic capacity, if generated under steady state. However, it is still debated whether a larger size alone contributes to this higher capacity (34), or if there are specific features in large platelets which over-proportionally increase their prohemostatic potential. **Table 1** provides an overview of functional comparisons between large and small human platelets. The majority of experiments included adjustments for cell size, suggesting a hyperproportional prohemostatic capacity of large platelets.

Steady-state large platelets have a higher capacity for glucose metabolism, resistance to osmotic shock (36), and lipid peroxidation (38). They aggregate faster and release more ATP and alpha granule proteins (34, 37), contain more fibrinogen, and serotonin (40), and express more human leukocyte antigen-I molecules (41) and membrane glycoproteins (43).

Platelets synthesize proteins (50) and large platelets have more ribosomes and incorporate more amino acids (35). Probably, large platelets have a higher capacity to translate mRNA. This needs to be demonstrated by future studies, which adequately control for residual leukocytes in the large platelet fraction.

Opper et al. found different patterns of cGMP synthesis and protein phosphorylation patterns after stimulating platelets of different size (44, 46), suggesting differences in signal transduction between large and small platelets.

The ability to mobilize Ca^{2+} in the cytosol is pivotal for platelet activation. Li et al. showed that the cytosolic Ca^{2+}-concentration is similar in resting large and small platelets, whereas higher amounts of Ca^{2+} are mobilized by large platelets (45).

Large platelets express more surface-bound fibrinogen, bind more von Willebrand factor, and metabolize more arachidonic acid (39), express more P-selectin, activate more integrin αIIbβ3 after ADP-stimulation (42, 47, 51), and release more thromboxane after collagen- and thrombin-induced aggregation in proportion to platelet size (39).

A recent study indicates that large-size platelets are functionally different compared to small platelets. Brambilla et al. found that large platelets express not only significantly higher amounts of tissue factor and tissue factor mRNA compared to small platelets. Large platelets also expose functionally active tissue factor on their cell membranes whereas the activity of tissue factor in small platelets is almost completely quenched by tissue factor pathway inhibitor (48). These results extent previous findings showing that platelets translate tissue factor (52) and point toward specific roles of large and small platelets in hemostasis.

Platelet Size during Increased Platelet Turnover

If platelet production is enhanced in healthy humans by application of thrombopoietin, the peripheral platelet concentration increases whereas platelet size measured by the mean platelet volume (MPV) slightly decreases without changes in platelet viability, platelet responsiveness to physiologic agonists, or expression of platelet activation markers (21).

In contrast, disease-related increased platelet turnover is often associated with an increase in platelet size (6, 53), e.g., in case of enhanced destruction of platelets by autoantibodies (54–56), during recovery after bone marrow suppression by chemotherapy (49), or in situations with increased consumption in patients with severe arterial disease (57, 58). These

TABLE 1 | Functional characterization of human large and small platelets.

Reference	Results	Size adjustment	Evidence for a hyperproportional difference between large and small platelets
Steady-state platelet production			
Booyse et al. (35)	Only large platelets contain ribosomes	Not performed	Yes
Karpatkin (36)	Large platelets: higher glycogen, higher orthophosphate, higher total adenine nucleotide, higher glucogenolysis capacity, higher glycolysis activity, higher protein synthesis, higher glycogen synthesis, higher resistance to osmotic shock	Ratios of analytes compared to ratios of platelet volumes	Yes
Karpatkin (37)	Large platelets: lag time to aggregation shorter; higher ATP release; following aggregation higher ADP release; higher release of platelet factor 4	Not performed	Not applicable
Karpatkin and Strick (38)	Large platelets: higher activity of glycolysis enzymes, less lipid peroxidation product, more resistant to lipid peroxidation	Equal amount of protein extract taken from large and small platelets	Yes
Thompson et al. (34)	Large platelets: maximal aggregation after activation by collagen or thrombin increased; contain larger amounts of ATP and beta-thromboglobulin	Relative change within each size fraction (aggregometry); relative comparison of ATP and beta-thromboglobulin before and after stimulation	Yes
Jakubowski et al. (39)	Large platelets: release more thromboxane after collagen or thrombin stimulation Platelet size correlates with the amount of metabolized arachidonic acid	Correlation to MPV	No
Mezzano et al. (40)	Large platelets: more fibrinogen, more serotonin and more absolute protein	Not performed	Not applicable
Pereira et al. (41)	Large platelets: more P1[a1] molecules; small platelets: more HLA-A2 molecules, more total HLA class I-molecules	Not performed	Not applicable
Frojmovic et al. (42)	Large platelets: more fibrinogen receptor expressed on membrane when activated; faster aggregation rate	Correlation of ratios large/small with size ratio large/small	No
Polanowska-Grabowska et al. (43)	Large platelets: faster adhesion to collagen, less sensitive to inhibition by prostacyclin, increased content of glycoprotein Ia/iia complex	Not performed	Not applicable
Opper et al. (44)	Large platelets: higher basal level of cgmp, higher cgmp synthesis rate after stimulation with sodium nitroprusside, lower activity of camp-dependent phosphodiesterases	Adjustment of protein content and platelet size	Yes
Li et al. (45)	Large platelets: higher maximal aggregation after stimulation with thrombin, increased ATP secretion, higher degree of calcium mobilization	Relative change within each size fraction (aggregometry)	Yes
Opper et al. (46)	Large platelets: higher degree of protein phosphorylation after thrombin stimulation, higher rate of ADP-ribosylation by cholera toxin; small platelets: higher basal phosphorylation levels of several proteins, higher ADP-Ribosylation by pertussis toxin and C3 exoenzyme, higher basal Ca^{2+}-level	Equal amount of protein extract taken from large and small platelets	Yes
Mangalpally et al. (47)	Large platelets: express more surface-bound fibrinogen, bind more von Willebrand factor after arachidonic acid- or ADP-stimulation, express more P-selectin, more activated glycoprotein iib/iiia after ADP stimulation; higher proportion of reticulated platelets	Adjustment to the platelet surface area	Yes
Brambilla et al. (48)	Large platelets: contain higher amounts of tissue factor and tissue factor mrna; mainly large platelets expose functionally active tissue factor	Not performed	Not applicable

(Continued)

TABLE 1 | Continued

Reference	Results	Size adjustment	Evidence for a hyperproportional difference between large and small platelets
Increased platelet turnover			
Balduini et al. (49)	Old platelets: MPV and P-LCR reduced; young platelets: MPV and P-LCR higher compared to old and to control; aggregation response faster in young platelets	Relative change within each size fraction (aggregometry)	Yes

MPV, mean platelet volume; P-LCR, platelet large cell ratio; HLA, human leukocyte antigen.

studies suggest that platelet size in disease is regulated by other mechanisms than the ones regulating platelet size during thrombopoietin-mediated megakaryocytopoiesis in healthy volunteers. Severe thrombocytopenia induced by disseminated intravascular coagulation in children is also associated with an increase in platelet size (59). However, in view of the findings of Nishimura et al. (32), this likely results from platelet production by the alternative pathway involving IL-1α induced fragmentation of megakaryocytes.

Platelet Size and Platelet Age

The first attempts to characterize young platelets were driven by the hypothesis, that large platelets are considerably younger than small platelets because they are more functionally active (37, 38). However, later studies did not reveal a direct relationship between platelet size and age. This was convincingly underscored by an experiment in baboons under conditions of steady-state platelet production. The animals received radioactively labeled methionine being incorporated by megakaryocytes (8). Radioactively labeled platelets were afterwards present in each assessed size fraction of platelets indicating that size and age of platelets do not correlate under steady-state conditions. Also in humans platelet size is likely not strongly associated with platelet age (7). After transfusion of radioactively labeled autologous platelets, the mean survival of a high-density platelet population was shorter than that of platelets with low density. The mean volumes of high- and low-density platelets were not different suggesting that platelet size is unrelated to platelet age under normal conditions, but implicating a role of platelet density for the age of circulating platelets.

Platelet Size as Risk Factor for Adverse Clinical Outcomes

Epidemiological studies in patients with cardiovascular disease found an association between an increased MPV and a higher prevalence of thromboembolic complications (12, 60–62). An increased platelet size due to increased platelet turnover also correlates with refractoriness to antiplatelet therapy (58) and predicts a higher incidence of adverse outcomes after coronary intervention (63).

It is unclear, whether the increased MPV is the cause or the consequence of an increased risk for thromboembolic outcomes (60, 64). An alternative explanation is that individuals with large platelets have *per se* an increased risk for thrombotic complications because genetic traits have been identified, which are at the same time associated with an increased MPV and an increased risk for cardiovascular disease (65).

An increased MPV also characterizes inherited bleeding disorders with dysfunctional large platelets (66).

PLATELET SUBPOPULATIONS

Reticulated Platelets

Ingram et al. first observed a unique population of newly formed platelets soon after the induction of acute blood loss in beagle dogs. They stained platelets with methylene blue and noticed coarse and punctate condensations in platelets similar to those seen in reticulocytes of red cells. Therefore, this platelet fraction was named "reticulated platelets" (67). Later, reticulated platelets were shown to contain more RNA, staining with nucleic acid-specific fluorescent dyes, such as thiazole orange (68).

Reticulated platelets likely represent the youngest platelet fraction. After *in vivo* biotinylation, freshly formed platelets carrying reduced levels of biotin were shown to be reticulated (69). These platelets are younger than 24 h (70) and decay their RNA during aging (71).

In healthy humans with steady-state platelet production around 8% of circulating platelets are reticulated (72). Furthermore, the proportion of reticulated platelets is enriched in the fraction of large platelets compared to the fraction of small platelets (47), suggesting a relationship between platelet size and age.

A limitation of studies applying thiazole orange to stain reticulated platelets is, however, the tendency of this dye to bind unspecifically to alpha-granule contents (73). Therefore, a higher proportion of thiazole orange positive platelets observed in larger platelets could in part result from unspecific binding and may not represent young platelets (74). This limitation may be overcome by more RNA-specific dyes (75), which may finally elucidate the relationship between the size and age of platelets under steady-state platelet production.

In patients with high platelet turnover, the MPV is increased and likewise the proportion of reticulated platelets (72, 76, 77). One example that these changes may have biological relevance is their response to antiplatelet therapy. Despite dual antiplatelet therapy, large platelets with a higher proportion of reticulated platelets show increased *in vitro* reactivity compared to small platelets (78). Moreover, newly formed reticulated platelets show increased thrombogenicity after stopping prasugrel (75). Both observations suggest consequences for individualized antiplatelet therapy.

Procoagulant Platelets

About 30% of circulating platelets (range of 15–55%) can exhibit a procoagulant phenotype after stimulation with the agonists *col*lagen *a*nd *t*hrombin (79, 80). They were named COAT-platelets, which was later changed to coated platelets. Coated platelets express high levels of functional α-granule derived Factor V (FV) (79) and other α-granule proteins on their surface, including fibrinogen, von Willebrand factor, thrombospondin, fibronectin, and α_2-antiplasmin (81). Furthermore, coated platelets expose procoagulant phosphatidylserine (PS) on their surfaces (79, 82). PS exposure on the outer platelet membrane is closely related to disruption of inner mitochondrial membranes in the cells (83). In platelets, this process is controlled by calpain and not by caspases as in other cells (84). Therefore, PS exposure on procoagulant platelets is not necessarily related to apoptosis (85, 86). As not all PS-exposing platelets show the typical features of coated platelets, coated platelets seem to represent a procoagulant subgroup of PS-exposing platelets (82, 87).

Activation of the protease activated receptor 1 with thrombin, SFLLRN, and AYPGKF had strong additional effect (80) on the collagen-induced calcium peak and induced a sustained cytoplasmatic elevation of Ca^{2+} which is crucial for the formation of procoagulant platelets (88). Differential phosphorylation of PKCalpha and p38MAPK may drive the different calcium fluxes in coated compared to non-coated platelets (89). Increased cytosolic Ca^{2+} levels result in the inactivation of adenylatecyclase and activation of phosphatidylinositol 3-kinase and Src tyrosine kinase which further promotes procoagulant platelet segregation (90). On the other hand, elevated cytosolic Ca^{2+} levels can reverse integrin αIIbβ3 activation by stimulating intracellular cleavage of the β3-chain *via* calpain (91). PAC-1 binding is reduced in coated platelets although surface expression of αIIbβ3 is not diminished (89). The underlying mechanism is displacement of PAC-1 a stronger bond rather than inactivation of αIIbβ3 (92). This may explain why coated platelets do not take part in the formation of aggregates mediated by αIIbβ3.

Thus, platelet subpopulations arrange differently in a thrombus (93). Within a thrombus platelets with activated αIIbβ3 integrins assemble to aggregates. Those with inactive αIIbβ3 integrins remain solitary and form blebs and shed microparticles (93–95), the typical features of coated platelets. Independently of αIIbβ3, coated platelets attach to aggregates by forming caps of colocalized fibrinogen and thrombospondin on the PS-positive platelet surface (96). This allows coated platelets to become incorporated into thrombi independently of activated αIIbβ3 integrins.

Interestingly, platelet size has not yet been directly investigated as a feature of procoagulant human platelets. In rabbits, young platelets showed a similar size and the same ability to form procoagulant platelets under steady state compared to older platelets (74). If size is associated with the procoagulant capability of human platelets, it could be applied to enrich or deplete procoagulant platelets in PCs.

Platelets Exposing Signals for Clearance

Platelets survive for up to 10 days under normal conditions (97, 98). Platelets exposing signals to induce their clearance may be seen as another subpopulation with a limited life span. It would be desirable to reduce the amount of these platelets in PCs to prolong survival of transfused platelets.

Three main mechanisms have been identified by which platelets mediate their clearance (99). First, degraded glycans appear as a signal on platelet membranes which are recognized by the hepatic Ashwell Morrel Receptor (100). This has been demonstrated for cold stored platelets (101) and for platelets in sepsis (102, 103). Concomitantly, the removal of glycan deprived platelets *via* the Ashwell Morell Receptor in the liver induces hepatic thrombopoietin-mRNA expression and leads to increased megakaryocyte numbers and *de novo* platelet production (100).

The second mechanism is platelet apoptosis. Platelet survival is extended if the proapoptotic proteins Bak and Bax are lacking and reduced if the prosurvival proteins Bcl-2, Bcl-xL, and Mcl-1 are absent (104). Recently, protein kinase A was identified as a mediator of platelet life span by regulating apoptosis (105). However, the exact signals on the platelet surface and the corresponding receptor recognizing apoptotic platelets for platelet clearance are not yet identified. It is also unknown whether apoptotic signals appear differently in platelets of different size.

Finally, platelets are cleared after being opsonized with antibodies, which can be autoantibodies in diseases such as autoimmune thrombocytopenia, or alloantibodies in case of feto-maternal incompatibility, or after platelet transfusion (106). This mechanism is likely independent of platelet size.

Of note, P-selectin is an adhesion receptor for leukocytes expressed by activated platelets and was suggested to mediate platelet clearance. Berger et al. demonstrated that P-selectin does not mediate platelet clearance but may modulate leukocyte recruitment or thrombus growth (107).

CONCLUSION AND PERSPECTIVES

Understanding features differentiating platelet subpopulations has greatly improved. For example, platelet size correlates with platelet reactivity and mRNA content, which may classify large platelets as a prohemostatic subpopulation. These large platelets could be enriched in blood centers by differential or density gradient centrifugation, or special apheresis techniques in order to produce more potent PCs, e.g., for trauma patients.

It remains unclear, if large platelet fractions also include more procoagulant platelets. To gain further insight, PS-exposure, Ca^{2+}-mobilization and the ability to form coated platelets should be assessed in large and small platelets. Additionally, no data exist whether immunological functions of platelets correlate with platelet size.

Highly relevant for the interpretation of any study on the association of platelet size and platelet function is the fact that platelet turnover is important for platelet formation. Large platelets under steady state are likely different from large platelets generated under conditions of increased platelet turnover. This difference may explain some of the conflicting results on large and small platelets reported in the literature. It will be mandatory for future studies to exactly define the conditions of platelet turnover under which the investigated platelet population is generated as well as the agonists mediating thrombopoiesis in health and disease (108).

Platelet turnover may also be relevant for the production of PCs. Platelets derived from whole blood donation are collected under steady-state conditions because the donation procedure routinely lasts ~5–15 min and will unlikely result in changes in the collected platelets. In contrast, repeated platelet apheresis procedures may stimulate platelet generation because it lowers the platelet content more rapidly over a period of 60–90 min (109) and can be performed up to 3 times a week. This may have an effect on the collected platelet population, as shown for the platelet proteome after repeated apheresis (33). Moreover, platelets collected from hypertensive donors may differ in phenotype and functionality compared to those from normotensive donors (110).

Finally, PCs are produced by differential centrifugation leading to a loss of very large and very small platelets. Recently it was shown that the preparation procedure of red cell concentrates is associated with mortality (111). Enrichment of a specific platelet subpopulation in PCs by different preparation methods might also be relevant for the outcomes of transfused patients.

In summary, there is increasing evidence on platelet subpopulations with different biological functions, which are particularly interesting for transfusion medicine. Better understanding of the characteristics and functions of platelet subpopulations may be applied to develop new or improved platelet products.

AUTHOR CONTRIBUTIONS

All authors listed have made a substantial, direct, and intellectual contribution to the work and approved it for publication.

REFERENCES

1. Mancuso ME, Santagostino E. Platelets: much more than bricks in a breached wall. *Br J Haematol* (2017) 178(2):209–19. doi:10.1111/bjh.14653
2. Morrell CN, Aggrey AA, Chapman LM, Modjeski KL. Emerging roles for platelets as immune and inflammatory cells. *Blood* (2014) 123(18):2759–67. doi:10.1182/blood-2013-11-462432
3. Cox D, Kerrigan SW, Watson SP. Platelets and the innate immune system: mechanisms of bacterial-induced platelet activation. *J Thromb Haemost* (2011) 9(6):1097–107. doi:10.1111/j.1538-7836.2011.04264.x
4. Gros A, Ollivier V, Ho-Tin-Noe B. Platelets in inflammation: regulation of leukocyte activities and vascular repair. *Front Immunol* (2014) 5:678. doi:10.3389/fimmu.2014.00678
5. Hamzeh-Cognasse H, Damien P, Chabert A, Pozzetto B, Cognasse F, Garraud O. Platelets and infections – complex interactions with bacteria. *Front Immunol* (2015) 6:82. doi:10.3389/fimmu.2015.00082
6. McDonald TP, Odell TT Jr, Gosslee DG. Platelet size in relation to platelet age. *Proc Soc Exp Biol Med* (1964) 115:684–9. doi:10.3181/00379727-115-29006
7. Mezzano D, Hwang K, Catalano P, Aster RH. Evidence that platelet buoyant density, but not size, correlates with platelet age in man. *Am J Hematol* (1981) 11(1):61–76. doi:10.1002/ajh.2830110108
8. Thompson CB, Love DG, Quinn PG, Valeri CR. Platelet size does not correlate with platelet age. *Blood* (1983) 62(2):487–94.
9. Agbani EO, Poole AW. Procoagulant platelets: generation, function and therapeutic targeting in thrombosis. *Blood* (2017) 130(20):2171–79. doi:10.1182/blood-2017-05-787259
10. Cognasse F, Sut C, Fromont E, Laradi S, Hamzeh-Cognasse H, Garraud O. Platelet soluble CD40-ligand level is associated with transfusion adverse reactions in a mixed threshold-and-hit model. *Blood* (2017) 130(11):1380–3. doi:10.1182/blood-2017-03-773945
11. Garraud O, Tariket S, Sut C, Haddad A, Aloui C, Chakroun T, et al. Transfusion as an inflammation hit: knowns and unknowns. *Front Immunol* (2016) 7:534. doi:10.3389/fimmu.2016.00534
12. Chu SG, Becker RC, Berger PB, Bhatt DL, Eikelboom JW, Konkle B, et al. Mean platelet volume as a predictor of cardiovascular risk: a systematic review and meta-analysis. *J Thromb Haemost* (2010) 8(1):148–56. doi:10.1111/j.1538-7836.2009.03584.x
13. Schick UM, Jain D, Hodonsky CJ, Morrison JV, Davis JP, Brown L, et al. Genome-wide association study of platelet count identifies ancestry-specific loci in Hispanic/Latino Americans. *Am J Hum Genet* (2016) 98(2):229–42. doi:10.1016/j.ajhg.2015.12.003
14. Soranzo N, Rendon A, Gieger C, Jones CI, Watkins NA, Menzel S, et al. A novel variant on chromosome 7q22.3 associated with mean platelet volume, counts, and function. *Blood* (2009) 113(16):3831–7. doi:10.1182/blood-2008-10-184234
15. Nurnberg ST, Rendon A, Smethurst PA, Paul DS, Voss K, Thon JN, et al. A GWAS sequence variant for platelet volume marks an alternative DNM3 promoter in megakaryocytes near a MEIS1 binding site. *Blood* (2012) 120(24):4859–68. doi:10.1182/blood-2012-01-401893
16. Shameer K, Denny JC, Ding K, Jouni H, Crosslin DR, de Andrade M, et al. A genome- and phenome-wide association study to identify genetic variants influencing platelet count and volume and their pleiotropic effects. *Hum Genet* (2014) 133(1):95–109. doi:10.1007/s00439-013-1355-7
17. Li J, Glessner JT, Zhang H, Hou C, Wei Z, Bradfield JP, et al. GWAS of blood cell traits identifies novel associated loci and epistatic interactions in Caucasian and African-American children. *Hum Mol Genet* (2013) 22(7):1457–64. doi:10.1093/hmg/dds534
18. Gieger C, Radhakrishnan A, Cvejic A, Tang W, Porcu E, Pistis G, et al. New gene functions in megakaryopoiesis and platelet formation. *Nature* (2011) 480(7376):201–8. doi:10.1038/nature10659
19. De Gabriele G, Penington DG. Regulation of platelet production: "thrombopoietin". *Br J Haematol* (1967) 13(2):210–5. doi:10.1111/j.1365-2141.1967.tb08733.x
20. Levin J, Levin FC, Hull DF III, Penington DG. The effects of thrombopoietin on megakaryocyte-cfc, megakaryocytes, and thrombopoiesis: with studies of ploidy and platelet size. *Blood* (1982) 60(4):989–98.
21. Harker LA, Roskos LK, Marzec UM, Carter RA, Cherry JK, Sundell B, et al. Effects of megakaryocyte growth and development factor on platelet production, platelet life span, and platelet function in healthy human volunteers. *Blood* (2000) 95(8):2514–22.
22. Patel SR, Hartwig JH, Italiano JE Jr. The biogenesis of platelets from megakaryocyte proplatelets. *J Clin Invest* (2005) 115(12):3348–54. doi:10.1172/JCI26891
23. Thon JN, Italiano JE. Platelet formation. *Semin Hematol* (2010) 47(3):220–6. doi:10.1053/j.seminhematol.2010.03.005
24. Dutting S, Gaits-Iacovoni F, Stegner D, Popp M, Antkowiak A, van Eeuwijk JMM, et al. A Cdc42/RhoA regulatory circuit downstream of glycoprotein Ib guides transendothelial platelet biogenesis. *Nat Commun* (2017) 8:15838. doi:10.1038/ncomms15838
25. Schwertz H, Koster S, Kahr WH, Michetti N, Kraemer BF, Weitz DA, et al. Anucleate platelets generate progeny. *Blood* (2010) 115(18):3801–9. doi:10.1182/blood-2009-08-239558
26. Larson MK, Watson SP. Regulation of proplatelet formation and platelet release by integrin alpha IIb beta3. *Blood* (2006) 108(5):1509–14. doi:10.1182/blood-2005-11-011957
27. Thon JN, Macleod H, Begonja AJ, Zhu J, Lee KC, Mogilner A, et al. Microtubule and cortical forces determine platelet size during vascular platelet production. *Nat Commun* (2012) 3:852. doi:10.1038/ncomms1838
28. Stegner D, vanEeuwijk JMM, Angay O, Gorelashvili MG, Semeniak D, Pinnecker J, et al. Thrombopoiesis is spatially regulated by the bone marrow vasculature. *Nat Commun* (2017) 8(1):127. doi:10.1038/s41467-017-00201-7
29. Machlus KR, Thon JN, Italiano JE Jr. Interpreting the developmental dance of the megakaryocyte: a review of the cellular and molecular processes mediating platelet formation. *Br J Haematol* (2014) 165(2):227–36. doi:10.1111/bjh.12758

30. Lefrancais E, Ortiz-Munoz G, Caudrillier A, Mallavia B, Liu F, Sayah DM, et al. The lung is a site of platelet biogenesis and a reservoir for haematopoietic progenitors. *Nature* (2017) 544(7648):105–9. doi:10.1038/nature21706
31. Kowata S, Isogai S, Murai K, Ito S, Tohyama K, Ema M, et al. Platelet demand modulates the type of intravascular protrusion of megakaryocytes in bone marrow. *Thromb Haemost* (2014) 112(4):743–56. doi:10.1160/TH14-02-0123
32. Nishimura S, Nagasaki M, Kunishima S, Sawaguchi A, Sakata A, Sakaguchi H, et al. IL-1alpha induces thrombopoiesis through megakaryocyte rupture in response to acute platelet needs. *J Cell Biol* (2015) 209(3):453–66. doi:10.1083/jcb.201410052
33. Thiele T, Braune J, Dhople V, Hammer E, Scharf C, Greinacher A, et al. Proteomic profile of platelets during reconstitution of platelet counts after apheresis. *Proteomics Clin Appl* (2016) 10(8):831–8. doi:10.1002/prca.201500134
34. Thompson CB, Jakubowski JA, Quinn PG, Deykin D, Valeri CR. Platelet size as a determinant of platelet function. *J Lab Clin Med* (1983) 101(2):205–13.
35. Booyse FM, Rafelson ME Jr. Studies on human platelets. I. Synthesis of platelet protein in a cell-free system. *Biochim Biophys Acta* (1968) 166(3):689–97. doi:10.1016/0005-2787(68)90376-6
36. Karpatkin S. Heterogeneity of human platelets. I. Metabolic and kinetic evidence suggestive of young and old platelets. *J Clin Invest* (1969) 48(6): 1073–82. doi:10.1172/JCI106063
37. Karpatkin S. Heterogeneity of human platelets. II. Functional evidence suggestive of young and old platelets. *J Clin Invest* (1969) 48(6):1083–7. doi:10.1172/JCI106064
38. Karpatkin S, Strick N. Heterogeneity of human platelets. V. Differences in glycolytic and related enzymes with possible relation to platelet age. *J Clin Invest* (1972) 51(5):1235–43. doi:10.1172/JCI106918
39. Jakubowski JA, Thompson CB, Vaillancourt R, Valeri CR, Deykin D. Arachidonic acid metabolism by platelets of differing size. *Br J Haematol* (1983) 53(3):503–11. doi:10.1111/j.1365-2141.1983.tb02052.x
40. Mezzano D, Aranda E, Foradori A. Comparative study of size, total protein, fibrinogen and 5-HT content of human and canine platelet density subpopulations. *Thromb Haemost* (1986) 56(3):288–92.
41. Pereira J, Cretney C, Aster RH. Variation of class I HLA antigen expression among platelet density cohorts: a possible index of platelet age? *Blood* (1988) 71(2):516–9.
42. Frojmovic M, Wong T. Dynamic measurements of the platelet membrane glycoprotein IIb-IIIa receptor for fibrinogen by flow cytometry. II. Platelet size-dependent subpopulations. *Biophys J* (1991) 59(4):828–37. doi:10.1016/S0006-3495(91)82295-0
43. Polanowska-Grabowska R, Raha S, Gear AR. Adhesion efficiency, platelet density and size. *Br J Haematol* (1992) 82(4):715–20. doi:10.1111/j.1365-2141.1992.tb06949.x
44. Opper C, Schrumpf E, Gear AR, Wesemann W. Involvement of guanylate cyclase and phosphodiesterases in the functional heterogeneity of human blood platelet subpopulations. *Thromb Res* (1995) 80(6):461–70. doi:10.1016/0049-3848(95)00201-4
45. Li BY, He SZ, Li WH. Heterogeneity of human platelet density subpopulations in aggregation, secretion of ATP, and cytosolic-free calcium concentration. *Zhongguo Yao Li Xue Bao* (1996) 17(2):152–5.
46. Opper C, Schuessler G, Kuschel M, Clement HW, Gear AR, Hinsch E, et al. Analysis of GTP-binding proteins, phosphoproteins, and cytosolic calcium in functional heterogeneous human blood platelet subpopulations. *Biochem Pharmacol* (1997) 54(9):1027–35. doi:10.1016/S0006-2952(97)00317-1
47. Mangalpally KK, Siqueiros-Garcia A, Vaduganathan M, Dong JF, Kleiman NS, Guthikonda S. Platelet activation patterns in platelet size sub-populations: differential responses to aspirin in vitro. *J Thromb Thrombolysis* (2010) 30(3):251–62. doi:10.1007/s11239-010-0489-x
48. Brambilla M, Rossetti L, Zara C, Canzano P, Giesen PLA, Tremoli E, et al. Do methodological differences account for the current controversy on tissue factor expression in platelets? *Platelets* (2017):1–9. doi:10.1080/09537104.2017.1327653
49. Balduini CL, Noris P, Spedini P, Belletti S, Zambelli A, Da Prada GA. Relationship between size and thiazole orange fluorescence of platelets in patients undergoing high-dose chemotherapy. *Br J Haematol* (1999) 106(1):202–7. doi:10.1046/j.1365-2141.1999.01475.x
50. Denis MM, Tolley ND, Bunting M, Schwertz H, Jiang H, Lindemann S, et al. Escaping the nuclear confines: signal-dependent pre-mRNA splicing in anucleate platelets. *Cell* (2005) 122(3):379–91. doi:10.1016/j.cell.2005.06.015
51. Frojmovic M, Wong T, van de Ven T. Dynamic measurements of the platelet membrane glycoprotein IIb-IIIa receptor for fibrinogen by flow cytometry. I. Methodology, theory and results for two distinct activators. *Biophys J* (1991) 59(4):815–27. doi:10.1016/S0006-3495(91)82294-9
52. Schwertz H, Tolley ND, Foulks JM, Denis MM, Risenmay BW, Buerke M, et al. Signal-dependent splicing of tissue factor pre-mRNA modulates the thrombogenicity of human platelets. *J Exp Med* (2006) 203(11):2433–40. doi:10.1084/jem.20061302
53. Blajchman MA, Senyi AF, Hirsh J, Genton E, George JN. Hemostatic function, survival, and membrane glycoprotein changes in young versus old rabbit platelets. *J Clin Invest* (1981) 68(5):1289–94. doi:10.1172/JCI110375
54. Adly AA, Ragab IA, Ismail EA, Farahat MM. Evaluation of the immature platelet fraction in the diagnosis and prognosis of childhood immune thrombocytopenia. *Platelets* (2015) 26(7):645–50. doi:10.3109/09537104.2014.969220
55. Kaito K, Otsubo H, Usui N, Yoshida M, Tanno J, Kurihara E, et al. Platelet size deviation width, platelet large cell ratio, and mean platelet volume have sufficient sensitivity and specificity in the diagnosis of immune thrombocytopenia. *Br J Haematol* (2005) 128(5):698–702. doi:10.1111/j.1365-2141.2004.05357.x
56. Ntaios G, Papadopoulos A, Chatzinikolaou A, Saouli Z, Karalazou P, Kaiafa G, et al. Increased values of mean platelet volume and platelet size deviation width may provide a safe positive diagnosis of idiopathic thrombocytopenic purpura. *Acta Haematol* (2008) 119(3):173–7. doi:10.1159/000135658
57. Bath PM, Butterworth RJ. Platelet size: measurement, physiology and vascular disease. *Blood Coagul Fibrinolysis* (1996) 7(2):157–61. doi:10.1097/00001721-199603000-00011
58. Freynhofer MK, Gruber SC, Grove EL, Weiss TW, Wojta J, Huber K. Antiplatelet drugs in patients with enhanced platelet turnover: biomarkers versus platelet function testing. *Thromb Haemost* (2015) 114(3):459–68. doi:10.1160/TH15-02-0179
59. Castle V, Coates G, Kelton JG, Andrew M. 111In-oxine platelet survivals in thrombocytopenic infants. *Blood* (1987) 70(3):652–6.
60. Lippi G. Genetic and nongenetic determinants of mean platelet volume. *Blood* (2016) 127(2):179–80. doi:10.1182/blood-2015-11-679852
61. Panova-Noeva M, Schulz A, Hermanns MI, Grossmann V, Pefani E, Spronk HM, et al. Sex-specific differences in genetic and nongenetic determinants of mean platelet volume: results from the Gutenberg Health Study. *Blood* (2016) 127(2):251–9. doi:10.1182/blood-2015-07-660308
62. Montoro-Garcia S, Schindewolf M, Stanford S, Larsen OH, Thiele T. The role of platelets in venous thromboembolism. *Semin Thromb Hemost* (2016) 42(3):242–51. doi:10.1055/s-0035-1570079
63. Freynhofer MK, Iliev L, Bruno V, Rohla M, Egger F, Weiss TW, et al. Platelet turnover predicts outcome after coronary intervention. *Thromb Haemost* (2017) 117(5):923–33. doi:10.1160/TH16-10-0785
64. Noris P, Melazzini F, Balduini CL. New roles for mean platelet volume measurement in the clinical practice? *Platelets* (2016) 27(7):607–12. doi:10.1080/09537104.2016.1224828
65. Eicher JD, Chami N, Kacprowski T, Nomura A, Chen MH, Yanek LR, et al. Platelet-related variants identified by exomechip meta-analysis in 157,293 individuals. *Am J Hum Genet* (2016) 99(1):40–55. doi:10.1016/j.ajhg.2016.05.005
66. Greinacher A, Pecci A, Kunishima S, Althaus K, Nurden P, Balduini CL, et al. Diagnosis of inherited platelet disorders on a blood smear: a tool to facilitate worldwide diagnosis of platelet disorders. *J Thromb Haemost* (2017) 15(7):1511–21. doi:10.1111/jth.13729
67. Ingram M, Coopersmith A. Reticulated platelets following acute blood loss. *Br J Haematol* (1969) 17(3):225–9. doi:10.1111/j.1365-2141.1969.tb01366.x
68. Fujii T, Shimomura T, Fujimoto TT, Kimura A, Fujimura K. A new approach to detect reticulated platelets stained with thiazole orange in thrombocytopenic patients. *Thromb Res* (2000) 97(6):431–40. doi:10.1016/S0049-3848(99)00182-6
69. Ault KA, Knowles C. In vivo biotinylation demonstrates that reticulated platelets are the youngest platelets in circulation. *Exp Hematol* (1995) 23(9):996–1001.
70. Dale GL, Friese P, Hynes LA, Burstein SA. Demonstration that thiazole-orange-positive platelets in the dog are less than 24 hours old. *Blood* (1995) 85(7):1822–5.

71. Angenieux C, Maitre B, Eckly A, Lanza F, Gachet C, de la Salle H. Time-dependent decay of mRNA and ribosomal RNA during platelet aging and its correlation with translation activity. *PLoS One* (2016) 11(1):e0148064. doi:10.1371/journal.pone.0148064
72. Kienast J, Schmitz G. Flow cytometric analysis of thiazole orange uptake by platelets: a diagnostic aid in the evaluation of thrombocytopenic disorders. *Blood* (1990) 75(1):116–21.
73. Robinson M, MacHin S, Mackie I, Harrison P. In vivo biotinylation studies: specificity of labelling of reticulated platelets by thiazole orange and mepacrine. *Br J Haematol* (2000) 108(4):859–64. doi:10.1046/j.1365-2141.2000.01939.x
74. Reddy EC, Wang H, Bang KWA, Packham MA, Rand ML. Young steady-state rabbit platelets do not have an enhanced capacity to expose procoagulant phosphatidylserine. *Platelets* (2017):1–7. doi:10.1080/09537104.2017.1295434
75. Baaten CC, Veenstra LF, Wetzels R, van Geffen JP, Swieringa F, de Witt SM, et al. Gradual increase in thrombogenicity of juvenile platelets formed upon offset of prasugrel medication. *Haematologica* (2015) 100(9):1131–8. doi:10.3324/haematol.2014.122457
76. Takubo T, Yamane T, Hino M, Ohta K, Koh KR, Tatsumi N. Clinical significance of simultaneous measurement of reticulated platelets and large platelets in idiopathic thrombocytopenic purpura. *Haematologia* (2000) 30(3):183–92. doi:10.1163/156855900300109189
77. Salvagno GL, Montagnana M, Degan M, Marradi PL, Ricetti MM, Riolfi P, et al. Evaluation of platelet turnover by flow cytometry. *Platelets* (2006) 17(3):170–7. doi:10.1080/09537100500437851
78. Guthikonda S, Alviar CL, Vaduganathan M, Arikan M, Tellez A, DeLao T, et al. Role of reticulated platelets and platelet size heterogeneity on platelet activity after dual antiplatelet therapy with aspirin and clopidogrel in patients with stable coronary artery disease. *J Am Coll Cardiol* (2008) 52(9):743–9. doi:10.1016/j.jacc.2008.05.031
79. Alberio L, Safa O, Clemetson KJ, Esmon CT, Dale GL. Surface expression and functional characterization of alpha-granule factor V in human platelets: effects of ionophore A23187, thrombin, collagen, and convulxin. *Blood* (2000) 95(5):1694–702.
80. Prodan CI, Joseph PM, Vincent AS, Dale GL. Coated-platelet levels are influenced by smoking, aspirin, and selective serotonin reuptake inhibitors. *J Thromb Haemost* (2007) 5(10):2149–51. doi:10.1111/j.1538-7836.2007.02691.x
81. Dale GL, Friese P, Batar P, Hamilton SF, Reed GL, Jackson KW, et al. Stimulated platelets use serotonin to enhance their retention of procoagulant proteins on the cell surface. *Nature* (2002) 415(6868):175–9. doi:10.1038/415175a
82. Heemskerk JW, Vuist WM, Feijge MA, Reutelingsperger CP, Lindhout T. Collagen but not fibrinogen surfaces induce bleb formation, exposure of phosphatidylserine, and procoagulant activity of adherent platelets: evidence for regulation by protein tyrosine kinase-dependent Ca2+ responses. *Blood* (1997) 90(7):2615–25.
83. Choo HJ, Kholmukhamedov A, Zhou C, Jobe S. Inner mitochondrial membrane disruption links apoptotic and agonist-initiated phosphatidylserine externalization in platelets. *Arterioscler Thromb Vasc Biol* (2017) 37(8):1503–12. doi:10.1161/ATVBAHA.117.309473
84. Wolf BB, Goldstein JC, Stennicke HR, Beere H, Amarante-Mendes GP, Salvesen GS, et al. Calpain functions in a caspase-independent manner to promote apoptosis-like events during platelet activation. *Blood* (1999) 94(5):1683–92.
85. Schoenwaelder SM, Yuan Y, Josefsson EC, White MJ, Yao Y, Mason KD, et al. Two distinct pathways regulate platelet phosphatidylserine exposure and procoagulant function. *Blood* (2009) 114(3):663–6. doi:10.1182/blood-2009-01-200345
86. Jackson SP, Schoenwaelder SM. Procoagulant platelets: are they necrotic? *Blood* (2010) 116(12):2011–8. doi:10.1182/blood-2010-01-261669
87. Mattheij NJ, Swieringa F, Mastenbroek TG, Berny-Lang MA, May F, Baaten CC, et al. Coated platelets function in platelet-dependent fibrin formation via integrin alphaIIbbeta3 and transglutaminase factor XIII. *Haematologica* (2016) 101(4):427–36. doi:10.3324/haematol.2015.131441
88. Keuren JF, Wielders SJ, Ulrichts H, Hackeng T, Heemskerk JW, Deckmyn H, et al. Synergistic effect of thrombin on collagen-induced platelet procoagulant activity is mediated through protease-activated receptor-1. *Arterioscler Thromb Vasc Biol* (2005) 25(7):1499–505. doi:10.1161/01.ATV.0000167526.31611.f6
89. Alberio L, Ravanat C, Hechler B, Mangin PH, Lanza F, Gachet C. Delayed-onset of procoagulant signalling revealed by kinetic analysis of COAT platelet formation. *Thromb Haemost* (2017) 117(6):1101–14. doi:10.1160/TH16-09-0711
90. Topalov NN, Kotova YN, Vasil'ev SA, Panteleev MA. Identification of signal transduction pathways involved in the formation of platelet subpopulations upon activation. *Br J Haematol* (2012) 157(1):105–15. doi:10.1111/j.1365-2141.2011.09021.x
91. Mattheij NJ, Gilio K, van Kruchten R, Jobe SM, Wieschhaus AJ, Chishti AH, et al. Dual mechanism of integrin alphaIIbbeta3 closure in procoagulant platelets. *J Biol Chem* (2013) 288(19):13325–36. doi:10.1074/jbc.M112.428359
92. Szasz R, Dale GL. Thrombospondin and fibrinogen bind serotonin-derivatized proteins on COAT-platelets. *Blood* (2002) 100(8):2827–31. doi:10.1182/blood-2002-02-0354
93. Munnix IC, Cosemans JM, Auger JM, Heemskerk JW. Platelet response heterogeneity in thrombus formation. *Thromb Haemost* (2009) 102(6):1149–56. doi:10.1160/TH09-05-0289
94. Heemskerk JW, Kuijpers MJ, Munnix IC, Siljander PR. Platelet collagen receptors and coagulation. A characteristic platelet response as possible target for antithrombotic treatment. *Trends Cardiovasc Med* (2005) 15(3):86–92. doi:10.1016/j.tcm.2005.03.003
95. Munnix IC, Kuijpers MJ, Auger J, Thomassen CM, Panizzi P, van Zandvoort MA, et al. Segregation of platelet aggregatory and procoagulant microdomains in thrombus formation: regulation by transient integrin activation. *Arterioscler Thromb Vasc Biol* (2007) 27(11):2484–90. doi:10.1161/ATVBAHA.107.151100
96. Abaeva AA, Canault M, Kotova YN, Obydennyy SI, Yakimenko AO, Podoplelova NA, et al. Procoagulant platelets form an alpha-granule protein-covered "cap" on their surface that promotes their attachment to aggregates. *J Biol Chem* (2013) 288(41):29621–32. doi:10.1074/jbc.M113.474163
97. Mustard JF, Rowsell HC, Murphy EA. Platelet economy (platelet survival and turnover). *Br J Haematol* (1966) 12(1):1–24. doi:10.1111/j.1365-2141.1966.tb00121.x
98. Najean Y, Ardaillou N, Dresch C. Platelet lifespan. *Annu Rev Med* (1969) 20:47–62. doi:10.1146/annurev.me.20.020169.000403
99. Grozovsky R, Giannini S, Falet H, Hoffmeister KM. Novel mechanisms of platelet clearance and thrombopoietin regulation. *Curr Opin Hematol* (2015) 22(5):445–51. doi:10.1097/MOH.0000000000000170
100. Grozovsky R, Begonja AJ, Liu K, Visner G, Hartwig JH, Falet H, et al. The Ashwell-Morell receptor regulates hepatic thrombopoietin production via JAK2-STAT3 signaling. *Nat Med* (2015) 21(1):47–54. doi:10.1038/nm.3770
101. Rumjantseva V, Grewal PK, Wandall HH, Josefsson EC, Sorensen AL, Larson G, et al. Dual roles for hepatic lectin receptors in the clearance of chilled platelets. *Nat Med* (2009) 15(11):1273–80. doi:10.1038/nm.2030
102. Grewal PK, Aziz PV, Uchiyama S, Rubio GR, Lardone RD, Le D, et al. Inducing host protection in pneumococcal sepsis by preactivation of the Ashwell-Morell receptor. *Proc Natl Acad Sci U S A* (2013) 110(50):20218–23. doi:10.1073/pnas.1313905110
103. Grewal PK, Uchiyama S, Ditto D, Varki N, Le DT, Nizet V, et al. The Ashwell receptor mitigates the lethal coagulopathy of sepsis. *Nat Med* (2008) 14(6):648–55. doi:10.1038/nm1760
104. Mason KD, Carpinelli MR, Fletcher JI, Collinge JE, Hilton AA, Ellis S, et al. Programmed anuclear cell death delimits platelet life span. *Cell* (2007) 128(6):1173–86. doi:10.1016/j.cell.2007.01.037
105. Zhao L, Liu J, He C, Yan R, Zhou K, Cui Q, et al. Protein kinase A determines platelet life span and survival by regulating apoptosis. *J Clin Invest* (2017) 127(12):4338–51. doi:10.1172/JCI95109
106. Curtis BR, McFarland JG. Human platelet antigens – 2013. *Vox Sang* (2014) 106(2):93–102. doi:10.1111/vox.12085
107. Berger G, Hartwell DW, Wagner DD. P-Selectin and platelet clearance. *Blood* (1998) 92(11):4446–52.
108. Alberio L. Do we need antiplatelet therapy in thrombocytosis? Pro. Diagnostic and pathophysiologic considerations for a treatment choice. *Hamostaseologie* (2016) 36(4):227–40. doi:10.5482/HAMO-14-11-0074
109. Heuft HG, Moog R, Fischer EG, Zingsem J. German, Austrian Plateletpheresis Study G. Donor safety in triple plateletpheresis: results from the German and

Austrian Plateletpheresis Study Group multicenter trial. *Transfusion* (2013) 53(1):211–20. doi:10.1111/j.1537-2995.2012.03714.x

110. Gebhard S, Steil L, Peters B, Gesell-Salazar M, Hammer E, Kuttler B, et al. Angiotensin II-dependent hypertension causes reversible changes in the platelet proteome. *J Hypertens* (2011) 29(11):2126–37. doi:10.1097/HJH.0b013e32834b1991
111. Heddle NM, Arnold DM, Acker JP, Liu Y, Barty RL, Eikelboom JW, et al. Red blood cell processing methods and in-hospital mortality: a transfusion registry cohort study. *Lancet Haematol* (2016) 3(5):e246–54. doi:10.1016/S2352-3026(16)00020-X

14

Disturbed Red Blood Cell Structure and Function: An Exploration of the Role of Red Blood Cells in Neurodegeneration

*Giel J. C. G. M. Bosman**

Department of Biochemistry, Radboud University Nijmegen Medical Centre, Nijmegen, Netherlands

Correspondence:
Giel J. C. G. M. Bosman
giel.bosman@radboudumc.nl

The structure of red blood cells is affected by many inborn and acquired factors, but in most cases this does not seem to affect their function or survival in physiological conditions. Often, functional deficits become apparent only when they are subjected to biochemical or mechanical stress *in vitro*, or to pathological conditions *in vivo*. Our data on the misshapen red blood cells of patients with neuroacanthocytosis illustrate this general mechanism: an abnormal morphology is associated with an increase in the susceptibility of red blood cells to osmotic and mechanical stress, and alters their rheological properties. The underlying mutations may not only affect red cell function, but also render neurons in specific brain areas more susceptible to a concomitant reduction in oxygen supply. Through this mechanism, an increased susceptibility of already compromised red blood cells to physiological stress conditions may constitute an additional risk factor in vulnerable individuals. Also, susceptibility may be induced or enhanced by systemic pathological conditions such as inflammation. An exploration of the literature suggests that disturbed red blood cell function may play a role in the pathophysiology of various neurodegenerative diseases. Therefore, interventions that reduce the susceptibility of red blood cells to physiological and pathological stress may reduce the extent or progress of neurodegeneration.

Keywords: aging, deformability, neuroacanthocytosis, neurodegeneration, red blood cell

INTRODUCTION

The statement that a healthy red blood cell is essential for organismal homeostasis may sound as a truism, but this depends on the functional definition of a healthy red blood cell. There are many genetically determined, structural abnormalities in the hemoglobin chains that, in most circumstances, do not affect red blood cell integrity and do not seem to affect transport of oxygen binding and release in lungs and tissues, respectively (1). Also, many obvious deviations of the classical discoid red blood cell shape, due to inborn errors in integral membrane proteins and cytoskeletal components, have no obvious clinical implications (2). In addition, there are hardly any data indicating that physiological aging *in vivo* or *in vitro* during storage in the blood bank has a notable effect on oxygen supply of the tissues and carbon dioxide removal (3).

The gas transport capacity of red blood cells is not only determined by the characteristics of hemoglobin, but also by the capacity to regulate intracellular pH, deformability, ATP production, redox status, resistance to osmotic and mechanical stress, and recognition and removal by the immune system. The role of most of these processes emerges mainly upon recognition of their putative involvement in pathophysiological mechanisms, and in most cases their molecular details become clear only after detailed study *in vitro*.

The absence of conspicuous clinical consequences, such as hemolysis and anemia, of many structural and functional flaws under physiological circumstances indicates that the red blood cell has considerable reserves to maintain structure and function. The limits of these reserves, in addition to the resilience provided by the erythropoietic system, may be reached when red blood cells are exposed to pathological processes, such as inflammation (4). Errors that are inborn or flaws that are acquired in the circulation in critical structural, functional, or metabolic red blood cell components are likely to increase the rate at which the weakest links in these defenses are breached. For example, a decrease in the capacity to maintain phospholipid asymmetry increases the likelihood of recognition by macrophages, that is mediated by the exposure of phosphatidylserine (PS) in the outer leaflet of the red blood cell membrane. Aging renders red blood cells more susceptible to PS exposure after osmotic stress (5, 6).

Here we explore the boundaries of these reserves, how they may be breached, and their pathological implications. The starting point of this exploration is the complex of structural and functional characteristics of the aging red blood cell, that was the foundation of our study of the misshapen red blood cells that accompany the neurological problems of patients with neuroacanthocytosis.

RED BLOOD CELL AGING

Physiological aging *in vivo*, as well as aging *in vitro* during storage in the blood bank, induces changes in the red cell membrane (7), in the activity of the main metabolic pathways (8, 9), and in hemoglobin (10). These changes not only affect function by decreasing deformability (11, 12), but also lead to the appearance of signals that trigger recognition and removal by the immune system. Especially the latter process is induced by the conditions that the cells normally encounter in their journey through the circulation, such as mechanical stress, oxidation and hyperosmotic conditions (5, 13, 14). A number of pathological conditions may trigger the same changes, as exemplified by the detrimental effects of inflammatory lipases on red blood cell structure and the association between inflammation and anemia (4, 15). Thus, the biophysical, biochemical, immunological, and functional characteristics of the healthy, aging red blood cell provide us with the tools to study the red blood cell structure-function relationship in a clinically relevant context.

NEUROACANTHOCYTOSIS

Neuroacanthocytosis (NA) is a family of rare neurodegenerative disorders, that includes chorea-acanthocytosis, McLeod syndrome, Huntington's disease-like 2, and panthothenate kinase-associated neurodegeneration. Patients with NA suffer from devastating movement disorders, caused by degeneration of spinal neurons in the basal ganglia. One hallmark of NA is the presence of acanthocytes, red blood cells with thorny protrusions, in the blood, but detailed morphological analysis shows the presence of many other misshapen red blood cells as well (16, 17). The presence of acanthocytes is mostly considered as an indication that the pathways that lead to the red blood cell abnormalities are the same as those involved in neuronal degeneration. The molecular similarities between the putative mechanisms inducing acanthocytosis in red blood cell membrane organization and in neurodegeneration in patients with NA have been discussed extensively (18, 19).

In patients with NA, the degree of acanthocytosis may vary over time. There are no clues for the identity of the processes that might cause a transition of mature discocytes to acanthocytes. A recent inventory of the available data has led us to the hypothesis that red blood cells with an acanthocyte shape may already be present in the final stages of erythropoiesis, and appear into the circulation as such (20). This is supported by the observation that an artificially induced, long-term disturbance of red blood cell membrane architecture had a lasting effect on erythropoiesis and caused the appearance of acanthocytes in the circulation (21).

Recent applications of various combinations of immunochemical, (phospho) proteomic, lipidomic and metabolomic approaches have provided indications for the mechanisms responsible for the acanthocyte shape. In acanthocytes, Lyn kinase-mediated phosphorylation and phosphatidylinositol-involving signaling pathways show altered activities. These pathways regulate the interaction between the main cytoskeletal and integral membrane proteins, and may be involved in autophagy during erythropoiesis (19, 20, 22, 23). As a band 3 plays a central role in multiprotein complex formation during erythropoiesis (24), disturbance of this process is likely to affect the stability of the binding of the cytoskeleton to the band 3-based ankyrin-complex and/or the junctional complex. A band 3-centered disturbance of this binding leads to various abnormal cell shapes, varying from spherocytosis to ovalocytosis and acanthocytosis (2, 25). Therefore, the processes that are affected in NA must have very specific, but a yet unknown characteristics in order to induce the characteristic acanthocyte shape. Band 3 does not only provide high-affinity binding sites for the actin-spectrin cytoskeleton, but also for deoxyhemoglobin and for key enzymes of the glycolytic enzyme complex. This interaction plays a regulatory role in red blood cell metabolism and function (26). Metabolomic analyses indicate that NA-associated alterations in band 3-centered protein-protein interactions may also affect the metabolism of red cells (16). The effect of the latter changes on red blood cell survival or function are presently unclear.

Clinical descriptions of patients with NA focus on the neurological symptoms, and in general do not provide clear indications for NA-specific red blood cell dysfunction. Measurement of deformability and relaxation *in vitro* shows that acanthocytes from NA-patients assume a normal bullet-like shape when passing through a microfluidic., capillary-mimicking system, and relax toward their original shape as quickly as cells with a normal morphology. However, acanthocytes have difficulties when passing through a spleen-mimicking device *in vitro* (16). Also, the misshapen red blood cells of NA patients show a decreased deformability as well as an abnormal aggregation behavior (**Figure 1**). Together, these data constitute strong indications for an altered rheology and decrease in deformability, that may not only be responsible for the splenomegaly and hemolysis described in patients with McLeod disease as well as in a patient with acanthocyte-associated band 3 mutations (18, 28), but may also contribute to the neurological problems (see below).

The abnormal cytoskelon/membrane associations that underly genetically determined alterations in red blood cell morphology are, in general, associated with a decreased deformability *in vitro* (12, 29). Decreased deformability is, in most cases, associated with a decrease in hematocrit and in hemoglobin concentration *in vivo*. Even at subclinical levels, these may not only induce an increased susceptibility to red blood cell-centered pathology, as exemplified by the anemia of aging (30), but also hypoperfusion and thereby hamper oxygen delivery. In the brain, deprivation of oxygen leads to excessive glutamate release and NMDA-receptor activation-induced neuronal cell death. The latter is stimulated by Lyn-related kinases, that are also implied in acanthocyte formation during erythropoiesis and neuronal dysfunction *in vitro* (23, 31). These data, together with sporadic clinical observations, led us to the hypothesis that, in patients with neuroacanthocytosis, the compromised function of acanthocytes and otherwise misshapen red blood cells contributes to the neuronal degeneration in the striatum (20). The most likely underlying mechanism would be a decrease in red blood cell rheology, resulting in a restricted perfusion of sensitive brain areas. More subtle metabolic effects of alterations in cell morphology on oxygen binding or release by hemoglobin may play a role as well. The former mechanism may primarily be caused by defective cytoskeleton-membrane interactions, the latter by defective, membrane-centered regulation of pH, ATP production, and/or redox status.

An etiological role of acanthocytosis has been postulated in the damage to the globus pallidus and development of choreoathetosis as rare complications of cardiopulmonary bypass during open-heart surgery, especially in young children (32). In this hypothesis, the mechanical stress exerted by the extracorporeal circulation system constitutes a mechanical

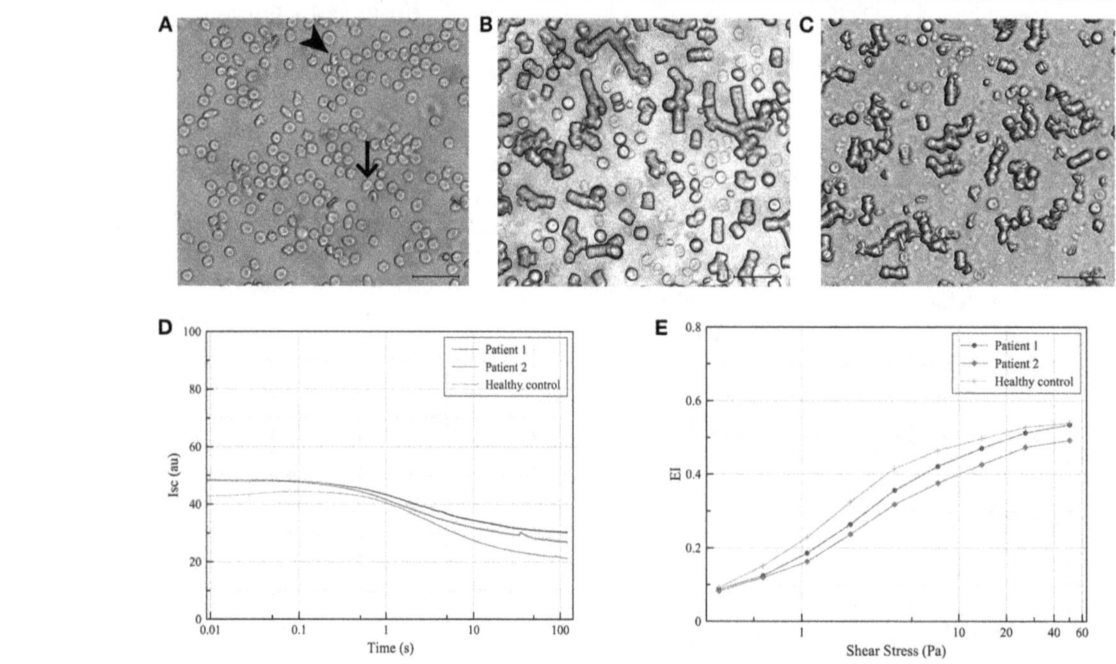

FIGURE 1 | Deformability and aggregation of red blood cells from patients with neuroacanthocytosis. Red blood cells were isolated from patients with neuroacanthocytosis as described before (16), and their morphology, aggregation and deformability were compared with those of a healthy control donor. **(A)** Bright-field microscopy of the red blood cells of one patient (0.1% hematocrit in phosphate-buffered saline), showing acanthocytes (arrowhead) and otherwise misshapen red blood cells (arrow); **(B)** Bright-field microscopy of the red blood cells of a healthy control donor (1% hematocrit in plasma), showing aggregates mostly as rouleaux after 2 to 3 min of incubation at room temperature; **(C)** Bright-field microscopy of red blood cells of an acanthocytosis patient showing smaller rouleaux and much more disordered aggregates; **(D)** Syllectograms of the red blood cells of a healthy control donor and two neuroacanthocytosis patients obtained in 40% hematocrit in plasma, showing altered aggregation characteristics of the patients' red blood cells; **(E)** Deformability curves of the red blood cells of one healthy control and two neuroacanthocytosis patients, showing a lower maximum elongation index (EI) in the patients' red blood cells. Aggregation and deformability were measured using a Lorrca (RR Mechatronics, Hoorn, The Netherlands) as described before (12, 27).

trigger that, in combination with hypothermia, spleen dysfunction, and/or altered pH regulation, may lead to the formation of misshapen red blood cells with a decreased deformability and to a hampered oxygen supply to the brain. A similar phenomenon may underlie the neurological problems following coronary-artery bypass surgery (33), and the higher risk of postoperative cognitive dysfunction in patients with diabetes (34). In most cases, the "postpump" chorea is transient (32). However, in NA patients a chronic acanthocytosis might lead to a chronic deficit in oxygen supply and thereby to a more severe and progressive neurodegeneration.

RED BLOOD CELLS AND NEURODEGENERATION

This hypothesis provided an additional trigger to explore the literature for indications that abnormal red blood cell function may be an etiological factor in neurodegeneration.

Acanthocytosis

Acanthocytes are present in patients with disorders of lipid metabolism such as abetalipoproteinemia and hypolipoproteinemia. However, these patients do not have any signs of NA-like neurodegeneration, and their red blood cells have a different molecular phenotype (25, 35). Acanthocytosis has been described in patients with aceruloplasminemia, and anemia has been reported to precede neurological symptoms in almost all patiens with this defect in copper transport and iron metabolism (36, 37). These data indicate that acanthocyte generation may be due to various causes, and that the functional properties of at least some types of acanthocytic red blood cells may contribute to the development of specific neurological deficits.

Anisocytosis

Abnormally shaped red blood cells display an increased heterogeneity in cell volume, due to impaired erythropoiesis or to excessive fragmentation or destruction. This heterogeneity, expressed as an increase in red blood cell distribution width (RDW), is associated with ischemic cerebrovascular disease (38), with increased odds of having dementia (39), with Alzheimer disease (40), and with the severity of leukoaraiosis (41). In related studies, we found indications for disturbed red blood cell aging, which is associated with changes in cell morphology, in patients with beginning demantia (42). Also, abnormal red blood cells were reported to be associated with cognitive performance in a large longitudinal aging study (43). Such associations may reflect the expression at different organs of a common pathological process. Alternatively, the abnormally shape of red blood cells in individuals with an increased RDW is likely to affect not only cellular deformability and thereby oxygen delivery (29), but may also be an indication for impaired red blood cell signaling-mediated vasodilation by NO, ATP and adenosine (44). In addition, correlations between RDW and sedentary behavior, and between RDW and muscle strength suggest that RDW may be a component of frailty in the elderly (45).

A closer look at red blood cell abnormalities in patients with various neurodegenerative diseases yields indications for abnormal cell morphology and/or red cell function in patients with Huntington's disease (46–48), Parkinson's disease (49), and Alzheimer's disease (50). These abnormalities may reflect peripheral phenomena of the major neurodegenerative mechanism, as indicated by the increased concentration of the *PARK7*-coded protein DJ-1 in red blood cells of early-stage Parkinson's disease patients (51) or by the alfa-synuclein levels in red blood cells with Parkinson's disease (52). Independent of the underlying mechanisms, the effects of these abnormalities on red blood cell function may constitute a risk factor, as has recently be argued for Alzheimer's disease (53).

Red Blood Cell-Centered Diseases and Neurological Problems

Various red blood cell-centered diseases have been reported to be associated with neurological problems. In patients with sickle cell disease and thalassemia, impaired cognitive and neuropsychological functioning are likely due to inadequate oxygen supply in the frontal, parietal and temporal lobes (54–56). In these hemoglobinopathies, decreased deformability and increased aggregation are likely to be the primary causes of the neurological problems. Also, some hereditary red blood cell enzymopathies that are accompanied by hemolytic anemia are associated with neurological problems (57). The latter may be due to the expression of the same mutated genes in the brain and in hematopoietic stem cells, but also to a functional impairment of the mature red blood cells.

In addition, treatment of anemia with red blood cell concentrates, especially in transfusion-dependent patients, may pose its own problems due to its effect on perturbed iron homeostasis, also in the brain [e.g., (58)]. The molecular interplay between red blood cell homeostasis, chronic transfusion and brain pathology remains to be established.

CONCLUSIONS

The data presented here indicate that physiological and pathological circumstances may affect red blood cell function, especially by diminishing their capacity to withstand pathophysiological stress conditions. In other words, in normal conditions, the characteristics of aging, stored, and genetically affected red blood cells may have only subclinical consequences. However, during periods of stress, for example during inflammation, already compromised cells may become less deformable, more fragile, or more prone to recognition by the immune system.

Our data on acanthocytosis illustrate that an abnormal red cell structure increases the susceptibility of the misshapen red cells to mechanical stress and alters their rheological properties. The underlying mutations may not only affect red cell shape and function, but also render neurons in vulnerable brain areas more susceptible to a concomitant reduction in oxygen supply.

Thus, interventions that reduce the susceptibility of red blood cells to pathological as well as physiological stress conditions may reduce the extent and/or progression of neurodegeneration.

ETHICS STATEMENT

The data shown here were obtained in a study that was approved by the Medical Ethical Committee of the Radboud University Medical Center and in accordance with the Declaration of Helsinki.

AUTHOR CONTRIBUTIONS

The author confirms being the sole contributor of this work and approved it for publication.

ACKNOWLEDGMENTS

I thank D. Lazari and J. K. Freitas Leal for the measurements of deformability and aggregation presented in **Figure 1**.

REFERENCES

1. Williamson D. The unstable haemoglobins. *Blood Rev.* (1993) 7:146–63.
2. An X, Mohandas, N. Disorders of red cell membrane. *Br J Haematol.* (2008) 141:367–75. doi: 10.1111/j.1365-2141.2008.07091.x
3. Gelderman MP, Yazer MH, Jia Y, Wood F, Alayash AI, Vostal JG. Serial oxygen equilibrium and kinetic measurements during RBC storage. *Transf Med.* (2010) 20:341–45. doi: 10.1111/j.1365-3148.2010.01016.x
4. Dinkla S, van Eijk LT, Fuchs B, Schiller J, Joosten I, Brock R, et al. Inflammation-associated changes in lipid composition and the organization of the erythrocyte membrane. *Biochim Biophys Acta Clin.* (2016) 5:186–92. doi: 10.1016/j.bbacli.2016.03.007
5. Bosman GJ, Cluitmans JC, Groenen YA, Were JM, Willekens FL, Novotny VM. Susceptibility to hyperosmotic stress-induced phosphatidylserine exposure increases during red blood cell storage. *Transfusion* (2011) 51:1072–8. doi: 10.1111/j.1537-2995.2010.02929.x
6. Ghasghaeinia M, Cluitmans JC, Akel A, Dreischer P, Toulany M, Köberle M, et al. The impact of erythrocyte age on eryptosis. *Brit J Haematol.* (2012) 157:606–14. doi: 10.1111/j.1365-2141.2012.09100.x
7. Bosman GJ. The proteome of the red blood cell: an auspicious source of new insights into membrane-centered regulation of homeostasis. *Proteomes* (2016) 4:E35. doi: 10.3390/proteomes4040035
8. D'Alessandro A, Kriebardis AG, Rinalducci S, Antonelou MH, Hansen KC, Papassideri IS, et al. An update on red blood cell storage lesions, as gleaned through biochemistry and omics technologies. *Transfusion* (2015) 55:205–19. doi: 10.1111/trf.12804
9. Bardyn M, Rappaz B, Jaferzadeh K, Crettaz D, Tissot JD, Moon I., et al. Red blood cell ageing markers: a multi-parametric analysis. *Blood Transf.* (2017) 15:239–48. doi: 10.2450/2017.0318-16
10. Willekens FL, Bosch FH, Roerdinkholder-Stoelwinder B, Groenen-Döpp YA, Werre JM. Quantification of loss of haemglobin components form the circulating red blood cell *in vivo*. *Eur J Haematol.* (1997) 58:246–50.
11. Bosch FH, Werre JM, Schipper L, Roerdinkholder-Stoelwinder B, Huls T, Willekens FL, et al. Determinants of red blood cell deformability in relation to cell age. *Eur J Haematol.* (1994) 42:35–41.
12. Cluitmans JC, Hardeman MR, Dinkla S, Brock R, Bosman GJ. Red blood cell deformability during storage: towards functional proteomics and metabolomics in the blood bank. *Blood Transf.* (2012) 10:s12–8. doi: 10.2450/2012.004S
13. Antonelou MH, Kriebardis AG, Stamoulis KE, Trougakos IP, Papassideri IS. Apoliprotein J/Clusterin is a novel structural component of human erythrocytes and a biomarker of cellular stress and senescence. *PLoS ONE* (2011) 6:e26032. doi: 10.1371/journal.pone.0026032
14. Mohanty JG, Nagababu E, Rifkind JM. Red blood cell oxidative stress impairs oxygen delivery and induced red blood cell aging. *Front Physiol.* (2014) 5:84. doi: 10.3389/fphys.2014.00084
15. Roy CN. Anemia of inflammation. *Hematol Am Soc Hematol Educ Program* (2010) 2010, 276–80. doi: 10.1182/asheducation-2010.1.276
16. Cluitmans JC, Tomelleri C, Yapici Z, Dinkla S, Bovee-Geurts P, Chokkalingam V, et al. Abnormal red cell structure and function in neuroacanthocytosis. *PLoS ONE* (2015) 10:e0125580. doi: 10.1371/journal.pone.0125580
17. Dulski J, Sołtan W, Schinwelski M, Rudzinska M, Wójcik-Pedziwiatr M, Wictore L, et al. Clinical variability of neuroacanthocytosis syndromes–a series of six patients with long follow-up. *Clin Neurol Neurosurg.* (2016) 147:78–83. doi: 10.1016/j.clineuro.2016.05.028
18. Jung HH, Danek A, Walker RH. Neuroacanthocytosis syndromes. *Orphanet J Rare Dis.* (2011) 6:68. doi: 10.1186/1750-1172-6-68
19. De Franceschi L, Bosman GJ, Mohandas N. Abnormal red cell features associated with hereditary neurodegenerative disorders: the neuroacanthocytosis syndromes. *Curr Opin Hematol.* (2014) 21:201–9. doi: 10.1097/MOH.0000000000000035
20. Adjobo-Hermans MJ, Cluitmans JC, Bosman GJ. Neuroacanthocytosis: observations, theories and perspectives on the origin and significance of acanthocytes. *Tremor Other Hyperkinet Mov.* (2015) 5:328. doi: 10.7916/D8VHftest2M
21. Florea A, Craciun C. Bee venom induced *in vivo* ultrastructural reactions of cells involved in the bone marrow erythropoiesis and of circulating red blood cells. *Microsc Microanal.* (2013) 19:393–405. doi: 10.1017/S14319276120 14195
22. Prohaska R, Sibon OC, Rudnicki DD, Danek A, Hayflick SJ, Verhaag EM, et al. Brain, blood and iron: perspectives on the roles of erythrocytes and iron in neurodegeneration. *Neurobiol Dis.* (2012) 46:607–24. doi: 10.1016/j.nbd.2012.03.006
23. Lupo F, Tibaldi E, Matte A, Sharma AK, Brunati AM, Alper SL, et al. A new molecular link between defective autophagy and erythroid abnormalities in chorea-acanthocytosis. *Blood* (2016) 128:2976–87. doi: 10.1182/blood-2016-07-727321
24. Satchwell TJ, Hawley BR, Bell AJ, Ribeiro ML, Toye AM. The cytoskeletal binding domain of band 3 is required for multiprotein complex formation and retention during erythropoiesis. *Haematologica* (2015) 100:133–42. doi: 10.3324/haematol.2014.114538
25. Kay MMB, Bosman GJ, Lawrence C. Functional topography of band 3: specific structural alteration linked to functional aberrations in human erythrocytes. *Proc Natl Acad Sci U.S.A.* (1988) 85:492–6.
26. Dzik WH. The air we breathe: three vital respiratory gases and the red blood cell: oxygen, nitric oxide, and carbon dioxide. *Transfusion* (2011) 51:676–85. doi: 10.1111/j.1537-2995.2011.03114.x
27. Hardeman MR, Goedhart PT, Dobbe JGG, Lettinga KP. Laser assisted optical rotational cell analyser. A new instrument for measurement of various structural hemorheological parameters. *Clin. Hemorheol.* (1994) 14:605–18.
28. Knox-Macaulay HH, Rehman JU, Al Zadjali S, Fawaz NA, Al Kindi S. Idiopathic thrombocytopenic purpura and hypokalaemic dRTA with compensated haemolysis and striking acanthocytosis in band 3 (SLC4A1/AE1) A858D homozygote. *Ann Hematol.* (2013) 92:553–4. doi: 10.1007/s00277-012-1590-3

29. Patel KV, Mohanty JG, Kanapuru B, Hesdorffer C, Ershler WB, Rifkind JM. Association of the red cell distribution width with red blood cell deformability. *Adv Exp Med.* (2013) 765:211–6. doi: 10.1007/978-1-4614-4989-8_29
30. Carmel R. Anemia and aging: an overview of clinical, diagnostic and biological issues. *Blood Rev.* (2001) 15:9–18. doi: 10.1054/blre.2001.0146
31. Stanlowsky N, Reinhardt P, Glass H, Kalmbach N, Naujock M, Hensel N, et al. Neuronal dysfunction in iPSC-derived medium spiny neurons from chorea-acanthocytosis patients is reversed by Src kinase inhibition and F-actin stabilization. *J Neurosci.* (2016) 36:12027–43. doi: 10.1523/JNEUROSCI.0456-16.2016
32. Popkirov S. Is postoperative encelopathy with choreoathetosis an acquired form of neuroacanthocytosis? *Med Hypotheses* (2016) 89:21–3. doi: 10.1016/j.mehy.2016.02.001
33. Newman MF, Kirchner JL, Phillips-Bute B, Gaver V, Grocott H, Jones RH, et al. Longitudinal assessment of neurocognitive function after coronary-artery bypass surgery. *N Engl J Med.* (2001) 344:395–402. doi: 10.1056/NEJM200102083440601
34. Feinkohl I, Winterer G, Pischon T. Diabetes is associated with risk of postoperative cognitive dysfunction: a meta-analysis. *Diabetes Metab Res Rev.* (2017) 33:e2884. doi: 10.1002/dmrr.2884
35. Stevenson VL, Hardie RJ. Acanthocytosis and neurological disorders. *J Neurol.* (2001) 248:87–94. doi: 10.1007/s004150170241
36. Vroegindeweij LH, van der Beek EH, Boon AJ, Hoogendoorn M, Kievit JA, Wilson JH, et al. Aceruloplasminemia presents as Type 1 diabetes in non-obese adults: a detailed case series. *Diabet Med.* (2015) 32:993–1000. doi: 10.1111/dme.12712
37. Kassubek R, Uttner I, Schönfeldt-Lecuona C, Kassubek J, Connemann BJ. Extending the aceruloplasminemia phenotype: NBIA on imaging and acanthocytosis, yet only minor neurological findings. *J Neurol Sci.* (2017) 376:151–2. doi: 10.1016/j.jns.2017.03.019
38. Danese E, Lippi G, Montagnana M. Red blood cell distribution width and cardiovascular diseases. *J Thorac Dis.* (2015) 7:E402–11. doi: 10.3978/j.issn.2072-1439.2015.10.04
39. Weuve J, Mendes de Leon CF, Bennett DA, Dong X, Evans DA. The red cell distribution width and anemia in association with prevalent dementia. *Alzheimer Dis Assoc Disord.* (2014) 28:99–105. doi: 10.1097/WAD.0b013e318299673c
40. Öztürk ZA, Ünal A, Yigiter R, Yesil Y, Kuyumcu ME, Neyal M, et al. Is increased red cell distribution width (RDW) indicating inflammation in Alzheimer's disease (AD)? *Arch Gerontol Geriatr.* (2013) 56:50–4. doi: 10.1016/j.archger.2012.10.002
41. Lee HB, Kim J, Oh SH, Kim SH, Kim HS, Kim WC, et al. Red blood cell distribution width is associated with severity of leukoaraiosis. *PLoS ONE* (2016) 11:e0150308. doi: 10.1371/journal.pone.0150308
42. Bosman GJ, Janzing JG, Bartholomeus IG, De Man AJ, Zitman FG, De Grip WJ. Erythrocyte aging characteristics in elderly individual with beginning dementia. *Neurobiol Aging* (1997) 18:291–5.
43. Gamaldo AA, Ferrucci L, Rifkind J, Longo DL, Zonderman AB. Relationship between mean corpuscular volume and cognitive performance in older adults. *J Am Geriatr Soc.* (2013) 61:84–9. doi: 10.1111/jgs.12066
44. Burnstock G. Purinergic signaling in the cardiovascular system. *Circ Res.* (2017) 120:207–28. doi: 10.1161/CIRCRESAHA.116.309726
45. Silva JC, Moraes ZV, Silva C, Mazon Sde B, Guariento ME, Fattori, A. Understanding red blood cell parameters in the context of the frailty phenotype: interpretations of the FIBRA (Frailty in Brazil Seniors) study. *Arch Gerontol Geriatr.* (2014) 59:636–41. doi: 10.1016/j.archger.2014.07.014
46. McCormack MK, Lazzarini A, Toke D, Lepore F. A genetic study of red cell osmotic fragility in Huntington's disease. *Am J Med Genet.* (1984) 18:5–11. doi: 10.1002/ajmg.1320180103
47. Olsson MG, Davidsson S, Muhammad ZD, Lahiri N, Tabrizi SJ, Akerstrom B, et al. Increased levels of hemoglobin an alpha1-microglobulin in Huntington's disease. *Front Biosci.* (2012) 4:950–7.
48. Zakharov SF, Shandala AM, Shcheglova MV, Gromov PS, Insarova NG, Sychova VA, et al. Comparative study of human erythrocyte membranes in normal people and in Huntington's chorea patients. *Vopr Med Khim.* (1990) 36:71–3.
49. Pretorius E, Swanepoel AC, Buys AV, Vermeulen N, Duim W, Kell DB. Eryptosis as a marker of Parkinson's disease. *Aging* (2014) 6:788–19. doi: 10.18632/aging.100695
50. Mohanty JG, Eckley DM, Williamson JD, Launer LJ, Rifkind JM. Do red blood cell-beta-amyloid interactions alter oxygen delivery in Alzheimer's disease? *Adv Exp Med Biol.* (2008) 614:29–35. doi: 10.1007/978-0-387-74911-2_4
51. Saito Y, Hamakubo T, Yoshida Y, Ogawa Y, Hara Y, Fujimura H, et al. Preparation and application of monoclonal antibodies against oxidized DJ-1. Significant elevation of oxidized DJ-1 in erythrocytes of early-stge Parkinson disease patients. *Neurosci Lett.* (2009) 465:1–5. doi: 10.1016/j.neulet.2009.08.074
52. Abd-Elhadi S, Honig A, Simhi-Haham D, Schechter M, Linetsky E, Ben-Hur T, et al. Total and proteinase K-resistant alpha-synuclein levels in erythrocytes, determined by their ability to bind phospholipids, associate with Parkinson's disease. *Sci Rep.* (2015) 5:11120. doi: 10.1038/srep11120
53. Kosenko EA, Tikhonova LA, Montoliu C, Barreto GE, Aliev K, Kaminsky YG. Metabolic abnormalities of erythrocytes as a risk factor for Alzheimer's disease. *Front Neurosci.* (2018) 11:728. doi: 10.3389/fnins.2017.00728
54. Choi S, Bush AM, Borzage MT, Joshi AA, Mack WJ, Coates TD, et al. Hemoglobin and mean platelet volume predicts diffuse T1-MRI white matter volume decrease in sickle cell disease patients. *Neuroimage Clin.* (2017) 15:239–46. doi: 10.1016/j.nicl.2017.04.023
55. Raz S, Koren A, Dan O, Levin C. Executive function and neural activation in adults with beta-thalassemia major: an event-related potentials study. *Ann N Y Acad Sci.* (2016) 1386:16–29. doi: 10.1111/nyas.13279
56. Pazgal I, Inbar E, Cohen M, Spilberg O, Stark P. High incidence of silent cerebral infarcts in adult patients with beta thalassemia major. *Thromb Res.* (2016) 144:119–22. doi: 10.1016/j.thromres.2016.06.010
57. Koralkova P, van Solinge WW, van Wijk R. Rare hereditary red blood cell enzymopathies associated with hemolytic anemia–pathophysiology, clinical aspects and laboratory diagnosis. *Int J Lab Hematol.* (2014) 36:388–97. doi: 10.1111/ijlh.12223
58. Ashraf A, Clark M, So PW. The aging of iron man. *Front Aging Neurosci.* (2018) 10:65. doi: 10.3389/finagi.2018.00065

15

Blood and Blood Components: From Similarities to Differences

Olivier Garraud[1,2]* *and Jean-Daniel Tissot*[3,4]

[1] *Faculty of Medicine, University of Lyon, Saint-Etienne, France,* [2] *Institut National de la Transfusion Sanguine, Paris, France,* [3] *Transfusion Interrégionale CRS, Epalinges, Switzerland,* [4] *Faculty of Biology and Medicine, University of Lausanne, Lausanne, Switzerland*

***Correspondence:**
Olivier Garraud
ogarraud@ints.fr

Blood transfusion is made possible because, in most countries and organizations, altruistic individuals voluntarily, anonymously, and generously donate (without compensation) either whole blood or separated components that are then processed and distributed by professionals, prior to being allocated to recipients in need. Being part of modern medicine, blood transfusion uses so-called standard blood components when relative to cellular fractions and fresh plasma. However, as will be discussed in this paper, strictly speaking, such so-called labile blood components are not completely standard. Furthermore, the prevalent system based on voluntary, non-remunerated blood donation is not yet universal and, despite claims by the World Health Organization that 100% of blood collection will be derived from altruistic donations by 2020 (postponed to 2025), many obstacles may hinder this ambition, especially when relative to the collection of the enormous amount of plasma destined for fractionation into plasma derivative or drugs. Finally, country organizations also vary due to the economy, sociology, politics, and epidemiology. This paper then, discusses the particulars (of which ethical considerations) of blood transfusion diversity and the consequences for donors, patients, and society.

Keywords: transfusion, blood donation, blood processing, blood components, ethics

INTRODUCTION

Blood and blood components (BCs) for transfusion chiefly originate from donations made by altruistic individuals. However, although 100% voluntary non-remunerated blood donation (VNRD) is the goal that has been set (by 2020 as publicized by the World Health Organization WHO—later revised to 2025 in some areas) (1, 2), it is far from being achieved at the present time for various reasons linked to contingency (3), and the emergence in low/middle-income countries of modern health-care services requiring more transfusion prescriptions. Blood for therapeutic use comes into two sets: (1) the one consists in labile blood components (LBCs) comprising essentially the cellular components [red blood cells concentrates (RBCCs) and platelet concentrates, PCs as well as part of therapeutic plasma, principally fresh frozen plasma FFP]; and (2) the other one consists in plasma derived or fractionated drugs, and occasionally in FFP obtained from large pools and subjected to stringent pathogen reduction. While the former is principally handled by blood establishments (BEs), many of them overruled by the public sector or Non Governmental, non-for-profit, organizations such as the Red-Cross/Red-Crescent, the latter is largely handled by the plasma fraction industry within the private, for-profit sector.

Labile blood components are usually labeled as "standard blood products," and thus refer to guidelines such as the Council of Europe's "Guide to the preparation, use and quality assurance of blood components" (4). However, all LBCs referring to the same label are, in fact, significantly different from each other: they depend on the donor, the process and the storage characteristics which are not consistent, as each consists either in single donor originating units or small pools (5 in mean, and >12 by all means); minipools apply to PCs and therapeutic plasma. Indeed, as each LBC reflects both the genetic and non-genetic-based characteristics of the donors (referred to as "storage lesions"), they all differ from one another despite considerable efforts made to minimize deviations in their process.

This paper will briefly outline the most visible community forms of and differences in LBCs, and the way in which differences can affect outcomes in: (1) recipients; (2) health policies and economics (as essential additional safety procedures can result in even more complex disparities between LBC inventories). The circumstances of blood collection and how ethics are concerned when blood supply does not meet demand or when marketing creates new markets will also be discussed.

AS THE ESSENTIAL DETERMINANT IN TRANSFUSION, BLOOD REPRESENTS A COMMON MATTER FOR HUMANS

Every human depends on nearly normal blood functions to survive. Moderate alterations may result in sub-physiological functioning, while more severe defects can be corrected by either drugs or blood derivatives (when available), or both, pending anticipated gene correction. Blood characterizes species and cannot be safely exchanged between species, even close ones such as humans and apes. Human blood transfusion can nevertheless be processed within the human species provided major compatibility rules are respected. This property first allowed blood transfusion to be performed in emergency situations, and later, with technological advances, to be applied almost routinely, despite the fact that "routine" is a word that never applies to blood transfusion from either the donor's or the recipient's perspective (5, 6).

Donated blood is humanity (7, 8) and ideally, VNRD blood is "pure" humanity, yet replacement donation shares the values of assistance and cannot be considered non-altruistic, even if a certain degree of social pressure cannot be ruled out (3). Maybe the lowest common denominator is the root symbol of blood, its sacred characteristic, whatever sacred may mean to people, ranging from religious to atheistic sentiments (9). Thanks to initiatives like Blood Donor Day on the 14th of June, it can be acknowledged on the highest scale that many people worldwide share the idealistic human view of blood donation for transfusion purposes (10). Ideally, this standpoint should make sure that such a process expands and infuses in areas where VNRD is not yet achievable. However, the situation is far from universal or exemplary. Three taints can be outlined as follows: (1) as the demand for BCs expands in many countries, BEs start applying marketing methods to attain prospective new blood donors, potentially altering the voluntary aspect of donation, or the benevolence (or the absence of profit) (11). The same holds true for plasma collectors within the industry (12–16). (2) The benefits of blood have been distorted to serve non-life-threatening medical conditions, and BCs have entered the for-profit market and business where blood is being increasingly used in welfare clinics for doping or cosmetic applications (17, 18). This merchandized blood may, therefore, no longer be available for therapeutic and medical indications, potentially worsening the shortage problem and ultimately leading BEs to use enhanced marketing tools and enter a vicious circle. (3) Blood and BCs for research now represent an expanding market, they can either be "conventional" as BEs trade left-overs from test tubes or residues from blood processing, or BCs purposefully processed, i.e., BEs collect blood from VNRDs not eligible for the therapeutic pathway or presenting characteristics required for specific research. In those cases, VNRDs are usually informed that all or part of their donation will be used for research programmes and they may object to this use. Moreover, some donors sell blood for specific research programmes, with the blood generally being collected outside of BEs; this is possible in some countries but is strictly forbidden in others. Research ethics committees would prevent these possibilities.

SIMILARITIES OF HUMAN BLOOD

As has already been outlined, one common platform for humans considering blood is the general anthropological consideration of this "fluid" which is both material (the blood tissue) and spiritual or the like (altruism, attraction/repulsion, life and death, genetics and lineages, war and peace, and so forth) (9). Regarding its materiality, human blood is unique to the species, and there is by no means any significant difference between ethnic groups, which refutes previous racist theories on the purity of blood. There are indeed certain variations that vary in their frequency in ethnic groups as will be presented in the next section of this paper, but none of them prevent donated blood from being issued to any other human, apart from major (ABH) blood (in fact, tissue) antigen group compatibility. These fundamental characteristics allow the principle of blood transfusion and, moreover, of universal blood transfusion, once the major restriction of the ABH system is taken care of.

DIVERSITIES IN HUMAN BLOOD AND BCs FOR TRANSFUSION

In contrast to what has been presented above, no siblings have identical blood. Indeed, even monozygotic twins display genetic and epigenetic differences. Whereas the Mendelian distribution of HLA antigens is transmitted in blocks (haplotypes), HLA diversity between humans ranges from between 10^6 and 10^7 (19). HLA polymorphism limits, to some extent, platelet and leukocyte availability and may also create complications such as immunization (20). Platelet antigens add diversity by bringing more than 30 additional groups often with two alleles each (about 5 matter essentially in transfusion) (21, 22). The diversity of erythrocyte antigenic alleles is not only huge (by the thousands) but is also non-haplotypic, offering a tremendous assortment of individual cell markers which is fascinating if we consider the uniqueness of each human, but limits the possibility of matching blood groups for transfusion (23). In fact, half a dozen such antigens are considered routine, allowing for wide-scale transfusion. It should be noted that not all individuals are equal and some individuals can be easily transfused (the vast majority) while others with rare blood groups cannot, requiring special programs with technical, ethical, and organizational problems. Similarly, there is diversity in people's propensity to become alloimmunized after blood transfusion, because HLA loci make people good or bad responders to RBC, platelet, or leukocyte antigens (a common law in innate and adaptive immune responses that varies in individuals) (24–26).

With respect to LBCs, despite being called "standard," and their largely similar appearance category by category, they are not, in fact, all the same. They are defined as standard because they fall within a range of maximum and minimum levels of either desired and undesired constituents, and only a few parameters are evaluated among the thousands of variables that make individuals' blood differ from another (4). Furthermore, for each category of LBC, besides the genetic variations between donors that transfer characteristics to the donated component (gender, tissue and HLA genotype, erythrocyte antigen genotype, platelet antigen genotype, protein variants, etc.), there are additional variation parameters that depend on the donors: the time of donation (morning, afternoon, after a meal or fasting, drug and dietary supplement intake, menstrual cycle for non-menopaused women, diet, hygiene habits, and many other parameters) (27–29). All of these parameters may influence the final characteristics of the LBC, though there is no evidence as yet of the effect apart from the presence of soluble antibodies against blood cell antigens (iso-anti-A or B; anti-HLA in females who have been pregnant). BEs extend the variety since the addition and diversification of devices, machines and automats multiply heterogeneity (**Table 1** aims to illustrate this). Finally, shelf-life duration multiplies LBC delivery diversity by 41 for RBCCs (in theory: 42 minus 1 day, as 1 day is needed to obtain all the parameters allowing the labeling and issue of the RBCC) (30) and 4 (5 minus 1 day) for PCs. It has further been noticed near two decades ago that RBCs do not recirculate the same depending on storage conditions of the component (one ¼ of the infused RBCs even never recirculate) (31).

What then is the clinical relevance of such diversity? The case of storage lesions has been extensively studied (32–34), having basically identified two sets of lesions: reversible and irreversible lesions (35). Conflicting data have been obtained from both experimental and clinical data, sparking disputes over the rationale for using fresh as opposed to old blood (36–38). In simple terms, it appears that neither fresh nor old blood is clearly defined, nor is the readout (patient outcome) providing conclusive information, and relevant clinical trials are still needed to resolve this issue (39–41). This issue is of utmost importance as it may revoke the current blood-banking paradigm (meaning that conflicts of interest when blood banks happen to be research principal investigators are non-negligible).

TABLE 1 | Parameters having proven or theoretical influence on the quality of the processed blood component (BC).

Main categories	Main items adding diversity	Level of diversity
Donor dependent parameters (genetically controlled)	• Sex/gender • Immunogenetic characteristics (blood groups) • Natural iso-antibodies • …	• Two • By the thousands (millions if applied also to HLA antigens) • Variable
Donor dependent parameters (only partly genetically controlled)	• Immunization status • Nutrition, metabolism • Hygiene and intoxications (therapeutic and recreational drugs, supplements, alcohol, tobacco) • Meal; or fast • Nycthemeral cycle • Genital cycle and periods • Outside temperature condition • …	Hundreds of influential parameters
Donor independent parameters (BC processing)	• Shipping time and temperature • Needles, plastics and bags, rotators, automats for collection and intermediate storage • Devices for cell separation • Working temperature • Additives (anticoagulant, solutions, pathogen inactivation, etc.) • Filtration steps (meshes, temperature, timing, etc.) • Pooling steps • Preservation conditions • Physical interactions in shelf-life conditions (stacking, shocks, thermic differences, shipping, etc.)	• Variable • Dozens influential parameters
Patient (recipient, beneficiary) dependent parameters	• Blood group • Immunization status • Matching conditions	• By the thousands

Each parameter being independent from the preceding one, diversity is created by the multiplication as opposed to the addition of all. The final diversity goes by the million or more. Not all parameters are equally influential but it clearly appears from the table that one given BC collected by one individual, despite being "standardized" to a norm, is unlikely to be "standard."

DISPARITIES IN PUBLIC HEALTH POLICIES

Labile blood components are not considered univocal in various countries and systems, though they are not considered to be drugs according to Directive 2002/98/EC (42), in contrast to plasma fractions or derivatives [Directive 2001/83/EC (43)], or industrially prepared and solvent-detergent secured therapeutic plasma originating from large pools. Some national regulations do, however, consider labile LBCs to be drugs, as is the case in Switzerland; and WHO recently (2015) added blood and blood derivatives to its list of essential medicines (44). Semantics between medicines and drugs are imprecise, however, and this decision has displeased a number of blood donor associations who are batting against confusion with LBCs and plasma derivatives (45). Furthermore, the logistics by which certified LBCs can be delivered to patients varies considerably between countries: according to the European directive, there are basically two main actors: BEs which collect, process, test, and distribute BCs, and Hospital Blood Banks or HBBs which acquire LBCs from BEs, build up an inventory and deliver selected LBCs to patients upon *ad hoc* immunohaematological matching (4). On some occasions, BE and HBB functions can be held by the same entity (as, e.g., in France).

In addition, Council of Europe directorate EDQM requests that BEs apply a minimum platform for blood testing, with additional options for BEs willing to raise the LBC safety level with, for example, the implementation of nucleic acid testing (NAT) (4). Some BEs perform NAT on each donation, even on frequent donors' donations, while others restrict it to new donations. NAT is applied to both pools and individuals, and some BEs that used NAT have reverted back to non-NAT because of its relatively low (and debatable) cost-effectiveness (46).

In short, there is significant heterogeneity in stances on the availability of LBCs to patients through organizations and countries' public health policies. Consistent efforts have been made by large bodies such as EDQM, the American Blood Bank Association or the International Society for Blood Transfusion ISBT to define safety and quality parameters that should apply to each issued LBC; however, this is still a range above and beyond which the LBC should not conform to standards; if testing is individual for most infectious markers (and even some are tested in pools), hematological markers are frequently tested by sampling to define quality (4). This is the reason why we call attention here on the false homogeneity of LBCs despite they go by the noun of "standard." This is in sharp contrast to the actual standardization of plasma derivatives obtained from 100 of 1000s of collections and subjected to an industrial processing (47).

DISPARITIES WITHIN ETHICAL CONSIDERATIONS

Ethics are largely cultural and it is difficult to establish a platform that fits all situations worldwide. Nevertheless, as early as 1975, WHO declared that sustainable efforts should be made by all countries to collect blood from VNRDs. WHO later set the objective of 100% VNRD by 2020 (the Melbourne Declaration, 2009) (1). The EDQM has also declared itself in favor of a generalized objective of 100% VNRD where possible (4). The Oviedo Convention (1997), set up under the auspices of the Council of Europe, has established standards for ethics in the field of human rights and dignity, with regard to the use of tissues of human origin (including blood) (48). Nonetheless, many states have been late in signing this convention and others have not yet ratified it. WHO, considering that many countries could not achieve the 2020 VNRD objective, postponed it to 2025 for certain Middle-Eastern countries. State WHO and ISBT in its revised code of Ethics, paid and compensated donations should no longer be acceptable; replacement donations remain questionable (49). The issue of paid versus unpaid plasma collection has been challenged by advocates for the plasma fractionation industry (13, 14, 16) (the case of paid cell donations is still existing in certain countries including Europe but apparently on the decline worldwide). It is worth noting that a very interesting study was published in 2012 questioning the ban on financial contracts with blood donors in Africa, with the declared objective to reduce the infectious burden on "donated" blood (50). This last example questions the universality of ethical values of blood donation when coming to strengthening safety in LBC beneficiaries, opening an additional ethical dilemma. Next, when this comes to plasma for fractionation, there have been requests that collection and fractionation are more equally dispatched in countries that prescribe most to do justice to patients in need in case there is shortage and to alleviate the burden of (paid) collection in countries hosting the majority of plasma collectors such as the USA (51).

We offer an opinion here: as opposed to normative ethics (the Oviedo Convention, the ISBT Code of Ethics), reflective ethics (anthropological and philosophical) are preferred in order to move forward with the safe use (for donors, recipients, stakeholders and society members, i.e. people, civilians and tax payers) of substances of human origin (41). In the meantime, there is clear evidence that ethics are extremely cultural and embedded with acknowledged or hidden religious sentiments with the populations concerned.

In short, it should be noticed that blood within the transfusion process offers an additional paradox: while the LBCs are relatively inhomogeneous relative to active constituents though relatively homogenous relative to the so-called ethicality of their collection, this is the other way around for plasma derivatives that are remarkably homogenous and standardized relative to active constituents but may be obtained both within the profit and the non-for-profit sectors. The latter case has been recently (2016) the subject of important debated in France and Switzerland and journalists reported both in the paper and the TV press on some potential malpractice with respect to donors' own safety and vulnerability.

CONCLUDING REMARKS

The transfusion process is at the crossroads of a multitude of paradoxes (42). It is one of the only medicines that rely on material outside the control of the pharmaceutical industry if we exclude plasma for fractionation. It professes to be precision medicine, yet the issued LBC comprises ±20% (or more) of the expected therapeutic constituent. It professes to be personalized medicine, but blood groups between donors and recipients match for the vast minority. It is prescribed for the most fragile patients, yet practitioners prove to have very limited knowledge on it (according to recent surveys, they usually know which is the target of a biosimilar drug or a therapeutic monoclonal antibody, but only largely relative to LBCs) (43). We believe it is important to advocate for prescribing doctors to receive further training on LBCs and transfusion medicine–setting apart the case of standardized plasma derivative or drugs—education and training are essential to understanding and respecting blood donors and donated LBCs, to making wise choices, and to the optimal management of patients' blood and donated LBCs, within the limitations of prevailing uncertainty (Garraud et al., in preparation). Being knowledgeable in the face of uncertainty would prevent a comparison of apples and oranges in published works, even in high-quality journals. It would be practical for prescribing doctors to forward their everyday questions to blood transfusion specialists; this would certainly be useful in establishing the most appropriate training programmes.

AUTHOR CONTRIBUTIONS

Both authors contributed equally to this manuscript and its revision.

ACKNOWLEDGMENTS

Both authors would like to thank the research groups to which they belong for their achievements in the fields of blood component characteristics and lesions. They also wish to thank their colleagues in the field of ethics applied to blood transfusion for their long-term collaboration, as well as the EMITm Think Tank. OG expresses his gratitude to the association Les Amis de Rémi, Savigneux, France, and the Association Recherche et Transfusion, Paris, France for their long-standing support.

REFERENCES

1. World Health Organization. *The Melbourne Declaration on 100% Voluntary Non-Remunerated Donation of Blood and Blood Components*. Available from: http://www.who.int/worldblooddonorday/MelbourneDeclarationWBDD09.pdf (Accessed: November 20, 2017).
2. World Health Organization, Regional Office for the Eastern Mediterranean. *Strategic Framework for Blood Safety and Availability 2016–2025*. (2016). Available from: http://www.who.int/iris/handle/10665/250402 (Accessed: November 20, 2017).
3. Haddad A, Bou Assi T, Garraud O. Can a decentralized blood system ensure self-sufficiency and blood safety? The Lebanese experience. *J Public Health Policy* (2017) 38:359–65. doi:10.1057/s41271-017-0076-x
4. EDQM (Council of Europe). *Guide to the Preparation, Use and Quality Assurance of Blood Components*. 19th ed. Strasbourg, France: EDQM Publishers (2017). 540 p.
5. Garraud O, Tissot JD. Theoretical and experimental ethics: advocacy for blood donors and beneficiaries of blood transfusions. *Transfus Med* (2017). doi:10.1111/tme.12457
6. Garraud O. "Transfusion clinique et biologique" – what makes transfusion medicine and biology so special? *Transfus Clin Biol* (2017) 24:403. doi:10.1016/j.tracli.2017.09.002
7. Tissot JD, Garraud O. Ethics and blood donation: a marriage of convenience. *Presse Med* (2016) 45:e247–52. doi:10.1016/j.lpm.2016.06.016
8. Garraud O, Politis C, Vuk T, Tissot JD. Rethinking transfusion medicine with a more holistic approach. *Transfus Clin Biol* (2017) 25:439–45. doi:10.1016/j.tracli.2017.10.005
9. Garraud O, Lefrère JJ. Blood and blood-associated symbols beyond medicine and transfusion: far more complex than first appears. *Blood Transfus* (2014) 12:14–21. doi:10.2450/2013.0131-13
10. World Health Organization. Available from: http://www.who.int/campaigns/world-blood-donor-day/2017/en/ (Accessed: November 20, 2017).
11. Aldamiz-Echevarria C, Aguirre-Garcia MS. A behavior model for blood donors and marketing strategies to retain and attract them. *Rev Lat Am Enfermagem* (2014) 22:467–75. doi:10.1590/0104-1169.3398.2439
12. Petrini C. Production of plasma-derived medicinal products: ethical implications for blood donation and donors. *Blood Transfus* (2014) 12(Suppl 1): s389–94. doi:10.2450/2013.0167-12
13. Farrugia A, Penrod J, Bult JM. The ethics of paid plasma donation: a plea for patient centeredness. *HEC Forum* (2015) 27:417–29. doi:10.1007/s10730-014-9253-5
14. Farrugia A, Del Bò C. Some reflections on the code of ethics of the International society of blood transfusion. *Blood Transfus* (2015) 13:551. doi:10.2450/2015.0266-14
15. Flanagan P. The code of ethics of the International society of blood transfusion. *Blood Transfus* (2015) 13:537–8. doi:10.2450/2015.0061-15
16. Farrugia A, Del Bò C. Reply to Flanagan "the code of ethics of the International society of blood transfusion" [blood transfus 2015; 13: 537-8]. *Blood Transfus* (2017) 15:286–8. doi:10.2450/2016.0013-16
17. Morkeberg J. Blood manipulation: current challenges from an anti-doping perspective. *Hematology Am Soc Hematol Educ Program* (2013) 1:627–31. doi:10.1182/asheducation-2013.1.627
18. Elghblawi E. Platelet-rich plasma, the ultimate secret for youthful skin elixir and hair growth triggering. *J Cosmet Dermatol* (2017). doi:10.1111/jocd.12404
19. Gourraud PA, Khankhanian P, Cereb N, Yang SY, Feolo M, Maiers M, et al. HLA diversity in the 1000 genomes dataset. *Plos One* (2014) 9:e97282. doi:10.1371/journal.pone.0097282
20. De Clippel D, Baeten M, Torfs A, Emonds MP, Feys HB, Compernolle V, et al. Screening for HLA antibodies in plateletpheresis donors with a history of transfusion or pregnancy. *Transfusion* (2014) 54:3036–42. doi:10.1111/trf.12727
21. McGuinn CE, Mitchell BW, Bussel JB. Chapter 91 – Fetal and neonatal alloimmune thrombocytopenia. In: Shaz BH, Hillyer CD, Abrams CS, Roshal M editors. *Transfusion medicine and hemostasis: clinical and laboratory aspects*. 2nd edn. (2013):609–13. doi:10.1016/B978-0-12-397164-7.00091-4
22. Brouk H, Bertrand G, Zitouni S, Djenouni A, Martageix C, Griffi F, et al. HPA antibodies in Algerian multitransfused patients: prevalence and involvement in platelet refractoriness. *Transfus Apher Sci* (2015) 52:295–9. doi:10.1016/j.transci.2014.12.028
23. International Societies for Blood Transfusion (ISBT) (2017). Available from: http://www.isbtweb.org/working-parties/red-cell-immunogenetics-and-blood-group-terminology/ISBT (Accessed: November 20, 2017).
24. Hendrickson JE, Eisenbarth SC, Tormey CA. Red blood cell alloimmunization: new findings at the bench and new recommendations for the bedside. *Curr Opin Hematol* (2016) 23:543–9. doi:10.1097/MOH.0000000000000277
25. Körmöczi GF, Mayr WR. Responder individuality in red blood cell alloimmunization. *Transfus Med Hemother* (2014) 41:446–51. doi:10.1159/000369179
26. Pavenski K, Freedman J, Semple JW. HLA alloimmunization against platelet transfusions: pathophysiology, significance, prevention and management. *Tissue Antigens* (2012) 79:237–45. doi:10.1111/j.1399-0039.2012.01852.x
27. Tzounakas VL, Kriebardis AG, Papassideri IS, Antonelou MH. Donor-variation effect on red blood cell storage lesion: a close relationship emerges. *Proteomics Clin Appl* (2016) 10:791–804. doi:10.1002/prca.201500128
28. Tzounakas VL, Georgatzakou HT, Kriebardis AG, Voulgaridou AI, Stamoulis KE, Foudoulaki-Paparizos LE, et al. Donor variation effect on red blood cell storage lesion: a multivariable, yet consistent, story. *Transfusion* (2016) 56:1274–86. doi:10.1111/trf.13582
29. Tzounakas VL, Georgatzakou HT, Kriebardis AG, Papageorgiou EG, Stamoulis KE, Foudoulaki-Paparizos LE, et al. Uric acid variation among regular blood donors is indicative of red blood cell susceptibility to storage lesion markers: a new hypothesis tested. *Transfusion* (2015) 55:2659–71. doi:10.1111/trf.13211
30. Acker JP, Marks DC, Sheffield WP. Quality assessment of established and emerging blood components for transfusion. *J Blood Transfus* (2016) 2016: 4860284. doi:10.1155/2016/4860284
31. Card RT, Mohandas N, Mollison PL. Relationship of post-transfusion viability to deformability of stored red cells. *Br J Haematol* (1983) 53:237–40. doi:10.1111/j.1365-2141.1983.tb02016.x
32. D'Alessandro A, Kriebardis AG, Rinalducci S, Antonelou MH, Hansen KC, Papassideri IS, et al. An update on red blood cell storage lesions, as gleaned through biochemistry and omics technologies. *Transfusion* (2015) 55:205–19. doi:10.1111/trf.12804
33. Burnouf T, Chou ML, Goubran H, Cognasse F, Garraud O, Seghatchian J. An overview of the role of microparticles/microvesicles in blood components: are they clinically beneficial or harmful? *Transfus Apher Sci* (2015) 53:137–45. doi:10.1016/j.transci.2015.10.010
34. Tissot JD, Bardyn M, Sonego G, Abonnenc M, Prudent M. The storage lesions: from past to future. *Transfus Clin Biol* (2017) 24:277–84. doi:10.1016/j.tracli.2017.05.012
35. Prudent M, Tissot JD, Lion N. The 3-phase evolution of stored red blood cells and the clinical trials: an obvious relationship. *Blood Transfus* (2017) 15:188. doi:10.2450/2017.0317-16
36. Klein HG, Cortés-Puch I, Natanson C. More on the age of transfused red cells. *N Engl J Med* (2015) 373:283. doi:10.1056/NEJMc1505699
37. Sanz CC, Pereira A. Age of blood and survival after massive transfusion. *Transfus Clin Biol* (2017) 24:449–53. doi:10.1016/j.tracli.2017.04.005
38. Gehrie EA, Tobian AAR. Finally, what we have been waiting for: evidence that transfusion of RBCs at the extreme of the storage spectrum is safe. *Lancet Haematol* (2017) 4:e504–5. doi:10.1016/S2352-3026(17)30179-5
39. Garraud O. Hemolysis in six week-old autologous red blood cell components questioned: worth addressing the issue of homologous components as well? *Transfus Apher Sci* (2017) 56:261–2. doi:10.1016/j.transci.2017.03.008

40. Garraud O, Tissot JD, Vlaar AP. Short-term versus long-term blood storage. *N Engl J Med* (2017) 376:1091. doi:10.1056/NEJMc1700464
41. Garraud O. Effect of "old" versus "fresh" transfused red blood cells on patients' outcome: probably more complex than appears. *J Thorac Dis* (2017) 9:E146–8. doi:10.21037/jtd.2017.02.03
42. Parliament of Europe. Directive 2002/98/Ec of the European parliament and of the council of 27 january 2003 setting standards of quality and safety for the collection, testing, processing, storage and distribution of human blood and blood components and amending directive2001/83/EC. *Off J Eur Union* (2003) L 33/30.
43. Parliament of Europe. Directive 2001/83/EC of the European parliament and of the council of 6 november 2001 on the community code relating to medicinal products for human use. *Off J Eur Union* (2002) L 311.
44. World Health Organisation. *19th WHO Model List of Essential Medicines*. (2015). Available from: http://www.who.int/medicines/publications/essentialmedicines/EML2015_8-May-15.pdf (Accessed: November 21, 2017).
45. Garraud O, Tissot JD. Les produits sanguins thérapeutiques: des médicaments ou des produits de santé à part ? *Transfus Clin Biol* (2016) 23:127–31. doi:10.1016/j.tracli.2016.06.001
46. Borkent-Raven BA, Janssen MP, van der Poel CL, Bonsel GJ, van Hout BA. Cost-effectiveness of additional blood screening tests in the Netherlands. *Transfusion* (2012) 52:478–88. doi:10.1111/j.1537-2995.2011.03319.x
47. Burnouf T. Current status and new developments in the production of plasma derivatives. *ISBT Sci Ser* (2015) 11:18–25. doi:10.1111/voxs.12269
48. Council of Europe. *The Oviedo Convention: Protecting Human Rights in the Biomedical Field (Convention on Human Rights and Biomedicine (ETS No 164))*. Strasbourg, France (1997). Available from: https://www.coe.int/en/web/conventions/full-list/-/conventions/treaty/164 (Accessed: November 21, 2017).
49. International Societies for Blood Transfusion (ISBT). *The Revised Code of Ethics*. (2017). Availale from: http://www.isbtweb.org/fileadmin/user_upload/ISBT_Code_Of_Ethics_English.pdf (Accessed: November 21, 2017).
50. Ala F, Allain JP, Bates I, Boukef K, Boulton F, Brandful J, et al. External financial aid to blood transfusion services in sub-Saharan Africa: a need for reflection. *PLoS Med* (2012) 9:e1001309. doi:10.1371/journal.pmed.1001309
51. Strengers PF, Klein HG. Plasma is a strategic resource. *Transfusion* (2016) 56:3133–7. doi:10.1111/trf.13913

16

Ultraviolet-Based Pathogen Inactivation Systems: Untangling the Molecular Targets Activated in Platelets

Peter Schubert[1,2], *Lacey Johnson*[3], *Denese C. Marks*[3,4] *and Dana V. Devine*[1,2*]

[1] Canadian Blood Services, Vancouver, BC, Canada, [2] Centre for Blood Research, University of British Columbia, Vancouver, BC, Canada, [3] Research and Development, Australian Red Cross Blood Service, Sydney, NSW, Australia, [4] Sydney Medical School, The University of Sydney, Sydney, NSW, Australia

Correspondence:
Dana V. Devine
dana.devine@blood.ca

Transfusions of platelets are an important cornerstone of medicine; however, recipients may be subject to risk of adverse events associated with the potential transmission of pathogens, especially bacteria. Pathogen inactivation (PI) technologies based on ultraviolet illumination have been developed in the last decades to mitigate this risk. This review discusses studies of platelet concentrates treated with the current generation of PI technologies to assess their impact on quality, PI capacity, safety, and clinical efficacy. Improved safety seems to come with the cost of reduced platelet functionality, and hence transfusion efficacy. In order to understand these negative impacts in more detail, several molecular analyses have identified signaling pathways linked to platelet function that are altered by PI. Because some of these biochemical alterations are similar to those seen arising in the context of routine platelet storage lesion development occurring during blood bank storage, we lack a complete picture of the contribution of PI treatment to impaired platelet functionality. A model generated using data from currently available publications places the signaling protein kinase p38 as a central player regulating a variety of mechanisms triggered in platelets by PI systems.

Keywords: platelets, pathogen inactivation, transfusion, mechanisms, signaling

THE CHALLENGES OF PLATELET TRANSFUSIONS

Platelets play an essential role in hemostasis, fibrinolysis, and vascular integrity, which are critical physiological processes to prevent and control bleeding (1–3). Platelet concentrates (PCs) are transfused to treat bleeding in thrombocytopenic, trauma, or surgery patients (4–6) as well as for prophylactic treatment of patients with hypoproliferative thrombocytopenia (7, 8). Over the last decades, development of improved therapies and the subsequent introduction of new transfusion guidelines have changed the practice of platelet transfusion (9, 10) which has, in turn, influenced the management of platelet inventories in the blood bank.

Additionally, the integrity and safety of platelet preparations could be compromised by the presence of pathogens, such as viruses, bacteria, and parasites (11). Serious complications or death due to bacterially contaminated units have been well documented, leading to several changes in the collection procedures, including stricter donor screening, improved skin disinfection methods and diversion of the first few milliliters of collected blood, and bacterial culture of PCs (12–16). However, the risk still exists, not only for undetected bacterial contamination but for the increasing number of emerging and re-emerging pathogens, particularly viruses for which screening tests may not be in place.

Finally, even with the use of pre-storage leukoreduction, the transfer of residual allogeneic donor leukocytes in PCs still occurs and can potentially cause adverse reactions in certain platelet recipients (17). All pathogen inactivation (PI) systems show inactivation capacity of these residual leukocytes (18, 19).

These challenges of platelet storage have led to the development and increasing implementation of PI technologies which are based on ultraviolet (UV) light-mediated damage of nucleic acids and subsequent inactivation of most pathogens as well as passenger white blood cells.

A BRIEF OVERVIEW OF CURRENT PI SYSTEMS

Currently, three PI systems to produce pathogen-reduced PCs are commercially available, utilizing UV in the presence or absence of a photosenzitizer. These technologies are extensively reviewed in the literature (20–29); therefore, only key points necessary for the context of this review are provided.

The INTERCEPT system (Cerus Corporation, Concord, CA, USA) uses amotosalen as photosensitzer in combination with UVA light (320–400 nm). Amotosalen penetrates the cellular membrane forming non-covalent links between pyrimidine residues in DNA and RNA. UV illumination induces a photochemical reaction that transforms the preexisting link into an irreversible covalent bond, preventing DNA replication and RNA transcription. Excess amotosalen and its photoproducts need to be removed by an in-line compound absorption device (30, 31).

The MIRASOL system (Terumo BCT, Lakewood, CO, USA) uses vitamin B2 (riboflavin) as the photosensitizer and UVA/UVB light (270–360 nm) (32, 33). In the presence of riboflavin, illumination generates free oxygen radicals causing irreversible damage to guanidine nucleotide bases. Riboflavin does not need to be removed following illumination as it is a common dietary element and generally considered to be safe.

The THERAFLEX-UV Platelets system (MacoPharma, Tourcoing, France) uses UVC light in combination with strong agitation which facilitates light penetration and does not require a photosensitizer. UVC acts directly on nucleic acids to induce pyrimidine dimers to block DNA replication (34, 35).

PATHOGEN-REDUCED PLATELET PRODUCTS

Pathogen-reduced PCs can be obtained by direct treatment of platelet components using a PI system, or they can be derived by treating whole blood with the MIRASOL (36, 37) or potentially the INTERCEPT system once a current trial turns out to be successful followed by processing into the (platelet) components (**Table 1**).

It is noteworthy to point out that the THERAFLEX system require PCs produced in platelet additive solution (PAS) while the MIRASOL and INTERCEPT systems can treat PCs in plasma or PAS.

TABLE 1 | Overview of pathogen inactivation (PI) treatment options to obtain pathogen-reduced platelet products.

Product treatment	Storage solution	PI system		
		INTERCEPT	MIRASOL	THERAFLEX
AP/PC	Plasma	+	+	–
	PAS	+	+	+
PRPC or BC/PC	Plasma	+	+	–
	PAS	+	+	+
WB (prior to PRPC or BC/PC production)	Plasma	–	+	–
	PAS	–	+	–

AP/PC, apheresis platelet concentrates; PRPC, platelet-rich plasma concentrate; BC/PC, buffy-coat-derived platelet concentrate; WB, whole blood; PAS, platelet additive solution.

ONGOING DEBATE: SAFETY VS EFFICACY OF PI

More than a decade ago, the interest in PI prompted many large-scale discussions (38–40). The outcome of these deliberations included the provision of information required for implementation of PI systems such as implementation criteria, component specifications, licensing requirements, and the impact in blood product inventories, as well as clinical issues such as transfusion efficacy, risk management issues, and cost–benefit assessments. Since then, numerous studies have been conducted to provide answers to questions on product safety, clinical efficacy, and quality.

In order to assess inactivation efficacy, studies spiking pathogens relevant to blood transfusion into PCs prior to illumination have been performed (34, 41–44). All PI systems currently on the market have demonstrated effectiveness in inactivating most tested pathogens with moderate to highly effective inactivation capacities for several emerging viruses including West Nile virus (45), chikungunyah virus (46), Zika virus (47, 48), dengue virus (49), and hepatitis-E-virus (50). Additionally, a comparative study (51) revealed that HIV-1 can be similarly inactivated by MIRASOL and INTERCEPT, however, less efficient compared to other viruses due to its resistance to UV light. Furthermore, INTERCEPT demonstrated a higher inactivation capacity for bovine viral diarrhea virus and pseudorabies virus compared to MIRASOL while both technologies showed similar log reductions for hepatitis-A-virus and porcine parvovirus. However, due to their chemistry, PI systems are only able to target pathogens that contain nucleic acids and consequently they are ineffective against prions and transmission of variant Creutzfeldt–Jakob disease (52).

In order to demonstrate clinical efficacy, several large clinical trials using these PI systems have been conducted or are underway (22, 53) and extensive hemovigilance studies have also been undertaken. The main message is that PI treatment damages the platelets in many ways including alterations in membrane integrity, signaling pathways and in some capacity functionality of miRNAs, which results in reduced recovery and survival in healthy volunteers (54, 55). Similarly, shorter transfusion intervals have been observed in patients receiving PI-treated platelets, but these observations for the most part have not been associated with increased World Health Organization grade 2 or greater bleeding in patients receiving pathogen-reduced platelets, as hemostatic efficacy seems to be maintained (22, 26). Furthermore, some evidence points toward the fact that transfusion of PI-treated platelets does not affect mortality, the risk of clinically significant or severe bleeding, or the risk of a serious adverse event (AE) (56). However, as pointed out by Kaiser-Guignard and colleagues, the results of the published clinical studies should be interpreted with caution, and their characteristics and possible biases should be taken into account (22), such that interpretation of clinical outcome data cannot be generalized across different PI systems (22). A recent systematic review presented strong evidence that transfusion of PI-treated platelets appears to increase the risk of platelet refractoriness and the frequency of platelet transfusions (56).

The majority of contributions to investigations of PIs are *in vitro* quality studies. Multiple analyses have been conducted to monitor potential changes in the platelet quality following illumination with the three different PI systems in combination with products of different characteristics (see **Table 1**). These studies have typically measured common blood banking parameters, including metabolic activities, platelet activation, and platelet function to evaluate product quality, and to determine whether quality control requirements of the individual jurisdictions were met. Comparisons of different studies; however, are hampered by the fact that these measures are influenced by the type and proportion of the platelet storage medium. PI treatment of platelets in different PAS differentially alters platelet quality features (57). Recent studies with the riboflavin/UV system (MIRASOL) revealed that the quality of platelets is similar whether stored in plasma or PAS; however, transfusion of treated PCs in PAS led to fewer transfusion reactions (58). This observation is corroborated by the finding that PAS seems to have a protective effect on platelets upon illumination (59).

Based on these diverse studies, in recent years, many (individual) opinions have been published outlining the pros and cons of PI in light of safety and efficacy (20, 60–64). Ongoing discussions are guided by experiences from blood centers that have implemented PI (65–67).

PLATELET STORAGE LESION (PSL): A GENERAL OVERVIEW

Many studies measuring changes to platelet *in vitro* quality indicate that PI treatment accelerates the progression of the PSL. This term describes the sum of all the deleterious changes in platelet structure and function that arise from the time the blood is withdrawn from the donor to the time the platelets are transfused to the recipient (68–73). It is mainly explained by triggering platelet activation during preparation and handling of PCs, especially the heightened metabolic activity and activation-specific changes to surface glycoproteins observed in stored platelets (74). Transient derangement of platelet metabolism can be rescued by plasma replacement, resulting in improved morphology scores, stabilized osmotic recovery, and completely restored platelet secretory responses (75).

THE IMPACT OF PI ON PLATELET FUNCTIONS

PLT Activation, Degranulation, and Protein Release

As mentioned above, the main feature of PSL seems to be platelet activation, which is commonly determined by the expression of P-selectin (CD62P) on the platelet surface, as a consequence of the release of the alpha-granule content. Many studies have shown that PI increases the surface expression of CD62P (58, 76–78).

Additional features of storage-mediated platelet activation are the increased phosphatidylserine (PS) externalization (79) and changes in the protein profile of platelet surface receptors (80, 81) which are further altered upon PI treatment (82).

Among other changes, the level of cytokines and chemokines also increases in the supernatant of the storage solution during platelet storage (83–85). Although some controversy continues in the literature (86), PI treatment appears to induce platelet degranulation, hence further increasing the levels of immune factors under some treatment conditions (86–91). The altered releasate composition may affect the immunomodulatory capacity of platelets. As a consequence of this accumulation, supernatants of MIRASOL PI-treated platelets can suppress LPS (lipopolysaccharide)-induced monocyte IL-12 production (92), as well as increase LPS-induced mononuclear cell production of IL-8 (93). A recent study has demonstrated that increased supernatant levels of pro-inflammatory molecules resulting from platelet granule release are associated with reactive oxygen species generation during storage (94). This finding is corroborated by an observed increased ROS production in MIRASOL PI-treated PCs (77, 95).

A brief summary is provided in **Table 2** highlighting the changes of platelet storage features by the individual PI systems.

Development of Platelet Apoptosis

There is an ongoing debate regarding the extent to which platelet activation and programmed cell death (apoptosis) in platelets overlap at the molecular level (113). Platelets contain most of the apoptotic machinery, including pro- and anti-apoptotic Bcl-protein family members as well as caspases (114). Activation of these pathways leads to microvesiculation with expression of PS in the outer layer of the platelet membrane (115). As PS exposure is believed to contribute to the development of inflammatory or immunomodulatory processes and ultimately regulates clearance of platelet from circulation, PS exposure monitored by annexin-V binding is commonly used to measure the development of platelet apoptosis.

Pathogen inactivation treatment also results in the externalization of PS (59, 116, 117). MIRASOL PI-treated PLTs exhibit an increased expression of proapoptotic proteins Bak and Bax, but not anti-apoptotic proteins Bcl-XL (109, 116). Additionally, MIRASOL PI-triggered activation of caspase cleavage leads to proteolytic cleavage of their respective substrate proteins (116). Similar results have recently been shown in INTERCEPT PI-treated platelets (118). However, these features are not prominent until later in storage (typically 5–7 days) and may only need to be considered in the context of extended platelet storage.

TABLE 2 | Summary of impact of pathogen inactivation (PI) treatment on platelet features compared to untreated control.

Platelet storage feature	PI system		
	INTERCEPT	MIRASOL	THERAFLEX
Metabolic activity	± (96); ↑ (97)	↑ (98)	↑ (99)
Platelet activation (CD62P expression)	↑ (96, 100)	↑ (98)	↑ (99)
Platelet adhesion (under flow)	± (101); ↑ (102)[a]	↓ (102); ±(103)	n.d.
Clot formation (thrombo-elastography)	↓ (104)	↑[b], ↓[c] (105)	↓ (99)
Responsiveness (to agonists)	↓ (102); ±↓[d] (106)[c]	↓ (98)	± (99)
Platelet apoptosis (PS exposure)	± (107); ↑ (108)[a]	↑ (109)	↑ (99)
Platelet microparticle release	↑ (110)	↑ (111)	↑ (112)
Free mitochondria release	n.d.	↑ (95)	n.d.

↓ = decrease; ± = similar; ↑ = increase; n.d. = not determined. The references are only examples of published studies, but are not comprehensive. Differences in some study outcomes could be due to variations in production methods used (platelet-rich plasma vs BC/PCs or apheresis PCs), composition in storage solution—plasma vs platelet additive solution (in different concentration)—and assay procedures.

[a]*At end of storage.*

[b]*Thrombus stability.*

[c]*Aggregation.*

[d]*Agonist-dependent.*

Microvesicle (MR) Release

Platelets are known to generate heterogeneous populations of cell-derived MVs (119). Platelet MVs have a bilayered phospholipid structure exposing procoagulant PS and expressing various membrane receptors, and they serve as cell-to-cell shuttles for bioactive molecules such as lipids, growth factors, microRNAs (miRNAs), and mitochondria (120). Further, the presence and quantity of MVs has been associated with the clinical severity of the atherosclerotic disease, diabetes, and cancer (6, 121). These features along with the observation that the number, function, and content of MVs in the components varies with age, gender, lipid, and hormone profiles of the blood donor (122) makes them one of the most discussed, controversial, and interesting topics in current blood banking and transfusion medicine (123). Different studies have demonstrated that all UV-based PI treatments increase the release of MVs from platelets compared to untreated controls (36, 95, 112, 124). To our knowledge, no study has directly addressed the impact of INTERCEPT on the release of MVs during PC storage; however, Kanzler et al. found a reduction of MVs in the platelet product immediate after INTERCEPT treatment (125).

Role of Platelets in Inflammation

Although once primarily recognized for their role in hemostasis and thrombosis, platelets have been increasingly recognized as a multipurpose cell. There is growing recognition of the critical role of platelets in inflammation and immune responses. Platelets release numerous inflammatory mediators such as RANTES or CD40L, modifying leukocyte and endothelial responses to a range of different inflammatory stimuli (88). Additionally, platelets form aggregates with leukocytes and form bridges between leukocytes and endothelium, largely mediated by platelet P-selectin. Through their interactions with monocytes, neutrophils, lymphocytes, and the endothelium, platelets are, therefore, important coordinators of inflammation and both innate and adaptive immune responses. As mentioned above, studies have shown that MIRASOL-treated platelets release such mediators (92, 93) and, therefore, might modulate inflammatory responses.

Mitochondria and Mitochondrial DNA (mtDNA) Release

Mitochondria are known as the powerhouse of cells and play a crucial role in maintaining platelet function throughout platelet storage (126). Mitochondria are released from activated platelets and upon hydrolysis of the mitochondrial membrane release mtDNA (127). MIRASOL-PI treatment also causes release of free mitochondria, mainly at the later stages of storage (95). Potentially associated with the mitochondria release, free mtDNA has been associated with AEs following platelet transfusion, and may be predictive of some types of AEs (128). mtDNA is a highly potent inflammatory trigger (128) that can be released from platelets during storage (129). Illumination of platelets with PI systems modifies mtDNA (129–131). Detection of PI-modified mtDNA using PCR assays can be used to monitor and confirm PI treatment (131). Furthermore, the relationship of mtDNA levels and AEs related to immunomodulation should also be considered; with a recent study showing an association between mtDNA and the incidence of respiratory distress posttransfusion (132).

MicroRNA

MicroRNAs are small (~20–24 nucleotides) RNA sequences generated by ribonucleases in the nucleus (by Drosha) and cytosol (by Dicer 1) through sequential enzymatic trimming of double stranded miRNA precursors. miRNAs are thought to fine tune gene expression through degradation of their mRNA targets (133). Although platelets are anucleate, high-throughput sequencing has revealed that human platelets harbor a complex array of miRNAs, which are key regulators of mRNA translation in different cell types (134). Activated platelets can deliver mRNA regulatory Argonaute-2 miRNA complexes to endothelial cells *via* MVs leading to modulation of cell function (135).

INTERCEPT, but not MIRASOL PI treatment has been shown to affect the platelet mRNA transcriptome (27, 136). However, miRNA synthesis and function were not affected and no cross-linking of miRNA-sized endogenous platelet RNA species was observed; rather miRNA levels were reduced (136, 137). Further, the reduction in the platelet miRNA levels induced by INTERCEPT correlated with platelet activation and an impaired platelet aggregation response to ADP (136). In contrast, a recent study presented by Arnason et al. (138) demonstrated that INTERCEPT treatment did not change the quality or significantly altered the miRNA profile of PCs. These controversial results prompted further investigations and as the clinical significance of MV-associated miRNAs is unknown, and speculation of a negative effect of PI-treated platelets including long-term consequences for recipients is as yet unwarranted. This is a relatively new area of research, and additional studies are required to fully understand the impact of PI treatment on miRNA synthesis and the resulting impact on platelet quality.

mRNA Levels and Protein Synthesis

Although anucleate, platelets have the capacity to synthesize biologically relevant proteins that are regulated *via* gene expression programs at the translational level in response to physiological stimuli (139–141). Recent studies have demonstrated that levels of specific mRNA species are reduced following MIRASOL PI treatment while others are less affected (142). Subsequent studies have revealed that this observation is mirrored in the platelet translatome, demonstrating that platelets are still capable of synthesizing proteins following PI treatment, suggesting that they may possess mechanism(s) to protect their mRNA from damage by the PI treatment (143). The clinical relevance of this finding, however, is still unknown.

Impact of PI Treatment on Platelet Lipidomics

Although the application of lipidomics to platelet biology is still in its infancy, seminal studies have shaped our knowledge of how lipids regulate key aspects of platelet biology, including aggregation, shape change, coagulation, and degranulation, as well as how lipids generated by platelets influence other cells, such as leukocytes and the vascular wall, and thus how they regulate hemostasis, vascular integrity, and inflammation, as well as contribute to pathologies, including arterial/deep vein thrombosis, and atherosclerosis (144). Mapping the human platelet lipidome revealed cytosolic phospholipase A2 as a regulator of mitochondrial bioenergetics during activation (145). A recent study has demonstrated that psoralen and UV light increased the order of lipid phases by covalent modification of phospholipids, thereby inhibiting membrane recruitment of effector kinases such as BTK and Akt and consequently affecting GPVI- and PAR1-mediated signal transduction (99).

FURTHER INVESTIGATIONS TOWARD UNDERSTANDING THE MOLECULAR MECHANISMS OF PI-INDUCED PLATELET ALTERATION: FROM PROTEOMICS TO SIGNALING

A variety of untargeted proteomic approaches have been used to assess the impact of PI systems on platelets (146–148). The effect of the PI treatment on the proteome appears to be different according to the particular technology. A comparative analysis of proteomic data revealed that MIRASOL seems to impact proteins involved mainly in platelet adhesion and shape change while INTERCEPT affects proteins of intracellular platelet activation pathways and THERAFLEX influences proteins linked to platelet shape change and aggregation (149). These conclusions are based on a relatively small number of studies and further analyses are required for verification.

A more targeted approach using a phospho-kinase antibody-based array demonstrated that a variety of kinases were activated by MIRASOL PI treatment (150). p38MAPK plays a central role in MIRASOL PI-mediated signaling by regulating a variety of platelet features, such as apoptosis (109), mitochondrial function, and release of free and MV-encapsulated mitochondria (95). The INTERCEPT system also triggers p38MAPK activation in platelets, and the phosphorylation of the p38MAPK substrate Tace is directly linked to GPIb cleavage possibly explaining the reduced adhesion of those platelets under flow conditions (118). The role of p38MAPK in mediating PI-triggered signaling linked to features

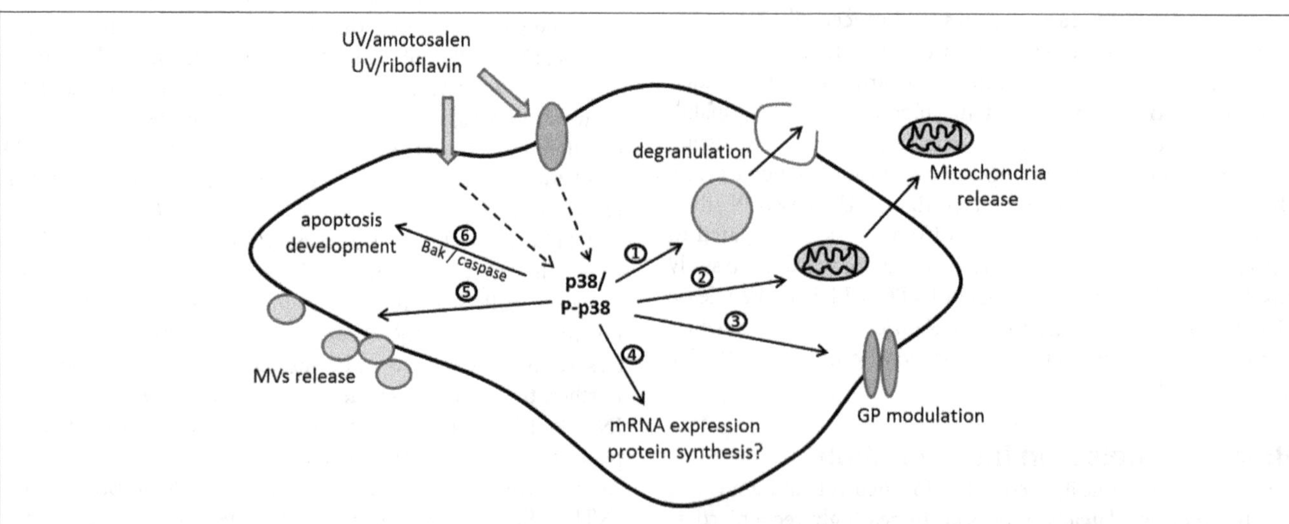

FIGURE 1 | Current molecular model of signaling triggered by ultraviolet (UV)/riboflavin (MIRASOL) and UV/amotosalen (INTERCEPT) in platelets: UV can penetrate either directly or *via* surface/receptor proteins to activate p38MAPK kinase as one of the central players in the signaling cascade. Thus far it has been shown that p38 activation/phosphorylation (P-p38) is involved in regulating (1) degranulation, (2) release of free mitochondria, (3) the modulation of glycoproteins (GPs), (4) the expression levels of mRNAs and potentially protein synthesis, (5) microvesicle (MVs) release, and (6) the development of apoptosis *via* proapoptotic protein expression and caspase activation. This figure was modified from Ref. (150).

of PSL is supported by studies demonstrating a regulatory role of p38MAPK in regulating PSL development (151) and platelet *in vivo* recovery and survival in mouse models (152). This body of work suggests that similar signaling pathways are activated by both of these PI systems as modeled in **Figure 1**. Although only a few studies to date have investigated the signaling aspect in platelets, it could be hypothesized that p38MAPK activation in response to the stress associated with the PI treatment may have a regulatory role in platelet life span (153) as inhibition of this protein leads to decreased apoptosis (109, 118).

CONCLUSION AND FUTURE DIRECTIONS

Although there are numerous studies in the literature assessing the impact of UV-based PI systems on platelet *in vitro* and *in vivo* function, only a few conclusions can be drawn. All technologies seem to accelerate the development of some form of the PSL but this likely results through different modes of action; therefore, it is likely that many divergent, as well as overlapping molecular mechanisms are triggered. Most of the functional studies conducted to decipher the role of signaling pathways in PI-treated platelets have been carried out using the INTERCEPT and MIRASOL system and thus the effects of the THERAFLEX system remain relatively unknown. However, it is clear that PI-treated platelets are different to untreated platelets, and the differences may go some way toward explaining some of the clinical observations following transfusion of PI-treated platelets. Proteomic analyses and in future other -omics approaches such as metabolomics (154) will likely shed more light into the specific effects of PI treatment. Additional targeted approaches will guide the formulation of signaling models, which may ultimately identify pathways known to impact platelet function upon illumination, and provide potential (protein) markers to assist with the fine-tuning of these technologies. We need to keep in mind, however, that the PI treatment does not only affect platelets *per se*, these procedures trigger the release of MVs, proteins, and nucleic acids in to the storage medium which also gets transfused. Whether any of these components will have deleterious effects on the recipients remains to be determined even though the initial clinical studies do not show significant clinical effects from PI treatment of PCs.

AUTHOR CONTRIBUTIONS

All authors contributed to this manuscript and approved the final version for submission.

ACKNOWLEDGMENTS

The authors received research funding from Cerus, Terumo, and MacoPharma. This study was supported in part by a grant from Health Canada and Canadian Blood Services. The views expressed herein do not necessarily represent the view of the federal government. The Australian governments fund the Australian Red Cross Blood Service to provide blood, blood products, and services to the Australian community.

REFERENCES

1. Packham MA. Role of platelets in thrombosis and hemostasis. *Can J Physiol Pharmacol* (1994) 72:278–84. doi:10.1139/y94-043
2. Ni H, Freedman J. Platelets in hemostasis and thrombosis: role of integrins and their ligands. *Transfus Apher Sci* (2003) 28:257–64. doi:10.1016/S1473-0502(03)00044-2
3. Wang Y, Andrews M, Yang Y, Lang S, Jin JW, Cameron-Vendrig A, et al. Platelets in thrombosis and hemostasis: old topic with new mechanisms. *Cardiovasc Hematol Disord Drug Targets* (2012) 12:126–32. doi:10.2174/1871529X11202020126
4. McCullough J. Overview of platelet transfusion. *Semin Hematol* (2010) 47:235–42. doi:10.1053/j.seminhematol.2010.04.001
5. McQuilten ZK, Crighton G, Engelbrecht S, Gotmaker R, Brunskill SJ, Murphy MF, et al. Transfusion interventions in critical bleeding requiring massive transfusion: a systematic review. *Transfus Med Rev* (2015) 29:127–37. doi:10.1016/j.tmrv.2015.01.001
6. Burnouf T, Elemary M, Radosevic J, Seghatchian J, Goubran H. Platelet transfusion in thrombocytopenic cancer patients: sometimes justified but likely insidious. *Transfus Apher Sci* (2017) 56:305–9. doi:10.1016/j.transci.2017.05.016
7. Slichter SJ. New thoughts on the correct dosing of prophylactic platelet transfusions to prevent bleeding. *Curr Opin Hematol* (2011) 18:427–35. doi:10.1097/MOH.0b013e32834babf4
8. Estcourt L, Stanworth S, Doree C, Hopewell S, Murphy MF, Tinmouth A, et al. Prophylactic platelet transfusion for prevention of bleeding in patients with haematological disorders after chemotherapy and stem cell transplantation. *Cochrane Database Syst Rev* (2012) 5:CD004269. doi:10.1002/14651858.CD004269.pub3
9. Annen K, Olson JE. Optimizing platelet transfusions. *Curr Opin Hematol* (2015) 22:559–64. doi:10.1097/MOH.0000000000000188
10. Kumar A, Mhaskar R, Grossman BJ, Kaufman RM, Tobian AA, Kleinman S, et al. Platelet transfusion: a systematic review of the clinical evidence. *Transfusion* (2015) 55:1116–27; quiz 1115. doi:10.1111/trf.12943
11. Morel P, Deschaseaux M, Bertrand X, Naegelen C, Thouverez M, Talon D. [Detection of bacterial contamination in platelet concentrates: perspectives]. *Transfus Clin Biol* (2002) 9:250–7. doi:10.1016/S1246-7820(02)00252-5
12. Dodd RY. Bacterial contamination and transfusion safety: experience in the United States. *Transfus Clin Biol* (2003) 10:6–9. doi:10.1016/S1246-7820(02)00277-X
13. Hillyer CD, Josephson CD, Blajchman MA, Vostal JG, Epstein JS, Goodman JL. Bacterial contamination of blood components: risks, strategies, and regulation: joint ASH and AABB educational session in transfusion medicine. *Hematology Am Soc Hematol Educ Program* (2003):575–89. doi:10.1182/asheducation-2003.1.575
14. Blajchman MA, Beckers EA, Dickmeiss E, Lin L, Moore G, Muylle L. Bacterial detection of platelets: current problems and possible resolutions. *Transfus Med Rev* (2005) 19:259–72. doi:10.1016/j.tmrv.2005.05.002
15. Alter HJ, Klein HG. The hazards of blood transfusion in historical perspective. *Blood* (2008) 112:2617–26. doi:10.1182/blood-2008-07-077370
16. Mathai J. Problem of bacterial contamination in platelet concentrates. *Transfus Apher Sci* (2009) 41:139–44. doi:10.1016/j.transci.2009.07.012
17. Garraud O, Tariket S, Sut C, Haddad A, Aloui C, Chakroun T, et al. Transfusion as an inflammation hit: knowns and unknowns. *Front Immunol* (2016) 7:534. doi:10.3389/fimmu.2016.00534
18. Fast LD, DiLeone G, Marschner S. Inactivation of human white blood cells in platelet products after pathogen reduction technology treatment in comparison to gamma irradiation. *Transfusion* (2011) 51:1397–404. doi:10.1111/j.1537-2995.2010.02984.x
19. Pohler P, Muller M, Winkler C, Schaudien D, Sewald K, Müller TH, et al. Pathogen reduction by ultraviolet C light effectively inactivates human white blood cells in platelet products. *Transfusion* (2015) 55:337–47. doi:10.1111/trf.12836
20. Lozano M, Cid J. Pathogen inactivation: coming of age. *Curr Opin Hematol* (2013) 20:540–5. doi:10.1097/MOH.0b013e328365a18f
21. Prowse CV. Component pathogen inactivation: a critical review. *Vox Sang* (2013) 104:183–99. doi:10.1111/j.1423-0410.2012.01662.x

22. Kaiser-Guignard J, Canellini G, Lion N, Abonnenc M, Osselaer JC, Tissot JD. The clinical and biological impact of new pathogen inactivation technologies on platelet concentrates. *Blood Rev* (2014) 28:235–41. doi:10.1016/j.blre.2014.07.005
23. Schlenke P. Pathogen inactivation technologies for cellular blood components: an update. *Transfus Med Hemother* (2014) 41:309–25. doi:10.1159/000365646
24. Kleinman S. Pathogen inactivation: emerging indications. *Curr Opin Hematol* (2015) 22:547–53. doi:10.1097/MOH.0000000000000186
25. Salunkhe V, van der Meer PF, de Korte D, Seghatchian J, Gutiérrez L. Development of blood transfusion product pathogen reduction treatments: a review of methods, current applications and demands. *Transfus Apher Sci* (2015) 52:19–34. doi:10.1016/j.transci.2014.12.016
26. Devine DV, Schubert P. Pathogen inactivation technologies: the advent of pathogen-reduced blood components to reduce blood safety risk. *Hematol Oncol Clin North Am* (2016) 30:609–17. doi:10.1016/j.hoc.2016.01.005
27. Osman A, Hitzler WE, Provost P. Peculiarities of studying the effects of pathogen reduction technologies on platelets. *Proteomics Clin Appl* (2016) 10:805–15. doi:10.1002/prca.201500124
28. Ramsey G. Hemostatic efficacy of pathogen-inactivated blood components. *Semin Thromb Hemost* (2016) 42:172–82. doi:10.1055/s-0035-1564845
29. Osman A, Hitzler WE, Provost P. The platelets' perspective to pathogen reduction technologies. *Platelets* (2017) 29(2):140–7. doi:10.1080/09537104.2017.1293806
30. Irsch J, Lin L. Pathogen inactivation of platelet and plasma blood components for transfusion using the INTERCEPT blood system. *Transfus Med Hemother* (2011) 38:19–31. doi:10.1159/000323937
31. Irsch J, Seghatchian J. Update on pathogen inactivation treatment of plasma, with the INTERCEPT blood system: current position on methodological, clinical and regulatory aspects. *Transfus Apher Sci* (2015) 52:240–4. doi:10.1016/j.transci.2015.02.013
32. Goodrich RP, Doane S, Reddy HL. Design and development of a method for the reduction of infectious pathogen load and inactivation of white blood cells in whole blood products. *Biologicals* (2010) 38:20–30. doi:10.1016/j.biologicals.2009.10.016
33. Marschner S, Goodrich R. Pathogen reduction technology treatment of platelets, plasma and whole blood using riboflavin and UV light. *Transfus Med Hemother* (2011) 38:8–18. doi:10.1159/000324160
34. Mohr H, Steil L, Gravemann U, Thiele T, Hammer E, Greinacher A, et al. A novel approach to pathogen reduction in platelet concentrates using short-wave ultraviolet light. *Transfusion* (2009) 49:2612–24. doi:10.1111/j.1537-2995.2009.02334.x
35. Seghatchian J, Tolksdorf F. Characteristics of the THERAFLEX UV-platelets pathogen inactivation system – an update. *Transfus Apher Sci* (2012) 46:221–9. doi:10.1016/j.transci.2012.01.008
36. Solheim BG. Pathogen reduction of blood components. *Transfus Apher Sci* (2008) 39:75–82. doi:10.1016/j.transci.2008.05.003
37. Allain JP, Goodrich R. Pathogen reduction of whole blood: utility and feasibility. *Transfus Med* (2017) 27(Suppl 5):320–6. doi:10.1111/tme.12456
38. Klein HG, Anderson D, Bernardi MJ, Cable R, Carey W, Hoch JS. Pathogen inactivation: making decisions about new technologies. Report of a consensus conference. *Transfusion* (2007) 47:2338–47. doi:10.1111/j.1537-2995.2007.01512.x
39. Webert KE, Cserti CM, Hannon J, Lin Y, Pavenski K, Pendergrast JM, et al. Proceedings of a consensus conference: pathogen inactivation-making decisions about new technologies. *Transfus Med Rev* (2008) 22:1–34. doi:10.1016/j.tmrv.2007.09.001
40. Klein HG, Glynn SA, Ness PM, Blajchman MA; NHLBI Working Group on Research Opportunities for the Pathogen Reduction/Inactivation of Blood Components. Research opportunities for pathogen reduction/inactivation of blood components: summary of an NHLBI workshop. *Transfusion* (2009) 49:1262–8. doi:10.1111/j.1537-2995.2009.02210.x
41. Keil SD, Bengrine A, Bowen R, Marschner S, Hovenga N, Rouse L, et al. Inactivation of viruses in platelet and plasma products using a riboflavin-and-UV-based photochemical treatment. *Transfusion* (2015) 55:1736–44. doi:10.1111/trf.13030
42. Keil SD, Hovenga N, Gilmour D, Marschner S, Goodrich R. Treatment of platelet products with riboflavin and UV light: effectiveness against high titer bacterial contamination. *J Vis Exp* (2015) 102:e52820. doi:10.3791/52820
43. Gowland P, Fontana S, Stolz M, Andina N, Niederhauser C. Parvovirus B19 passive transmission by transfusion of intercept(R) blood system-treated platelet concentrate. *Transfus Med Hemother* (2016) 43:198–202. doi:10.1159/000445195
44. Taha M, Culibrk B, Kalab M, Schubert P, Yi QL, Goodrich R, et al. Efficiency of riboflavin and ultraviolet light treatment against high levels of biofilm-derived *Staphylococcus epidermidis* in buffy coat platelet concentrates. *Vox Sang* (2017) 112:408–16. doi:10.1111/vox.12519
45. Ruane PH, Edrich R, Gampp D, Keil SD, Leonard RL, Goodrich RP. Photochemical inactivation of selected viruses and bacteria in platelet concentrates using riboflavin and light. *Transfusion* (2004) 44:877–85. doi:10.1111/j.1537-2995.2004.03355.x
46. Vanlandingham DL, Keil SD, Horne KM, Pyles R, Goodrich RP, Higgs S. Photochemical inactivation of chikungunya virus in plasma and platelets using the Mirasol pathogen reduction technology system. *Transfusion* (2013) 53:284–90. doi:10.1111/j.1537-2995.2012.03717.x
47. Fryk JJ, Marks DC, Hobson-Peters J, Watterson D, Hall RA, Young PR, et al. Reduction of Zika virus infectivity in platelet concentrates after treatment with ultraviolet C light and in plasma after treatment with methylene blue and visible light. *Transfusion* (2017) 57:2677–82. doi:10.1111/trf.14256
48. Santa Maria F, Laughhunn A, Lanteri MC, Aubry M, Musso D, Stassinopoulos A. Inactivation of zika virus in platelet components using amotosalen and ultraviolet A illumination. *Transfusion* (2017) 57:2016–25. doi:10.1111/trf.14161
49. Faddy HM, Fryk JJ, Watterson D, Young PR, Modhiran N, Muller DA, et al. Riboflavin and ultraviolet light: impact on dengue virus infectivity. *Vox Sang* (2016) 111:235–41. doi:10.1111/vox.12414
50. Owada T, Kaneko M, Matsumoto C, Sobata R, Igarashi M, Suzuki K, et al. Establishment of culture systems for genotypes 3 and 4 hepatitis E virus (HEV) obtained from human blood and application of HEV inactivation using a pathogen reduction technology system. *Transfusion* (2014) 54:2820–7. doi:10.1111/trf.12686
51. Kwon SY, Kim IS, Bae JE, Kang JW, Cho YJ, Cho NS, et al. Pathogen inactivation efficacy of Mirasol PRT system and intercept blood system for non-leucoreduced platelet-rich plasma-derived platelets suspended in plasma. *Vox Sang* (2014) 107:254–60. doi:10.1111/vox.12158
52. Lescoutra-Etchegaray N, Sumian C, Culeux A, Durand V, Gurgel PV, Deslys JP, et al. Removal of exogenous prion infectivity in leukoreduced red blood cells unit by a specific filter designed for human transfusion. *Transfusion* (2014) 54:1037–45. doi:10.1111/trf.12420
53. McClaskey J, Xu M, Snyder EL, Tormey CA. Clinical trials for pathogen reduction in transfusion medicine: a review. *Transfus Apher Sci* (2009) 41:217–25. doi:10.1016/j.transci.2009.09.008
54. Snyder E, Raife T, Lin L, Cimino G, Metzel P, Rheinschmidt M, et al. Recovery and life span of 111indium-radiolabeled platelets treated with pathogen inactivation with amotosalen HCl (S-59) and ultraviolet A light. *Transfusion* (2004) 44:1732–40. doi:10.1111/j.0041-1132.2004.04145.x
55. AuBuchon JP, Herschel L, Roger J, Taylor H, Whitley P, Li J, et al. Efficacy of apheresis platelets treated with riboflavin and ultraviolet light for pathogen reduction. *Transfusion* (2005) 45:1335–41. doi:10.1111/j.1537-2995.2005.00202.x
56. Estcourt LJ, Malouf R, Hopewell S, Trivella M, Doree C, Stanworth SJ, et al. Pathogen-reduced platelets for the prevention of bleeding. *Cochrane Database Syst Rev* (2017) 7:CD009072. doi:10.1002/14651858.CD009072.pub3
57. Leitner GC, List J, Horvath M, Eichelberger B, Panzer S, Jilma-Stohlawetz P. Additive solutions differentially affect metabolic and functional parameters of platelet concentrates. *Vox Sang* (2016) 110:20–6. doi:10.1111/vox.12317
58. Ignatova AA, Karpova OV, Trakhtman PE, Rumiantsev SA, Panteleev MA. Functional characteristics and clinical effectiveness of platelet concentrates treated with riboflavin and ultraviolet light in plasma and in platelet additive solution. *Vox Sang* (2016) 110:244–52. doi:10.1111/vox.12364
59. van der Meer PF, Bontekoe IJ, Daal BB, de Korte D. Riboflavin and UV light treatment of platelets: a protective effect of platelet additive solution? *Transfusion* (2015) 55:1900–8. doi:10.1111/trf.13033
60. Hervig T, Seghatchian J, Apelseth TO. Current debate on pathogen inactivation of platelet concentrates – to use or not to use? *Transfus Apher Sci* (2010) 43:411–4. doi:10.1016/j.transci.2010.10.012
61. Lozano M, Cid J. Analysis of reasons for not implementing pathogen inactivation for platelet concentrates. *Transfus Clin Biol* (2013) 20:158–64. doi:10.1016/j.tracli.2013.02.017

62. Hess JR, Pagano MB, Barbeau JD, Johannsson PI. Will pathogen reduction of blood components harm more people than it helps in developed countries? *Transfusion* (2016) 56:1236–41. doi:10.1111/trf.13512
63. Lozano M, Cid J. Platelet concentrates: balancing between efficacy and safety? *Presse Med* (2016) 45:e289–98. doi:10.1016/j.lpm.2016.06.020
64. Magron A, Laugier J, Provost P, Boilard E. Pathogen reduction technologies: the pros and cons for platelet transfusion. *Platelets* (2017) 29(1):2–8. doi:10.1080/09537104.2017.1306046
65. Murphy WG. Pathogen reduction: state of reflection in Ireland. *Transfus Clin Biol* (2011) 18:488–90. doi:10.1016/j.tracli.2011.05.004
66. Jimenez-Marco T, Mercant C, Lliteras E, Cózar M, Girona-Llobera E. Practical issues that should be considered when planning the implementation of pathogen reduction technology for plateletpheresis. *Transfus Apher Sci* (2015) 52:84–93. doi:10.1016/j.transci.2014.12.004
67. Devine DV. Implementation of pathogen inactivation technology: how to make the best decisions? *Transfusion* (2017) 57:1109–11. doi:10.1111/trf.14117
68. Seghatchian J, Krailadsiri P. The platelet storage lesion. *Transfus Med Rev* (1997) 11:130–44. doi:10.1053/tm.1997.0110130
69. Thon JN, Schubert P, Devine DV. Platelet storage lesion: a new understanding from a proteomic perspective. *Transfus Med Rev* (2008) 22:268–79. doi:10.1016/j.tmrv.2008.05.004
70. Shrivastava M. The platelet storage lesion. *Transfus Apher Sci* (2009) 41:105–13. doi:10.1016/j.transci.2009.07.002
71. Devine DV, Serrano K. The platelet storage lesion. *Clin Lab Med* (2010) 30:475–87. doi:10.1016/j.cll.2010.02.002
72. Bennett JS. Shedding new light on the platelet storage lesion. *Arterioscler Thromb Vasc Biol* (2016) 36:1715–6. doi:10.1161/ATVBAHA.116.308095
73. Tissot JD, Bardyn M, Sonego G, Abonnenc M, Prudent M. The storage lesions: from past to future. *Transfus Clin Biol* (2017) 24:277–84. doi:10.1016/j.tracli.2017.05.012
74. Bode AP. Platelet activation may explain the storage lesion in platelet concentrates. *Blood Cells* (1990) 16:109–25; discussion 125–6.
75. Rinder HM, Snyder EL, Tracey JB, Dincecco D, Wang C, Baril L, et al. Reversibility of severe metabolic stress in stored platelets after in vitro plasma rescue or in vivo transfusion: restoration of secretory function and maintenance of platelet survival. *Transfusion* (2003) 43:1230–7. doi:10.1046/j.1537-2995.2003.00484.x
76. Johnson L, Winter KM, Reid S, Hartkopf-Theis T, Marschner S, Goodrich RP, et al. The effect of pathogen reduction technology (Mirasol) on platelet quality when treated in additive solution with low plasma carryover. *Vox Sang* (2011) 101:208–14. doi:10.1111/j.1423-0410.2011.01477.x
77. Johnson L, Marks D. Treatment of platelet concentrates with the Mirasol pathogen inactivation system modulates platelet oxidative stress and NF-kappaB activation. *Transfus Med Hemother* (2015) 42:167–73. doi:10.1159/000403245
78. Tynngård N, Trinks M, Berlin G. In vitro function of platelets treated with ultraviolet C light for pathogen inactivation: a comparative study with non-irradiated and gamma-irradiated platelets. *Transfusion* (2015) 55:1169–77. doi:10.1111/trf.12963
79. Shapira S, Friedman Z, Shapiro H, Presseizen K, Radnay J, Ellis MH. The effect of storage on the expression of platelet membrane phosphatidylserine and the subsequent impacton the coagulant function of stored platelets. *Transfusion* (2000) 40:1257–63. doi:10.1046/j.1537-2995.2000.40101257.x
80. Thon JN, Devine DV. Translation of glycoprotein IIIa in stored blood platelets. *Transfusion* (2007) 47:2260–70. doi:10.1111/j.1537-2995.2007.01455.x
81. Rijkers M, van der Meer PF, Bontekoe IJ, Daal BB, de Korte D, Leebeek FW, et al. Evaluation of the role of the GPIb-IX-V receptor complex in development of the platelet storage lesion. *Vox Sang* (2016) 111:247–56. doi:10.1111/vox.12416
82. Terada C, Mori J, Okazaki H, Satake M, Tadokoro K. Effects of riboflavin and ultraviolet light treatment on platelet thrombus formation on collagen via integrin alphaIIbbeta3 activation. *Transfusion* (2014) 54:1808–16. doi:10.1111/trf.12566
83. Rinder HM, Snyder EL. Activation of platelet concentrate during preparation and storage. *Blood Cells* (1992) 18:445–56; discussion 457–60.
84. Rinder HM, Snyder EL, Bonan JL, Napychank PA, Malkus H, Smith BR. Activation in stored platelet concentrates: correlation between membrane expression of P-selectin, glycoprotein IIb/IIIa, and beta-thromboglobulin release. *Transfusion* (1993) 33:25–9. doi:10.1046/j.1537-2995.1993.33193142305.x
85. Aye MT, Palmer DS, Giulivi A, Hashemi S. Effect of filtration of platelet concentrates on the accumulation of cytokines and platelet release factors during storage. *Transfusion* (1995) 35:117–24. doi:10.1046/j.1537-2995.1995.35295125733.x
86. Apelseth T, Hervig T. Comments on "Release of immune modulation factors from platelet concentrates during storage after photochemical pathogen inactivation treatment". *Transfusion* (2009) 49:603–4; author reply 604–5. doi:10.1111/j.1537-2995.2008.02047.x
87. Apelseth TO, Hervig TA, Wentzel-Larsen T, Bruserud O. Cytokine accumulation in photochemically treated and gamma-irradiated platelet concentrates during storage. *Transfusion* (2006) 46:800–10. doi:10.1111/j.1537-2995.2006.00800.x
88. Cognasse F, Osselaer JC, Payrat JM, Chavarin P, Corash L, Garraud O. Release of immune modulation factors from platelet concentrates during storage after photochemical pathogen inactivation treatment. *Transfusion* (2008) 48:809–13. doi:10.1111/j.1537-2995.2008.01655.x
89. Picker SM, Steisel A, Gathof BS. Evaluation of white blood cell- and platelet-derived cytokine accumulation in MIRASOL-PRT-treated platelets. *Transfus Med Hemother* (2009) 36:114–20. doi:10.1159/000203359
90. Tauszig ME, Picker SM, Gathof BS. Platelet derived cytokine accumulation in platelet concentrates treated for pathogen reduction. *Transfus Apher Sci* (2012) 46:33–7. doi:10.1016/j.transci.2011.10.025
91. Sandgren P, Berlin G, Tynngård N. Treatment of platelet concentrates with ultraviolet C light for pathogen reduction increases cytokine accumulation. *Transfusion* (2016) 56:1377–83. doi:10.1111/trf.13601
92. Loh YS, Dean MM, Johnson L, Marks DC. Treatment of platelets with riboflavin and ultraviolet light mediates complement activation and suppresses monocyte interleukin-12 production in whole blood. *Vox Sang* (2015) 109:327–35. doi:10.1111/vox.12283
93. Loh YS, Johnson L, Kwok M, Marks DC. Pathogen reduction treatment alters the immunomodulatory capacity of buffy coat-derived platelet concentrates. *Transfusion* (2014) 54:577–84. doi:10.1111/trf.12320
94. Ghasemzadeh M, Hosseini E. Platelet granule release is associated with reactive oxygen species generation during platelet storage: a direct link between platelet pro-inflammatory and oxidation states. *Thromb Res* (2017) 156:101–4. doi:10.1016/j.thromres.2017.06.016
95. Chen Z, Schubert P, Bakkour S, Culibrk B, Busch MP, Devine DV. p38 mitogen-activated protein kinase regulates mitochondrial function and microvesicle release in riboflavin- and ultraviolet light-treated apheresis platelet concentrates. *Transfusion* (2017) 57:1199–207. doi:10.1111/trf.14035
96. van Rhenen DJ, Vermeij J, Mayaudon V, Hind C, Lin L, Corash L. Functional characteristics of S-59 photochemically treated platelet concentrates derived from buffy coats. *Vox Sang* (2000) 79:206–14. doi:10.1046/j.1423-0410.2000.7940206.x
97. Picker SM, Speer R, Gathof BS. Functional characteristics of buffy-coat PLTs photochemically treated with amotosalen-HCl for pathogen inactivation. *Transfusion* (2004) 44:320–9. doi:10.1111/j.1537-2995.2003.00590.x
98. Schubert P, Culibrk B, Coupland D, Scammell K, Gyongyossy-Issa M, Devine DV. Riboflavin and ultraviolet light treatment potentiates vasodilator-stimulated phosphoprotein Ser-239 phosphorylation in platelet concentrates during storage. *Transfusion* (2012) 52:397–408. doi:10.1111/j.1537-2995.2011.03287.x
99. Van Aelst B, Devloo R, Vandekerckhove P, Compernolle V, Feys HB. Ultraviolet C light pathogen inactivation treatment of platelet concentrates preserves integrin activation but affects thrombus formation kinetics on collagen in vitro. *Transfusion* (2015) 55:2404–14. doi:10.1111/trf.13137
100. Apelseth TØ, Bruserud Ø, Wentzel-Larsen T, Bakken AM, Bjørsvik S, Hervig T. In vitro evaluation of metabolic changes and residual platelet responsiveness in photochemical treated and gamma-irradiated single-donor platelet concentrates during long-term storage. *Transfusion* (2007) 47:653–65. doi:10.1111/j.1537-2995.2007.01167.x
101. Lozano M, Galan A, Mazzara R, Corash L, Escolar G. Leukoreduced buffy coat-derived platelet concentrates photochemically treated with amotosalen HCl and ultraviolet A light stored up to 7 days: assessment of hemostatic function under flow conditions. *Transfusion* (2007) 47:666–71. doi:10.1111/j.1537-2995.2007.01169.x

102. Picker SM, Schneider V, Gathof BS. Platelet function assessed by shear-induced deposition of split triple-dose apheresis concentrates treated with pathogen reduction technologies. *Transfusion* (2009) 49:1224–32. doi:10.1111/j.1537-2995.2009.02092.x
103. Li J, Lockerbie O, de Korte D, Rice J, McLean R, Goodrich RP. Evaluation of platelet mitochondria integrity after treatment with Mirasol pathogen reduction technology. *Transfusion* (2005) 45:920–6. doi:10.1111/j.1537-2995.2005.04381.x
104. Tynngård N, Johansson BM, Lindahl TL, Berlin G, Hansson M. Effects of intercept pathogen inactivation on platelet function as analysed by free oscillation rheometry. *Transfus Apher Sci* (2008) 38:85–8. doi:10.1016/j.transci.2007.12.012
105. Terada C, Shiba M, Nagai T, Satake M. Effects of riboflavin and ultraviolet light treatment on platelet thrombus formation and thrombus stability on collagen. *Transfusion* (2017) 57:1772–80. doi:10.1111/trf.14114
106. Abonnenc M, Sonego G, Kaiser-Guignard J, Crettaz D, Prudent M, Tissot JD, et al. In vitro evaluation of pathogen-inactivated buffy coat-derived platelet concentrates during storage: psoralen-based photochemical treatment step-by-step. *Blood Transfus* (2015) 13:255–64. doi:10.2450/2014.0082-14
107. Jansen GA, van Vliet HH, Vermeij H, Beckers EA, Leebeek FW, Sonneveld P, et al. Functional characteristics of photochemically treated platelets. *Transfusion* (2004) 44:313–9. doi:10.1111/j.1537-2995.2003.00588.x
108. Picker SM, Oustianskaia L, Schneider V, Gathof BS. Functional characteristics of apheresis-derived platelets treated with ultraviolet light combined with either amotosalen-HCl (S-59) or riboflavin (vitamin B2) for pathogen-reduction. *Vox Sang* (2009) 97:26–33. doi:10.1111/j.1423-0410.2009.01176.x
109. Chen Z, Schubert P, Culibrk B, Devine DV. p38MAPK is involved in apoptosis development in apheresis platelet concentrates after riboflavin and ultraviolet light treatment. *Transfusion* (2015) 55:848–57. doi:10.1111/trf.12905
110. Diquattro M, De Francisci G, Bonaccorso R, Tagliavia AM, Marcatti M, Palma B, et al. Evaluation of amotosalem treated platelets over 7 days of storage with an automated cytometry assay panel. *Int J Lab Hematol* (2013) 35:637–43. doi:10.1111/ijlh.12102
111. Ostrowski SR, Bochsen L, Salado-Jimena JA, Ullum H, Reynaerts I, Goodrich RP, et al. In vitro cell quality of buffy coat platelets in additive solution treated with pathogen reduction technology. *Transfusion* (2010) 50:2210–9. doi:10.1111/j.1537-2995.2010.02681.x
112. Johnson L, Hyland R, Tan S, Tolksdorf F, Sumian C, Seltsam A, et al. In vitro quality of platelets with low plasma carryover treated with ultraviolet C light for pathogen inactivation. *Transfus Med Hemother* (2016) 43:190–7. doi:10.1159/000441830
113. Seghatchian J, Krailadsiri P. Platelet storage lesion and apoptosis: are they related? *Transfus Apher Sci* (2001) 24:103–5. doi:10.1016/S0955-3886(00)00134-X
114. Lebois M, Josefsson EC. Regulation of platelet lifespan by apoptosis. *Platelets* (2016) 27:497–504. doi:10.3109/09537104.2016.1161739
115. Leytin V. Apoptosis in the anucleate platelet. *Blood Rev* (2012) 26:51–63. doi:10.1016/j.blre.2011.10.002
116. Reid S, Johnson L, Woodland N, Marks DC. Pathogen reduction treatment of buffy coat platelet concentrates in additive solution induces proapoptotic signaling. *Transfusion* (2012) 52:2094–103. doi:10.1111/j.1537-2995.2011.03558.x
117. Bashir S, Cookson P, Wiltshire M, Hawkins L, Sonoda L, Thomas S, et al. Pathogen inactivation of platelets using ultraviolet C light: effect on in vitro function and recovery and survival of platelets. *Transfusion* (2015) 53:990–1000. doi:10.1111/j.1537-2995.2012.03854.x
118. Stivala S, Gobbato S, Infanti L, Reiner MF, Bonetti N, Meyer SC, et al. Amotosalen/ultraviolet A pathogen inactivation technology reduces platelet activatability, induces apoptosis and accelerates clearance. *Haematologica* (2017) 102:1650–60. doi:10.3324/haematol.2017.164137
119. Burnouf T, Goubran HA, Chou ML, Devos D, Radosevic M. Platelet microparticles: detection and assessment of their paradoxical functional roles in disease and regenerative medicine. *Blood Rev* (2014) 28:155–66. doi:10.1016/j.blre.2014.04.002
120. Marcoux G, Duchez AC, Rousseau M, Lévesque T, Boudreau LH, Thibault L, et al. Microparticle and mitochondrial release during extended storage of different types of platelet concentrates. *Platelets* (2017) 28:272–80. doi:10.1080/09537104.2016.1218455
121. Badimon L, Suades R, Fuentes E, Palomo I, Padró T. Role of platelet-derived microvesicles as crosstalk mediators in atherothrombosis and future pharmacology targets: a link between inflammation, atherosclerosis, and thrombosis. *Front Pharmacol* (2016) 7:293. doi:10.3389/fphar.2016.00293
122. Enjeti AK, Ariyarajah A, D'Crus A, Seldon M, Lincz LF. Circulating microvesicle number, function and small RNA content vary with age, gender, smoking status, lipid and hormone profiles. *Thromb Res* (2017) 156:65–72. doi:10.1016/j.thromres.2017.04.019
123. Burnouf T, Chou ML, Goubran H, Cognasse F, Garraud O, Seghatchian J. An overview of the role of microparticles/microvesicles in blood components: are they clinically beneficial or harmful? *Transfus Apher Sci* (2015) 53:137–45. doi:10.1016/j.transci.2015.10.010
124. Maurer-Spurej E, Larsen R, Labrie A, Heaton A, Chipperfield K. Microparticle content of platelet concentrates is predicted by donor microparticles and is altered by production methods and stress. *Transfus Apher Sci* (2016) 55:35–43. doi:10.1016/j.transci.2016.07.010
125. Kanzler P, Mahoney A, Leitner G, Witt V, Maurer-Spurej E. Microparticle detection to guide platelet management for the reduction of platelet refractoriness in children – a study proposal. *Transfus Apher Sci* (2017) 56:39–44. doi:10.1016/j.transci.2016.12.016
126. Hayashi T, Tanaka S, Hori Y, Hirayama F, Sato EF, Inoue M. Role of mitochondria in the maintenance of platelet function during in vitro storage. *Transfus Med* (2011) 21:166–74. doi:10.1111/j.1365-3148.2010.01065.x
127. Boudreau LH, Duchez AC, Cloutier N, Soulet D, Martin N, Bollinger J, et al. Platelets release mitochondria serving as substrate for bactericidal group IIA-secreted phospholipase A2 to promote inflammation. *Blood* (2014) 124:2173–83. doi:10.1182/blood-2014-05-573543
128. Cognasse F, Aloui C, Anh Nguyen K, Hamzeh-Cognasse H, Fagan J, Arthaud CA, et al. Platelet components associated with adverse reactions: predictive value of mitochondrial DNA relative to biological response modifiers. *Transfusion* (2016) 56:497–504. doi:10.1111/trf.13373
129. Bakkour S, Chafets DM, Wen L, van der Meer PF, Mundt JM, Marschner S, et al. Development of a mitochondrial DNA real-time polymerase chain reaction assay for quality control of pathogen reduction with riboflavin and ultraviolet light. *Vox Sang* (2014) 107:351–9. doi:10.1111/vox.12173
130. Bruchmüller I, Lösel R, Bugert P, Corash L, Lin L, Klüter H, et al. Effect of the psoralen-based photochemical pathogen inactivation on mitochondrial DNA in platelets. *Platelets* (2005) 16:441–5. doi:10.1080/09537100500129300
131. Bakkour S, Chafets DM, Wen L, Dupuis K, Castro G, Green JM, et al. Assessment of nucleic acid modification induced by amotosalen and ultraviolet A light treatment of platelets and plasma using real-time polymerase chain reaction amplification of variable length fragments of mitochondrial DNA. *Transfusion* (2016) 56:410–20. doi:10.1111/trf.13360
132. Simmons JD, Lee YL, Pastukh VM, Capley G, Muscat CA, Muscat DC, et al. Potential contribution of mitochondrial DNA damage associated molecular patterns in transfusion products to the development of acute respiratory distress syndrome after multiple transfusions. *J Trauma Acute Care Surg* (2017) 82:1023–9. doi:10.1097/TA.0000000000001421
133. Boilard E, Belleannee C. (Dicer)phering roles of microRNA in platelets. *Blood* (2016) 127:1733–4. doi:10.1182/blood-2016-01-694893
134. Plé H, Landry P, Benham A, Coarfa C, Gunaratne PH, Provost P. The repertoire and features of human platelet microRNAs. *PLoS One* (2012) 7:e50746. doi:10.1371/journal.pone.0050746
135. Laffont B, Corduan A, Plé H, Duchez AC, Cloutier N, Boilard E, et al. Activated platelets can deliver mRNA regulatory Ago2*microRNA complexes to endothelial cells via microparticles. *Blood* (2013) 122:253–61. doi:10.1182/blood-2013-03-492801
136. Osman A, Hitzler WE, Meyer CU, Landry P, Corduan A, Laffont B, et al. Effects of pathogen reduction systems on platelet microRNAs, mRNAs, activation, and function. *Platelets* (2015) 26:154–63. doi:10.3109/09537104.2014.898178
137. Osman A, Hitzler WE, Ameur A, Provost P. Differential expression analysis by RNA-seq reveals perturbations in the platelet mRNA transcriptome triggered by pathogen reduction systems. *PLoS One* (2015) 10:e0133070. doi:10.1371/journal.pone.0133070
138. Arnason NA, Landro R, Harðarson B, Guðmundsson S, Sigurjónsson ÓE. *Effect of Pathogen Inactivation on MicroRNA Profile of Platelet Concentrates During Storage Under Standard Blood Banking Condition in: ISBT 2017.* Copenhagen: Wiley (2017).
139. Weyrich AS, Lindemann S, Tolley ND, Kraiss LW, Dixon DA, Mahoney TM, et al. Change in protein phenotype without a nucleus: translational control

in platelets. *Semin Thromb Hemost* (2004) 30:491–8. doi:10.1055/s-2004-833484

140. Zimmerman GA, Weyrich AS. Signal-dependent protein synthesis by activated platelets: new pathways to altered phenotype and function. *Arterioscler Thromb Vasc Biol* (2008) 28:s17–24. doi:10.1161/ATVBAHA.107.160218
141. Weyrich AS, Schwertz H, Kraiss LW, Zimmerman GA. Protein synthesis by platelets: historical and new perspectives. *J Thromb Haemost* (2009) 7:241–6. doi:10.1111/j.1538-7836.2008.03211.x
142. Klein-Bosgoed C, Schubert P, Devine DV. Riboflavin and ultraviolet illumination affects selected platelet mRNA transcript amounts differently. *Transfusion* (2016) 56:2286–95. doi:10.1111/trf.13715
143. Schubert P, Culibrk B, Karwal S, Goodrich RP, Devine DV. Protein translation occurs in platelet concentrates despite riboflavin/UV light pathogen inactivation treatment. *Proteomics Clin Appl* (2016) 10:839–50. doi:10.1002/prca.201500139
144. O'Donnell VB, Murphy RC, Watson SP. Platelet lipidomics: modern day perspective on lipid discovery and characterization in platelets. *Circ Res* (2014) 114:1185–203. doi:10.1161/CIRCRESAHA.114.301597
145. Slatter DA, Aldrovandi M, O'Connor A, Allen SM, Brasher CJ, Murphy RC, et al. Mapping the human platelet lipidome reveals cytosolic phospholipase A2 as a regulator of mitochondrial bioenergetics during activation. *Cell Metab* (2016) 23:930–44. doi:10.1016/j.cmet.2016.04.001
146. Prudent M, Crettaz D, Delobel J, Tissot JD, Lion N. Proteomic analysis of intercept-treated platelets. *J Proteomics* (2012) 76 Spec No:316–28. doi:10.1016/j.jprot.2012.07.008
147. Thiele T, Sablewski A, Iuga C, Bakchoul T, Bente A, Görg S, et al. Profiling alterations in platelets induced by amotosalen/UVA pathogen reduction and gamma irradiation – a LC-ESI-MS/MS-based proteomics approach. *Blood Transfus* (2012) 10(Suppl 2):s63–70. doi:10.2450/2012.010S
148. Marrocco C, D'Alessandro A, Girelli G, Zolla L. Proteomic analysis of platelets treated with gamma irradiation versus a commercial photochemical pathogen reduction technology. *Transfusion* (2013) 53:1808–20. doi:10.1111/trf.12060
149. Prudent M, D'Alessandro A, Cazenave JP, Devine DV, Gachet C, Greinacher A, et al. Proteome changes in platelets after pathogen inactivation – an inter-laboratory consensus. *Transfus Med Rev* (2014) 28:72–83. doi:10.1016/j.tmrv.2014.02.002
150. Schubert P, Coupland D, Culibrk B, Goodrich RP, Devine DV. Riboflavin and ultraviolet light treatment of platelets triggers p38MAPK signaling: inhibition significantly improves in vitro platelet quality after pathogen reduction treatment. *Transfusion* (2015) 53:3164–73. doi:10.1111/trf.12173
151. Skripchenko A, Awatefe H, Thompson-Montgomery D, Myrup A, Turgeon A, Wagner SJ. An inhibition of p38 mitogen activated protein kinase delays the platelet storage lesion. *PLoS One* (2013) 8:e70732. doi:10.1371/journal.pone.0070732
152. Canault M, Duerschmied D, Brill A, Stefanini L, Schatzberg D, Cifuni SM, et al. p38 mitogen-activated protein kinase activation during platelet storage: consequences for platelet recovery and hemostatic function in vivo. *Blood* (2010) 115:1835–42. doi:10.1182/blood-2009-03-211706
153. Josefsson EC, White MJ, Dowling MR, Kile BT. Platelet life span and apoptosis. *Methods Mol Biol* (2012) 788:59–71. doi:10.1007/978-1-61779-307-3_5
154. Nemkov T, Hansen KC, Dumont LJ, D'Alessandro A. Metabolomics in transfusion medicine. *Transfusion* (2016) 56:980–93. doi:10.1111/trf.13442

17

Pathogen Inactivation of Cellular Blood Products—An Additional Safety Layer in Transfusion Medicine

*Axel Seltsam**

German Red Cross Blood Service NSTOB, Institute Springe, Springe, Germany

Correspondence:
Axel Seltsam
axel.seltsam@bsd-nstob.de

In line with current microbial risk reduction efforts, pathogen inactivation (PI) technologies for blood components promise to reduce the residual risk of known and emerging infectious agents. The implementation of PI of labile blood components is slowly but steadily increasing. This review discusses the relevance of PI for the field of transfusion medicine and describes the available and emerging PI technologies that can be used to treat cellular blood products such as platelet and red blood cell units. In collaboration with the French medical device manufacturer Macopharma, the German Red Cross Blood Services developed a new UVC light-based PI method for platelet units, which is currently being investigated in clinical trials.

Keywords: transfusion, platelets, pathogen inactivation, ultraviolet light, red blood cells

INTRODUCTION

From the late 1970s to the mid-1980s, contaminated hemophilia blood products were a serious public health problem, resulting in the infection of large numbers of hemophiliacs with the human immunodeficiency virus (HIV). If safety measures had been implemented in a timely and consistent manner after identification of the acquired immune deficiency syndrome (AIDS) epidemic in 1981 and isolation of the HIV in 1983, the transmission of HIV infection by these blood products could have been prevented in most cases. This contaminated blood scandal made the community aware that new pathogens may emerge and threaten blood safety at any time. However, there was a significant delay in the introduction of HIV detection systems in some countries and in some cases, the detection tests that were implemented proved to be unreliable. In addition, the plasma products used for therapy were not even treated by heat inactivation—a pathogen inactivation (PI) method that was readily available and approved at that time. Consequently, blood and blood components became subject to drug law in some countries (1, 2).

Increasingly stringent donor eligibility criteria and more sensitive virus detection methods have reduced the risk of transfusion-transmitted infection (TTI) by blood products significantly, but a residual risk of TTI with viruses, bacteria, protozoa, and prions remains. False-negative test results due to test failures, very low-pathogen concentrations in the peripheral blood or escaped mutants can result in TTI in spite of negative screening tests (e.g., for *Treponema pallidum*, hepatitis B, hepatitis C, and HIV). In addition, transfusion recipients may be infected by pathogens not targeted in regular blood donor screening programs (e.g., hepatitis A and bacteria). Transfusion safety is particularly susceptible to pathogens that enter regions in which they are not yet endemic. The fact that viruses that are usually endemic in tropical regions have recently caused outbreaks in Western countries demonstrates that these pathogens can arise and threaten transfusion safety at any time (3, 4).

Blood safety is still mainly based on the reactive principle of introducing new test systems or new donor election criteria after a threat to transfusion recipients has been identified. In other words, infections by contaminated blood products must first occur before appropriate counter-measures are established. At the beginning of the last decade, a number of cases of West Nile virus occurred in the USA through the transmission of blood components before the first detection system for donor testing was implemented (3). The recent Zika virus outbreak on the American continent has heightened concerns over this reactive approach to blood supply safety (5, 6).

During an international consensus conference, transfusion experts and other stakeholders in the field of transfusion medicine recommended a change from the hitherto reactive strategy toward a proactive, preventive approach to blood safety (7). Recently, developed and approved PI technologies for cellular blood products, such as red blood cell (RBC) and platelet units, are considered key measures for closing or at least reducing the safety gap caused by emerging pathogens. While virus reduction procedures are an integral part of the process of manufacturing plasma derivatives from plasma pools, and although the methylene blue system has been used for PI of single donor plasma units for nearly two decades (8), a new generation of PI methods for platelet units have recently become available (9, 10). PI technologies for the treatment of RBC units are still in development and have not received market authorization yet.

TECHNOLOGIES

The use of PI technologies for blood products has a number of advantages. Because they inactivate most clinically relevant viruses, bacteria, and protozoa, they can help to eliminate the residual risk of infection during the "window period" when transfusion-relevant pathogens (e.g., HIV) cannot be detected by donor screening tests. Their broad activity against pathogens also helps to reduce the risk of recognizable infectious agents (e.g., bacteria), which still cannot be prevented completely. In contrast to screening tests for transfusion-borne pathogens, PI proactively protects against emerging infectious agents entering the blood supply in a given community.

All PI methods used to treat cellular blood products work by impairing the target pathogen's ability to replicate. When used alone or in combination, ultraviolet (UV) light and alkylating agents cause irreversible damage to the nucleic acids of pathogens. Therefore, they effectively eliminate classical pathogens such as viruses, bacteria, fungi, and protozoa, but are ineffective against prions. The latter protein-based pathogenic agents can cause sporadic and variant Creutzfeldt–Jakob disease in humans.

The following PI technologies for cellular products are currently available or in the pipeline.

INTERCEPT Blood System for Platelets and Plasma

The INTERCEPT Blood System for platelets and plasma is manufactured by Cerus Corporation (Concord, CA, USA). The mechanism of action of this PI technology is based on the properties of amotosalen HCl (S-59), a photoactive compound which penetrates cellular and nuclear membranes and binds to the double-stranded regions of DNA and RNA. When activated by low-energy UVA light (320–400 nm), amatosalen cross-links nucleic acids and thus irreversibly blocks the replication of DNA and RNA (11). After illumination, residual amotosalen and its photoproducts must be removed during an incubation step lasting up to 16 h. The amatosalen/UVA procedure is not suitable for RBCs because of UVA light absorption by hemoglobin.

MIRASOL PRT System for Platelets and Plasma

The MIRASOL system was developed by TerumoBCT (Lakewood, CO, USA). This photodynamic procedure employs riboflavin (vitamin B2) and broad spectrum UV light (mainly UVA und UVB, 285–365 nm). On exposure to UVA and UVB light, riboflavin associates with nucleic acids and mediates oxygen-independent electron transfer, causing irreversible damage to the nucleic acids (12). Because naturally occurring vitamin B2 and its photodegradation products are non-toxic and non-mutagenic, they do not need to be removed prior to transfusion. In addition to plasma and platelets, protocols for extension of the MIRASOL system to whole blood are now in development.

THERAFLEX System for Platelets

THERAFLEX UV-Platelets is a novel UVC-based PI technology that works without photoactive substances. It is the product of a joint venture between Macopharma (Mouvaux, France) and the German Red Cross Blood Service NSTOB in Springe, Germany. Shortwave UVC light (254 nm) directly interacts with nucleic acids to form pyrimidine dimers that block the elongation of nucleic acid transcripts (13). UVC irradiation mainly affects the nucleic acids of pathogens and leukocytes and does not impair plasma and platelet quality. As no photoactive substances are involved, UVC treatment is just as simple but faster (takes less than 1 min) than gamma irradiation, and can easily be integrated into the manufacturing processes at blood banks (**Figure 1**). The THERAFLEX system was originally developed for platelets but is also suitable for plasma and RBC units.

S-303 PI System for RBCs

The S-303 PI system (INTERCEPT RBC system, Cerus Corporation, Concord, CA, USA) was specifically developed for RBC units. S-303 is a modular compound that prevents nucleic acid replication by targeting and cross-linking nucleic acids. Once added to the RBC unit, this amphipathic compound rapidly passes through cell and viral envelope membranes and intercalates into the helical regions of nucleic acids. S-300, the non-reactive byproduct of this reaction, is subsequently removed by incubation and centrifugation, which can take up to 20 h (14). In contrast to the other PI technologies described here, the S-303 system does not require UV light. However, glutathione (GSH), a naturally occurring antioxidant, must be used to prevent non-specific reactions between S-303 and other nucleophiles present in the RBC unit. These may include small

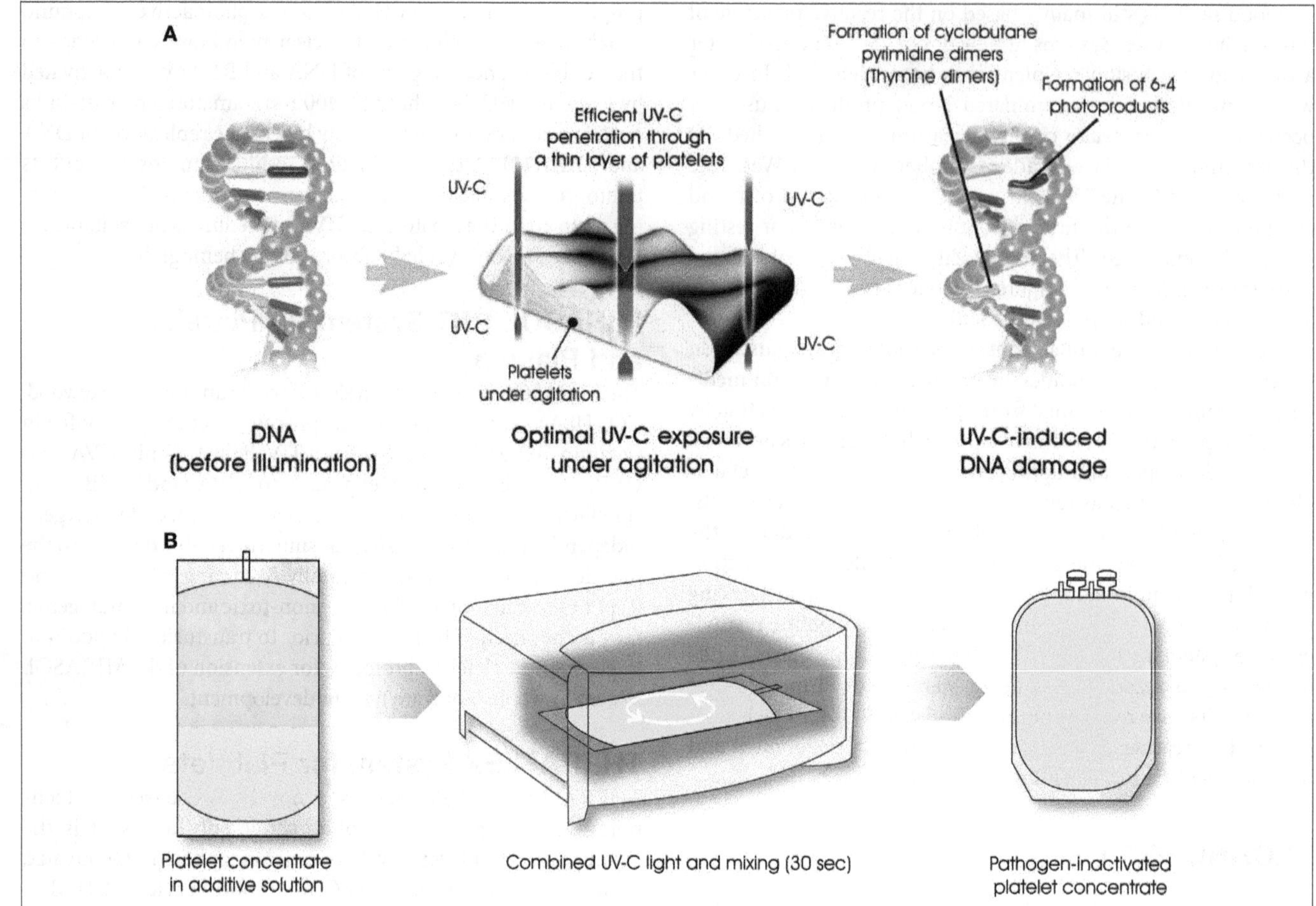

FIGURE 1 | The THERAFLEX ultraviolet (UV)-Platelets pathogen inactivation system uses UVC light to induce irreversible damage to the nucleic acids of viruses, bacteria, fungi, protozoa, and leukocytes. Intense agitation of the platelet bag during UVC illumination results in efficient mixing, ensuring the uniform treatment of all blood compartments **(A)**. For the illumination step of this simple and rapid procedure, platelet units are placed in the irradiation device for a period of less than 1 min **(B)**. Afterward, the pathogen-reduced platelet product can be used for transfusion.

TABLE 1 | Pathogen inactivation technologies.

	Technology			
	INTERCEPT blood system	**MIRASOL PRT system**	**THERAFLEX UV-Platelets**	**S-303 system**
Mechanism of action	UVA plus amotosalen (alkylating agent)	UV plus riboflavin (vitamin B2 = photosensitizer)	UVC alone	Alkylating agent
Blood products	Plasma and platelets	Plasma and platelets (in development for whole blood)	Plasma and platelets (in development for RBCs)	RBCs
Status	Approved in some countries	Approved in some countries	In clinical development	In clinical development

UV, ultraviolet light; UVA, wavelength A; UVC, wavelength C; RBC, red blood cell.

molecules, such as phosphate and water, and macromolecules, such as proteins.

The INTERCEPT and MIRASOL systems for platelets and plasma have already been approved in the USA and some European and Asian countries, while both the THERAFLEX system and the S-303 system are still in clinical development. The UVC-based THERAFLEX system is expected to receive marketing authorization within the next few years (**Table 1**).

CLINICAL STUDIES

Platelets

Clinical studies show that platelets retain their hemostatic efficacy after PI treatment. Following prophylactic transfusion, there was no difference in the ability of pathogen-reduced and untreated platelet units to prevent severe bleeding (15). However, almost all clinical trials demonstrated that post-transfusion survival and recovery rates were consistently lower in patients receiving platelets treated with PI technology than in those transfused with untreated platelets (16–19). Accordingly, the transfusion of pathogen-reduced platelets resulted in lower platelet count increments (CIs), lower corrected count increments, shorter intervals between platelet transfusions, and a higher number of platelet transfusions per patient. However, observational studies showed no evidence of increased product consumption rates when pathogen-reduced platelet units were used in a routine setting (20).

Interestingly, the rate of acute transfusion reactions may be lower after the transfusion of pathogen-reduced versus untreated platelets. However, there have been concerns over acute respiratory distress associated with amatosalen/UVA-treated platelets (15). While the results of animal studies suggest that UV light-treated platelets mediated a higher risk of pulmonary toxicity (21), an analysis of clinical data by an expert panel does not confirm significant differences in the rates of acute lung disorders between PI-treated and untreated platelets (22). The results of ongoing large-scale phase III and hemovigilance studies will help to further clarify open questions with respect to therapeutic efficacy and potential side effects of pathogen-reduced platelets (23).

Red Blood Cells

The S-303 system, which is in clinical development, is the only PI technology available for RBCs. Current studies are investigating the second-generation S-303 PI process. The first-generation S-303 procedure only marginally affected RBC quality and function, but after reports of immunization against pathogen-inactivated RBCs in transfused patients emerged, a new generation of the S-303 system had to be developed. In the second-generation S-303 system, the quencher concentration of GSH was increased from 2 to 20 mmol/l in order to decrease the affinity of S-303 for proteins and thus to avoid the formation of neoantigens on the surface of erythrocytes (24). However, recent studies show that immunization against S-303-coated RBCs still occurs after modification of the S-303 system (25). In particular, the fact that antibodies against S-303-treated cells were also detected in healthy blood donors who had never been transfused with pathogen-reduced RBCs suggests that some individuals may be immunized by S-303-like substances in the environment (e.g., food or air) or may have naturally occurring antibodies against epitopes on the S-303 molecule. These data clearly show that the use of chemical agents for PI of cellular products increases the risk of immune responses against blood components in transfusion recipients. Various phase III clinical trials to test the second-generation S-303 PI system for RBCs in acute and chronic anemia patients are currently ongoing or planned.

IMPLEMENTATION IN ROUTINE USE

The INTERCEPT and MIRASOL PI systems for platelets and plasma are used in some parts of Asia, Europe, and the USA. In Europe, the willingness to use pathogen-reduced platelet units varies between countries and regions. PI technologies are implemented nationwide in some countries (e.g., Switzerland and Belgium), but only regionally in others (e.g., Poland). Evaluation of PI technologies for platelets is under way at some blood centers in Germany. In 2011, the Swiss national authority (Swissmedic) ordered the nationwide implementation of PI of platelet units. This measure was mainly aimed at preventing or at least minimizing the risk of fatal transfusion reactions caused by bacterially contaminated platelet units. Analysis of Swiss hemovigilance data revealed that without PI, one fatal case of transfusion-transmitted sepsis by contaminated platelet units would occur in Switzerland every 2 years. The US Food and Drug Administration (FDA) recently recommended the use of approved PI technologies as an alternative to bacterial detection methods in order to adequately control the risk of bacterial contamination of platelets (26, 27).

The preventive potential of PI of cellular blood components first became apparent during a chikungunya virus epidemic on the French island of La Reunion in the Indian Ocean in 2006 (28). Because more than 30% of the inhabitants were infected, local blood donation was suspended to prevent TTI. To sustain the availability of platelet components, the French national blood service (Etablissement Français du Sang) implemented universal PI of platelet components on the island. The success of this measure demonstrated that PI can effectively support the availability of safe labile blood components during an epidemic.

The West Nile virus epidemic in the USA was the first example of a large-scale arboviral threat to the blood supply of a Western country that required an urgent response across government agencies and non-governmental organizations. The dramatic spread of Zika virus in the Americas since 2015 has generated a sense of public health urgency akin to AIDS, along with immediate concerns over blood safety. In areas of active transmission, "FDA guidance recommends that blood be outsourced from unaffected areas, unless there are measures to screen donations using a laboratory test, or unless the blood components are subjected to PI technology" with an approved method (29). The INTERCEPT system was approved by the FDA in 2014 and has already been implemented at a number of US blood centers.

OUTLOOK

Despite the increasing and profound safety and efficacy record of pathogen-reduced blood cellular products, there are still concerns that impede the introduction of PI technology in hemotherapy. The INTERCEPT protocol includes incubation and adsorption steps that result in a significant loss of platelets (up to 15%) during preparation and PI treatment. However, this loss could be offset by performing PI with higher platelet counts in the starting products. The platelet yields could be increased by using more buffy coats (e.g., five instead of four) to manufacture pooled platelets, or by collecting higher numbers of platelets during the apheresis process. Moreover, this measure could compensate for reduced platelet CIs in transfusion recipients and thus lower the possible need for increased platelet unit utilization.

All PI technologies mentioned in this review exhibit gaps in their PI efficacy. The amatosalen/UVA-based system (INTERCEPT) is ineffective for non-enveloped viruses such as hepatitis A, hepatitis E, and parvovirus B19 (30). The riboflavin/UV-based system (MIRASOL) has only weakly effects against bacteria and some viruses (31). The UVC light-based system (THERAFLEX) is highly effective against bacteria and most transfusion-relevant viruses, but only moderately effective against HIV (32). However, when highly sensitive screening tests for HIV are performed, UVC-based PI could further reduce the risk of virus transmission during the "window period" in which the pre-nucleic acid testing can be negative and in patients with occult infections. Despite these weaknesses, PI systems generally have the potential to significantly add an additional layer of safety to blood transfusion.

Major concerns surrounding the implementation of PI have to do with its impact on the integrity of blood components and the toxicity of the chemicals used in these systems. In particular, acute and chronic toxicities may be caused by PI technologies that use active chemicals. Although only small quantities of photochemical compounds are used in PI technologies and they appear to provide sufficient safety margins, it cannot be excluded that alkylating agents such as amatosalen may be carcinogenic in the long term in a subset of transfused patients. A major advantage of the THERAFLEX system is that it works without photoactive substances, thus eliminating the risk of photoreagent-related adverse events (10, 13).

According to various stakeholders in the field of transfusion medicine, it is crucial to inactivate pathogens in all blood components in order to increase the safety margin of the entire blood supply. As long as PI is not routinely implemented in the production of RBC units (the most commonly used blood components), PI cannot achieve its full potential to enhance blood safety. Experts and health authorities are increasingly recommending the implementation of PI systems for platelets and plasma as an important step toward improving blood safety. A Canadian risk-benefit analysis suggests that if a new pathogen entered the blood supply, the use of pathogen-reduced plasma and platelets would reduce the risk of TTI by 40% (33).

The additional costs of PI implementation may be responsible for the hesitant acceptance of this technology by hospitals and funding agencies. Although based on assumptions and simplifications, the available cost-effectiveness analyses suggest that PI implementation, like other measures for the improvement of blood safety, has an acceptable cost–benefit ratio in this specific application (34, 35). The potential cost savings from PI implementation could offset some costs associated with the technology (e.g., production costs); however, the amount of potential offsetting cost reductions may vary considerably between different countries and regions and must be evaluated on an individual basis for blood centers and hospitals (36). Finally, the available resources influence how politicians and health authorities decide on how to meet public concerns for safety in transfusion medicine. If emerging evidence continues to demonstrate the efficacy of PI, it will be difficult to explain to individuals with severe transfusion-associated infections why this readily available risk mitigation and safety measure was not implemented.

AUTHOR CONTRIBUTIONS

The author confirms being the sole contributor of this work and approved it for publication.

REFERENCES

1. Engelfriet CP, Reesink HW, Snyder EL, Dzik WH, Masse M, Naegelen C, et al. The official requirements for platelet concentrates. *Vox Sang* (1998) 75(4):308–17. doi:10.1046/j.1423-0410.1998.75403081.x
2. Devine DV, Bradley AJ, Maurer E, Levin E, Chahal S, Serrano K, et al. Effects of prestorage white cell reduction on platelet aggregate formation and the activation state of platelets and plasma enzyme systems. *Transfusion* (1999) 39(7):724–34. doi:10.1046/j.1537-2995.1999.39070724.x
3. Harrington T, Kuehnert MJ, Kamel H, Lanciotti RS, Hand S, Currier M, et al. West Nile virus infection transmitted by blood transfusion. *Transfusion* (2003) 43(8):1018–22. doi:10.1046/j.1537-2995.2003.00481.x
4. Bianco C. Dengue and chikungunya viruses in blood donations: risks to the blood supply? *Transfusion* (2008) 48(7):1279–81. doi:10.1111/j.1537-2995.2008.01806.x
5. Lanteri MC, Kleinman SH, Glynn SA, Musso D, Keith Hoots W, Custer BS, et al. Zika virus: a new threat to the safety of the blood supply with worldwide impact and implications. *Transfusion* (2016) 56(7):1907–14. doi:10.1111/trf.13677
6. Motta IJ, Spencer BR, Cordeiro da Silva SG, Arruda MB, Dobbin JA, Gonzaga YB, et al. Evidence for transmission of Zika virus by platelet transfusion. *N Engl J Med* (2016) 375(11):1101–3. doi:10.1056/NEJMc1607262
7. Klein HG, Anderson D, Bernardi MJ, Cable R, Carey W, Hoch JS, et al. Pathogen inactivation: making decisions about new technologies. Report of a consensus conference. *Transfusion* (2007) 47(12):2338–47. doi:10.1111/j.1537-2995.2007.01512.x
8. Pereira A. Methylene-blue-photoinactivated plasma and its contribution to blood safety. *Transfusion* (2004) 44(6):948–50; author reply 950. doi:10.1111/j.0041-1132.2004.359_6.x
9. Pelletier JP, Transue S, Snyder EL. Pathogen inactivation techniques. *Best Pract Res Clin Haematol* (2006) 19(1):205–42. doi:10.1016/j.beha.2005.04.001
10. Seltsam A, Muller TH. Update on the use of pathogen-reduced human plasma and platelet concentrates. *Br J Haematol* (2013) 162(4):442–54. doi:10.1111/bjh.12403
11. Irsch J, Lin L. Pathogen inactivation of platelet and plasma blood components for transfusion using the INTERCEPT blood system. *Transfus Med Hemother* (2011) 38(1):19–31. doi:10.1159/000323937
12. Marschner S, Goodrich R. Pathogen reduction technology treatment of platelets, plasma and whole blood using riboflavin and UV light. *Transfus Med Hemother* (2011) 38(1):8–18. doi:10.1159/000324160
13. Seltsam A, Muller TH. UVC irradiation for pathogen reduction of platelet concentrates and plasma. *Transfus Med Hemother* (2011) 38(1):43–54. doi:10.1159/000323845
14. Henschler R, Seifried E, Mufti N. Development of the S-303 pathogen inactivation technology for red blood cell concentrates. *Transfus Med Hemother* (2011) 38(1):33–42. doi:10.1159/000324458
15. McCullough J, Vesole DH, Benjamin RJ, Slichter SJ, Pineda A, Snyder E, et al. Therapeutic efficacy and safety of platelets treated with a photochemical process for pathogen inactivation: the SPRINT trial. *Blood* (2004) 104(5):1534–41. doi:10.1182/blood-2003-12-4443
16. van Rhenen D, Gulliksson H, Cazenave JP, Pamphilon D, Ljungman P, Kluter H, et al. Transfusion of pooled buffy coat platelet components prepared with photochemical pathogen inactivation treatment: the euroSPRITE trial. *Blood* (2003) 101(6):2426–33. doi:10.1182/blood-2002-03-0932
17. Kerkhoffs JL, van Putten WL, Novotny VM, Te Boekhorst PA, Schipperus MR, Zwaginga JJ, et al. Clinical effectiveness of leucoreduced, pooled donor platelet concentrates, stored in plasma or additive solution with and without pathogen reduction. *Br J Haematol* (2010) 150(2):209–17. doi:10.1111/j.1365-2141.2010.08227.x
18. Mirasol Clinical Evaluation Study Group. A randomized controlled clinical trial evaluating the performance and safety of platelets treated with MIRASOL

pathogen reduction technology. *Transfusion* (2010) 50(11):2362–75. doi:10.1111/j.1537-2995.2010.02694.x

19. Rebulla P, Vaglio S, Beccaria F, Bonfichi M, Carella A, Chiurazzi F, et al. Clinical effectiveness of platelets in additive solution treated with two commercial pathogen-reduction technologies. *Transfusion* (2017) 57(5):1171–83. doi:10.1111/trf.14042
20. Cazenave JP, Isola H, Waller C, Mendel I, Kientz D, Laforet M, et al. Use of additive solutions and pathogen inactivation treatment of platelet components in a regional blood center: impact on patient outcomes and component utilization during a 3-year period. *Transfusion* (2011) 51(3):622–9. doi:10.1111/j.1537-2995.2010.02873.x
21. Gelderman MP, Chi X, Zhi L, Vostal JG. Ultraviolet B light-exposed human platelets mediate acute lung injury in a two-event mouse model of transfusion. *Transfusion* (2011) 51(11):2343–57. doi:10.1111/j.1537-2995.2011.03135.x
22. Corash L, Lin JS, Sherman CD, Eiden J. Determination of acute lung injury after repeated platelet transfusions. *Blood* (2011) 117(3):1014–20. doi:10.1182/blood-2010-06-293399
23. Ypma PF, van der Meer PF, Heddle NM, van Hilten JA, Stijnen T, Middelburg RA, et al. A study protocol for a randomised controlled trial evaluating clinical effects of platelet transfusion products: the pathogen reduction evaluation and predictive analytical rating score (PREPAReS) trial. *BMJ Open* (2016) 6(1):e010156. doi:10.1136/bmjopen-2015-010156
24. Benjamin RJ, McCullough J, Mintz PD, Snyder E, Spotnitz WD, Rizzo RJ, et al. Therapeutic efficacy and safety of red blood cells treated with a chemical process (S-303) for pathogen inactivation: a phase III clinical trial in cardiac surgery patients. *Transfusion* (2005) 45(11):1739–49. doi:10.1111/j.1537-2995.2005.00583.x
25. North AK, Henschler R, Geisen C, Garratty G, Arndt PA, Kattamis A, et al. Evaluation of naturally occurring antibodies to pathogen inactivated red blood cells. *Transfusion* (2010) 50(Suppl):38A.
26. *Bacterial Risk Control Strategies for Blood Collection Establishments and Transfusion Services to Enhance the Safety and Availability of Platelets for Transfusion. Draft Guidance for Industry.* U.S. Department of Health and Human Services, Food and Drug Administration, Center for Biologics Evaluation and Research (2016).
27. Sachais BS, Paradiso S, Strauss D, Shaz BH. Implications of the US Food and Drug Administration draft guidance for mitigating septic reactions from platelet transfusions. *Blood Adv* (2017) 1(15):1142–7. doi:10.1182/bloodadvances.2017008334
28. Rasongles P, Angelini-Tibert MF, Simon P, Currie C, Isola H, Kientz D, et al. Transfusion of platelet components prepared with photochemical pathogen inactivation treatment during a chikungunya virus epidemic in Ile de La Reunion. *Transfusion* (2009) 49(6):1083–91. doi:10.1111/j.1537-2995.2009.02111.x
29. Kuehnert MJ, Epstein JS. Assuring blood safety and availability: Zika virus, the latest emerging infectious disease battlefront. *Transfusion* (2016) 56(7):1669–72. doi:10.1111/trf.13673
30. Hauser L, Roque-Afonso AM, Beyloune A, Simonet M, Deau Fischer B, Burin des Roziers N, et al. Hepatitis E transmission by transfusion of Intercept blood system-treated plasma. *Blood* (2014) 123(5):796–7. doi:10.1182/blood-2013-09-524348
31. Goodrich RP, Gilmour D, Hovenga N, Keil SD. A laboratory comparison of pathogen reduction technology treatment and culture of platelet products for addressing bacterial contamination concerns. *Transfusion* (2009) 49(6):1205–16. doi:10.1111/j.1537-2995.2009.02126.x
32. Mohr H, Steil L, Gravemann U, Thiele T, Hammer E, Greinacher A, et al. A novel approach to pathogen reduction in platelet concentrates using short-wave ultraviolet light. *Transfusion* (2009) 49(12):2612–24. doi:10.1111/j.1537-2995.2009.02334.x
33. Kleinman S, Cameron C, Custer B, Busch M, Katz L, Kralj B, et al. Modeling the risk of an emerging pathogen entering the Canadian blood supply. *Transfusion* (2010) 50(12):2592–606. doi:10.1111/j.1537-2995.2010.02724.x
34. Postma MJ, van Hulst M, De Wolf JT, Botteman M, Staginnus U. Cost-effectiveness of pathogen inactivation for platelet transfusions in the Netherlands. *Transfus Med* (2005) 15(5):379–87. doi:10.1111/j.1365-3148.2005.00609.x
35. Custer B, Agapova M, Martinez RH. The cost-effectiveness of pathogen reduction technology as assessed using a multiple risk reduction model. *Transfusion* (2010) 50(11):2461–73. doi:10.1111/j.1537-2995.2010.02704.x
36. McCullough J, Goldfinger D, Gorlin J, Riley WJ, Sandhu H, Stowell C, et al. Cost implications of implementation of pathogen-inactivated platelets. *Transfusion* (2015) 55(10):2312–20. doi:10.1111/trf.13149

On the Way to *in vitro* Platelet Production

Catherine Strassel*, Christian Gachet and François Lanza

Université de Strasbourg, INSERM, EFS Grand Est, BPPS UMR-S 1255, FMTS, Strasbourg, France

****Correspondence:***
Catherine Strassel
catherine.strassel@efs.sante.fr

The severely decreased platelet counts (10–30. 10^3 platelets/µL) frequently observed in patients undergoing chemotherapy, radiation treatment, or organ transplantation are associated with life-threatening increased bleeding risks. To circumvent these risks, platelet transfusion remains the treatment of choice, despite some limitations which include a limited shelf-life, storage-related deterioration, the development of alloantibodies in recipients and the transmission of infectious diseases. A sustained demand has evolved in recent years for controlled blood products, free of infectious, inflammatory, and immune risks. As a consequence, the challenge for blood centers in the near future will be to ensure an adequate supply of blood platelets, which calls for a reassessment of our transfusion models. To meet this challenge, many laboratories are now turning their research efforts toward the *in vitro* and customized production of blood platelets. In recent years, there has been a major enthusiasm for the cultured platelet production, as illustrated by the number of reviews that have appeared in recent years. The focus of the present review is to critically asses the arguments put forward in support of the culture of platelets for transfusion purposes. In light of this, we will recapitulate the main advances in this quickly evolving field, while noting the technical limitations to overcome to make cultured platelet a transfusional alternative.

Keywords: platelets, *in vitro* production, megakaryocytes, biomanufacturing, hematopoietic stem cells

INTRODUCTION

Blood platelets are small anucleate cells (2–4 µm in diameter) derived from the cytoplasmic fragmentation of their MK precursor (1). MKs are produced in the bone marrow through a highly orchestrated process (2). Hematopoietic stem cells (HSCs) lie at the apex of this process and give rise to progenitors which progressively commit to the megakaryocytic lineage to produce immature MKs (3). MK maturation involves an increase in DNA content (up to 64N) through endomitosis accompanied by massive enlargement of the cytoplasm, the emergence of numerous alpha and dense granules and the development of an extensive membrane network, the demarcation membrane system (DMS) (4–6). Terminally differentiated MKs are intimately associated with the sinusoidal endothelium of the bone marrow. Following extensive cytoskeletal remodeling, fully mature MKs extend cytoplasmic projections called proplatelets into the vessel lumen, where platelets are released under shear forces produced by the circulating blood (7, 8). The entire sequence is strongly influenced by cytokines, extracellular matrix components, surface topography, matrix stiffness, and blood flow (9). This efficient procedure generates 10^{11} functional platelets per day to sustain an average count of 3.10^{11} platelets/L in man (10).

THE CULTURED PLATELETS IN THE TRANSFUSIONAL CONTEXT

More than 100 million blood donations are collected each year, but the transfusion situation varies greatly in different parts of the world. Nearly half of the donations are made in high-income countries, where < 20% of the world's population lives (WHO). In industrialized countries, blood banks operate on a just-in-time basis. Maintaining an adequate platelet supply, ensuring their appropriate use and guaranteeing transfusion safety, together with the prevention of the transmission of infectious diseases, are the main concerns of these blood banks.

In this context, the field of platelet and transfusion research has witnessed an increasing interest in producing platelets *in vitro*. A number of arguments are frequently put forward to justify this research on the grounds of three main threats: i) a risk of shortage, ii) the contamination hazard, and iii) the immunological risk.

i) The shortage threat: Maintaining appropriate stocks of platelet concentrates is becoming a major concern worldwide, due to the ever increasing number of patients experiencing long periods of severe thrombocytopenia related to bone marrow failure, anti-cancer therapy, bone marrow grafts, or immune-related or drug-induced thrombocytopenia (11). The short *in vivo* half-life of human platelets imposes regular platelet transfusions for these patients, while a maximum shelf-life of 5 days further increases the demand for platelets. In the USA, platelet transfusion rose by 7.3% from 2008 to 2011 and the market for platelets is expected to grow at a rate of 5.3% per annum over the next decade (12). This enhanced need has been cited to advocate the development of *in vitro* platelet production, although these figures might not apply equally to all countries. In France, for example, platelet transfusion increased by only 0.5% from 2012 to 2016 and has remained stable since, principally due to new guidelines allowing a reduction in the number of transfused platelets per unit body weight (13). Whereas this has shelved the prospect of a short term shortage, the long term trend merits surveillance. In any event, all countries are facing situations with peak demands and/or periods of low blood donation (vacations, public holidays…) where cultured platelets could represent a real alternative to maintain optimal stocks of platelet concentrates.

ii) The contamination hazard: Platelet transfusion has been routine practice for over five decades (14) but is however not devoid of potential risks. A bacterial contamination remains the major cause of platelet transfusion-related morbidity and mortality (15). Fortunately, the introduction of pathogen inactivation systems and bacterial detection tests, together with careful donor screening and rigorous skin disinfection, has raised transfusion safety to levels never achieved before (16). Nevertheless, the risks of biological hazards and contamination of blood products cannot be totally eliminated and also vary widely between countries. Platelets can capture emergent pathogens which remain undetectable or possibly resistant to inactivation, leading to a residual risk of infection (17). To circumvent these drawbacks and reach conditions of absolute safety, cultured platelets could be an attractive alternative.

iii) The immunological risk: Alloimmunization and platelet refractoriness remain major complications associated with platelet transfusion, despite the introduction of leukodepletion methods (18). The selection of HLA-compatible platelets and/or crossmatch-negative donors can solve these problems but is often difficult to achieve (19). In addition to alloimmunization, ABO-incompatibility can result in weaker transfusion efficacy (20). These problems could be resolved by the generation of universal cultured platelets lacking HLA class I and expressing preferably 0 antigens to improve their compatibility (21).

In summary, although platelet transfusion remains self-sustainable and safe, transfusion practices are destined to evolve, justifying as a precautionary measure research focusing on the efficient culture of platelets. The availability of cultured platelets, free of infectious, inflammatory, and immune risks, would undoubtedly be a real step forward for patients requiring frequent blood transfusions or lacking suitable compatible donors.

OVERVIEW OF THE CHALLENGE

Platelet culture for transfusion will be quite a challenging task. It will require their production in amounts equivalent to one unit ($2–5.10^{11}$) of apheresis- or buffy coat-derived platelets and with the quality and functionality of native platelets. In essence, the *in vitro* conditions need to reproduce as closely as possible the *in vivo* environment. Assuming that each bone marrow megakaryocyte (MK) generates 2000–3000 platelets, 250.10^6 mature MKs will be needed to produce one unit of platelet concentrate. However, despite an increasing knowledge of the molecular and cellular mechanisms governing platelet production and the development of innovative bioreactor technologies, the current yields have remained limited to 100 to 150 platelets/MK over the past several years (22, 23). To meet the challenge still ahead, there is a need to develop further knowledge (**Figure 1**).

1. To reach sufficient MK progenitor amplification efficiencies to obtain the equivalent of one unit of platelets ($\sim 5.10^{11}$ platelets);
2. To obtain a level of MK maturation closely matching that of the bone marrow;
3. To efficiently release platelets from mature MKs;
4. To demonstrate native hemostatic properties and functionality following transfusion.

IMPROVING MK AMPLIFICATION EFFICIENCIES

The source of hematopoietic progenitors/stem cells is of paramount importance and conditions the strategies and expansion capacities. Two main sources have been used i) pluripotent stem cells, including human embryonic stem cells

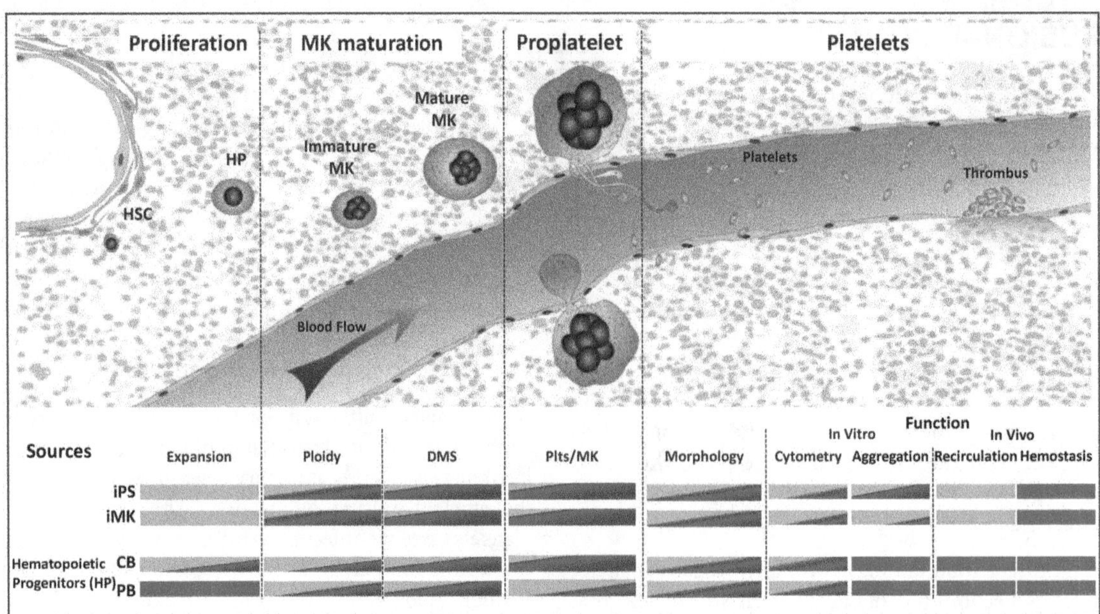

FIGURE 1 | Schematic representation of the major stages of platelet biogenesis coupled with an overview of the main technical or biological hurdles that have either been overcome (green) or need to be met (red) to consider cultured platelet as a clinical alternative. HSC, hematopoietic stem cells; HP, hematopoietic progenitors; MK, megakaryocytes; DMS, demarcation membrane system; Plts, platelets; iPS, induced pluripotent stem cells; iMK, immortalized megakaryocytes.

(hESCs) and induced pluripotent stem cells (iPSCs), and ii) hematopoietic progenitors derived from bone marrow (BM), cord blood (CB) and peripheral blood (PB) (CD34+ cells). Each of these offers advantages and disadvantages for the development of a transfusion product.

i) Pluripotent stem cells: hESCs and iPSCs both possess the significant advantage of a self-renewal capacity. iPSCs offer the additional benefit of avoiding the ethical concerns raised by hESCs and therefore constitute the most attractive pluripotent stem cells (24). The reader can refer to two previous excellent reviews on this subject (25, 26). Significant progress has been made in iPSC engineering to enhance platelet production. A promising development has undoubtedly been the generation of two types of expandable MK line (25). One type was obtained following several optimization steps resulting in the sequential introduction of c-MYC, BMI1, and BCL-XL (27). The second was developed by overexpressing the transcription factors GATA-1, FLI1, and TAL1 under chemically defined conditions (28). Both cell lines tolerate cryopreservation and can be expanded upon demand to generate platelets with higher efficiency and in shorter times as compared to iPSC-derived MKs. In the objective of avoiding platelet transfusion refractoriness, another remarkable achievement has been the generation of iPSC-derived HLA class I-silenced MKs and platelets using RNA-interference TALEN or *CRISPR/Cas9* editing strategies (29–31).

   Although the above arguments speak in favor of iPSCs, this source still faces a number of drawbacks. The yield of platelets remains low with < 10 platelets/MK, possibly due to some immaturity of iPSC-derived MKs (low ploidy and a less well developed DMS) (25, 27, 28, 32). Another drawback for clinical applications is the potential tumorigenicity of these cells. This risk is considered to be minor on the grounds that platelets lack replication and can be irradiated before transfusion (22, 25). However, caution might prevail and impede their acceptance by regulatory authorities. In any case, careful separation of the *bona fide* platelets from other cellular elements, such as nucleated cells including immature MK, large fragments with remnant nuclear material (DNA, RNA), in the final culture suspension will be required to minimize gene-related risks.

ii) Hematopoietic progenitors: As compared to hESCs and iPSCs, hematopoietic progenitors, conventionally isolated through their CD34 positivity, are technologically easier to manage for platelet generation. They can be derived from cord blood (CB), bone marrow (BM) or peripheral blood (PB) and their harvest is easy and rapid with no ethical concerns and low cost (33). The major advantage of CD34+ cells is their platelet yield, usually around 100–150 platelets/MK, while several studies have mentioned that platelets derived from these progenitors share ultrastructural and functional characteristics with circulating platelets (34, 35).

One limitation often evoked to oppose the use of CD34+ cells is their finite expansion. However, large numbers of safe CB-derived HSCs are stored around the world and could be used for the bio-manufacture of platelets. Similarly, PB-derived CD34+ cells eluted from leukoreduction filters (LRFs) represent a source with strong potential. Around $0.4.10^6$ PB-derived CD34+ cells can be eluted from one LRF and the French Blood Bank, for example, destroys more than 3.10^6 LRFs/year (36). LRFs are an easily available and safe source of cells submitted to a stringent quality control process. Automation and standardization of the process would allow the constitution of large homogeneous and safe CD34+ cell pools. Even if these cells do not possess the theoretical unlimited expansion potential of iPSCs, recent studies indicate that this could be partly overcome by the use of novel agents like StemRegenin 1 (SR1) (37), nicotinamide (NAM) (38), mesenchymal stromal cell (MSC) coculture (39), or notch ligands (40). Moreover, CD34+ cells harbor the same potential as iPSCs to produce HLA-deficient platelets, since both CB- and PB-derived HSCs could be selected and pooled according to their HLA/ABO phenotype to generate compatible platelets for transfusion. Altogether, the availability of safe, HLA/ABO-pooled, CB-, and LRF-derived CD34+ cells combined with new strategies favoring their proliferation could lead to a regain of the use of CD34+ cells for platelet production.

Choosing between iPSCs and hematopoietic progenitors will be a matter of compromise taking into account the proliferation and maturation potentials of the cells when planning large-scale cultures. Despite undeniable technological advances, platelet production from iPSCs requires relatively complex and sophisticated methods, which might complicate the industrial-scale generation of cultured platelets. We postulate that CD34+ cells derived from PB, which are presently underexploited, could represent an interesting trade-off in terms of their availability, cost, and MK maturation and platelet yields (35).

OBTAINING A LEVEL OF MK MATURATION CLOSELY MATCHING THAT OF THE BM

Efficient platelet production requires a high degree of MK maturation, which is itself dependent on i) efficient endomitosis and ii) DMS expansion (2). Endomitosis contributes to the production of large amounts of proteins and to organelle development within a single MK (6). DMS expansion provides the reservoir of membranes required to feed the extension of numerous proplatelets and *in fine* the release of individual platelets. To reach an optimal degree of MK maturation *in vitro* we have to faithfully mimic these processes, which are influenced by specific microenvironments in the bone marrow (cytokines, stiffness) and depend on efficient lipid biosynthesis.

i) Ploidization. So far, even under optimal conditions, MKs derived from adult progenitors or iPSCs present lower ploidy levels than MKs resident in the bone marrow, indicating a certain lack of maturity. Consistent with this finding, it has been observed that smaller and less polyploid MKs produce fewer platelets than larger MKs (41). This has also been documented in fetal and neonatal MKs, which are significantly smaller and of lower ploidy than adult MKs and produce fewer platelets than their adult counterparts (42). Whereas the mechanisms underlying the small size and low ploidy of neonatal MKs remain unclear, Elagib et al. recently identified an RNA-binding protein, IGF2BP3, regulating the human fetal-adult MK transition (43). These authors demonstrated that downregulation of IGF2BP3 using a lentiviral strategy enhanced neonatal MK enlargement, growth arrest, and polyploidization. In addition, use of a pharmacological inhibitor of IGF2BP3 expression elicited adult features in neonatal MKs. This could open the way to the development of new strategies to enhance MK maturation and platelet production. Other molecules favoring endomitosis have been identified, such as actin polymerization inhibitors and Rho kinase inhibitors (44–46), but these agents did not significantly improve platelet yields.

ii) DMS expansion. The production by a single MK of thousands of platelets requires considerable membrane synthesis and its folding into a well-organized DMS. The DMS is fueled by invagination from the outer membrane with further contributions from internal golgi-derived membranes and contacts with the endoplasmic reticulum, which together provide a continuous membrane supply (4). It has been reported that immature MKs have a high capacity for cholesterol and phospholipid synthesis and are also able to capture fatty acids (47). The importance of cholesterol uptake is further suggested by studies showing that hypercholesterolemia positively influences platelet production (48). A better knowledge of the lipid pathways involved in MK maturation could help us to devise culture media supplements favoring platelet production.

Bone marrow is a complex and dynamic cellular tissue where MKs interact with other cells and protein matrices in a 3-dimensional (3D) configuration (49). Recent findings have highlighted the environmental stiffness of the bone marrow as a key regulator of MK maturation, whereby adaptation of the cells to the surrounding physical constraints favors higher ploidy and proplatelet formation (34, 50). These observations can be applied directly to *in vitro* platelet production. Thus, Aguilar et al. recently showed that MKs grown in 2% methylcellulose (30–60 Pa) exhibited enhanced DMS expansion leading to increased platelet production. Mechanistically, these authors demonstrated the increased nuclear translocation of an important regulator of MK maturation, megakaryoblastic leukemia factor-1 (MKL1), which was triggered by the physical constraints (51). Identifying the stiffness-mediated factors involved in MK maturation should provide an important means of improving the production of platelets in culture.

EFFICIENTLY RELEASING PLATELETS FROM MATURE MKS

In vivo, under physiological conditions, efficient platelet release requires i) the transmigration of proplatelets/MK fragments through the endothelial barrier and ii) their exposure to the blood flow (8).

i) Endothelial cells. Upon reaching the sinusoids, mature MKs come into contact with endothelial cells. A seminal study conducted by Rafii et al. demonstrated that human BM microvascular endothelial cells (BMECs) specifically supported the MK differentiation of CD34+ progenitors

(52). More recently, the interplay between MKs and the sinusoidal barrier has been examined in more detail. It could be shown that MKs form podosomes which are able to degrade the extracellular matrix, allowing elongation of proplatelets into the lumen (53). The importance of podosomes in thrombopoiesis is further suggested by the occurrence of thrombocytopenia in primary genetic deficiencies affecting podosome formation (WASP, CDc42, α-actinin, or CD44) (54, 55). Work by Antkowiack et al. also indicates that EC contacts triggering podosome formation could participate in the DMS polarization preceding proplatelet extension (56).

Current efforts in bioreactor development will require additional research to reveal the specific mechanisms involved in the transmigration of mature MKs into the lumen. Endothelial cells have already been introduced into 3D flow systems but did not appear to positively affect proplatelet elongation or platelet numbers (34, 57). The positive impact of EC might depend on the additional presence of soluble factors such as Il1b, an inflammatory cytokine reported to enhance MK and EC interactions (58). Stimulating the endothelium through the VEGFR1-mediated pathway also increased platelet production (59). Finally, a signaling lipid circulating in the blood, S1P, has been proposed as a new key regulator of platelet release, *in vitro* and under flow conditions (60).

ii) Blood flow. When left under static conditions, MKs extending proplatelets liberate individual platelets with a very low efficiency (61). Thus, to mimic *in vivo* conditions where platelet release depends heavily on shear forces (8, 60), a number of laboratories have integrated flow into newly developed scalable microfluidic platelet bioreactors. Baruch et al. have designed a bioreactor comprising a multitude of staggered pillars covered with von Willebrand factor. MKs adhering to the pillars and subjected to hydrodynamic forces stretch out long extensions and release platelet-like elements (62). Another microchamber developed by Thon et al. consists of one channel separated by a series of 2 μm diameter gaps from another channel where flow is applied. Trapped MKs extend proplatelets and release platelets into the second channel more efficiently than in the absence of flow (63). Nakagawa et al. have designed original gaps where trapped MKs are submitted to a bidirectional flow, applied at a 60° angle reported to be 3.6 times more effective than a 90° platelet release angle (64). Although this is an attractive variant, incorporation of this geometry into future devices will require thorough morphological and functional analysis of the platelets released. The development of these bioreactors has established proof of the feasibility of *ex vivo* platelet production. However, despite taking into account extracellular matrix proteins, stiffness, and flow, the platelet yields obtained are only of the order of 30–50 platelets/MK.

DEMONSTRATING NATIVE FUNCTIONALITY AND HEMOSTATIC PROPERTIES FOLLOWING TRANSFUSION

If cultured platelets are to be considered as a clinical alternative, they must equal the quality of donor-derived platelets in terms of i) morphology and ultrastructure and ii) *in vitro*, and iii) *in vivo* functionality (65). So far, studies of the quality and functionality of cultured platelets are still fragmentary.

i) Morphology and ultrastructure. Native platelets are typically anucleate, exhibit a characteristic discoid shape and are filled with secretory granules (α, δ, lysosomes) which contain endogenously synthesized or endocytosed molecules.

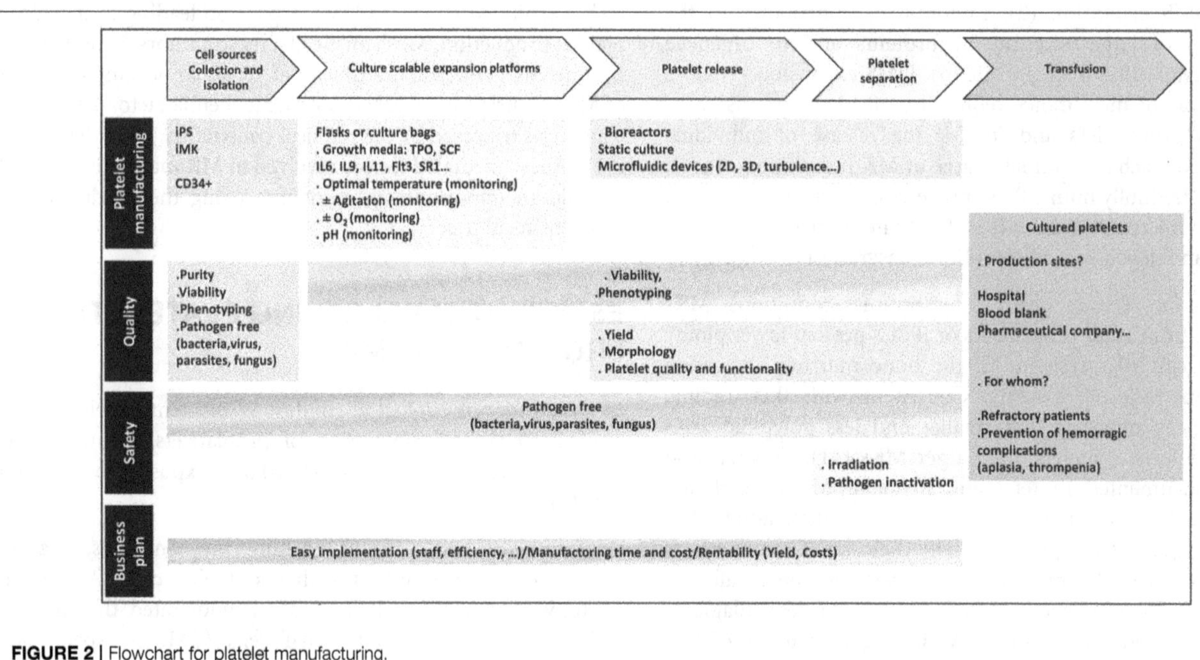

FIGURE 2 | Flowchart for platelet manufacturing.

Microscopic analyses have revealed that cultured platelets are typically larger than native ones and have an increased RNA content, two characteristic features of "young" platelets (27, 32, 35, 57). This raises the question of whether such immaturity is useful or detrimental for platelet recirculation after transfusion. In addition, platelet functions are largely dependent on the molecules stored in their granules. Culture media do not usually contain certain components required for platelet function such as fibrinogen or serotonin. Studies will be required to determine whether we need to load platelets with proteins they lack during culture, or whether they are capable of filling their granules during recirculation to ensure their normal function.

ii) *In vitro* evaluation of platelet function. In the majority of studies, the functionality of the platelets generated *in vitro* has only been incompletely addressed. The tests have mostly relied on flow cytometric measurement of P-selectin exposure and PAC-1 binding to detect GPIIb-IIIa activation. Usually, a large proportion of cultured platelets express these activation markers upon stimulation by agonists such as ADP or thrombin (27, 32, 34). One may note that a state of pre-activation, visualized by P-selectin expression, is often observed in the absence of any agonist (66, 67). In itself, this positivity does not inevitably predict poor transfusion properties. Indeed, in one study it was reported that circulating degranulated platelets rapidly lose surface P-selectin to the plasma pool but continue to circulate and function *in vivo* (68). The demonstration of platelet aggregation has often been restricted to a flow cytometric approach (2 color assays), due to the limited numbers of purified platelets obtained in culture (27, 34). However, as shown by Feng et al., this should not routinely exempt us from standard aggregometry testing as a quality control for transfusion applications (32).

iii) *In vivo* evaluation of platelet function. The *in vivo* functionality of cultured platelets has mainly been attested on the basis of their ability to participate in a developing thrombus after vessel injury in the mouse (27, 32, 35). Concerning their capacity to recirculate, this has only been demonstrated in a few studies. A quite similar half-life to that of native platelets was observed after transfusion into immune-deficient mice (27, 28, 32). Although these results are encouraging, they do not provide a definitive answer to the question of the true ability of cultured platelets to fulfill their functions. Finally, there are to date no available data concerning the *in vivo* hemostatic properties of the cells, i.e., their capacity to correct a bleeding tendency in thrombocytopenic individuals. With the declared ambition of being a transfusion substitute, it is now time to move on in the area of the functionality of cultured platelets with an accurate evaluation of their hemostatic potential in thrombocytopenic mice.

CONCLUSION AND PERSPECTIVES

Over the past 5 years, considerable efforts have been made to improve the production of platelets *in vitro,* mainly in relation to iPSC generation and the availability of universal platelets, together with the design of original and scalable bioreactors. A dozen dedicated teams around the world are competing to achieve *ex vivo* platelet production. However, in addition to their important research efforts, it is also important to consider production costs which have to be greatly reduced to make cultured platelet an economic reality (**Figure 2**). In this respect, optimization of the crucial steps of platelet generation (MK maturation and platelet release) and a better understanding of the molecular and cellular mechanisms governing platelet production will be required to make cultured platelets a clinical alternative in certain situations. In any case, one must recall that despite the technical advances and enthusiasm underlying this challenge, nothing will ever replace the voluntary, free and anonymous donation of blood.

AUTHOR CONTRIBUTIONS

All authors listed have made a substantial, direct and intellectual contribution to the work, and approved it for publication.

REFERENCES

1. Kaushansky K. Historical review: megakaryopoiesis and thrombopoiesis. *Blood* (2008) 111:981–6. doi: 10.1182/blood-2007-05-088500
2. Machlus KR, Thon JN, Italiano JEJr. Interpreting the developmental dance of the megakaryocyte: a review of the cellular and molecular processes mediating platelet formation. *Br J Haematol.* (2014) 165:227–36. doi: 10.1111/bjh.12758
3. Woolthuis CM, Park CY. Hematopoietic stem/progenitor cell commitment to the megakaryocyte lineage. *Blood* (2016) 127:1242–8. doi: 10.1182/blood-2015-07-607945
4. Eckly A, Heijnen H, Pertuy F, Geerts W, Proamer F, Rinckel JY, et al. Biogenesis of the demarcation membrane system (DMS) in megakaryocytes. *Blood* (2014) 123:921–30. doi: 10.1182/blood-2013-03-492330
5. Guo T, Wang X, Qu Y, Yin Y, Jing T, Zhang Q. Megakaryopoiesis and platelet production: insight into hematopoietic stem cell proliferation and differentiation. *Stem Cell Investig.* (2015) 2:3. doi: 10.3978/j.issn.2306-9759.2015.02.01
6. Mazzi S, Lordier L, Debili N, Raslova H, Vainchenker W. Megakaryocyte and polyploidization. *Exp Hematol.* (2018) 57:1–13. doi: 10.1016/j.exphem.2017.10.001
7. Patel SR, Hartwig JH, Italiano JEJr. The biogenesis of platelets from megakaryocyte proplatelets. *J Clin Invest.* (2005) 115:3348–54. doi: 10.1172/JCI26891
8. Junt T, Schulze H, Chen Z, Massberg S, Goerge T, Krueger A, et al. Dynamic visualization of thrombopoiesis within bone marrow. *Science* (2007) 317:1767–70. doi: 10.1126/science.1146304
9. Leiva O, Leon C, Kah Ng S, Mangin P, Gachet C, Ravid K. The role of extracellular matrix stiffness in megakaryocyte and platelet development and function. *Am J Hematol.* (2018) 93:430–41. doi: 10.1002/ajh.25008
10. Daly ME. Determinants of platelet count in humans. *Haematologica* (2011) 96:10–3. doi: 10.3324/haematol.2010.035287
11. Tiberghien P, Follea G, Muller JY. Platelet Transfusions in Acute Leukemia. *N Engl J Med.* (2016) 375:96–7. doi: 10.1056/NEJMc1515066

12. Thon JN, Medvetz DA, Karlsson SM, Italiano JEJr. Road blocks in making platelets for transfusion. *J Thromb Haemost.* (2015) 13 (Suppl. 1):S55–62. doi: 10.1111/jth.12942
13. Slichter SJ, Kaufman RM, Assmann SF, Mccullough J, Triulzi DJ, Strauss RG, et al. Dose of prophylactic platelet transfusions and prevention of hemorrhage. *N Engl J Med.* (2010) 362:600–13. doi: 10.1056/NEJMoa0904084
14. Han T, Stutzman L, Cohen E, Kim U. Effect of platelet transfusion on hemorrhage in patients with acute leukemia: an autopsy study. *Cancer* (1966) 19:1937–42. doi: 10.1002/1097-0142(196612)19:12<1937::AID-CNCR2820191221>3.0.CO;2-G
15. Frazier SK, Higgins J, Bugajski A, Jones AR, Brown MR. Adverse reactions to transfusion of blood products and best practices for prevention. *Crit Care Nurs Clin North Am.* (2017) 29:271–90. doi: 10.1016/j.cnc.2017.04.002
16. Stormer M, Vollmer T. Diagnostic methods for platelet bacteria screening: current status and developments. *Transfus Med Hemother.* (2014) 41:19–27. doi: 10.1159/000357651
17. Assinger A. Platelets and infection - an emerging role of platelets in viral infection. *Front Immunol.* (2014) 5:649. doi: 10.3389/fimmu.2014.00649
18. Slichter SJ. Platelet refractoriness and alloimmunization. *Leukemia* (1998) 12 (Suppl. 1):S51–3.
19. Salama OS, Aladl DA, El Ghannam DM, Elderiny WE. Evaluation of platelet cross-matching in the management of patients refractory to platelet transfusions. *Blood Transfus.* (2014) 12:187–94. doi: 10.2450/2014.0120-13
20. Valsami S, Dimitroulis D, Gialeraki A, Chimonidou M, Politou M. Current trends in platelet transfusions practice: the role of ABO-RhD and human leukocyte antigen incompatibility. *Asian J Transfus Sci.* (2015) 9:117–23. doi: 10.4103/0973-6247.162684
21. Baigger A, Blasczyk R, Figueiredo C. Towards the manufacture of megakaryocytes and platelets for clinical application. *Transfus Med Hemother.* (2017) 44:165–73. doi: 10.1159/000477261
22. Heazlewood SY, Nilsson SK, Cartledge K, Be CL, Vinson A, Gel M, et al. Progress in bio-manufacture of platelets for transfusion. *Platelets* (2017) 28:649–56. doi: 10.1080/09537104.2016.1257783
23. Thon JN, Dykstra BJ, Beaulieu LM. Platelet bioreactor: accelerated evolution of design and manufacture. *Platelets* (2017) 28:472–7. doi: 10.1080/09537104.2016.1265922
24. Takahashi K, Tanabe K, Ohnuki M, Narita M, Ichisaka T, Tomoda K, et al. Induction of pluripotent stem cells from adult human fibroblasts by defined factors. *Cell* (2007) 131:861–72. doi: 10.1016/j.cell.2007.11.019
25. Sugimoto N, Eto K. Platelet production from induced pluripotent stem cells. *J Thromb Haemost.* (2017) 15:1717–27. doi: 10.1111/jth.13736
26. Karagiannis P, Eto K. Manipulating megakaryocytes to manufacture platelets *ex vivo*. *J Thromb Haemost.* (2015) 13 (Suppl. 1):S47–53. doi: 10.1111/jth.12946
27. Nakamura S, Takayama N, Hirata S, Seo H, Endo H, Ochi K, et al. Expandable megakaryocyte cell lines enable clinically applicable generation of platelets from human induced pluripotent stem cells. *Cell Stem Cell* (2014) 14:535–48. doi: 10.1016/j.stem.2014.01.011
28. Moreau T, Evans AL, Vasquez L, Tijssen MR, Yan Y, Trotter MW, et al. Large-scale production of megakaryocytes from human pluripotent stem cells by chemically defined forward programming. *Nat Commun.* (2016) 7:11208. doi: 10.1038/ncomms11208
29. Liu Y, Wang Y, Gao Y, Forbes JA, Qayyum R, Becker L, et al. Efficient generation of megakaryocytes from human induced pluripotent stem cells using food and drug administration-approved pharmacological reagents. *Stem Cells Transl Med.* (2015) 4:309–19. doi: 10.5966/sctm.2014-0183
30. Borger AK, Eicke D, Wolf C, Gras C, Aufderbeck S, Schulze K, et al. Generation of HLA-universal iPSCs-derived megakaryocytes and platelets for survival under refractoriness conditions. *Mol Med.* (2016) 22:274–285. doi: 10.2119/molmed.2015.00235
31. Zhang N, Zhi H, Curtis BR, Rao S, Jobaliya C, Poncz M, et al. CRISPR/Cas9-mediated conversion of human platelet alloantigen allotypes. *Blood* (2016) 127:675–80. doi: 10.1182/blood-2015-10-675751
32. Feng Q, Shabrani N, Thon JN, Huo H, Thiel A, Machlus KR, et al. Scalable generation of universal platelets from human induced pluripotent stem cells. *Stem Cell Rep.* (2014) 3:817–31. doi: 10.1016/j.stemcr.2014.09.010
33. Lee EJ, Godara P, Haylock D. Biomanufacture of human platelets for transfusion: rationale and approaches. *Exp Hematol.* (2014) 42:332–46. doi: 10.1016/j.exphem.2014.02.002
34. Di Buduo CA, Wray LS, Tozzi L, Malara A, Chen Y, Ghezzi CE, et al. Programmable 3D silk bone marrow niche for platelet generation *ex vivo* and modeling of megakaryopoiesis pathologies. *Blood* (2015) 125:2254–64. doi: 10.1182/blood-2014-08-595561
35. Strassel C, Brouard N, Mallo L, Receveur N, Mangin P, Eckly A, et al. Aryl hydrocarbon receptor-dependent enrichment of a megakaryocytic precursor with a high potential to produce proplatelets. *Blood* (2016) 127:2231–40. doi: 10.1182/blood-2015-09-670208
36. Peytour Y, Villacreces A, Chevaleyre J, Ivanovic Z, Praloran V. Discarded leukoreduction filters: a new source of stem cells for research, cell engineering and therapy? *Stem Cell Res.* (2013) 11:736–42. doi: 10.1016/j.scr.2013.05.001
37. Boitano AE, Wang J, Romeo R, Bouchez LC, Parker AE, Sutton SE, et al. Aryl hydrocarbon receptor antagonists promote the expansion of human hematopoietic stem cells. *Science* (2010) 329:1345–8. doi: 10.1126/science.1191536
38. Horwitz ME, Chao NJ, Rizzieri DA, Long GD, Sullivan KM, Gasparetto C, et al. Umbilical cord blood expansion with nicotinamide provides long-term multilineage engraftment. *J Clin Invest.* (2014) 124:3121–8. doi: 10.1172/JCI74556
39. De Lima M, Mcniece I, Robinson SN, Munsell M, Eapen M, Horowitz M, et al. Cord-blood engraftment with *ex vivo* mesenchymal-cell coculture. *N Engl J Med.* (2012) 367:2305–15. doi: 10.1056/NEJMoa1207285
40. Delaney C, Heimfeld S, Brashem-Stein C, Voorhies H, Manger RL, Bernstein ID. Notch-mediated expansion of human cord blood progenitor cells capable of rapid myeloid reconstitution. *Nat Med.* (2010) 16:232–6. doi: 10.1038/nm.2080
41. Mattia G, Vulcano F, Milazzo L, Barca A, Macioce G, Giampaolo A, et al. Different ploidy levels of megakaryocytes generated from peripheral or cord blood CD34+ cells are correlated with different levels of platelet release. *Blood* (2002) 99:888–97. doi: 10.1182/blood.V99.3.888
42. De Alarcon PA, Graeve JL. Analysis of megakaryocyte ploidy in fetal bone marrow biopsies using a new adaptation of the feulgen technique to measure DNA content and estimate megakaryocyte ploidy from biopsy specimens. *Pediatr Res.* (1996) 39:166–70. doi: 10.1203/00006450-199601000-00026
43. Elagib KE, Lu CH, Mosoyan G, Khalil S, Zasadzinska E, Foltz DR, et al. Neonatal expression of RNA-binding protein IGF2BP3 regulates the human fetal-adult megakaryocyte transition. *J Clin Invest.* (2017) 127:2365–77. doi: 10.1172/JCI88936
44. Baatout S. Megakaryocytopoiesis: growth factors, cell cycle and gene expression. *Anticancer Res.* (1998) 18:1871–82.
45. Avanzi MP, Mitchell WB. *Ex vivo* production of platelets from stem cells. *Br J Haematol.* (2014) 165:237–47. doi: 10.1111/bjh.12764
46. Avanzi MP, Oluwadara OE, Cushing MM, Mitchell ML, Fischer S, Mitchell WB. A novel bioreactor and culture method drives high yields of platelets from stem cells. *Transfusion* (2016) 56:170–8. doi: 10.1111/trf.13375
47. Schick PK, Williams-Gartner K, He XL. Lipid composition and metabolism in megakaryocytes at different stages of maturation. *J Lipid Res.* (1990) 31:27–35.
48. Wang N, Tall AR. Cholesterol in platelet biogenesis and activation. *Blood* (2016) 127:1949–53. doi: 10.1182/blood-2016-01-631259
49. Malara A, Abbonante V, Di Buduo CA, Tozzi L, Currao M, Balduini A. The secret life of a megakaryocyte: emerging roles in bone marrow homeostasis control. *Cell Mol Life Sci.* (2015) 72:1517–36. doi: 10.1007/s00018-014-1813-y
50. Ivanovska IL, Shin JW, Swift J, Discher DE. Stem cell mechanobiology: diverse lessons from bone marrow. *Trends Cell Biol.* (2015) 25:523–32. doi: 10.1016/j.tcb.2015.04.003
51. Aguilar A, Pertuy F, Eckly A, Strassel C, Collin D, Gachet C, et al. Importance of environmental stiffness for megakaryocyte differentiation and proplatelet formation. *Blood* (2016) 128:2022–32. doi: 10.1182/blood-2016-02-699959
52. Rafii S, Shapiro F, Pettengell R, Ferris B, Nachman RL, Moore MA, et al. Human bone marrow microvascular endothelial cells support long-term proliferation and differentiation of myeloid and megakaryocytic progenitors. *Blood* (1995) 86:3353–63.
53. Schachter H. Complex N-glycans: the story of the "yellow brick road". *Glycoconj J.* (2014) 31:1–5. doi: 10.1007/s10719-013-9507-5

54. Kunishima S, Okuno Y, Yoshida K, Shiraishi Y, Sanada M, Muramatsu H, et al. ACTN1 mutations cause congenital macrothrombocytopenia. *Am J Hum Genet.* (2013) 92:431–8. doi: 10.1016/j.ajhg.2013.01.015
55. Di Martino J, Henriet E, Ezzoukhry Z, Goetz JG, Moreau V, Saltel F. The microenvironment controls invadosome plasticity. *J Cell Sci.* (2016) 129:1759–68. doi: 10.1242/jcs.182329
56. Antkowiak A, Viaud J, Severin S, Zanoun M, Ceccato L, Chicanne G, et al. Cdc42-dependent F-actin dynamics drive structuration of the demarcation membrane system in megakaryocytes. *J. Thromb. Haemost.* (2016) 14:1268–84. doi: 10.1111/jth.13318
57. Thon JN, Italiano JE. Platelets: production, morphology and ultrastructure. *Handb Exp Pharmacol.* (2012) 210:3–22. doi: 10.1007/978-3-642-29423-5_1
58. Beaulieu LM, Lin E, Mick E, Koupenova M, Weinberg EO, Kramer CD, et al. Interleukin 1 receptor 1 and interleukin 1beta regulate megakaryocyte maturation, platelet activation, and transcript profile during inflammation in mice and humans. *Arterioscler Thromb Vasc Biol.* (2014) 34:552–64. doi: 10.1161/ATVBAHA.113.302700
59. Pitchford SC, Lodie T, Rankin SM. VEGFR1 stimulates a CXCR4-dependent translocation of megakaryocytes to the vascular niche, enhancing platelet production in mice. *Blood* (2012) 120:2787–95. doi: 10.1182/blood-2011-09-378174
60. Zhang L, Orban M, Lorenz M, Barocke V, Braun D, Urtz N, et al. A novel role of sphingosine 1-phosphate receptor S1pr1 in mouse thrombopoiesis. *J Exp Med.* (2012) 209:2165–81. doi: 10.1084/jem.20121090
61. Dunois-Larde C, Capron C, Fichelson S, Bauer T, Cramer-Borde E, Baruch D. Exposure of human megakaryocytes to high shear rates accelerates platelet production. *Blood* (2009) 114:1875–83. doi: 10.1182/blood-2009-03-209205
62. Blin A, Le Goff A, Magniez A, Poirault-Chassac S, Teste B, Sicot G, et al. Microfluidic model of the platelet-generating organ: beyond bone marrow biomimetics. *Sci Rep.* (2016) 6:21700. doi: 10.1038/srep21700
63. Thon JN, Mazutis L, Wu S, Sylman JL, Ehrlicher A, Machlus KR, et al. Platelet bioreactor-on-a-chip. *Blood* (2014) 124:1857–67. doi: 10.1182/blood-2014-05-574913
64. Nakagawa Y, Nakamura S, Nakajima M, Endo H, Dohda T, Takayama N, et al. Two differential flows in a bioreactor promoted platelet generation from human pluripotent stem cell-derived megakaryocytes. *Exp Hematol.* (2013) 41:742–8. doi: 10.1016/j.exphem.2013.04.007
65. Sim X, Poncz M, Gadue P, French DL. Understanding platelet generation from megakaryocytes: implications for *in vitro*-derived platelets. *Blood* (2016) 127:1227–33. doi: 10.1182/blood-2015-08-607929
66. Sullenbarger B, Bahng JH, Gruner R, Kotov N, Lasky LC. Prolonged continuous *in vitro* human platelet production using three-dimensional scaffolds. *Exp Hematol.* (2009) 37:101–10. doi: 10.1016/j.exphem.2008.09.009
67. Pallotta I, Lovett M, Kaplan DL, Balduini A. Three-dimensional system for the *in vitro* study of megakaryocytes and functional platelet production using silk-based vascular tubes. *Tissue Eng Part C Methods* (2011) 17:1223–32. doi: 10.1089/ten.tec.2011.0134
68. Michelson AD, Barnard MR, Hechtman HB, Macgregor H, Connolly RJ, Loscalzo J, et al. *In vivo* tracking of platelets: circulating degranulated platelets rapidly lose surface P-selectin but continue to circulate and function. *Proc Natl Acad Sci USA.* (1996) 93:11877–82. doi: 10.1073/pnas.93.21.11877

19

Hepatitis B Virus Blood Screening: Need for Reappraisal of Blood Safety Measures?

Daniel Candotti* and Syria Laperche

Department of Blood-Transmitted Pathogens, National Transfusion Infectious Risk Reference Laboratory, National Institute of Blood Transfusion, Paris, France

***Correspondence:** Daniel Candotti dcandotti@ints.fr*

Over the past decades, the risk of HBV transfusion–transmission has been steadily reduced through the recruitment of volunteer donors, the selection of donors based on risk-behavior evaluation, the development of increasingly more sensitive hepatitis B antigen (HBsAg) assays, the use of hepatitis B core antibody (anti-HBc) screening in some low-endemic countries, and the recent implementation of HBV nucleic acid testing (NAT). Despite this accumulation of blood safety measures, the desirable zero risk goal has yet to be achieved. The residual risk of HBV transfusion–transmission appears associated with the preseroconversion window period and occult HBV infection characterized by the absence of detectable HBsAg and extremely low levels of HBV DNA. Infected donations tested false-negative with serology and/or NAT still persist and derived blood components were shown to transmit the virus, although rarely. Questions regarding the apparent redundancy of some safety measures prompted debates on how to reduce the cost of HBV blood screening. In particular, accumulating data strongly suggests that HBsAg testing may add little, if any HBV risk reduction value when HBV NAT and anti-HBc screening also apply. Absence or minimal acceptable infectious risk needs to be assessed before considering discontinuing HBsAg. Nevertheless, HBsAg remains essential in high-endemic settings where anti-HBc testing cannot be implemented without compromising blood availability. HBV screening strategy should be decided according to local epidemiology, estimate of the infectious risk, and resources.

Keywords: hepatitis B virus, transfusion, blood safety, nucleic acid testing, HBsAg, anti-HBc, residual risk

INTRODUCTION

Despite a vaccine and antiviral treatments being available, hepatitis B infection remains a global serious public health issue that affects more than two billion people worldwide. Hepatitis B virus belongs to the Hepadnaviridae family, which genome is a ~3.2-kb partially double-stranded circular DNA enclosed in an icosahedral capsid composed of HBV core (HBc) protein and an outer lipid envelope constituting the 30–42 nm in diameter viral particle. Three viral glycosylated surface proteins (large, middle, and small) embedded in the lipid envelop and are involved in virus binding of and entry into susceptible hepatocytes. During the viral life cycle, non-infectious subviral particles, designed HBV surface antigen (HBsAg), that lack the nucleocapsid and are composed of lipids and small surface proteins are produced in 1,000–10,000 excess compared with infectious virions (1). Due to its limited size, the HBV genome has a highly compact structure consisting in four overlapping reading frames for P, S, C, and X genes, which code for the reverse transcriptase/DNA polymerase, surface, core, and X proteins, respectively. The reverse transcription of a pre-genomic RNA intermediate during HBV replication contributes to a significant natural genetic diversity among viral strains. According to this genetic heterogeneity, HBV variants are classified currently into nine genotypes (A–I), some of them being further subdivided in subgenotypes (2). HBV genotypes and subgenotypes have different geographical distributions and are increasingly associated with differences in the natural history, clinical outcome of the infection, and detection. HBV chronic carriage prevalence varies according to geographical regions. Sub-Saharan Africa, South East Asia, China, and the Amazon Basin are highly endemic (≥8% HBsAg seroprevalence) or of higher intermediate endemicity (5–7.99%). Countries from the Mediterranean area, Eastern Europe, the Middle East, and North-West of South America are of lower intermediate endemicity (2–4.99%). Western and Northern Europe, North America, part of South America, India, and Australia have mostly low endemicity levels (<2%) (3).

HBV is transmitted through direct exposure to infected blood or organic fluids. The main routes of infection are sexual, vertical from an infected mother to her child during birth or shortly after, and parenteral including blood transfusion. Before 1970, approximately 6% of multi-transfused patients acquired HBV infection through transfusion. Over the past decades, the risk of HBV transfusion–transmission has been steadily reduced by the successive implementation of various safety measures that include donor selection based on risk-behavior evaluation, serological screening for HBsAg and antibodies against the core protein (anti-HBc), and nucleic acid testing (NAT) for HBV DNA. Nevertheless, hepatitis B remains a viral infection transmissible by transfusion with a residual risk varying according to HBV epidemiology, donor populations, and screening strategies (4). The HBV calculated residual risk estimate ranged between <1 and 1.4 per million donations in low-endemic countries and 16 and >100 in high-endemic countries (5–11). These estimates depend on the mathematical models used and are limited by the lack of recent published reports especially from sub-Saharan Africa. Nevertheless, the residual risk of HBV transfusion–transmission is associated mainly with blood donations tested negative for HBsAg and/or HBV DNA and collected during the early phase of primary infection or during the late stages of infection. Success or failure to intercept such potentially infectious donations may depend on the screening strategy and the performance of both serological and molecular assays used. Despite the existence of this residual risk, questions regarding the apparent redundancy of some of the safety measures implemented over the years (i.e., testing for two direct markers HBsAg and viral DNA) prompted debates on how to reduce the cost of HBV blood screening. However, it appears essential to consider carefully the potential negative impact on blood safety before considering removing any safety procedure, especially in high HBV prevalence settings.

The aim of this review is to examine the intrinsic limits and complementarity of HBV screening strategies of blood donations according to the epidemiologic situation.

BLOOD DONOR SELECTIVE RECRUITMENT

In recent years, careful selection of blood donors became an essential and pragmatic element of blood safety management. In that respect, WHO actively promotes the recruitment of voluntary non-remunerated donors (VNRDs) (12). The generally high prevalence of bloodborne pathogens observed in paid donors supported this strategy. Blood safety is improved further by encouraging VNRDs to become regular donors who show considerably lower prevalence of viral markers (13). This policy was successfully implemented in most of high-income countries but might have negative consequences by excluding traditional family/replacement donors (FRDs) that constitute 4–100% of the blood supply in middle- and low-income countries (mainly in Latin America, Africa, and Central Asia), and therefore perpetuating blood shortage and increasing the cost of blood transfusion (14). Exclusion of FRDs relied mainly on the assumption that these donors could not be differentiated from unsafe paid donors. However, during the past few years, a wealth of evidence has been collected that showed no epidemiological and social difference between FRDs and first-time VNRDs (13, 15–17).

A second level of donor selection based on risk-behavior evaluation and at-risk exposure is used by most blood services worldwide to refuse high-risk individuals to donate blood temporarily or permanently. This procedure generally involves pre-donation risk assessment that requires first-time and regular donors to self-declare or self-complete a questionnaire every time before donation followed by a confidential interview with a medical counselor. However, the effectiveness of this donor self-deferral system strongly depends on donor education and accurate and truthful risk disclosure. Despite limited comprehensive data, the prevalence of overall non-compliance with transfusion-transmitted infection (TTI) risk-related deferral criteria was estimated between 1.65 and 13% in general donor populations, irrespective of blood screening results (18, 19). Studies exploring the rate of non-compliance reported substantially higher rates (~25%) among donors tested positive for viral infection(s) post-donation (20, 21). Recently, an overall 10% non-compliance rate was reported in HBV-infected blood donors from the Netherlands (21). Multiple and complex factors were found associated with non-compliance varying from deliberate (e.g., test seeking, social discomfort, disagreement with deferral criteria, and misunderstanding of the pre-donation screening purpose since donations are tested further) to genuine (e.g., misinterpretation of questions, failure of recall, and erroneous no-risk belief associated with temporally remote exposure) non-disclosures. Furthermore, a main risk factor associated with HBV infection in donors is to originate from an endemic region, and this cannot constitute selection criteria for obvious ethical and practical reasons. It would be unethical to consider this criterion for selection. Albeit the efficacy of donor risk-behavior selection is reflected by the significant lower prevalence of TTIs commonly reported among eligible donors compared with general populations, donor non-compliance may compromise transfusion safety and still needs to be minimized (22).

SERUM ALANINE AMINOTRANSFERASE LEVEL TESTING

Serum alanine aminotransferase (ALT) level testing was initially introduced in blood services as a surrogate marker for what was then called "non-A non-B" hepatitis and was later identified as hepatitis C. Elevated ALT level in an asymptomatic donor may constitute an unspecific marker for a wide range of active and potentially transmissible viral hepatitis infections (i.e., HBV, HAV, HCV, and HEV) (23). Therefore, exclusion of donors with elevated ALT is still used in several middle- and low-income countries, particularly where alternative molecular screening remains not affordable due to cost and technical constraints. However, ALT elevation could be mainly caused by various heterogeneous life style factors that are not related to viral infections and do not constitute a direct threat to blood safety. Unnecessary deferral of donors with elevated ALT might exacerbate the problem of blood shortage as debated in Japan and China where the ALT exclusion threshold was raised to 60 and 50 IU/L, respectively, in an attempt to mitigate the problem (24, 25). Following the implementation of effective serological and NAT for HCV and HBV, most of Western countries discontinued ALT routine donor screening as it was reported to have no significant added value in preventing HBV or HCV TTI (26, 27).

HBsAg TESTING

HBsAg is the first serological marker to appear during the course of HBV infection and remains the first line of HBV screening in blood donors. However, HBsAg screening required an optimal analytical sensitivity to limit the so-called "window period" (WP) phase, commonly defined as the time between infection and detection of the viral antigen, and to enhance the ability to detect the smallest amount of HBsAg during the asymptomatic late stage of chronic infection. Since the first assay available in 1970, the sensitivity and specificity of HBsAg testing has been steadily improving with the development of enzyme immunoassays (EIAs) including enzyme-linked immunoabsorbent assays that use chemoluminescence and polyclonal antibodies. A comparative evaluation of 70 HBsAg assays (51 EIAs and 19 rapid tests) from around the world indicated sensitivities ranging between 0.013 and 1 IU/mL for 84% of the EIAs tested (28). The pre-HBsAg WP was estimated to 32.5 days when using assays with <0.13 IU/mL sensitivity (**Figure 1**). Recently, an

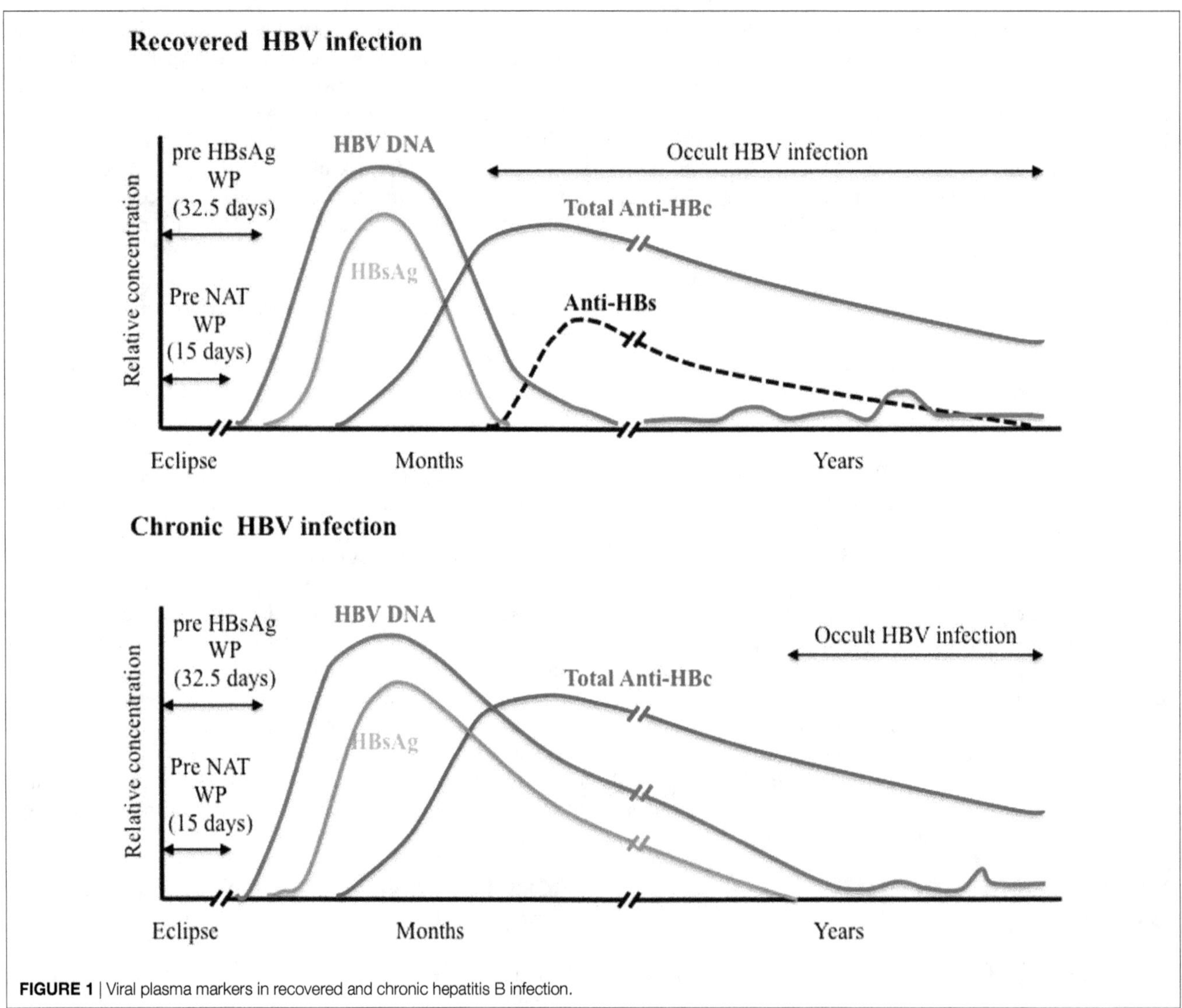

FIGURE 1 | Viral plasma markers in recovered and chronic hepatitis B infection.

enhanced HBsAg chemiluminescent EIA (HBsAg-HQ) and an ultra-high sensitive HBsAg assay employing a semi-automated immune complex transfer chemiluminescence enzyme technique (ICT-CLEIA) were developed that showed 5 and 0.5 mIU/mL sensitivities, respectively (29, 30). These highly sensitive assays were reported to detect HBsAg before HBV DNA in few cases and to possibly reduce the WP to ~14 days (30, 31). However, they were developed mainly to monitor HBV reactivation in treated patients, and their suitability regarding blood donor screening has not been evaluated so far.

Although HBsAg EIAs proved to be effective in blood donor screening, they have many limitations in endemic low/middle-income countries that include high cost, need for sophisticated equipment and trained technicians, continuous supply of electricity, and long turnaround times. Despite showing reduced sensitivity ranging between 1.5 and >4 IU/mL compared with EIAs, rapid tests offer the advantage of low cost and rapid delivery of results and may constitute the only available HBV screening alternative in some resource-limited regions (28, 32–34).

Aside from the WP, HBsAg screening may fail to identify donors infected with HBV variants (35). Mutations within and outside the immunodominant regions of the S protein have been functionally associated with HBsAg structural changes that may lead to impaired detection by the current immunoassays (36, 37). These mutations may arise from escaping the host immune response during infection, vaccine, or HBV immunoglobulin treatment (36, 38). Because of the overlap of P and S ORFs, drug-selected changes in the reverse transcriptase/polymerase may also influence HBsAg detection (39). Recently, chronic HBV infection with antigen levels below the detection threshold of HBsAg assays was increasingly identified in donors and was defined as occult HBV infection (OBI) (40). Studies suggested that undetected HBsAg levels might be associated with mutations in the surface promoter impairing S gene expression or to mutations in the S protein and deletions in the pre-S1/S2 region that reduced HBsAg production and secretion from infected hepatocytes (41–44). In addition, the impact of HBV genotypes on the efficiency of HBsAg detection remains unclear. Albeit the most sensitive and commonly used HBsAg assays showed similar sensitivity in detecting all genotypes, some others had impaired sensitivity for genotypes D–F (28, 45). To overcome the risk of HBsAg false-negative results related to HBV variants, monoclonal antibodies were replaced by polyclonal antibodies against both "wild-type" and variant viruses. HBsAg assays using multiple monoclonal antibodies for capture together with a polyclonal conjugate for detection appear to be the most efficient in detecting a wide range of HBsAg epitopes. Another cause of HBsAg detection failure may be the formation of immune complexes in the presence of HBV surface antibodies (anti-HBs) (46). Furthermore, few studies described unusual cases of acute asymptomatic infections in blood donors detected by HBV NAT that, in contrast to overt acute HBV infection, never showed detectable HBsAg despite seroconverting to anti-HBc overtime and therefore were so-called acute primary OBI (47).

Generally, blood donor samples that initially reacted on a primary screening are retested either in duplicate with the same assay or with an alternative immunoassay. Despite a ≥99.5% specificity level estimated for the majority of HBsAg assays, repeat reactive samples not confirmed by further testing may represent either biological false-reactive or true positive with indeterminate testing results raising issues for donor management and unnecessary loss of blood components (28, 48). An Australian study reported similar HBsAg false-reactive rates of 0.02 and 0.03% in first-time and repeat donors, respectively (49). The causes of HBsAg false reactivity remain unclear but there were reports that HBV vaccination could result in a transient antigenemia in vaccinees (50). False reactivity appeared to be specific for an assay, mostly transient with ~85% of these donors found consistently negative at subsequent donations, and partially associated with low sample-to-cutoff (s/co) ratios (51). This predictive value of s/co ratios should be considered with caution as the s/co ratio distributions for false-reactive and confirmed-positive HBsAg results showed some overlap. Therefore, it is advisable that donors initially testing HBsAg repeat reactive are subject to serologic confirmation using a second immunoassay and a neutralization assay.

ANTI-HBc TESTING

Anti-HBc antibodies usually appear 6–12 weeks after infection are considered non-protective and remain detectable lifelong in immunocompetent subjects constituting the most sensitive marker for exposure to HBV irrespective of the current infection state (**Figure 1**). Anti-HBc may be the only serological marker of HBV infection at the end of a resolving infection when anti-HBs decline to undetectable levels or in OBI where HBsAg may be undetectable and HBV DNA only intermittently detectable (52–55). Recently, increasing evidence of HBV transmission by anti-HBc-reactive donors who repeatedly tested HBsAg and HBV individual donation (ID)-NAT negative with the most sensitive assays available has been reported (56–59).

Since it was first introduced in the late 1980s as a surrogate marker for non-A non-B hepatitis, anti-HBc screening for blood donors remains controversial. It is generally admitted that deferring anti-HBc reactive units would too severely affect blood supply and at a non-affordable cost in medium- and high-endemic areas where anti-HBc prevalence in blood donors ranges between 8 and >50% (i.e., Mediterranean area, East Asia, and sub-Saharan Africa). By contrast, the donor loss caused by universal anti-HBc screening was considered sustainable in some medium/low-endemic countries including Canada, France, Germany, Ireland, the Netherlands, Lebanon, and USA (60, 61). To limit potential donor loss associated with a ~5% anti-HBc prevalence, Japan implemented a complex screening algorithm that includes anti-HBs testing of anti-HBc only donations (56). Donations anti-HBc-reactive only that contain anti-HBs levels >100–500 IU/L are considered eligible for apheresis plasma donation for fractionation while red blood cells and platelets are discarded, and donations with low anti-HBc and anti-HBs levels are rejected. Plasmas from recovered anti-HBc-reactive individuals containing high levels of anti-HBs (e.g., >8,000 IU/L in France) still are needed to supply human hepatitis B immunoglobulin (HIBG) essential to prevent infection in immunosuppressed transplant patients and newborns from HBV-infected mothers. Setting of a minimum limit in anti-HBs titer (usually 500 IU/L) by plasma fractionators and/or national regulatory bodies and implementation of virus reduction procedures assure viral safety of products produced from anti-HBc positive plasmas (http://www.who.int/bloodproducts/publications/en/).

Blood products containing low levels of HBV DNA were found poorly infectious when transfused in the presence of anti-HBs (54). However, the protective level of anti-HBs remains a matter of debates as cases of HBV transfusion–transmission despite concomitant detectable anti-HBs were documented (56, 62, 63). Furthermore, the frequency of anti-HBs carriers among anti-HBc only donors may vary according to HBV epidemiology and vaccine coverage. Studies conducted in Europe, Japan, and North America reported that approximately 90% of anti-HBc-reactive donors carried also anti-HBs and 63–70% of them had titers >100 IU/L (56, 61, 64–66). By contrast, in Ghana, a country with high HBV endemicity, anti-HBs was detected in 24.5% of anti-HBc-reactive donors (67). Caution is required when comparing seroprevalences between studies due to differences in screening algorithms and methodology.

There are still limitations to anti-HBc screening even in low-endemic countries. Albeit recently improved, the specificity of anti-HBc testing is not optimal with reported false-reactivity rates of 16–75% according to assays and screening algorithms (60, 65, 66, 68–70). Recombinant/peptide antigen-based confirmatory assays being not available, secondary testing with an alternative EIA is needed to distinguish between true- and false-positivity and to confirm borderline reactive results that might be associated with low avidity or low titer of antibodies (65, 71). Additional testing for anti-HBs, anti-HBe, and/or HBeAg was considered to have confirmatory value for anti-HBc (56, 65, 66, 68). These complex confirmatory algorithms add economic and organizational constraints to blood services, but it is beneficial for the donor not to be permanently deferred due to false-positive outcome. Another limitation is that anti-HBc screening does not identify WP infections. In addition, simultaneous detection of HBV DNA and anti-HBs in the absence of detectable anti-HBc has been described. These cases were mostly associated with various degree of immunosuppression in patients, core regions deletion, and immunotolerance to HBc antigen in children born from HBeAg-positive mothers (45, 72, 73). However, rare anti-HBc negative/HBV DNA positive cases were also identified in immunocompetent blood donors irrespective of the presence of anti-HBs (53, 74, 75). The frequency of this unusual serological profile seems to vary according to the geographical origin of the donors and possibly vaccine coverage as it was detected in approximately 2 and 13% of OBI donors from Europe and Southeast Asia, respectively (53, 75).

HBV NAT

Nucleic acid testing for HBV DNA was introduced initially in Austria, Germany, and Japan in the late 1900s. After 2004, its implementation for routine blood donation screening was extended worldwide when high-throughput commercial multiplexed NAT assays that included HBV DNA detection in addition to HIV and HCV RNAs were developed and licensed (76). The fully automated commercial multiplex (HBV/HCV/HIV) NAT assays mainly used in transfusion laboratories are the PCR-based cobas TaqScreen MPX version 1 or 2 assays (Roche Diagnostics), and the Procleix Ultrio or Ultrio Plus/Elite assays (Grifols Ltd.) that employ transcription-mediated amplification. The most recent cobas TaqScreen MPX v2 and Procleix Ultrio Plus assays showed specificity of 99.9% and similar 95% limit of detection (LOD) of 2–4 IU/mL for HBV DNA when applied to ID testing (77, 78). This high sensitivity allowed HBV NAT to reduce significantly the WP left by HBsAg testing to an estimated eclipse phase of ~15 days following infection (**Figure 1**) (79). In addition, HBV NAT uncovered a relatively large number of HBsAg-negative occult HBV infection (OBI) among blood donors who tested anti-HBc and/or anti-HBs positive (40). The majority of OBI donors are characterized by a viral load <50 IU/mL and, in some cases, the presence of a high amino acid variability within the S protein that might impair recognition by HBsAg assays (37, 53, 80). The sensitivity of HBV NAT not only depends on the efficiency of the amplification and detections methods used but also on the input plasma volume and the efficiency of the nucleic acid extraction (81). Moreover, the NAT analytical sensitivity may vary considerably between HBV genotypes and between strains of the same genotype, especially genotype D that is the most polymorphic types of HBV (82).

HBV NAT implementation may be limited by the considerable cost of high-throughput fully automated commercial platforms and reagents, especially in low- or medium-income countries of Africa, Asia, and South America. In high-income countries with usually low HBV prevalence, the clinical risk reduction benefit of NAT was associated with an extremely low cost-effectiveness (83). In addition to multiplexing, testing for viral genomes in plasma pools of various sizes was implemented to reduce the cost of NAT. However, there has been a constant progression toward screening smaller pools of six to eight plasmas and to ID. Indeed, the dilution factor introduced by the pooling process reduces the sensitivity of HBV NAT and its ability to detect the low levels of HBV DNA observed in the majority of OBI donors (9, 76, 78). Nevertheless, even ID-NAT may not be sensitive enough to detect potentially infectious blood products with extremely low levels of HBV DNA (56–58).

Discrepancies between serological and molecular testing and the increasing sensitivity of NAT assays make difficult to distinguish between true- and false-positive HBV DNA results. While the commercial multiplex cobas TaqScreen MPX v2 assay allows the simultaneous detection and direct identification of HBV, HCV, and HIV by using virus-specific probes labeled with different dyes, the cobas TaqScreen MPX v1 and Procleix Ultrio Plus assays indicate the presence of viral genomes with a single consensual signal that does not discriminate between these viruses. Therefore, three additional separate virus-specific discriminatory NAT assays are necessary to identify the virus in the originally reactive sample. Discriminatory assays do not fully qualify for confirmation since they are using the same technology and reagents as the initial screening assay. Furthermore, 0.09–0.29% of tested donations reactive in the initial multiplex assay might be non-reactive in the discriminatory assays and/or in the multiplex assay when repeated and were designed non-repeat-reactive

(NRR) (55, 84–87). The reasons of these discrepancies remained unclear but probably reflect Poisson distribution statistics of HBV DNA levels around the assay's LOD, especially in OBI donors, since multiplex and discriminatory assays showed no significant difference in sensitivity according to manufacturers (81, 85). Therefore, ID-NAT screened NRR donations are not released for transfusion in most countries, but donors may remain eligible to donate again as false-positive results cannot be totally excluded.

In the absence of serological investigations or detectable serological markers (i.e., WP), false-positive NAT results due to cross-contamination may be ruled out by retesting a clean sample from the initial plasma bag and by donor follow-up. However, caution should apply when considering the intermittently detectable HBV DNA levels observed in some OBI donors over time (53). NRR donations might be tested for anti-HBc to identify occult HBV carriers (88). NRR donations were reported more frequently reactive for anti-HBc than HBV DNA-negative donations (57 versus 7%, respectively) (85). However, this is not applicable in high-endemic countries such as China that showed an anti-HBc detection rate of 48% in HBV DNA non-reactive donations implicated in reactive minipools of 6 and 68% in ID-NAT NRR donations (86, 87). Alternatively, most ID-NAT users have adopted a serology-like algorithm to discriminate true from false initial reactive results. Multiple repeat tests are performed to identify NRR donations with low viral load using either the multiplex assay or a second independent commercial or in-house assay preferentially targeting a different region of the viral genome. This approach has its drawbacks as it is costly and NAT assays show different levels of sensitivity. Even the most sensitive assays may fail to detect extremely low levels of HBV DNA consistently (81). NAT sensitivity can be enhanced by several non-exclusive changes in the standard procedures aiming to increase the number of HBV DNA templates in the amplification reaction. This can be achieved by purifying viral DNA from larger volumes of plasma and/or by concentrating viral particles with high-speed centrifugation (84). Nevertheless, these approaches are not suitable for large-scale blood donation screening.

HBV SCREENING STRATEGY: ARE ALL VIRAL MARKERS OF VALUE?

Blood donation screening for multiple HBV markers showed discrepant results. The frequency of these discrepancies is difficult to evaluate as they largely depend on the performance of the assays used. Nevertheless, a recent large-scale multiregional study using a comparable HBV screening algorithm showed that among 9,455 confirmed HBV-infected donors, 84.8% were consistently reactive for the three markers, 5.9% were anti-HBc and HBV ID-NAT reactive (OBI), and 2.65% were HBV DNA reactive only [WP (2.25%), primary OBI (0.13%), and anti-HBs only OBI (2.27%)] (89). In addition, 6.45% of donors were HBsAg and anti-HBc reactive but ID-NAT non-reactive. Previous studies reported absence of detectable HBV DNA in 2–20% of HBsAg reactive/anti-HBc reactive donors depending on the LOD of the molecular assays used (67, 76, 78, 82, 90). No confirmed HBV-infected donation testing HBsAg only has been identified so far.

In low-endemic affluent countries, the implementation of both HBsAg, anti-HBc, and HBV NAT provides the optimal level of blood safety by allowing detection of both the early phase of acute infection, persistent occult infection with potential transient detectable viremia, and genetic and/or antigenic viral variants. In addition, ID-NAT should be preferred, as it appeared more efficient in reducing the transmission risk by both WP and occult infections compared with MP-NAT (91). A residual risk would be left by the remaining early infection eclipse phase before HBV DNA becomes detectable. However, questions regarding the apparent redundancy of testing, especially for the two direct markers HBsAg and HBV DNA, prompted debates on how to reduce the cost of HBV blood screening without compromising blood safety. Accumulating data suggests that the apparently efficient combination of NAT and anti-HBc to detect both WP donations and low viremic chronic carriers precludes the need for HBsAg testing. There is increasing evidence that anti-HBc screening, if applied, would have interdicted infectious donations containing extremely low HBV DNA level undetectable with the most sensitive NAT (56–58). Despite being recommended by WHO and included in the European directive, the question of maintaining HBsAg testing might be raised but the absence of potential negative impact on blood safety needs to be assessed before considering discontinuing HBsAg. Therefore, the infectivity of such donations needs to be investigated. However, HBV infectivity studies are limited by the lack of physiologically reliable *in vitro* cell culture and susceptible animal models that generally require high doses of virus for infection (92). An alternative approach might be to isolate and amplify the viral genome present in HBsAg positive/HBV DNA negative donations and to use it in *in vitro* transfection experiments to study the virus replicative properties as a surrogate of infectivity. Dropping a screening test is highly challenging because it is politically sensitive and must not be perceived by the public as exposing recipients to higher risk. Solid scientific evidence about absence or minimal acceptable infectious risk should be provided to regulatory agencies and decision-makers who have the final decision.

In moderate- and high-endemic countries, anti-HBc testing cannot be implemented without compromising blood availability. Therefore, HBsAg testing in combination with NAT would be preferable when resource is available. Highly sensitive ID-NAT only might be considered, as it appears more efficient in detecting HBV chronic carriers than even enhanced sensitivity HBsAg assays. However, the existence of HBsAg reactive/HBV DNA non-reactive donations comforts maintaining HBsAg screening. In high-endemic countries with limited resource, HBV blood safety still relies essentially on HBsAg testing with inexpensive rapid tests as mentioned earlier. Pre-donation viral screening of blood donors using such rapid tests was shown effective and cost-effective, particularly in high-endemic areas (i.e., sub-Saharan Africa and China) where their use reduced wastage of collecting infected blood (93, 94). Additional testing of rapid test-negative donations with a different and more sensitive serological assay and/or expensive NAT still is needed to ensure an acceptable level of safety. The cost limitation of NAT may be addressed by developing in-house multiplex assays and/or by adapting assays using less expensive technologies that have been recently developed for monitoring viral infection at the point-of-care (93, 95, 96). In addition, quality assurance (QA) issues may persist in some resource-limited settings even with relatively simple serological assays such as HBsAg EIAs (33). Possible implementation of sophisticated but non-standardized in-house NAT assays may be prone to even bigger QA problems. Cheaper and well-validated commercial NAT assays may still be preferable to avoid false sense of biosecurity. However, the suitability of these new molecular methods for high-throughput blood screening remains to be evaluated. Discussions on the cost of NAT implementation must also take into account the multiplex format of the currently available systems that include HCV and HIV testing.

Decisions on screening strategy face the dilemma between cost-effectiveness and clinical benefit in terms of HBV TTI risk reduction. The HBV residual transmission risk depends essentially on the infectivity of the blood products from undetected HBV-infected donations. The minimum 50% infectious dose by transfusion was estimated between 20 and 200 IU (100–1,000 virions) in the absence of anti-HBs antibodies (54, 58). The HBV residual TTI risk may also vary according to the donation testing algorithms, the sensitivity of the serological and NAT assays used, and the HBV epidemiology. A recently developed mathematical model estimated this residual risk based on the probability distribution of the HBV DNA load in randomly selected OBI donors, the probability that a given DNA load remains undetected by NAT, and the probability that this DNA load causes infection in the recipient (4). According to this model, 3 and 14% of ID-NAT undetected OBI donations might cause infection by red blood cell concentrates and fresh-frozen plasmas, respectively. Another model based on lookback data reported similar 2–3% residual estimates of OBI transmission (58). When HBsAg and anti-HBc serology in combination with ID-NAT are used, the residual risk may be associated essentially with the remaining DNA-negative eclipse phase in early acute infection and the rare cases of anti-HBs only OBI with intermittent detectable DNA, albeit the infectivity of corresponding blood products is still unknown (75, 79).

Pathogen reduction technologies (PRTs) might represent an attractive strategy. Although PRTs are currently used to complement current testing, there are still limitations to overcome before considering it as a full alternative to testing. Indeed, PRTs were reported not 100% effective against infectious agents present in high loads (97). Efficacy of 2 to >5 log reduction in HBV infectivity has been reported using different PRTs (98). Therefore, the HBV infectious risk may be diminished but not eliminated since HBV viral loads ranging between undetectable to $>10^9$ IU/mL are observed in blood donors (99, 100). In developed countries, PRTs are applied currently to fresh-frozen plasmas and platelet concentrates but remain unavailable for red cell concentrates. Some controversies also persist regarding their impact on the functional aspects of the treated components, albeit the clinical efficacy of treated products is generally satisfactory [see Ref. (98) for review]. Recently, the ability of pathogen reduction of whole blood to provide safer products at an affordable cost for low- and middle-income countries while retaining the ability to prepare functional components was raised (98, 101). The benefits of PRTs might be amplified in low-resource and high-risk countries due to the efficacy against different types of local bloodborne pathogens, including major TTIs (e.g., HBV, HCV, and HIV) and others widely endemic but yet unaddressed (e.g., malaria and bacterial infections). Few reports demonstrated that implementation of PRTs in resource-limited settings was feasible (98, 101). More studies are needed to assess the practical sustainability in terms of infrastructures, supplies, and cost-utility of PRTs implementation in settings where serology and NAT are already limited.

Finally, effective HBV vaccines have been available since the early 1980s, and vaccination has led to a 70–90% decrease in chronic HBV carrier rates in the countries where it has been implemented (102). Therefore, the extension of HBV vaccine coverage in both donor and recipient populations has the potential to reduce significantly the residual risk of HBV transfusion–transmission. However, 5–10% of healthy vaccinees failed to mount an adequate antibody response, vaccination alone failed to protect 10–30% of newborns from HBsAg/HBeAg-positive mothers, and occult HBV infection was frequently reported in individuals with protective anti-HBs levels. Suboptimal protection might be due to heterologous HBsAg (sub)genotypes or to the decline of anti-HBs level over time in vaccinees (63, 102). Nevertheless, a recently developed new generation of recombinant HBV vaccines that contain correctly folded HBsAg and additional neutralizing epitopes of the preS antigens was shown to be highly immunogenic, inducing faster and higher seroprotection rates against HBV compared with conventional vaccines. With optimal vaccines and vaccination coverage, eradication of HBV might be possible but that is another story.

AUTHOR CONTRIBUTIONS

DC and SL contributed equally to the conception and writing of the work and approved it for publication.

REFERENCES

1. Jaroszewicz J, Calle Serrano B, Wursthorn K, Deterding K, Schlue J, Raupach R, et al. Hepatitis B surface antigen (HBsAg) levels in the natural history of hepatitis B virus (HBV)-infection: an European perspective. *J Hepatol* (2010) 52:514–22. doi:10.1016/j.jhep.2010.01.014
2. Kramvis A. Genotypes and genetic variability of hepatitis B virus. *Intervirology* (2014) 57:141–50. doi:10.1159/000360947
3. Schweitzer A, Horn J, Mikolajczyk RT, Krause G, Ott JJ. Estimations of worldwide prevalence of chronic hepatitis B virus infection: a systematic review of data published between 1965 and 2013. *Lancet* (2015) 386:1546–55. doi:10.1016/S0140-6736(15)61412-X
4. Weusten J, van Drimmelen H, Vermeulen M, Lelie N. A mathematical model for estimating residual transmission risk of occult hepatitis B virus infection with different blood safety scenarios. *Transfusion* (2017) 57:841–9. doi:10.1111/trf.14050
5. Shang G, Seed CR, Wang F, Nie D, Farrugia A. Residual risk of transfusion-transmitted viral infections in Shenzhen, China, 2001 through 2004. *Transfusion* (2007) 47:529–39. doi:10.1111/j.1537-2995.2006.01146.x
6. Jayaraman S, Chalabi Z, Perel P, Guerriero C, Roberts I. The risk of transfusion-transmitted infections in sub-Saharan Africa. *Transfusion* (2010) 50:433–42. doi:10.1111/j.1537-2995.2009.002402.x
7. Niederhauser C. Reducing the risk of hepatitis B virus transfusion-transmitted infection. *J Blood Med* (2011) 2:91–102. doi:10.2147/JBM.S12899

8. Kim MJ, Park Q, Min HK, Kim HO. Residual risk of transfusion-transmitted infection with human immunodeficiency virus, hepatitis C virus, and hepatitis B virus in Korea from 2000 through 2010. *BMC Infect Dis* (2012) 12:160. doi:10.1186/1471-2334-12-160
9. Vermeulen M, Coleman C, Mitchel J, Reddy R, van Drimmelen H, Ficket T, et al. Sensitivity of individual-donation and minipool nucleic acid amplification test options in detecting window period and occult hepatitis B virus infections. *Transfusion* (2013) 53:2459–66. doi:10.1111/trf.12218
10. Mapako T, Janssen MP, Mvere DA, Emmanuel JC, Rusakaniko S, Postma MJ, et al. Impact of using different blood donor subpopulations and models on the estimation of transfusion transmission residual risk of human immunodeficiency virus, hepatitis B virus, and hepatitis C virus in Zimbabwe. *Transfusion* (2016) 56:1520–8. doi:10.1111/trf.13472
11. Seed CR, Kiely P, Hoad VC, Keller AJ. Refining the risk estimate for transfusion-transmission of occult hepatitis B virus. *Vox Sang* (2017) 112:3–8. doi:10.1111/vox.12446
12. WHO Expert Group. Expert Consensus Statement on achieving self-sufficiency in safe blood and blood products, based on voluntary non-remunerated blood donation (VNRBD). *Vox Sang* (2012) 103:337–42. doi:10.1111/j.1423-0410.2012.01630.x
13. Asenso-Mensah K, Achina G, Appiah R, Owusu-Ofori S, Allain J-P. Can family or replacement blood donors become regular volunteer donors? *Transfusion* (2014) 54:797–804. doi:10.1111/trf.12216
14. Allain J-P, Sibinga CT. Family donors are critical and legitimate in developing countries. *Asian J Transfus Sci* (2016) 10:5–11. doi:10.4103/0973-6247.164270
15. Loua A, Nze Nkoure G. Relative safety of first-time volunteer and replacement donors in Guinea. *Transfusion* (2010) 50:1850–1. doi:10.1111/j.1537-2995.2010.02718.x
16. Mbanya DN, Feunou F, Tayou TC. Volunteer or family/replacement donations: are the tides changing? *Transfusion* (2010) 50:1849–50. doi:10.1111/j.1537-2995.2010.02656.x
17. Allain J-P. Moving on from voluntary non-remunerated donors: who is the best donor? *Br J Haematol* (2011) 154:763–9. doi:10.1111/j.1365-2141.2011.08708.x
18. Lucky TT, Seed CR, Waller D, Lee JF, McDonald A, Wand H, et al. Understanding noncompliance with selective donor deferral criteria for high-risk behaviors in Australian blood donors. *Transfusion* (2014) 54:1739–49. doi:10.1111/trf.12554
19. Wong HT, Lee SS, Lee CK, Chan DP. Failure of self-disclosure of deferrable risk behaviors associated with transfusion-transmissible infections in blood donors. *Transfusion* (2015) 55:2175–83. doi:10.1111/trf.13106
20. Polizzotto MN, Wood EM, Ingham H, Keller AJ; Australian Red Cross Blood Service Donor and Product Safety Team. Reducing the risk of transfusion-transmissible viral infection through blood donor selection: the Australian experience 2000 through 2006. *Transfusion* (2008) 48:55–63. doi:10.1111/j.1537-2995.2007.01482.x
21. Slot E, Janssen MP, Marijt-van der Kreek T, Zaaijer HL, van de Laar TJ. Two decades of risk factors and transfusion-transmissible infections in Dutch blood donors. *Transfusion* (2016) 56:203–14. doi:10.1111/trf.13298
22. van der Bij AK, Coutinho RA, Van der Poel CL. Surveillance risk profiles among new and repeat blood donors with transfusion-transmissible infections from 1995 through 2003 in the Netherlands. *Transfusion* (2006) 46:1729–36. doi:10.1111/j.1537-2995.2006.00964.x
23. Wang M, He M, Wu B, Ke L, Han T, Wang J, et al. The association of elevated alanine aminotransferase levels with hepatitis E virus infections among blood donors in China. *Transfusion* (2017) 57:273–9. doi:10.1111/trf.13991
24. Shi L, Wang JX, Stevens L, Ness P, Shan H. Blood safety and availability: continuing challenges in China's blood banking system. *Transfusion* (2014) 54:471–82. doi:10.1111/trf.12273
25. Furuta RA, Sakamoto H, Kuroishi A, Yasiui K, Matsukura H, Hirayama F. Metagenomic profiling of the viromes of plasma collected from blood donors with elevated serum alanine aminotransferase levels. *Transfusion* (2015) 55:1889–99. doi:10.1111/trf.13057
26. Busch MP, Korelitz JJ, Kleinman SH, Lee SR, AuBuchon JP, Schreiber GB. Declining value of alanine aminotransferase in screening of blood donors to prevent posttransfusion hepatitis B and C virus infection. The Retrovirus Epidemiology Donor Study. *Transfusion* (1995) 35:903–10. doi:10.1046/j.1537-2995.1995.351196110893.x
27. Ren FR, Wang JX, Huang Y, Yao FZ, Lv YL, Li JL, et al. Hepatitis B virus nucleic acid testing in Chinese blood donors with normal and elevated alanine aminotransferase. *Transfusion* (2011) 51:2588–95. doi:10.1111/j.1537-2995.2011.03215.x
28. Scheiblauer H, El-Nageh M, Diaz S, Nick S, Zeichhardt H, Grunert H-P, et al. Performance evaluation of 70 hepatitis B virus (HBV) surface antigen (HBsAg) assays from around the world by a geographically diverse panel with an array of HBV genotypes and HBsAg subtypes. *Vox Sang* (2010) 98:403–14. doi:10.1111/j.1423-0410.2009.01272.x
29. Matsubara N, Kusano O, Sugamata Y, Itoh T, Mizuii M, Tanaka J, et al. A novel hepatitis B virus surface antigen immunoassay as sensitive as hepatitis B virus nucleic acid testing in detecting early infection. *Transfusion* (2009) 49:585–95. doi:10.1111/j.1537-2995.2008.02026.x
30. Shinkai N, Kusumoto S, Murakami S, Ogawa S, Ri M, Matsui T, et al. Novel monitoring of hepatitis B reactivation based on ultra-high sensitive hepatitis B surface antigen assay. *Liver Int* (2017) 37:1138–47. doi:10.1111/liv.13349
31. Deguchi M, Kagita M, Yoshioka N, Tsukamoto H, Takao M, Tahara K, et al. Evaluation of the highly sensitive chemiluminescent enzyme immunoassay "Lumipulse HBsAg-HQ" for hepatitis B virus screening. *J Clin Lab Anal* (2017). doi:10.1002/jcla.22334
32. Laperche S; Francophone African Group for Research in Blood Transfusion. Multinational assessment of blood-borne virus testing and transfusion safety on the African continent. *Transfusion* (2013) 53:816–26. doi:10.1111/j.1537-2995.2012.03797.x
33. Bloch EM, Shah A, Kaidarova Z, Laperche S, Lefrere JJ, van Hasselt J, et al. A pilot external quality assurance study of transfusion screening for HIV, HCV and HBsAG in 12 African countries. *Vox Sang* (2014) 107:333–42. doi:10.1111/vox.12182
34. Pruett CR, Vermeulen M, Zacharias P, Ingram C, Tayou Tagny C, Bloch EM. The use of rapid diagnostic tests for transfusion infectious screening in Africa: a literature review. *Transfus Med Rev* (2015) 29:35–44. doi:10.1016/j.tmrv.2014.09.003
35. Servant-Delmas A, Mercier-Darty M, Ly TD, Wind F, Alloui C, Sureau C, et al. Variable capacity of 13 hepatitis B virus surface antigen assays for the detection of HBsAg mutants in blood samples. *J Clin Virol* (2012) 53:338–45. doi:10.1016/j.jcv.2012.01.003
36. Hollinger FB. Hepatitis B virus genetic diversity and its impact on diagnostic assays. *J Viral Hepat* (2007) 14(Suppl 1):11–5. doi:10.1111/j.1365-2893.2007.00910.x
37. El Chaar M, Candotti D, Crowther RA, Allain J-P. Impact of HBV surface proteins mutations on the diagnosis of occult HBV infection. *Hepatology* (2010) 52:1600–10. doi:10.1002/hep.23886
38. Gerlich WH. Breakthrough of hepatitis B virus escape mutants after vaccination and virus reactivation. *J Clin Virol* (2006) 36(Suppl 1):S18–22. doi:10.1016/S1386-6532(06)80004-1
39. Pollicino T, Isgrò G, Di Stefano R, Ferraro D, Maimone S, Brancatelli S, et al. Variability of reverse transcriptase and overlapping S gene in hepatitis B virus isolates from untreated and lamivudine-resistant chronic hepatitis B patients. *Antivir Ther* (2009) 14:649–54.
40. Raimondo G, Allain J-P, Brunetto MR, Buendia MA, Chen DS, Colombo M, et al. Statements from the Taormina expert meeting on occult hepatitis B virus infection. *J Hepatol* (2008) 49:652–7. doi:10.1016/j.jhep.2008.07.014
41. Chaudhuri V, Tayal R, Nayak B, Acharya SK, Panda SK. Occult hepatitis B virus infection in chronic liver disease: full-length genome and analysis of mutant surface promoter. *Gastroenterology* (2004) 127:1356–71. doi:10.1053/j.gastro.2004.08.003
42. Fang Y, Teng X, Xu WZ, Li D, Zhao HW, Fu LJ, et al. Molecular characterization and functional analysis of occult hepatitis B virus infection in Chinese patients infected with genotype C. *J Med Virol* (2009) 81:826–35. doi:10.1002/jmv.21463
43. Martin CM, Welge JA, Rouster SD, Shata MT, Sherman KE, Blackard JT. Mutations associated with occult hepatitis B virus infection result in decreased surface antigen expression in vitro. *J. Viral Hepat* (2012) 19:716–23. doi:10.1111/j.1365-2893.2012.01595.x
44. Biswas S, Candotti D, Allain J-P. Specific amino acid substitutions in the S protein prevent its excretion in vitro and may contribute to occult hepatitis B infection. *J Virol* (2013) 87:7882–92. doi:10.1128/JVI.00710-13
45. Gerlich WH, Glebe D, Schüttler CG. Deficiencies in the standardization and sensitivity of diagnostic tests for hepatitis B virus. *J Viral Hepat* (2007) 14(Suppl 1):16–21. doi:10.1111/j.1365-2893.2007.00912.x
46. Zhang JM, Xu Y, Wang XY, Yin YK, Wu XH, Weng XH, et al. Coexistence of hepatitis B surface antigen (HBsAg) and heterologous subtype-specific

antibodies to HBsAg among patients with chronic hepatitis B virus infection. *Clin Infect Dis* (2007) 44:1161–9. doi:10.1086/513200

47. Manzini P, Abate ML, Valpreda C, Milanesi P, Curti F, Rizzetto M, et al. Evidence of acute primary occult hepatitis B virus infection in an Italian repeat blood donor. *Transfusion* (2009) 49:757–64. doi:10.1111/j.1537-2995.2008.02041.x
48. Dow BC. 'Noise' in microbiological screening assays. *Transfus Med* (2000) 10:97–106. doi:10.1046/j.1365-3148.2000.00248.x
49. Kiely P, Stewart Y, Castro L. Analysis of voluntary blood donors with biologic false reactivity on chemiluminescent immunoassays and implications for donor management. *Transfusion* (2003) 43:584–90. doi:10.1046/j.1537-2995.2003.00386.x
50. Dow BC, Yates P, Galea G, Munro H, Buchanan I, Ferguson K. Hepatitis B vaccines may be mistaken for confirmed hepatitis B surface antigen-positive blood donors. *Vox Sang* (2002) 82:15–7. doi:10.1046/j.0042-9007.2001.00125.x
51. Kiely P, Walker K, Parker S, Cheng A. Analysis of sample-to-cutoff ratios on chemiluminescent immunoassays used for blood donor screening highlights the need for serologic confirmatory testing. *Transfusion* (2010) 50:1344–51. doi:10.1111/j.1537-2995.2009.02572.x
52. Allain J-P, Candotti D. Diagnostic algorithm for HBV safe transfusion. *Blood Transfus* (2009) 7:174–82. doi:10.2450/2008.0062-08
53. Candotti D, Lin CK, Belkhiri D, Sakuldamrongpanich T, Biswas S, Lin S, et al. Occult hepatitis B infection in blood donors from South East Asia: molecular characterization and potential mechanisms of occurrence. *Gut* (2012) 61:1744–53. doi:10.1136/gutjnl-2011-301281
54. Allain J-P, Mihaljevic I, Gonzalez-Fraile MI, Gubbe K, Holm-Harritshøj L, Garcia JM, et al. Infectivity of blood products from donors with occult hepatitis B virus infection. *Transfusion* (2013) 53:1405–15. doi:10.1111/trf.12096
55. Kiely P, Margaritis AR, Seed CR, Yang H. Australian Red Cross Blood Service NAT Study Group. Hepatitis B virus nucleic acid amplification testing of Australian blood donors highlights the complexity of confirming occult hepatitis B virus infection. *Transfusion* (2014) 54:2084–91. doi:10.1111/trf.12556
56. Taira R, Satake M, Momose S, Hino S, Suzuki Y, Murokawa H, et al. Residual risk of transfusion-transmitted hepatitis B virus (HBV) infection caused by blood components derived from donors with occult HBV infection in Japan. *Transfusion* (2013) 53:1393–404. doi:10.1111/j.1537-2995.2012.03909.x
57. Vermeulen M, Coleman C, Walker E, Koppleman M, Lelie N, Reddy R. Transmission of occult HBV infection by ID-NAT screened blood. *Vox Sang* (2014) 107(Suppl 1):146.
58. Seed CR, Maloney R, Kiely P, Bell B, Keller A, Pink J, et al. Infectivity of blood components from donors with occult hepatitis B infection – results from an Australian lookback programme. *Vox Sang* (2015) 108:113–22. doi:10.1111/vox.12198
59. Candotti D, Assennato S, Laperche S, Allain J-P, Levicnic-Stezinar S. HBV transfusion-transmission despite the use of highly sensitive HBV NAT. *Vox Sang* (2017) 112(Suppl 1):19.
60. van de Laar TJ, Marijt-van der Kreek T, Molenaar-de Backer MW, Hogema BM, Zaaijer HL. The yield of universal antibody to hepatitis B core antigen donor screening in the Netherlands, a hepatitis B virus low-endemic country. *Transfusion* (2015) 55:1206–13. doi:10.1111/trf.12962
61. Esposito A, Sabia C, Iannone C, Nicoletti GF, Sommese L, Napoli C. Occult hepatitis infection in transfusion medicine: screening policy and assessment of current use of anti-HBc testing. *Transfus Med Hemother* (2017) 44:263–72. doi:10.1159/000460301
62. Levicnic-Stezinar S, Rahne-Potokar U, Candotti D, Lelie N, Allain J-P. Anti-HBs positive occult hepatitis B virus carrier blood infectious in two transfusion recipients. *J Hepatol* (2008) 48:1022–5. doi:10.1016/j.jhep.2008.02.016
63. Stramer SL, Wend U, Candotti D, Foster GA, Hollinger FB, Dodd RY, et al. Nucleic acid testing to detect HBV infection in blood donors. *N Engl J Med* (2011) 364:236–47. doi:10.1056/NEJMoa1007644
64. Kleinman SH, Kuhns MC, Todd DS, Glynn SA, McNamara A, DiMarco A, et al. Frequency of HBV DNA detection in US blood donors testing positive for the presence of anti-HBc: implications for transfusion transmission and donor screening. *Transfusion* (2003) 43:696–704. doi:10.1046/j.1537-2995.2003.00391.x
65. Schmidt M, Nübling CM, Scheiblauer H, Chudy M, Walch LA, Seifried E, et al. Anti-HBc screening of blood donors: a comparison of nine anti-HBc tests. *Vox Sang* (2006) 91:237–43. doi:10.1111/j.1423-0410.2006.00818.x
66. Katz L, Strong M, Tegtmeier G, Stramer S. Performance of an algorithm for the reentry of volunteer blood donors deferred due to false-positive test results for antibody to hepatitis core antigen. *Transfusion* (2008) 48:2315–22. doi:10.1111/j.1537-2995.2008.01844.x
67. Allain J-P, Candotti D, Soldan K, Sarkodie F, Phelps B, Giachetti C, et al. The risk of hepatitis B virus infection by transfusion in Kumasi, Ghana. *Blood* (2003) 101:2419–25. doi:10.1182/blood-2002-04-1084
68. Laperche S, Maniez M, Barlet V, El Ghouzzi MH, Le Vacon F, Levayer T, et al. A revised method for estimating hepatitis B virus transfusion residual risk based on antibody to hepatitis B core antigen incident cases. *Transfusion* (2008) 48:2308–14. doi:10.1111/j.1537-2995.2008.01873.x
69. Hourfar MK, Walch LA, Geusendam G, Dengler T, Janetzko K, Gubbe K, et al. Sensitivity and specificity of Anti-HBc screening assays – which assay is best for blood donor screening? *Int J Lab Hematol* (2009) 31:649–56. doi:10.1111/j.1751-553X.2008.01092.x
70. Juhl D, Knobloch JK, Görg S, Hennig H. Comparison of two test strategies for clarification of reactive results for anti-HBc in blood donors. *Transfus Med Hemother* (2016) 43:37–43. doi:10.1159/000441676
71. Ollier L, Laffont C, Kechkekian A, Doglio A, Giordanengo V. Detection of antibodies to hepatitis B core antigen using the Abbott ARCHITECT anti-HBc assay: analysis of borderline reactive sera. *J Virol Methods* (2008) 154:206–9. doi:10.1016/j.jviromet.2008.09.006
72. Lai MW, Lin TY, Liang KH, Lin WR, Yeh CT. Hepatitis B viremia in completely immunized individuals negative for anti-hepatitis B core antibody. *Medicine (Baltimore)* (2016) 95:e5625. doi:10.1097/MD.0000000000005625
73. Anastasiou OE, Widera M, Verheyen J, Korth J, Gerken G, Helfritz FA, et al. Clinical course and core variability in HBV infected patients without detectable anti-HBc antibodies. *J Clin Virol* (2017) 93:46–52. doi:10.1016/j.jcv.2017.06.001
74. Laperche S, Guitton C, Smilovici W, Courouce A-M. Blood donors infected with the hepatitis B virus but persistently lacking antibodies to the hepatitis B core antigen. *Vox Sang* (2001) 80:90–4. doi:10.1046/j.1423-0410.2001.00016.x
75. Deng X, Candotti D, Wang D, Wang X, Chen H, Laperche S, et al. Concomitant presence of HBV DNA and anti-HBs as only markers of HBV infection in donors with occult hepatitis B in Dalian, China. *Vox Sang* (2016) 111 (Suppl 1):57.
76. Roth WK, Busch MP, Schuller A, Ismay S, Cheng A, Seed CR, et al. International survey on NAT testing of blood donations: expanding implementation and yield from 1999 to 2009. *Vox Sang* (2012) 102:82–90. doi:10.1111/j.1423-0410.2011.01506.x
77. Müller MM, Fraile MI, Hourfar MK, Peris LB, Sireis W, Rubin MG, et al. Evaluation of two, commercial, multi-dye, nucleic acid amplification technology tests, for HBV/HCV/HIV-1/HIV-2 and B19V/HAV, for screening blood and plasma for further manufacture. *Vox Sang* (2013) 104:19–29. doi:10.1111/j.1423-0410.2012.01635.x
78. Stramer SL, Krysztof DE, Brodsky JP, Fickett TA, Reynolds B, Dodd RY, et al. Comparative analysis of triplex nucleic acid test assays in United States blood donors. *Transfusion* (2013) 53:2525–37. doi:10.1111/trf.12178
79. Lelie N. Occult HBV infection and blood safety: a review. In: Allain J-P, Fu Y, Li C, Raimondo G, editors. *Occult Hepatitis B Infection*. Beijing: Science Press (2015). p. 210–32.
80. Candotti D, Grabarczyk P, Ghiazza P, Roig R, Casamitjana N, Iudicone P, et al. Characterization of occult hepatitis B virus from blood donors carrying genotype A2 or genotype D strains. *J Hepatol* (2008) 49:537–47. doi:10.1016/j.jhep.2008.04.017
81. Enjalbert F, Krysztof DE, Candotti D, Allain J-P, Stramer SL. Comparison of seven hepatitis B virus (HBV) nucleic acid testing assays in selected samples with discrepant HBV marker results from United States blood donors. *Transfusion* (2014) 54:2485–95. doi:10.1111/trf.12653
82. Grabarczyk P, van Drimmelen H, Kopacz A, Gdowska J, Liszewski G, Piotrowski D, et al. Head-to-head comparison of two transcription-mediated amplification assay versions for detection of hepatitis B virus, hepatitis C virus, and human immunodeficiency virus Type 1 in blood donors. *Transfusion* (2013) 53:2512–24. doi:10.1111/trf.12190
83. Janssen MP, van Hulst M, Custer B; ABO RBDM Health Economics and Outcomes Working Group & Collaborators. An assessment of differences in costs and health benefits of serology and NAT screening of donations for blood transfusion in different Western countries. *Vox Sang* (2017) 112:518–25. doi:10.1111/vox.12543
84. Candotti D, Allain J-P. Molecular virology in transfusion medicine laboratory. *Blood Transfus* (2013) 11:203–16. doi:10.2450/2012.0219-12

85. Charlewood R, Flanagan P. Ultrio and Ultrio Plus non-discriminating reactives: false reactives or not? *Vox Sang* (2013) 104:7–11. doi:10.1111/j.1423-0410.2012.01624.x
86. Wang L, Chang L, Xie Y, Huang C, Xu L, Qian R, et al. What is the meaning of a nonresolved viral nucleic acid test-reactive minipool? *Transfusion* (2015) 55:395–404. doi:10.1111/trf.12818
87. Gou H, Pan Y, Ge H, Zheng Y, Wu Y, Zeng J, et al. Evaluation of an individual-donation nucleic acid amplification testing algorithm for detecting hepatitis B virus infection in Chinese blood donors. *Transfusion* (2015) 55:2272–81. doi:10.1111/trf.13135
88. Cable R, Lelie N, Bird A. Reduction of the risk of transfusion-transmitted viral infection by nucleic acid amplification testing in the Western Cape of South Africa: a 5-year review. *Vox Sang* (2013) 104:93–9. doi:10.1111/j.1423-0410.2012.01640.x
89. Lelie N, Bruhn R, Busch M, Vermeulen M, Tsoi WC, Kleinman S, et al. Detection of different categories of hepatitis B virus (HBV) infection in a multi-regional study comparing the clinical sensitivity of hepatitis B surface antigen and HBV-DNA testing. *Transfusion* (2017) 57:24–35. doi:10.1111/trf.13819
90. Kuhns MC, Kleinman SH, McNamara AL, Rawal B, Glynn S, Busch MP. Lack of correlation between HBsAg and HBV DNA levels in blood donors who test positive for HBsAg and anti-HBc: implications for future HBV screening policies. *Transfusion* (2004) 44:1332–9. doi:10.1111/j.1537-2995.2004.04055.x
91. Vermeulen M, van Drimmelen H, Coleman C, Mitchel J, Reddy R, Lelie N. A mathematical approach to estimate the efficacy of individual-donation and minipool nucleic acid amplification test options in preventing transmission risk by window period and occult hepatitis B virus infections. *Transfusion* (2014) 54:2496–504. doi:10.1111/trf.12657
92. Allweiss L, Dandri M. Experimental *in vitro* and *in vivo* models for the study of human hepatitis B virus infection. *J Hepatol* (2016) 64(Suppl 1):S17–31. doi:10.1016/j.hep.2016.02.012
93. Owusu-Ofori S, Temple J, Sarkodie F, Anokwa M, Candotti D, Allain J-P. Predonation screening of blood donors with rapid tests: implementation and efficacy of a novel approach to blood safety in resource-poor settings. *Transfusion* (2005) 45:133–40. doi:10.1111/j.1537-2995.2004.04279.x
94. Li L, Li KY, Yan K, Ou G, Li W, Wang J, et al. The history and challenges of blood donor screening in China. *Transfus Med Rev* (2017) 31:89–93. doi:10.1016/j.tmrv.2016.11.001
95. Cai Z, Lou G, Cai T, Yang J, Wu N. Development of a novel genotype-specific loop-mediated isothermal amplification technique for Hepatitis B virus genotypes B and C genotyping and quantification. *J Clin Virol* (2011) 52:288–94. doi:10.1016/j.jcv.2011.08.013
96. Ondiek J, Namukaya Z, Mtapuri-Zinyowera S, Balkan S, Elbireer A, Ushiro Lumb I, et al. Multicountry validation of SAMBA – a novel molecular point-of-care test for HIV-1 detection in resource-limited setting. *J Acquir Immune Defic Syndr* (2017) 76:e52–7. doi:10.1097/QAI.0000000000001476
97. Hauser L, Roque-Afonso AM, Beylouné A, Simonet M, Deau Fischer B, Burin des Roziers N, et al. Hepatitis E transmission by transfusion of Intercept blood system-treated plasma. *Blood* (2014) 123:796–7. doi:10.1182/blood-2013-09-524348
98. Ware AD, Jacquot C, Tobian AAR, Gehrie EA, Ness PM, Bloch EM. Pathogen reduction and blood transfusion safety in Africa: strengths, limitations and challenges of implementation in low-resource settings. *Vox Sang* (2018) 113:3–12. doi:10.1111/vox.12620
99. Garmiri P, Loua A, Haba N, Candotti D, Allain J-P. Deletions and recombinations in the core region of hepatitis B virus genotype E strains from asymptomatic blood donors in Guinea, west Africa. *J Gen Virol* (2009) 90:2444–51. doi:10.1099/vir.0.012013-0
100. Grabarczyk P, Garmiri P, Liszewski G, Doucet D, Sulkowska E, Brojer E, et al. Molecular and serological characterization of hepatitis B virus genotype A and D infected blood donors in Poland. *J Viral Hepat* (2010) 17:444–52. doi:10.1111/j.1365-2893.2009.01192.x
101. Allain J-P, Goodrich R. Pathogen reduction of whole blood: utility and feasibility. *Transfus Med* (2017) 27(Suppl 5):320–6. doi:10.1111/tme.12456
102. Gerlich WH. Prophylactic vaccination against hepatitis B: achievements, challenges and perspectives. *Med Microbiol Immunol* (2015) 204:39–55. doi:10.1007/s00430-014-0373-y

An Original Approach to Evaluating the Quality of Blood Donor Selection: Checking Donor Questionnaires and Analyzing Donor Deferral Rate

Philippe Gillet and Esther Neijens*

Service du Sang, Belgian Red-Cross, Suarlée, Belgium

Correspondence:
Philippe Gillet
philippe.gillet@croix-rouge.be

Blood donor selection is a cornerstone for blood transfusion safety, designed to safeguard the health of both donors and recipients. In the Service du Sang, Belgian Red Cross, French and German-speaking part of Belgium (SFS), health professionals (HPs) are allowed to interview donors on their own after formal qualification. This qualification is afterward evaluated by means of two complementary quality indicators: monitoring of donor health questionnaires (DHQs) and analysis of donor deferral rate. The study aims to evaluate the degree to which both quality indicators may be useful and appropriate tools to evaluate the quality of blood donor selection. An analysis performed on 2016 data showed that noncompliance detected by means of DHQ monitoring seems to be more frequent in HPs who conduct a low number of interviews compared to all HPs as a group (5.67 vs. 3.23%; $p < 0.001$). Deferral rates are also higher in HPs with a lower activity compared to HPs who interview more donors (14.80 vs. 13.00%, $p < 0.001$). Furthermore, statistically differences are observed between the type of blood donation venue in terms of the global deferral rate (for instance fixed site vs. schools: 11.9 vs. 19.5%; $p < 0.001$), and specific reasons for deferral (such as sexual risk behavior and travel in at-risk areas, the differences being highly significant between each category of blood donation venue; $p < 0.001$). Providing the HPs with feedback on these findings was an opportunity to draw their attention to some aspects of the selection process in order to improve it.

Keywords: blood donor selection, transfusion safety, evaluation, donor health questionnaire, donor deferral rate

INTRODUCTION

Blood donor selection is a cornerstone for blood transfusion safety, designed to safeguard the health of both donors and recipients. Donor safety (1, 2) is targeted by reducing the risk of complications associated with blood donation (rare but not absent) (3) and, in order to improve recipient safety, blood donor selection attempts to reduce the risk of transfusion-transmitted infections (TTI). A recent study conducted in Senegal confirmed what is globally accepted based on epidemiological data, i.e., the efficacy of blood donor selection in reducing the prevalence of HIV seropositive donors (4).

Abbreviations: DHQ, Donor Health Questionnaire; HP, health professional; QCF, Questionnaire Control Form; SFS, Service du Sang, Belgian Red Cross, French and German-speaking part of Belgium; TTI, transfusion-transmitted infections.

The European Directive 2005/62/EC (5) recommends entrusting the responsibility for blood donor selection to qualified health professionals (HPs). Training in blood donor selection encompasses both a theoretical and a practical approach: the HP has to be able to take the right decision (knowledge of blood donor selection criteria) and to communicate this decision to donors in an appropriately understanding manner (professional relationship with each donor based on trust).

The blood donor selection process usually encompasses four main steps (6):

- Pre-donation information and advice: this is usually provided in a leaflet, especially about transfusion-transmitted infections (and the associated risk factors) and the potential risks of donation.
- Donor Health Questionnaire (DHQ): filled out by the donor alone (before the pre-donation interview) or with the HP (during the pre-donation interview).
- Donor interview: conducted by a qualified HP.
- Donor health assessment: at the end of the interview, the donor is declared eligible to give blood or deferred temporarily or permanently; this decision also takes into account physical and biological parameters, such as hemoglobin level, blood pressure, heart rate, and weight.

Before an HP is allowed to conduct donor interviews and selection alone, qualification must be acquired.

In the Service du Sang, Belgian Red Cross, French and German-speaking part of Belgium (SFS), the following qualification criteria are used and as recommended in terms of training objectives (7), communicated to the HPs at the start of the training session:

- Theoretical training is provided (possibly *via* e-learning) focusing on blood donor selection criteria: a predefined grade must be achieved in order to continue the training,
- the ability to take the right decision is assessed in simulated cases by a senior HP/supervisor,
- a certain number of donor interviews is overseen by a senior HP/supervisor in order to assess the trainee's ability to take the right decision and to communicate properly with donor, especially when the donor is deferred,
- the supervisor monitors the first interviews performed alone by checking the donor health questionnaires (DHQs) (see below).

Each step must be successfully completed before the next step is taken. When all steps are completed, the HP is qualified for donor selection.

After this initial qualification, HPs are allowed to interview donors alone, but their qualification is not infinite. It is nevertheless difficult to evaluate the quality of this activity. As confidentiality is a prerequisite for the pre-donation interview, regular attendance by a third person (supervisor) is not recommended even with a view to evaluating the competency of each HP. Furthermore, the presence of a third person could influence the behavior of both the donor, who might hesitate to disclose all the relevant data [donors' compliance is not always achieved (8, 9)] and the HP, who might be more inclined to apply all the procedures than when conducting the interviews alone.

Blood donor selection by qualified HPs can be evaluated in various ways. For example, the quality of the decision taken by a trainee (nurse, technician, or physician) can be assessed by comparison with the decision taken by a senior physician, the latter being considered as the reference (10). In the SFS, the qualification of each HP is formally monitored through two main quality indicators, the monitoring of DHQs and the donor deferral rate:

- A sample of DHQs filled in by donors and analyzed by the HPs during the pre-donation interview are monitored yearly for each HP in order to assess whether the HP in question collected the relevant data and used them properly.
- The donor deferral rate observed for each individual HP is compared to the overall rate for all HPs within the SFS in order to detect differences that might reflect different ways of selecting donors.

Both quality indicators are used routinely by the SFS. The study aims to analyze their adequacy to evaluate the quality of blood donor selection and to possibly improve blood transfusion safety.

Results of both indicators are provided to each individual HP to improve their blood donor selection, and, as a consequence, to improve blood transfusion safety.

Evaluations performed on blood donor selections, which took place in 2016 in the SFS are analyzed and the results reported in the study that provides some examples of issues detected and thoughts about the further development of these tools.

MATERIALS AND METHODS

The study was conducted as an audit of blood donor medical selection analyzing two indicators: DHQs monitoring and blood donor deferral rate. This audit was submitted to the Erasme-ULB Ethics Committee (Brussels, Belgium), which determined that full review and approval was not required.

DHQs Monitoring

In the SFS, each HP ideally undergoes one annual monitoring by a senior HP (supervisor). The paper version of the DHQ filled in by the donor and checked by the HP with the donor during the face-to-face interview, the data entry in the data-base (eProgesa® software, MAK systems, Paris, France) and the decision taken are checked for a series of DHQs, typically all the DHQs for one blood collection session for this HP.

The DHQ used by the SFS is made up of 43 questions, of which 42 are to be answered by ticking a yes/no box. One text answer is mandatory, i.e., country of birth. The DHQ must mandatorily be dated and signed by both the donor and the HP. In addition, HPs are asked to document the interview and their reading and checking of the DHQ with the donor by writing a comment and/or additional info and/or "ok" or at least by adding a checkmark next to the answer provided by the donor, if this answer could be a potential reason for deferral or when the "yes" answer generates a specific laboratory analysis request when entered into the database. This is the case for example for the question "Have you ever had a malaria attack?" which induces the detection of malaria antibodies.

Blood Donor Deferral Rate

Data collected in eProgesa from January to December 2016 involving all donations and including HPs identification, decision taken by the HP (donor acceptance or deferral), reason for deferral (when the donor is deferred), and type of blood donation venue (fixed site or mobile site, i.e., village, school, office, or special) were analyzed.

Statistical Analysis

In order to evaluate HPs' compliance in donor selection, the following items are checked, according to the DHQ used by the SFS. These items are listed in a standardized questionnaire control form (QCF) used by supervisors in order to document the control:

- Donor signature
- HP signature
- Donor's "Yes" answers documented
- Answers to all questions
- Coherent answer on DHQ and entry into data-base
- Donor selection.

Data from all QCFs collected in 2016 were recorded in an Excel data-base and analyzed by descriptive statistics (mean, median, and percentiles), including the identification of HPs, the blood donation venue, the category of donor (first-time vs. regular or repeat donor), and the six types of noncompliance listed above.

Blood donor deferral rates were calculated globally and for each specific deferral category for the whole group of HPs, for HPs who conducted fewer than 500 interviews during the research period and for those who conducted 500 interviews or more. Deferral rates in the various blood donation venues were compared. The statistical analysis was performed by using the chi square test in order to evaluate the degree to which observed differences were statistically significant.

RESULTS

During the study period, 209,617 pre-donation interviews were conducted by 125 HPs (**Table 1**).

Out of these 125 HPs, 57 (46%) were assessed with a total of 2,063 DHQs. More HPs may have been monitored but were not included in the study because the QCFs were not provided on time.

Deferral rates were calculated and analyzed for all donations.

Donor Health Questionnaires

This study reports data from 2,063 DHQ checks carried out within the SFS, i.e., 0.98% of all DHQs for 2016.

Table 2 provides data analyzed from the 57 monitored HPs. The proportion of DHQs assessed for first-time donors is 12.4% (256 out of 2,063).

Noncompliances for the various parameters checked by means of the QCF, as described above, are displayed in absolute numbers and in percentages of the total number of DHQs checked for all HPs as a group. The distribution according to median and P10, 75 and 90 shows great inter-individual variability.

Table 3 provides data analyzed from a total of 1,610 DHQs from HPs who interviewed more than 500 donors during the study period ($N = 47$), i.e., a selection of HPs who performed donor selection most regularly.

For the whole group of HPs (**Table 2**), 5.67% of the DHQs were rejected by the supervisor.

The most frequent noncompliance issue was a missing answer, i.e., no box ticked by the donor and no comment provided by the HCP: 3.01% of the checked DHQs.

The second most frequent noncompliance was missing HP signature (2.76%).

The least frequently reported noncompliance was missing donor signature: 5 times out of 2,063, i.e., 0.24%.

Overall, the quality of the decision (donor acceptance or deferral) was considered as being wrong in 0.92% of the cases.

TABLE 1 | Activity of health professionals (HPs).

2016	SFS	Fewer than 500 pre-donation interviews	500 or more pre-donation interviews
HP	125	34	91
Pre-donation interviews	209,617	10,861	198,756
Interview/HP	1,677	319	2,184

TABLE 2 | Monitoring of donor health questionnaires.

	No. of health professionals (HPs)	No. of questionnaires	No. of first-time donors	Questionnaires not OK	Donor's signature missing	HP's signature missing	Response not documented	No response to at least one question	Discrepancy between questionnaire and decision	Quality of decision
SFS	57	2,063	256	117	5	57	22	62	10	19
%				5.67%	0.24%	2.76%	1.07%	3.01%	0.48%	0.92%
Median				0.00%	0.00%	0.00%	0.00%	0.00%	0.00%	0.00%
P10				0.00%	0.00%	0.00%	0.00%	0.00%	0.00%	0.00%
P75				4.76%	0.00%	2.94%	0.00%	1.69%	0.00%	0.00%
P90				8.09%	0.00%	5.91%	4.46%	4.86%	0.00%	3.02%

Data were analyzed from 57 HPs whose questionnaires were monitored in 2016.

TABLE 3 | Monitoring of donor health questionnaires (more than 500 pre-donation interviews).

	No. of health professionals (HPs)	No. of questionnaires	No. of first-time donors	Questionnaires not OK	Donor's signature missing	HPs signature missing	Response not documented	No response to at least one question	Discrepancy between questionnaire and decision	Quality of decision
SFS	47	1,610	193	52	3	34	14	22	2	9
%				3.23%	0.19%	2.11%	0.87%	1.37%	0.12%	0.56%
Median				0.00%	0.00%	0.00%	0.00%	0.00%	0.00%	0.00%
P10				0.00%	0.00%	0.00%	0.00%	0.00%	0.00%	0.00%
P75				4.27%	0.00%	1.14%	0.00%	0.00%	0.00%	0.00%
P90				8.09%	0.00%	5.08%	3.02%	4.63%	0.00%	2.56%

Data were analyzed from HPs who have interviewed more than 500 donors during the study period.

The HP subgroup who interviewed most donors on an annual basis (more than 500) had lower percentages of noncompliance than the whole group for all parameters checked (**Table 3**).

A great variability was observed for the various criteria in both the whole group of HPs and in the group of HPs who interviewed more than 500 donors during the study period.

Blood Donor Deferral Rate

A total of 13.09% of the 209,617 donors interviewed by the 125 HPs were deferred for blood donation (**Table 4**).

The deferral reason was recorded by the HPs in the data-base during the pre-donation interview for 85.12% of donors.

The main reasons were:

- Exposure to potential transfusion-transmitted infectious agents within the deferral period, due to surgery, endoscopy, tattoo, piercing, potentially contaminating accident, acupuncture, mesotherapy, or blood transfusion: 1.60% (traveling and sexual risk behavior are not included in this item).
- Traveling in a region where transfusion-transmitted infectious agents are present, mainly malaria, Chagas disease, and West Nile Virus infection: 1.57%.
- Sexual risk behavior, i.e., new sexual partner within the deferral period, men having sex with men, or sexual partner infected with HIV, HBV, or HCV: 1.09%.

Other deferral reasons, such as current infection or serious medical condition were less frequent.

Quite a number of donors (4.5%) were not allowed to give blood, but blood analyses were performed in order to check previous results. The main reason is probably low hemoglobin level, but this information is not available for analysis.

Table 4 provides data on deferral rates for the group of HPs as a whole, for HPs who interviewed fewer than 500 donors and for HPs who interviewed at least 500 donors during the same study period. SDs suggest major inter-individual differences.

In HPs who interview more donors (at least 500/year) overall deferral rates were lower and, more interestingly, variability tended to decrease, particularly for the global deferral rate (SD: 9.84% compared to 3.28%).

Furthermore, statistically significant differences are observed between the type of blood donation venue, i.e., fixed or the various types of mobile sites (**Table 5**). For instance, there is a significant difference in global deferral rates (**Table 5**) between fixed and mobile sites, such as schools, offices, and special campaigns (for instance, during periods requiring a call to potential donors by media). Differences between each category (fixed sites, villages, schools, offices, and special drives) are highly significant with respect to sexual risk behavior and travel in at-risk areas (**Table 5**).

TABLE 4 | Comparison of deferral rates between health professionals (HPs) who conducted fewer than or at least 500 pre-donation interviews during 2016.

2016		SFS (%)	Fewer than 500 pre-donation interviews (%)	500 or more pre-donation interviews (%)	*p*
Deferral rate	μ	13.09	14.80	13.00	<0.001
	σ	5.95	9.84	3.28	
Recording rate	μ	85.12	78.47	85.54	<0.001
	σ	12.72	14.33	11.50	
Sexual risk behavior deferral rate	μ	1.09	1.25	1.08	NS
	σ	0.68	0.80	0.64	
Travel deferral rate	μ	1.57	1.25	1.59	<0.01
	σ	1.01	0.89	1.05	
Exposure to potential TTI	μ	1.60	1.58	1.60	NS
	σ	0.56	0.73	0.48	

TTI, transfusion-transmitted infections; NS, not significant.

Data for each individual HP are compared with those of the group as a whole and to those of HPs working in the same type of venue as the monitored HPs. This comparison allowed to identify differences that were discussed with the HP, an opportunity to assess their blood donor selection activity and, when needed, to provide additional training.

DISCUSSION

The analysis of the data suggests that checking DHQs and analyzing blood donor deferral rate on an individual basis may be used as quality indicators of blood donor selection and as a basis for improvement of this activity.

Donor Health Questionnaires

The completion of DHQs is a useful tool to provide HPs with adequate data to take the right decision. Using a DHQ reduces the risk of transmission of blood-borne infectious agents by transfusion. A study showed a significant reduction in Gabonese seropositive donors (hepatitis B, hepatitis C, and syphilis) who

TABLE 5 | Comparison of donors' deferral rate between fixed and mobile sites.

2016	Fixed sites (%)	Villages (%)	Schools (%)	Offices (%)	Special (%)	Comments
Overall deferral rate	11.9	12.3	19.5	16.0	19.5	No difference between schools and special drives $p < 0.05$ between fixed sites and villages $p < 0.001$ between all other categories
Sexual risk behavior	0.92	0.66	4.03	1.39	2.32	$p < 0.001$ between all categories
Travel	1.40	0.98	1.79	3.91	2.82	$p < 0.001$ between all categories
Exposure to potential transfusion-transmitted infections	1.19	1.70	2.78	1.83	2.82	$p < 0.001$ between all categories (except between villages and offices, and between schools and special: not significant)

completed a DHQ (11), although this encouraging finding was not observed in all studies (12), probably partly because of differences in the prevalence of pathogens.

One limitation of the DHQ is its understanding by all donors; its form has to be regularly analyzed and reviewed (13, 14), in particular, to ensure donors' compliance with respect to questions about sexual risk behaviors (15, 16); nevertheless, direct questions pinpointing sexual behavior may reduce donor's intention to return for a further donation (especially in the case of experienced blood donors) (16).

Another limitation of the DHQ is the noncompliance on the part of some donors when it comes to responding properly and honestly to all questions. To improve donors satisfaction and probably to make donors more compliant when it comes to filling out the DHQ honestly, an abbreviated questionnaire may be an alternative at least for repeat and regular donors (17).

A standardized DHQ is used by most blood services to collect relevant data in order to evaluate the donor's eligibility to give blood. Each blood service uses its own standardized DHQ. Exceptions are the USA and Canada, where uniform DHQs have been used since 2005. In Germany, a national DHQ has been recently tested (16).

An automated computer-assisted pre-donation interview could improve the collection of relevant data (14, 18) but in most countries, the pre-donation interview is conducted without the assistance of a computer and remains a human activity. An evaluation of this activity could, therefore, be useful to improve donor selection.

These critical findings highlight the importance of analyzing DHQs as a means to evaluate the quality of the blood donor selection, confidentiality required by the donor interview conflicting with the attendance of a supervisor.

In this study, monitoring DHQs by means of the QCF allowed to identify a number of issues which otherwise would have gone unnoticed and adapted feedback was provided to the HPs concerned.

Some issues occured only once, as for any human activity: one HP for example, forgot to make sure that an answer was given to one question in the set of DHQs checked. This HP was then reminded of the importance of staying focused. If several questions remained unanswered, the HP received different feedback and was possibly monitored for a certain period until they improved.

An issue such as a missing HP signature is major, but was mostly due to simple forgetfulness on the part of the HP who made an adequate donor selection. In fact, as HPs are asked to comment/sign off on all "yes" answers that might be a reason for deferral, tracking their comments made it possible to confirm whether the DHQ has been checked during donor selection. Missing signatures could, therefore, be noticed by the supervisor in most cases.

The same type of noncompliance issues detected during the DHQ checks may have a very different impact on transfusion safety. The impact may be possible transmission of a TTI, a health consequence for the donor, or rather noncompliance with the legal framework which may have no immediate consequences for safety in a specific case, but should of course be avoided.

Therefore, it is important that the supervisor who performs the checks have thorough knowledge of the consequences of all issues, and give appropriate feedback to the HP involved.

The supervisor adapts their evaluation of the HP when performing DHQ controls accordingly. The examples below illustrate this individualized approach:

- A not documented "yes" answer or no answer to the question: When the question involves antecedents of allergy or asthma, the consequence is rather minor, whereas when it concerns contact with a person suffering from hepatitis or another infectious disease, this may have major consequences. In fact, the HP may have missed a reason for deferral or for requesting additional laboratory analyses, with potential transmission of a TTI.
- Discrepancies between DHQ completion and data entry: For instance, it is more important to enter the actual "yes" answer in the data-base for the question "Have you ever had a malaria attack?" in the case of a first-time donor than for "Have you ever been operated on since you were born?" Indeed, a positive answer to antecedents of malaria automatically generates an analysis request and possibly deferral of the donor. Therefore, if the appropriate answer is not entered, the opportunity for an analysis request and/or donor deferral will be missed.
- Donor selection: Missing deferral of a donor who is at risk of having been infected with a blood-borne agent, such as a donor who has a new sexual partner within the deferral period, can have a safety impact. On the other hand, accepting a donor whose hemoglobin level is 0.1 g/dL below the legal threshold for giving blood is wrong, but has no safety consequences for either the recipient or the donor.

The least frequent noncompliance issue observed in this study, the missing donor signature, is a major one as without this confirmation from the donor, the blood bag cannot be used.

Sometimes systematic or very frequent issues were detected in some or all of the HPs in a group, or in an individual HP. For the supervisor, this was an opportunity to remind the HPs of the rules to be followed in order to improve blood collection quality and safety. In some cases, the issue was a subject for a continued education session.

Examples:

- The majority of HPs in a group understood the question involving a "donor born in a malaria region, who has lived in this region for the 5 first years of their life?" as living in a malaria region for the *full* first 5 years. Therefore, if the donor has only lived in this region for 1 year, the answer entered was "no," resulting in the malaria analysis request not being automatically generated on the first blood donation. Not testing for malaria could miss a reason for deferral and transmission of malaria. How to answer this question correctly was explained to the HP group twice by the supervisor, first by email when it became obvious that this was a recurrent error, and then included in the next continued education session. After these two steps, there was a marked improvement.
- One HP did not check properly in which countries Chagas disease is present and forgot to record the relevant journey. As a result, the analysis request was not generated.

The reminder to this HP to check whether a country is affected by Chagas disease had an obvious impact on their data entry.

In some situations, incorrect documentation has no impact on blood quality or safety, but can give the wrong impression of noncompliance. This may induce the presence of findings during an audit or inspection.

For instance, one HP always entered the date of the interview as the start date for a temporary contra-indication (e.g., following a tattoo) instead of the actual date; the end date, however, was correctly calculated. The donor was thus deferred for the correct duration and there was no safety issue whatsoever. However, a *post hoc* administrative check would identify the duration of the deferral as being too short and consider it to be a failure to comply with legal requirements. The HP was thus reminded to enter the actual start date and subsequent checks confirmed that this was being done correctly.

Noncompliance seems to be more frequent in HPs who conduct fewer interviews (5.67 vs. 3.23%; $p < 0.001$). This information is interesting and should be analyzed further in order to assess whether there is a threshold in the number of interviews to be conducted over a specific period.

This finding is also of use for adapting the frequency of DHQ controls to the number of interviews performed, HPs with a high number of interviews needing less frequent controls than those with a low number of interviews.

The variability between all of the HPs as a group and those who interviewed more than 500 donors during the study period encourages individual analysis of the data and the use of the analysis to set up specific strategies for each HP. Even if an HP is well-graded they can potentially improve their competency toward a better grade and continue to reduce the transfusion risk, even it will never be zero.

Blood Donor Deferral Rate

Analysis of deferral rates is another efficient way of evaluating HP donor interviews and provides a different type of information than DHQ monitoring.

Deferral affects the supply of blood components because a blood bag is not collected and because the return rate for a further donation is reduced (19, 20), in particular, for first-time donors.

The comparison of individual deferral rates of an HP with the whole group allowed to identify discrepancies that were discussed with the monitored HP.

Examples:

- An HP had a much higher overall deferral rate than the group as a whole. Discussion with the supervisor revealed that this HP was very anxious about making mistakes, and preferred to defer donors if there was any doubt whatsoever.
- An HP had a much lower deferral rate for new sexual partners than the group as a whole. It appeared that this HP did not feel comfortable asking the question on this topic and relied entirely on the answer provided by the donor on the DHQ. Nevertheless, it is a well-known fact that quite a number of donors misunderstand or ignore the question and answer "no," when in fact they should answer "yes." Therefore, asking the question orally is important. Detection of this deviation was an opportunity to discuss this particular topic with the HP and provide additional training.

These two issues would not have been detected by means of DHQ monitoring; they illustrate the complementarity of the two blood donor selection evaluation tools used by the SFS.

These great inter-individual differences emphasize the importance of providing each HP with personal data in order to give individual advice and plan specific training.

It is important to take into account the various parameters, which may have an effect, such as the type of blood donation venue (**Table 5**). For instance, a frequent observation is that the number of deferrals due to sexual risk behavior is higher in blood collections organized in schools than in other types of venues, most probably due to the younger donor population (students). When an HP performs more donor selections in schools than average, it is logical for them to have a higher deferral rate than the HP group as a whole. On the other hand, the number of deferrals due to sexual risk behavior in blood collections organized in villages is below average. An HP who works mainly in village venues will, therefore, show a lower deferral rate for this risk factor. Donors' deferral rates being statistically different among the types of donation venues, individual data have to be given to each HP with global data as a reference and with the distribution of their interviews in terms of donation venue. When these are considered, unexpected deviations can be selected and discussed with each individual HP, where applicable.

No hard data are available about the impact of the feedback provided by the supervisor to the HPs, but clear improvements were reported. An objective analysis of this impact may be valuable to validate the monitoring tools.

CONCLUSION

In the SFS as in most blood transfusion centers, donor selection is the result of a pre-donation interview performed confidentially by an HP who has had full *ad hoc* training and has been qualified accordingly. The quality of the selection process is difficult to assess, but is important in the context of blood transfusion safety.

Having a supervisor present during the interview introduces a bias in itself, as both the donor and the HP may act differently compared to a plain face-to-face interview. Therefore, two complementary methods have been developed in the SFS to assess the quality of the selection process, i.e., *post hoc* control of the DHQs and analysis and comparison of deferral rates. Even if the number of DHQs checked was low compared to the total amount of donors selected, it made it possible to identify a number of mistakes made in donor selection, both at individual HP level as well as in a group of HPs. Deferral rates analyses also pinpointed the difficulties experienced by HPs in specific selection situations.

Providing the HPs with feedback on these findings is an opportunity to talk to them and draw their attention to some aspects of the selection process in order to improve it. In certain situations, the topic was included in a continued education session. Clear improvements were reported when further controls and/or deferral analyses were performed.

A comparison of the results for HPs according to the number of interviews conducted on an annual basis showed that for both the control of DHQs and the deferral rates, HPs with a greater number of interviews made fewer mistakes.

In conclusion, controls of DHQs and analyses of donor deferral rate seem to be useful tools to improve the quality of donor selection. It may be interesting to assess whether there is a threshold number of interviews, a HP should conduct per year in order to achieve optimal donor selection quality.

AUTHOR CONTRIBUTIONS

PG collected data recorded by HPs and performed a preliminary analysis of these data in order to develop figures and tables. EN and PG enhanced a deeper analysis of the data, and EN exploited the data with a view to planning individual and overall actions. EN and PG wrote the article.

ACKNOWLEDGMENTS

The authors thank the donors for their confidence, their generosity, and their colleagues for their collaboration, especially Micheline Lambermont and André Rapaille for their inspiring comments.

REFERENCES

1. Beauplet A, Danic B, Aussant-Bertel F; et les médecins de l'EFS Bretagne. Sélection médicale des candidats à un don de sang: prévention des risques pour le donneur. *Transfus Clin Biol* (2003) 10:433–67. doi:10.1016/j.tracli.2003.07.002
2. Eder A. Evidence-based selection criteria to protect blood donors. *J Clin Apher* (2010) 25(6):331–7. doi:10.1002/jca.20257
3. Sorensen BS, Johnsen SP, Jorgensen J. Complications related to blood donation: a population-based study. *Vox Sang* (2008) 94:132–7. doi:10.1111/j.1423-0410.2007.01000.x
4. Seck M, Dièye B, Guèye YB, Fayec BF, Senghor AB, Toure SA, et al. Évaluation de l'efficacité de la sélection médicale des donneurs de sang dans la prévention des agents infectieux. *Transfus Clin Biol* (2016) 23:98–102. doi:10.1016/j.tracli.2015.11.001
5. *Commission Directive 2005/62/EC of 30 September 2005 Implementing Directive 2002/98/EC of the European Parliament and of the Council as Regards Community Standards and Specifications Relating to a Quality System for Blood Establishments.*
6. Follea G, Sideras Z, Carter M. Collection (donor selection). In: De Kort W, editor. *Donor Management Manual.* The Netherlands: DOMAINE Project (2010). p. 137–44.
7. University of Adelaïde. *Writing Course Learning Outcomes.* Available from: https://www.adelaide.edu.au/learning/teaching/curriculum/outcomes/writing-course-learning-outcomes.pdf. Accessed September 8, 2017
8. Lucky TTA, Seed CR, Waller D, Lee JF, McDonald A, Wand H, et al. Understanding noncompliance with selective donor deferral criteria for high-risk behaviors in Australian blood donors. *Transfus Clin Biol* (2014) 54(7):1739–49. doi:10.1111/trf.12554
9. Lee SS, Cheung EKH, Leung JNS, Lee CK. Noncompliance to infectious disease deferral criteria among Hong Kong's blood donors. *Vox Sang* (2017) 112(5):425–33. doi:10.1111/vox.12520
10. Coffe C, Romieu B, Adjou C, Giraudeau B, Bastard B, Danic B, et al. Entretien prédon par un personnel paramédical formé et habilité: faisabilité, fiabilité et sécurité. *Transfus Clin Biol* (2011) 18(2):206–17. doi:10.1016/j.tracli.2011.02.001
11. Kouegnigan Rerambiah L, Biyoghe AS, Bengone C, Djoba Siawaya JF. Evaluation of blood donors questionnaire in a developing country: the case of Gabon. *Transfus Clin Biol* (2014) 21(3):116–9. doi:10.1016/j.tracli.2014.03.003
12. Zou S, Eder AF, Musavi F, Notari EP IV, Fang CT, Dodd RY, et al. Implementation of the Uniform Donor History Questionnaire across the American Red Cross Blood Services: increased deferral among repeat presenters but no measurable impact on blood safety. *Transfusion* (2007) 47:1990–8. doi:10.1111/j.1537-2995.2007.01422.x
13. Goldman M, Ram SS, Yi Q-L, O'Brien SH. The Canadian donor health assessment questionnaire: can it be improved? *Transfusion* (2006) 46:2169–75. doi:10.1111/j.1537-2995.2006.01048.x
14. Goldman M, Ram SS, Yi Q-L, Mazerall J, O'Brien SF. The donor health assessment questionnaire: potential for format change and computer-assisted self-interviews to improve donor attention. *Transfus Clin Biol* (2007) 47:1595–600. doi:10.1111/j.1537-2995.2007.01329.x
15. Sümnig H, Lembcke H, Weber R, Deitenbeck K, Greffin K, Bux J, et al. Evaluation of a New German blood donor questionnaire. *Vox Sang* (2014) 106:55–60. doi:10.1111/vox.12088
16. Offergeld R, Heiden M. Selecting the right donors – still a challenge: development of a Uniform Donor Questionnaire in Germany. *Transfus Med Hemother* (2017) 44:255–62. doi:10.1159/000479193
17. Kamel HT, Bassett MB, Custer B, Paden CJ, Strollo AM, McEvoy P, et al. Safety and donor acceptance of an abbreviated donor history questionnaire. *Transfusion* (2006) 46:1745–53. doi:10.1111/j.1537-2995.2006.00967.x

21

Transfusion-Transmitted Hepatitis E: NAT Screening of Blood Donations and Infectious Dose

Jens Dreier, Cornelius Knabbe and Tanja Vollmer*

Institut für Laboratoriums- und Transfusionsmedizin, Herz- und Diabeteszentrum Nordrhein- Westfalen, Universitätsklinik der Ruhr-Universität Bochum, Bad Oeynhausen, Germany

***Correspondence:**
Jens Dreier
jdreier@hdz-nrw.de

The risk and importance of transfusion-transmitted hepatitis E virus (TT-HEV) infections by contaminated blood products is currently a controversial discussed topic in transfusion medicine. The infectious dose, in particular, remains an unknown quantity. In the present study, we illuminate and review this aspect seen from the viewpoint of a blood donation service with more than 2 years of experience in routine HEV blood donor screening. We systematically review the actual status of presently known cases of TT-HEV infections and available routine NAT-screening assays. The review of the literature revealed a significant variation regarding the infectious dose causing hepatitis E. We also present the outcome of six cases confronted with HEV-contaminated blood products, identified by routine HEV RNA screening of minipools using the highly sensitive RealStar HEV RT-PCR Kit (95% LOD: 4.7 IU/mL). Finally, the distribution of viral RNA in different blood components [plasma, red blood cell concentrate (RBC), platelet concentrates (PC)] was quantified using the first WHO international standard for HEV RNA for NAT-based assays. None of the six patients receiving an HEV-contaminated blood product from five different donors (donor 1: RBC, donor 2–5: APC) developed an acute hepatitis E infection, most likely due to low viral load in donor plasma (<100 IU/mL). Of note, the distribution of viral RNA in blood components depends on the plasma content of the component; nonetheless, HEV RNA could be detected in RBCs even when low viral plasma loads of 100–1,000 IU/mL are present. Comprehensive retrospective studies of TT-HEV infection offered further insights into the infectivity of HEV RNA-positive blood products. Minipool HEV NAT screening (96 samples) of blood donations should be adequate as a routine screening assay to identify high viremic donors and will cover at least a large part of viremic phases.

Keywords: hepatitis E virus, blood donor, blood safety, NAT testing, transfusion–transmission

INTRODUCTION

Hepatitis E virus (HEV) is an emerging infectious threat to blood safety. In the recent decade, there have been several reports of transfusion-transmitted hepatitis E virus (TT-HEV) infection [for review, see Ref. (1)], although the risk of infection through consumption of raw or undercooked pork and wild boar is even greater (2). In industrialized countries, HEV infection, mainly with genotype 3, usually causes an acute, self-limiting, asymptomatic, or mild hepatitis. However, the significance of HEV genotype 3 infections has changed because chronic hepatitis with rapidly progressive cirrhosis in organ transplant recipients and patients with hematological malignancy, as well as fulminant hepatitis in patients with chronic liver disease, have been observed (1, 3). HEV-infected immunocompromised patients develop chronic hepatitis E in approximately 60% of cases (4).

Since 2004, HEV has gained importance as a transfusion transmissible infectious agent, although earlier reports pointed to the risk of infection (5, 6). HEV has been transmitted in samples of red blood cells, platelet preparations, pooled granulocytes, and fresh frozen plasma (FFP) (solvent-detergent treated, amotosalen-treated, secured by quarantine). As a result, the public health implications of HEV in Europe have gained greater momentum due to an increasing number of hepatitis E cases and recent reports of chronic, persistent HEV infections associated with progression to cirrhosis in immunosuppressed patients. The question of hepatitis E and contribution of NAT screening on blood safety is currently extensively discussed, not only by several European committees and local blood authorities but also internally by a large number of blood transfusion facilities. Domanovic questioned the situation as "a shift to screening" and summarized the epidemiology of HEV infections among blood donors and outlined strategies to prevent TT-HEV in 11 European countries (7). A nationwide HEV RNA screening of blood donations was introduced in Ireland, the UK, and recently the Netherlands. Several blood establishments in Germany, France, and recently Switzerland perform selective screening intended for use in high-risk patients or universal screening for HEV RNA. Blood authorities in Greece, Portugal, Italy, and Spain are evaluating the situation (7). Regardless of the risk of HEV transmission *via* blood products, most authorities have recommended HEV monitoring of immunosuppressed patients. The implementation of a HEV run control for screening human plasma pools requested by the Ph. Eur. 1646 (8) is another indication toward a transfusion relevance of HEV. So far, there have been only specific case reports of HEV transmission by SD-treated plasma (SDP) but not by other plasma-derived medicinal products. However, it is not unlikely that cases might have been overlooked due to diagnostic failure (9). Past serologic investigations in Japan implicated coagulation factors in the transmission of HEV. The conclusion was based on the significantly higher prevalence of HEV antibody in hemophilia patients receiving coagulation factors that were not subjected to virus inactivation or removal, compared with patients who received virus-inactivated coagulation factors (10). Cost-effectiveness analyses were carried out in the Netherlands to assess whether an appropriate measure should be implemented for blood donor screening (11). The analysis led to the conclusion that the prevention of HEV transmission through the screening of blood donations is not markedly expensive compared with other blood-screening measures. However, the key issue of these cost-effectiveness analyses is the minimum viral load required to be detected in the donor blood. Thus, attention is now focused on the limit of detection of NAT (ID versus pool NAT), which is primary influenced by the minimum infectious dose of a blood product triggering an infection in the recipient. The German Advisory Committee on Blood (Arbeitskreis Blut) recommended a NAT sensitivity of 100 IU HEV RNA/mL [per single donation (12)], which is difficult to achieve with the currently available NAT assays using minipool NAT. For these reasons, the ongoing discussions address the question of the most appropriate and effective strategy to minimize the risk of TT-HEV infection, taking into account the costs, the logistics of testing, and the infection risk and outcome of HEV-infected blood recipients. The present review provides a comprehensive view of the various aspects of TT-HEV infection and a discussion on the current status on the issue of screening for this virus.

MATERIALS AND METHODS

HEV RNA Screening, Serological Testing, and Measurement of Liver-Specific Parameters in Blood Donors and Transfusion Recipients

Routine HEV RNA screening of therapeutic blood products was introduced in our blood donation service in January 2015. From January 2015 to July 2017, a total of 235,524 donations from 86,933 donors were screened for the presence of HEV RNA revealing 182 HEV RNA-positive donors. For four of these HEV RNA-positive donors, a lookback procedure need to be initiated, and a total of nine viremic previous donations of these donors were identified, which were transfused to six different recipients (**Table 1**).

Hepatitis E virus RNA-positive blood donors were identified using the RealStar HEV RT-PCR Kit (Altona Diagnostics, Hamburg, Germany), as described previously (13). Total nucleic acid (RNA/DNA) was extracted from 500 µL of donor and recipient samples using the NucliSens easyMAG (bioMerieux, Nürtingen, Germany) automated RNA/DNA extraction system followed by HEV RNA detection using the RealStar HEV RT-PCR Kit (13). HEV titer of positive samples was quantified using the first WHO international standard for HEV RNA for NAT-based assays (Paul Ehrlich Institute, Langen, Germany). The linear range of quantification was from 25 to 10E+07 IU/mL.

Screening for the presence of HEV-specific IgM and IgG antibodies was performed using the Anti-HEV ELISA (IgM and IgG, Euroimmun, Lübeck, Germany) according to the manufacturer's instructions. Serum concentrations of glutamate dehydrogenase (GLDH), aspartate aminotransferase (AST), alanine aminotransferase (ALT), and total bilirubin were measured in plasma samples using the respective enzymatic assays on the Architect system (Abbott Diagnostics Europe, Wiesbaden, Germany). All HEV-infected donors underwent pre-donation medical examination and negated current diseases or any known risk factors for viral infection. The study protocol followed the ethical guidelines of the Ruhr University, Bochum, and was approved by the institutional review board; donors provided informed consent.

Processing of Blood Products and Quantification of the Viral Load

Apheresis-derived single-donor PCs (APCs) were prepared after standard processing with the Haemonetics MCS + (Haemonetics GmbH, München, Germany). The final product consisted

TABLE 1 | Cases of transfusion of blood products containing hepatitis E virus (HEV) RNA from this study.

Donor					Recipient				Outcome			
Donor	**Blood product**	**Viral load (IU/mL), genotype**	**Infectious dose (IU)**	**Anti-HEV IgM/IgG**	**Recipient, sex and age**	**Anti-HEV IgG[a]**	**Primary disease**	**Immuno-compromised**	**Follow-up period (days)**	**Outcome**	**HEV-PCR**	**Anti-HEV IgG**
1	RBC (314 mL)	<25 GT 3	<2.50E+02	Negative	1 M, 23 years	Negative	Heart transplantation	Yes	134 days	No HEV infection	Negative	Negative
2	PC 1 (234 mL)	<25 GT 3	<4.68E+03	Negative	2 M, 76 years	Negative	Heart valve failure, atrial fibrillation	No	35 days	No HEV infection, died sepsis	Negative	Negative
	PC 2 (243 mL)		<4.86E+03		3 M, 54 years		Left ventricular heart failure	No	50 days	No HEV infection	Negative	Negative
3 donation 1	PC 1 (230 mL) PC 2 (254 mL) Total	27.8 GT 3	5.12E+03 5.65E+03 1.08E+04	Negative	4 F, 26 years	Negative	Hypertrophic cardiomyopathy	No	16 days	No HEV infection[b]	Negative	Negative
3 donation 2	PC 1 (244 mL) PC 2 (244 mL) Total	69.4 GT 3	1.35E+04 1.35E+04 2.71E+04	Negative	5 M, 72 years	Negative	Arrhythmia	No	NA	Died arrhythmia	NA	NA
4	PC 1 (242 mL) PC 2 (244 mL) Total	<25 GT 3	<3.97E+03 <4.00E+03 7.97E+03	Negative	6 F, 79 years	Negative	Leukemia	Yes	NA	Died leukemia	NA	NA

[a] *At the date of transfusion.*
[b] *Patient no longer available.*

of 2.0–4.0 × 10E+11 platelets/unit (205–295 mL) containing 0.76–0.84 mL/mL human plasma and 0.16–0.24 mL/mL ACD-A stabilizer. For the preparation of RBC, whole blood donations were collected into a multiple bag system with inline filtration for leukoreduction (CompoFlow quadruple 4F, 70-mL CPD/100-mL PAGGS-M—WB + PDS-V, Fresenius Kabi Deutschland GmbH, Bad Homburg, Germany), followed by centrifugation of the filtered whole blood unit at 4,182 × *g* and 22°C for 45 min. Automated fractionation was carried out using the CompoMat G5 separator (Fresenius Kabi), and RBCs were stored directly at 4 ± 2°C. The final product volume averaged from 200 to 400 mL. The residual plasma volume was estimated to be 10 mL per RBC. The corresponding plasma products (FFP) contained a total volume of 180–380 mL with 0.75–0.82 mL/mL human plasma.

Viral RNA in the different blood components (FFP, RBC, RBC supernatant, PC) was extracted from 4.8-mL sample with the Chemagic Viral DNA/RNA reagent kit (Viral 5k, PerkinElmer Chemagen Technology GmbH, Baesweiler, Germany) combined with the automated Chemagic magnetic separation module MSMI (PerkinElmer Chemagen Technology GmbH) according to the manufacturer's instructions. For the recovery of RBC supernatant, 50 mL of RBC were transferred to EDTA-containing monovettes followed by centrifugation for 10 min at 5,000 rpm. Therefore, the RBC supernatant contained CPD/PAGGS-M stabilizator and a minimal proportion of residual plasma. For RNA extraction of RBCs, the alternative lysis buffer CMG-825 (lysis buffer blood, PerkinElmer Chemagen Technology GmbH) was used. The 95% lower limit of detection was calculated by Probit analysis to 4.7 IU/mL [confidence interval: 3.6–7.5 IU/mL (13)] for FFP, PC, and RBC supernatant and to 8.9 IU/mL (confidence interval: 6.5–21.1 IU/mL) for RBCs.

Searching Criteria

For the systematic review of HEV cases, the PubMed database (http://www.ncbi.nlm.nih.gov/pubmed/), a public search engine maintained by the United States National Library of Medicine (NLM) at the National Institutes of Health (NIH) that provides access to over 24 million citations in all fields of life sciences, mostly from the MEDLINE (Medical Literature Analysis and retrieval System Online), was searched for publications between 2004 and 2017 (publications dates) using specific search strings including "hepatitis E/HEV infection," "transfusion transmitted hepatitis E/HEV infection," and "hepatitis E/HEV blood donor screening."

Statistical Analysis

All values are given as mean ± SD. Median values and SD were calculated and Spearman's rank correlation analysis was performed using the GraphPad Prism 5.0 software (GraphPad Software, San Diego, CA, USA). Statistical analysis to assess differences between values was performed using the Mann–Whitney *U* test.

RESULTS

A systematic review of individual case reports regarding the transfusion of HEV-contaminated blood products from 2004 to

2017 is summarized in chronological order of occurrence in Table S1 in Supplementary Material. Cases including those patients who died shortly after transfusion for reasons other than HEV infection were excluded. We further describe six new cases of patients transfused with HEV-contaminated blood products, and none of the recipients developed HEV infection.

Case Description

Table 1 summarizes the donor and recipient information of all six cases. Anti-HEV IgM and IgG antibodies were not detected in any HEV RNA-positive donor and serum concentrations of GLDH, AST, ALT, and total bilirubin were all within normal range (data not shown). The presence of HEV RNA was confirmed in a secondary sample. Additionally, the corresponding plasma product of the RBC of donor 1 was available and the presence of HEV RNA was further confirmed. Donors 1 and 4 did not return for blood donation after HEV infection. For the other two donors, anti-HEV IgG seroconversion was observed after 149 days (donor 2) and 116 days (donor 3) after the first HEV RNA-positive donation. For HEV genotyping of all donor samples, HEV-nucleotide sequence, corresponding to a 242-bp fragment of the ORF1 region, was amplified and sequenced. Phylogenetic analysis showed that the samples clustered together and were related to HEV genotype 3, which is prevalent in Germany.

All recipients were anti-HEV IgM and anti-HEV IgG negative at the time of transfusion of HEV RNA-positive blood products. The viral load in plasma samples of donors 1, 2, and 4 was determined to be 17, 12, and 20 IU/mL, respectively. These values were below the linear range of quantification (<25 IU/mL), and therefore a maximum infectious dose was calculated assuming a viral load of 25 IU/mL. Recipient 1, an immunocompromised man after heart transplantation, received one RBC. Assuming a residual plasma volume of 10 mL per RBC, the maximum corresponding infectious dose was calculated as 250 IU. This patient did not develop HEV infection within the follow-up period of 134 days, and neither HEV RNA nor anti-HEV antibodies were detectable.

Each apheresis platelet donation resulted in two APCs. The two immunocompetent recipients R2 and R3 received APCs from donor 2 with infectious doses of 4.68E+03 IU (APC1) and 4.86E+03 IU (APC2), assuming an average residual plasma volume of 0.8 mL per APC. Neither patients developed an HEV infection within the follow-up period of 35 days (recipient R2) or 50 days (recipient R3); moreover, no HEV RNA or anti-HEV antibodies were detectable. Accordingly, recipient R6 received two apheresis platelets (APC1: 242 mL, APC2: 244 mL) from donor 4 with a total maximum infectious dose of 7.97E+03 IU (total volume transfused: 486 mL), but she died shortly after transfusion for reasons other than HEV infection.

Donor 3 donated platelets regularly approximately every 14 days and showed the highest viral load compared with the other donors. The first viremic donation (donation 1) contained 27.8 IU/mL HEV RNA, and the second donation, 18 days later (donation 2), contained 69.4 IU/mL HEV RNA. The double APCs were transfused to two immunocompetent recipients (recipients R4 and R5). Recipient 4 received a total infectious dose of 1.08E+04 IU HEV RNA (donation 1, total volume of 484 mL, APC1: 230 mL, APC2: 254 mL). This patient did not develop an acute HEV infection within 16 days after transfusion, and neither HEV RNA nor anti-HEV antibodies were detectable. However, the observation period was short and the possibility that HEV infection may have occurred later could not be ruled out. This patient was released from hospital and unfortunately no follow-up samples were sent to our laboratory for further follow-up. The second HEV-positive donation of donor 3 had a total infectious dose corresponding to 2.71E+04 IU HEV RNA (donation 2, transfusion of a total volume of 488-mL APC, APC1, and APC2: 244 mL). The recipient (R5) of these two apheresis platelets died shortly after transfusion for reasons other than HEV infection.

The cases of recipients 4–6 were excluded from the subsequent overview due to the short follow-up period.

Distribution of Viral RNA in Different Blood Products

In order to determine if a reduction of the viral load occurs during the manufacturing process of blood products, e.g., by centrifugation or by adsorption to components of the blood bag system, including the filter used for leukoreduction, viral loads were quantified in the plasma of HEV RNA-positive donors and additionally quantified in the corresponding blood products, FFP and RBC. Results from the respective blood products were correlated with the expected viral loads calculated with quantified results for plasma of HEV RNA-positive donors, assuming no removal during the production process. Calculation of virus titer assumed a mean plasma content of 0.80 mL/mL human plasma (80%) for FFP. For RBCs, the remaining plasma volume of 10 mL per RBC was assumed for consideration of the total volume of each individual RBC after processing. A total of 73 value pairs were available for correlation analysis of FFPs (**Figure 1A**), of which three were excluded due to low viral load (<25 IU/mL). Likewise, a total of 73 value pairs were available for RBC (**Figure 1B**), of which 31 with low viral load (<25 IU/mL) were excluded. Spearman's correlation analysis revealed a good correlation of $r = 0.9418$ (95% CI: 0.9065–0.9641) for FFP and a good correlation of $r = 0.9290$ (95% CI: 0.8538–0.9663) for RBC. The wider distribution between the measured and calculated HEV titer in RBC is based on the considerably lower plasma amount of only 10 mL per RBC (mean RBC volume 268 mL, mean plasma proportion 3.7%) and the resultant higher method-specific quantification error.

In order to determine if HEV RNA or virus particles are bound to the surface of red blood cells, HEV RNA was quantified in 20 different RBCs as well as in the cell-free supernatants of RBCs (**Figure 1C**). Spearman's correlation analysis again revealed a good correlation of $r = 0.9390$ (95% CI: 0.8492–0.9760), indicating that no specific binding to red blood cell surfaces had occurred.

Figure 2 displays the distribution of viral RNA in FFP and RBC depending on the viral load, quantified in the plasma of HEV RNA-positive donors. HEV RNA was detected in the RBCs of all donations where the viral load in plasma was quantified as >1,000 IU/mL (**Figure 2A**). Quantified FFPs contained a total mean volume of 287 mL, corresponding to a total plasma volume of 230 mL. Comparison of the quantified mean values for FFP

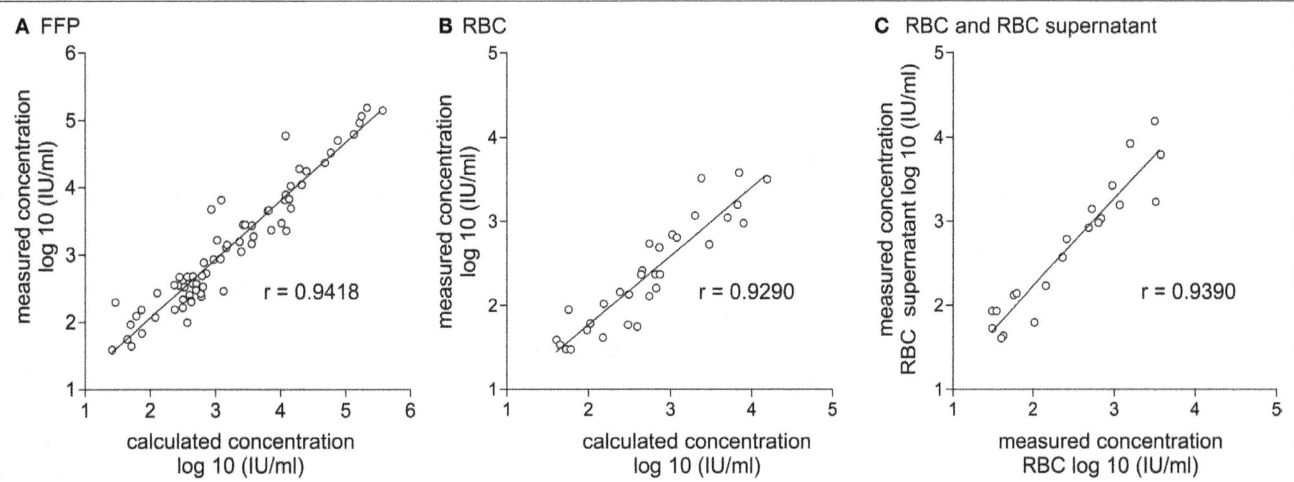

FIGURE 1 | Correlation of calculated and effectively quantified viral load in fresh frozen plasma (FFP) and red blood cell concentrate (RBC) and correlation of viral load in RBC and RBC supernatant. Displayed is the correlation between the effectively quantified hepatitis E virus (HEV) titer and the expected viral load in FFP **(A)** and RBC **(B)**. Calculation of the expected viral load in FFP is based on quantification results of HEV viral load in plasma of donors assuming a mean plasma content of 0.8 mL/mL plasma in the corresponding plasma product. Calculation of the expected viral load in RBC is based on quantification results of HEV viral load in plasma of donors assuming a residual plasma content of 10 mL/RBC. **(C)** Correlation of the effectively quantified HEV titer in RBC and RBC supernatant. The linear range of quantification was from 25 to 10E+07 IU/mL. Therefore, all values <25 IU/mL were excluded.

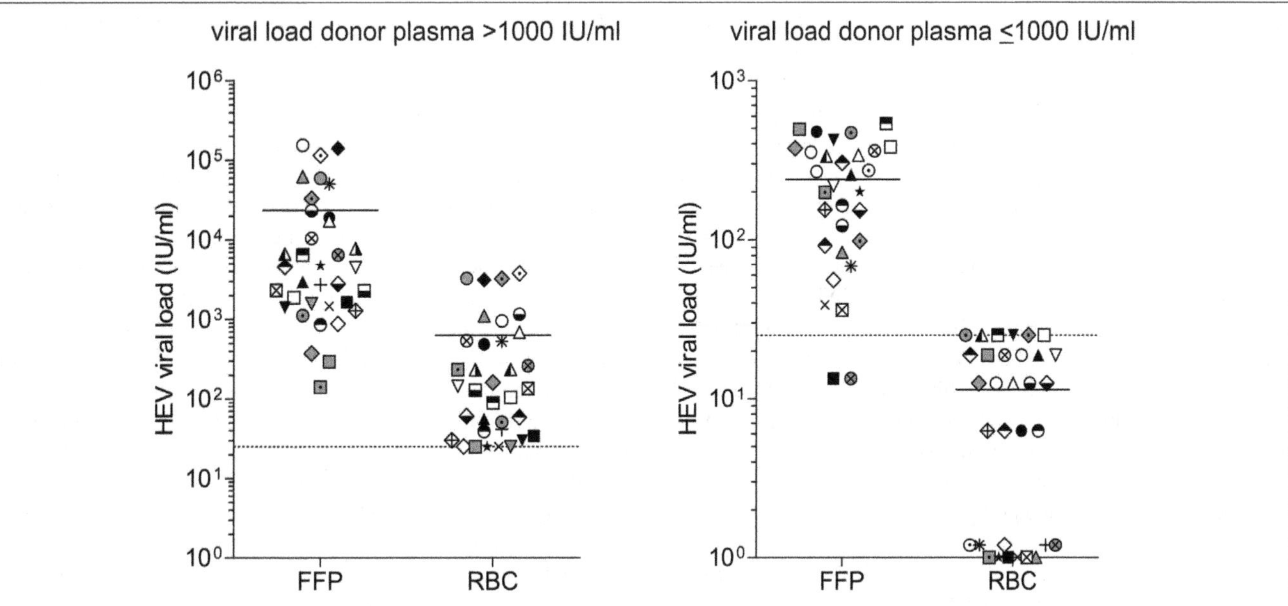

FIGURE 2 | Distribution of viral load in different blood products. The hepatitis E virus (HEV) titer in plasma of donors and the corresponding blood products fresh frozen plasma (FFP) and red blood cell concentrates (RBCs) was quantified using the first WHO international standard for HEV RNA for NAT-based assays. The distinction of viral loads >1,000 IU/mL **(A)** and ≤1,000 IU/mL **(B)** is based on quantification results of HEV viral load in plasma of donors, not in the corresponding blood products. Equal symbols present quantification results in different blood products from the same donor, quantification was performed in quadruplicate. The linear range of quantification was from 25 to 10E+07 IU/mL. Values <25 IU/mL were displayed as 25 IU/mL. For RBCs with low viral loads, not all replicates were positive for HEV RNA. Results were displayed as follows: 0 IU/mL: 0/4 positive replicates; 6.25 IU/mL: 1/4 positive replicates; 12.5 IU/mL: 2/4 positive replicates; 18.75 IU/mL: 3/4 positive replicates; and 25 IU/mL: 4/4 positive replicates (quantification results <25 IU/mL). The solid horizontal line represents mean values, and the dotted horizontal line is representative for the value 25 IU/mL.

(2.34E+04 ± 4.08E+04 IU/mL) with those obtained for RBCs (6.29E+02 ± 1.05E+03 IU/mL) revealed the percentage proportion of 2.7% for RBCs, essentially corresponding to the calculated mean plasma proportion of 3.7%.

For RBCs, where the viral load in plasma was quantified >1,000 IU/mL (**Figure 2B**), a maximum viral load of 25 IU/mL was detected and often not all replicates were positive for HEV RNA. Negative results might either indicate that RBC contains no viral RNA or the viral load is below the detection limit of the assay (8.9 IU/mL).

DISCUSSION

German public health authorities have recognized an increasing number of acute HEV infections, which is probably due to higher clinical awareness but more likely due to detection of HEV-infected asymptomatic blood donors identified through NAT screening by blood donation establishments. A high frequency of HEV viremic donors have been reported in recent large screening studies in several European countries (13–17). The asymptomatic infection is mostly characterized by a period of asymptomatic viremia, with an estimated duration of 68 days (18). The typical serological course of an acute HEV infection showed detectable IgM antibodies following an incubation period of 2–6 weeks, decline to baseline levels within three to 6 month, followed by longer lasting IgG antibodies which remains detectable for up to 15 years (19–21). The progression of anti-HEV immunoglobulins in asymptomatic cases is comparable with symptomatic cases (22). However, the factual incidence of TT-HEV infection and the real clinical importance is currently unknown. The rate of reported TT-HEV infections is very small, probably due to underreporting, failure to recognize or misinterpretation of symptoms (23), or development of HEV infection long after transfusion, hampering any association with an earlier transfusion event (24). Moreover, the occurrence of primary asymptomatic infection in recipients is certainly an option. Besides a recent large study in England (24), only a small number of individual cases of TT-HEV infection (Table S1 in Supplementary Material) and cases of transfusion of HEV-containing blood without TT-HEV infection (Table S2 in Supplementary Material) have been described (14, 23, 25–46). The large 2012–2013 study in England retrospectively screened 225,000 English blood donors for HEV by NAT. Follow-up of the recipients who had received HEV genotype 3-contaminated blood components indicated that 42% had evidence of TT-HEV infection, with transmission possibly linked to the absence of HEV-specific antibodies (24). A high virus load in the donor, corresponding with the volume of plasma transfused with the final blood component, rendered infection more likely. Moreover, multiple different kinds of blood products were involved, but the transmission rates varied. Of all transfused RBC, only 25% caused HEV infection, whereas 40% of transfused PPCs, 50% of transfused APCs, and 100% of transfused FFPs or pooled granulocytes caused HEV infection (24).

Analysis of 19 Japanese cases of TT-HEV infection by Satake et al. found a comparable rate of infection of 50% (29). All TT-HEV cases present in the Satake's study were included in our case analysis (Table S1 in Supplementary Material). The studies by Satake et al. and Hewitt et al. [18 patients (24)] also identified several patients transfused with HEV-contaminated components without the development of HEV infection [5 patients (29), 18 patients (24)], but these cases were not considered in Table S2 in Supplementary Material because no detailed case descriptions are available.

Unfortunately, some cases only revealed poor data sets, missing important facts for both, the recipients of contaminated blood products or the respective donors. For example, the pretransfusion serostatus in recipients is often only assumable based on the posttransfusion status, or the serostatus is entirely absent. The serological status of the blood donors is also often missing. Additionally, the duration between transfusion, determination of infection, and follow-up of patients including the accompanying therapy and laboratory parameters is often incomplete or untraceable. Most important, the viral HEV load and the resulting infectious dose is not determined. Taken into consideration only the individual cases included in Tables S1 and S2 where the viral load infused is available, 39 patients received blood products containing HEV, of whom 28 patients develop TT-HEV infection.

Tedder and colleagues performed an estimation of the infectious dose of the individual blood product types involved in the UK study in a subsequent analysis, demonstrating that components causing TT-HEV infection had a considerably higher median infectious dose of 1.44E+06 IU than components not causing TT-HEV infection [median total viral load transfused: 2.40E+04 IU (2, 24)]. Accordingly to this study, our systematic case review analysis showed a significant difference in the median viral load transfused between HEV-infected (median: 5.20E+05 IU, this study) and non-infected patients (median: 1.91E+03 IU, $p < 0.0001$, **Figure 3A**). Statistical significant differences in the median viral load transfused were also observed between HEV-infected (median: 4.40E+05 IU) and non-infected non-immunocompromised patients (median: 1.91E+03 IU, $p = 0.0002$), whereas no differences were observed between HEV-infected (median: 4.80E+05 IU) and non-infected immunocompromised patients (median: 1.55+04 IU, $p = 0.1006$). When the immune status of the recipient, which was mentioned to have a major impact on the actual risk of TT-HEV infection, was also taken into account, no differences were observed in the median viral load transfused between immunocompromised and non-immunocompromised patients, independently from the infection outcome (HEV-infected, $p = 0.6286$; non-HEV-infected, $p = 0.5044$). The lowest infectious dose resulting in TT-HEV infection observed in general was 7.05E+03 IU. When the type of blood product was considered, the lowest infectious dose transfused was 7.05E+03 IU for PCs without subdivision of APC and PPCs, 3.16E+04 IU for RBCs, and 3.60E+04 IU for FFPs (**Figure 3B**). Tedder et al. demonstrated that the lowest dose of virus resulting in an infection was 2.00E+04 IU, whereby only 55% of the components containing this dose transmitted an infection (2). Among non-transmitting components, 60% contained or exceeded this infectious dose. Satake et al. summarized that infusion of total viral loads between 2.00E+04 IU and 2.60E+05 IU can occur without HEV transmission (29). In our systematic case review analysis, all components with a viral load >5.00E+04 IU caused infection (**Figure 3A**), independently from the immune status of the recipient; however, only one of the non-transmitting components exceeded this value. Furthermore, the pretransfusion serostatus of recipients receiving HEV-contaminated blood products might have an impact on the development of HEV infection. With the exception of three cases in the study by Hewitt et al. (24) and two additional cases (29, 38, 39, 46), all described cases had a seronegative pretransfusion status. Future studies including IgG positive pretransfusion cases might contribute to

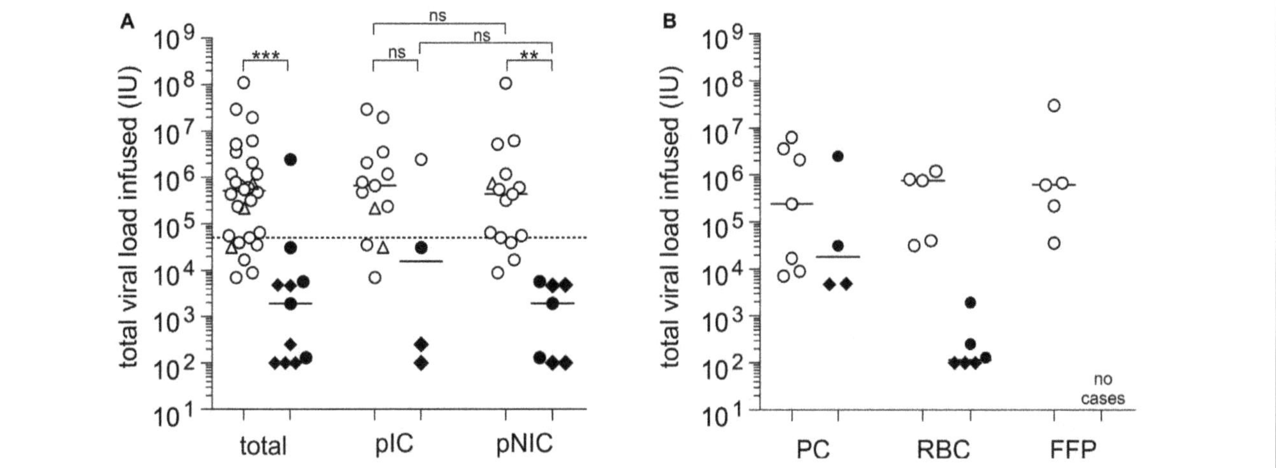

FIGURE 3 | Systematic case review analysis of the total viral load transfused observed in individual case studies (Tables S1 and S2). **(A)** Displayed is the total viral load transfused resulting in posttransfusion hepatitis E virus (HEV) infection or no posttransfusion HEV infection, independently from and depending on the immune status of the recipients ($n = 39$). pIC, possibly immunocompromised; pNIC, possibly not immuno-compromised. **(B)** Displayed is the total viral load transfused resulting in posttransfusion HEV infection or no posttransfusion HEV infection depending on the transfused blood product ($n = 25$). RBC, red blood cell concentrates; PC, apheresis or pooled PCs; FFP, fresh frozen plasma. ◊: values specified with <IU/mL, viral loads for these cases are placed at the maximum possible value, Δ: estimated infectious dose, solid bars indicate median viral load. The solid horizontal line represents median values, and the dotted horizontal line represents the minimum infectious dose. White symbols: HEV infection and black symbols: no HEV infection. ***$p < 0.0001$, **$p = 0.0002$, and *$p < 0.05$, ns, not significant.

the assessment of a protective effect of previous experienced HEV infection or the effectiveness of future available vaccination of donors and/or at risk recipients.

In addition to the cases mentioned in Table S1 in Supplementary Material, Arankalle et al. described two cases of putative, but in our opinion unlikely, posttransfusion hepatitis. HEV infection was assumed due to seroconversion of both patients within weeks after transfusion, but no HEV RNA was detected in patients for comparative sequence analysis. Additionally, donor screening of five of the six involved donations revealed no HEV RNA (6). In Japan, seven further posttransfusion hepatitis E cases (six cases of RBC transfusion, one case of PC transfusion) were detected, according to the official announcement of the Japanese Red Cross Society, but no information on either donor or patient antibody status or the infectious dose were available (26). The German authorities also announced four further posttransfusion hepatitis E cases (two RBC, two PC) in their actual hemovigilance report so far, without detailed case information (47).

The lack of a small animal model and efficient cell culture system has hampered the study of HEV replication, pathogenesis, and infectious dose determination. HEV isolates of genotypes 3 and 4 have been adapted to grow *in vitro*, but HEV cell culture is inefficient and limited, and requires genetic modifications of the HEV isolates (48–51). Experimental HEV infection in the rhesus monkey model led to acute hepatitis E after transfusion of 10 mL plasma from a HEV-infected donor (52). Immune-deficient human-liver chimeric mouse also serves as an appropriate model to study HEV genotype 1 and 3 infection, virus–host interactions, and drug efficacy (53, 54). For example, chronic HEV infection was observed after intrasplenic injection of HEV-GT1-containing preparation with an infectious dose of 2.5E+05 IU (53). These models could serve as a starting point to determine the infectivity and pathogenicity of HEV. However, it is currently questionable whether these models are faithful representation of human infection and could answer the question of infectious dose in humans.

The plasma proportion of the transfused blood product seemed to affect the risk for TT-HEV at most, but so far no information is available on the partitioning of HEV into the different components from a single blood donation (9). It is conceivable that manufacturing processes during the fractionation of whole blood might result in lower viral loads than what is expected on the basis of viral plasma load of blood donors and the assumed residual plasma content. We have shown that the fractionation process in our blood transfusion facility does not considerably reduce the concentration of viral RNA, but this may not generally valid for other production processes.

The question remains as to which screening strategy is necessary and practicable. Screening may constitute a universal approach to include all blood products or a selective screening can be performed for only the products that would be used in at-risk patients. This issue is primarily influenced by two sides: the hospital-sided clear definition of at-risk patients and the logistic implications for the order of blood products, and supply and availability, managed by the blood establishment. The second question is whether minipool screening of up to 96 samples or ID testing is necessary. We would submit that the required detection limit, which need to be derived from the infectious dose, plays an important role for the second issue. Thus, the decision for ID or pool NAT depends on logistic and costs, which are in part dictated by the required sensitivity. **Table 2** summarizes the currently available commercially HEV NAT-screening assays including the analytical sensitivities. The analytical sensitivity (95% LOD) of HEV NAT assays ranges from 4.7 to 18.6 IU/mL, and all assays used for blood screening detected positive donations of all genotypes 1 to 4 and demonstrated a good

TABLE 2 | Overview of currently commercially available hepatitis E virus (HEV) NAT-screening methods.

Kit name	RealStar HEV RT-PCR Kit 1.0	Cobas HEV test	Procleix HEV assay	HEV NAT kit
Manufacturer	**Altona Diagnostics**	**Roche Diagnostics**	**Grifols**	**GFE Blut**
Automation	No	Full automation cobas® 6800/8800 Systems	Full automation Procleix® Panther® System	Full automation PoET System
FDA/CE-IVD	No/yes	No/yes	No/yes	No/yes
Sample preparation/nucleic-acid extraction				
Virus enrichment pre-extraction	No	No	No	No
Maximal MP size	96	Depending on regional regulation	12	Up to 96
Nucleic-acid extraction procedure	Chemagic Viral RNA/DNA Kit on MSM-I (4.8-mL protocol)	Magnetic glass particles for fully automated NA-extraction	Target-specific extraction—magnetic microparticles capture viral nucleic acids with viral-specific capture oligonucleotides	Fully automated magnetic bead extraction
Processed sample volume (plasma mL)	4.8	0.85	0.525	1.3
Elution volume (μL)	100	50	n.a., single-tube format	90
Plasma-equivalents (mL)/PCR (%)	1.2 (100)	0.425 (35)	0.525 (44)	0.433 (36)
NAT/detection				
Principle of NAT detection	RT-PCR, TaqMan probes	RT-PCR, TaqMan probes	Transcription-mediated amplification	RT-PCR, TaqMan probes
NAT instrument	Rotorgene Q	cobas® 6800/8800 Systems	Procleix® Panther® System	PoET System
Target (gene region)	ORF3	5′UTR	n.a.	n.a.
Eluat/PCR volume (μL/μL)	25/50	25/50	100% of the sample is processed and used in the amplification reaction	30/75 or 10/25
Test specifications				
Analytical sensitivity (95% LOD IU/mL)	4.7 (451.2–96 pool)	18.6	7,88	8.2 (787.2–96 pool, 75-μL PCR)
Specificity	100% Genotype 1–4	100% Genotype 1–4	99,98% Genotype 1–4	100% Genotype 1–4
Accomplishment				
Hands on time	30 min	15 min	15 min	n.a.
Time to result	4 h	3 h	3.5 h	5 h
Throughput	960 results (10 pools of 96 samples) in 4 h	96 results (94 pools plus 2 controls) in 3 h 384 results (376 pools plus 8 controls) in 8 h shift (cobas® 6800 System)	5,775 results (275 pools of 16 samples) in 8 h 10,500 results (500 pools of 16 samples) in 12 h	Depending on configuration. e.g., 8,448 in 5 h, 16,896 in 9 h (176 pools of 96 samples)
Remarks	Automation on AltoStar system for ID NAT pending		Intended use includes cadaveric (non-heart beating) donors	Preliminary data; IVD certification pending.

performance in routine testing (**Table 2**). In most settings, the Procleix HEV (Grifols) is used in individual testing (ID NAT), where the 95% LOD was determined to be 5.5–12.78 IU/mL, which is slightly different than that of the manufacturer's value (15, 55). The disadvantage of current commercial HEV NAT assays is their requirement of special screening platforms that are fully integrated and automated, and not as flexible as open NAT platforms. For this reason, we introduced routine minipool HEV NAT screening (96 donations) using an in-house testing regime in our transfusion facility in January 2015. The setting of HEV NAT using RealStar HEV RT-PCR Kit 1.0 [Altona Diagnostics, 95% LOD 4.7 IU/mL (CI: 3.6–7.6, 452 IU/mL) per single donation] is compatible to the virus NAT screening used in our blood transfusion service (13, 56). Our HEV NAT is comparable with commercial HEV NAT-screening methods (**Table 2**) in spite of a lower level of automation and throughput. The novel automation platform AltoStar allows ID NAT testing or alternatively a higher automation grade for pool NAT. It is to be noted that the sensitivity of the RealStar HEV RT-PCR Kit strongly depends on the nucleic-acid extraction method used, ranging from 4.7 to 37.8 IU/mL (13, 55, 56). In our screening setting, we use the fully automated nucleic-acid extraction method Chemagic Viral DNA/RNA Kit that allows the processing of large plasma volumes (4.8 mL). Compared with the other commercial HEV NAT-screening methods from GFE Blut, Roche, and Grifols, the processed sample volume of our method is 3.7-fold, 5.6-fold, and 9.1-fold higher, respectively, resulting in a considerably higher number of HEV plasma-equivalents per PCR reaction. Therefore, this combination is, to the best of our knowledge, the most sensitive HEV NAT. It does not fully meet the sensitivity of 100 IU HEV RNA/mL recommended by the German authorities, but at present, it is not clear whether this sensitivity is absolutely necessary. Our minipool screening strategy aims to identify high viremic donors and will cover at least a large part of viremic phases (22, 57). The European medicine agency so far has also recommended minipool screening in their reflection paper on hepatitis E (9). However, it remains to be seen in the future whether all relevant viremic phases that could result in TT-HEV infections will be detected.

AUTHOR CONTRIBUTIONS

JD and TV designed the study, analyzed and interpreted the data, and drafted the manuscript. CK designed the study and revised the manuscript critically. All authors contributed to drafting the text and approved the manuscript.

REFERENCES

1. Ankcorn MJ, Tedder RS. Hepatitis E: the current state of play. *Transfus Med* (2017) 27(2):84–95. doi:10.1111/tme.12405
2. Tedder RS, Ijaz S, Kitchen A, Ushiro-Lumb I, Tettmar KI, Hewitt P, et al. Hepatitis E risks: pigs or blood-that is the question. *Transfusion* (2017) 57(2):267–72. doi:10.1111/trf.13976
3. Xin S, Xiao L. Clinical manifestations of hepatitis E. *Adv Exp Med Biol* (2016) 948:175–89. doi:10.1007/978-94-024-0942-0_10
4. Izopet J, Lhomme S, Chapuy-Regaud S, Mansuy JM, Kamar N, Abravanel F. HEV and transfusion-recipient risk. *Transfus Clin Biol* (2017) 24(3):176–81. doi:10.1016/j.tracli.2017.06.012
5. Dreier J, Juhl D. Autochthonous hepatitis E virus infections: a new transfusion-associated risk? *Transfus Med Hemother* (2014) 41(1):29–39. doi:10.1159/000357098
6. Arankalle VA, Chobe LP. Retrospective analysis of blood transfusion recipients: evidence for post-transfusion hepatitis E. *Vox Sang* (2000) 79(2):72–4. doi:10.1159/000031215
7. Domanović D, Tedder R, Blümel J, Zaaijer H, Gallian P, Niederhauser C, et al. Hepatitis E and blood donation safety in selected European countries: a shift to screening? *Euro Surveill* (2017) 22(16):1–8. doi:10.2807/1560-7917.ES.2017.22.16.30514
8. European Pharmacopeia Chapter 8.3: Human plasma (pooled and treated for virus inactivation). *Eur Pharmacopoeia* (2014):4353–5.
9. European Medicines Agency. *Reflection Paper on Viral Safety of Plasma-Derived Medicinal Products with Respect to Hepatitis E Virus* (2015). Available from: http://www.ema.europa.eu/docs/en_GB/document_library/Scientific_guideline/2015/07/WC500189012.pdf
10. Toyoda H, Honda T, Hayashi K, Katano Y, Goto H, Kumada T, et al. Prevalence of hepatitis E virus IgG antibody in Japanese patients with hemophilia. *Intervirology* (2008) 51(1):21–5. doi:10.1159/000118792
11. de Vos AS, Janssen MP, Zaaijer HL, Hogema BM. Cost-effectiveness of the screening of blood donations for hepatitis E virus in the Netherlands. *Transfusion* (2017) 57(2):258–66. doi:10.1111/trf.13978
12. Pauli G, Aepfelbacher M, Bauerfeind U, Blümel J, Burger R, Gärtner B, et al. Hepatitis E virus. *Transfus Med Hemother* (2015) 42(4):247–65. doi:10.1159/000431191
13. Vollmer T, Diekmann J, Johne R, Eberhardt M, Knabbe C, Dreier J. Novel approach for the detection of hepatitis E virus infection in German blood donors. *J Clin Microbiol* (2012) 50(8):2708–13. doi:10.1128/JCM.01119-12
14. Harritshøj LH, Holm DK, Saekmose SG, Jensen BA, Hogema BM, Fischer TK, et al. Low transfusion transmission of hepatitis E among 25,637 single-donation, nucleic acid-tested blood donors. *Transfusion* (2016) 56(9):2225–32. doi:10.1111/trf.13700
15. O'Riordan J, Boland F, Williams P, Donnellan J, Hogema BM, Ijaz S, et al. Hepatitis E virus infection in the Irish blood donor population. *Transfusion* (2016) 56(11):2868–76. doi:10.1111/trf.13757
16. Gallian P, Couchouron A, Dupont I, Fabra C, Piquet Y, Djoudi R, et al. Hepatitis E virus infections in blood donors, France. *Emerg Infect Dis* (2014) 20(11):1914–7. doi:10.3201/eid2011.140516
17. Sauleda S, Ong E, Bes M, Janssen A, Cory R, Babizki M, et al. Seroprevalence of hepatitis E virus (HEV) and detection of HEV RNA with a transcription-mediated amplification assay in blood donors from Catalonia (Spain). *Transfusion* (2015) 55(5):972–9. doi:10.1111/trf.12929
18. Hogema BM, Molier M, Sjerps M, de Waal M, van Swieten P, van de Laar T, et al. Incidence and duration of hepatitis E virus infection in Dutch blood donors. *Transfusion* (2016) 56(3):722–8. doi:10.1111/trf.13402
19. Kamar N, Dalton HR, Abravanel F, Izopet J. Hepatitis E virus infection. *Clin Microbiol Rev* (2014) 27(1):116–38. doi:10.1128/CMR.00057-13
20. Dalton HR, Bendall R, Ijaz S, Banks M. Hepatitis E: an emerging infection in developed countries. *Lancet Infect Dis* (2008) 8(11):698–709. doi:10.1016/S1473-3099(08)70255-X
21. Purcell RH, Emerson SU. Hepatitis E: an emerging awareness of an old disease. *J Hepatol* (2008) 48(3):494–503. doi:10.1016/j.jhep.2007.12.008
22. Vollmer T, Diekmann J, Eberhardt M, Knabbe C, Dreier J. Hepatitis E in blood donors: investigation of the natural course of asymptomatic infection, Germany, 2011. *Euro Surveill* (2016) 21(35):1–9. doi:10.2807/1560-7917.ES.2016.21.35.30332
23. Haïm-Boukobza S, Ferey MP, Vétillard AL, Jeblaoui A, Pélissier E, Pelletier G, et al. Transfusion-transmitted hepatitis E in a misleading context of autoimmunity and drug-induced toxicity. *J Hepatol* (2012) 57(6):1374–8. doi:10.1016/j.jhep.2012.08.001
24. Hewitt PE, Ijaz S, Brailsford SR, Brett R, Dicks S, Haywood B, et al. Hepatitis E virus in blood components: a prevalence and transmission study in southeast England. *Lancet* (2014) 384:1766–73. doi:10.1016/S0140-6736(14)61034-5
25. Khuroo MS, Kamili S, Yattoo GN. Hepatitis E virus infection may be transmitted through blood transfusions in an endemic area. *J Gastroenterol Hepatol* (2004) 19(7):778–84. doi:10.1111/j.1440-1746.2004.03437.x
26. Fuse K, Matsuyama Y, Moriyama M, Miyakoshi S, Shibasaki Y, Takizawa J, et al. Late onset post-transfusion hepatitis E developing during chemotherapy for acute promyelocytic leukemia. *Intern Med* (2015) 54(6):657–61. doi:10.2169/internalmedicine.54.2332
27. Mitsui T, Tsukamoto Y, Yamazaki C, Masuko K, Tsuda F, Takahashi M, et al. Prevalence of hepatitis E virus infection among hemodialysis patients in Japan: evidence for infection with a genotype 3 HEV by blood transfusion. *J Med Virol* (2004) 74(4):563–72. doi:10.1002/jmv.20215
28. Tamura A, Shimizu YK, Tanaka T, Kuroda K, Arakawa Y, Takahashi K, et al. Persistent infection of hepatitis E virus transmitted by blood transfusion in a patient with T-cell lymphoma. *Hepatol Res* (2007) 37(2):113–20. doi:10.1111/j.1872-034X.2007.00024.x
29. Satake M, Matsubayashi K, Hoshi Y, Taira R, Furui Y, Kokudo N, et al. Unique clinical courses of transfusion-transmitted hepatitis E in patients with immunosuppression. *Transfusion* (2017) 57(2):280–8. doi:10.1111/trf.13994
30. Andonov A, Rock G, Lin L, Borlang J, Hooper J, Grudeski E, et al. Serological and molecular evidence of a plausible transmission of hepatitis E virus through pooled plasma. *Vox Sang* (2014) 107(3):213–9. doi:10.1111/vox.12156
31. Matsubayashi K, Nagaoka Y, Sakata H, Sato S, Fukai K, Kato T, et al. Transfusion-transmitted hepatitis E caused by apparently indigenous hepatitis E virus strain in Hokkaido, Japan. *Transfusion* (2004) 44(6):934–40. doi:10.1111/j.1537-2995.2004.03300.x
32. Matsubayashi K, Kang JH, Sakata H, Takahashi K, Shindo M, Kato M, et al. A case of transfusion-transmitted hepatitis E caused by blood from a donor infected with hepatitis E virus via zoonotic food-borne route. *Transfusion* (2008) 48(7):1368–75. doi:10.1111/j.1537-2995.2008.01722.x
33. Matsui T, Kang JH, Matsubayashi K, Yamazaki H, Nagai K, Sakata H, et al. Rare case of transfusion-transmitted hepatitis E from the blood of a donor infected with the hepatitis E virus genotype 3 indigenous to Japan: viral dynamics from onset to recovery. *Hepatol Res* (2015) 45(6):698–704. doi:10.1111/hepr.12390
34. Colson P, Coze C, Gallian P, Henry M, De Micco P, Tamalet C. Transfusion-associated hepatitis E, France. *Emerg Infect Dis* (2007) 13(4):648–9. doi:10.3201/eid1304.061387

35. Boxall E, Herborn A, Kochethu G, Pratt G, Adams D, Ijaz S, et al. Transfusion-transmitted hepatitis E in a 'nonhyperendemic' country. *Transfus Med* (2006) 16(2):79–83. doi:10.1111/j.1365-3148.2006.00652.x
36. Kimura Y, Gotoh A, Katagiri S, Hoshi Y, Uchida S, Yamasaki A, et al. Transfusion-transmitted hepatitis E in a patient with myelodysplastic syndromes. *Blood Transfus* (2014) 12(1):103–6. doi:10.2450/2013.0081-13
37. Miyoshi M, Kakinuma S, Tanabe Y, Ishii K, Li TC, Wakita T, et al. Chronic hepatitis E infection in a persistently immunosuppressed patient unable to be eliminated after ribavirin therapy. *Intern Med* (2016) 55(19):2811–7. doi:10.2169/internalmedicine.55.7025
38. Inagaki Y, Oshiro Y, Tanaka T, Yoshizumi T, Okajima H, Ishiyama K, et al. A nationwide survey of hepatitis E virus infection and chronic hepatitis E in liver transplant recipients in Japan. *EBioMedicine* (2015) 2(11):1607–12. doi:10.1016/j.ebiom.2015.09.030
39. Tanaka T, Akamatsu N, Sakamoto Y, Inagaki Y, Oshiro Y, Ohkohchi N, et al. Treatment with ribavirin for chronic hepatitis E following living donor liver transplantation: a case report. *Hepatol Res* (2016) 46(10):1058–9. doi:10.1111/hepr.12641
40. Hauser L, Roque-Afonso AM, Beyloune A, Simonet M, Fischer BD, des Roziers NB, et al. Hepatitis E transmission by transfusion of Intercept blood system-treated plasma. *Blood* (2014) 123(5):796–7. doi:10.1182/blood-2013-09-524348
41. Coilly A, Haim-Boukobza S, Roche B, Antonini TM, Pause A, Mokhtari C, et al. Posttransplantation hepatitis E: transfusion-transmitted hepatitis rising from the ashes. *Transplantation* (2013) 96(2):e4–6. doi:10.1097/TP.0b013e318296c9f7
42. Huzly D, Umhau M, Bettinger D, Cathomen T, Emmerich F, Hasselblatt P, et al. Transfusion-transmitted hepatitis E in Germany, 2013. *Euro Surveill* (2014) 19(21):1–4. doi:10.2807/1560-7917.ES2014.19.21.20812
43. Kurihara T, Yoshizumi T, Itoh S, Harimoto N, Harada N, Ikegami T, et al. Chronic hepatitis E virus infection after living donor liver transplantation via blood transfusion: a case report. *Surg Case Rep* (2016) 2(1):32. doi:10.1186/s40792-016-0159-0
44. Hoad VC, Gibbs T, Ravikumara M, Nash M, Levy A, Tracy SL, et al. First confirmed case of transfusion-transmitted hepatitis E in Australia. *Med J Aust* (2017) 206(7):289–90. doi:10.5694/mja16.01090
45. Riveiro-Barciela M, Sauleda S, Quer J, Salvador F, Gregori J, Pirón M, et al. Red blood cell transfusion-transmitted acute hepatitis E in an immunocompetent subject in Europe: a case report. *Transfusion* (2017) 57(2):244–7. doi:10.1111/trf.13876
46. Pischke S, Hiller J, Lutgehetmann M, Polywka S, Rybczynski M, Ayuk F, et al. Blood-borne hepatitis E virus transmission: a relevant risk for immunosuppressed patients. *Clin Infect Dis* (2016) 63(4):569–70. doi:10.1093/cid/ciw309
47. Paul-Ehrlich-Institut. *Haemovigilance report of the Paul-Ehrlich-Institut 2015: Assessment of the reports of serious adverse transfusion reactions pursuant to section 63i AMG (Arzneimittelgesetz, German Medicines Act).* Available from: https://www.pei.de/SharedDocs/Downloads/vigilanz/haemovigilanz/publikationen/haemovigilance-report-2015.pdf;jsessionid=BFAF09FD4B6089DDE655202CB737AD58.2_cid354?__blob=publicationFile&v=3
48. Shukla P, Nguyen HT, Torian U, Engle RE, Faulk K, Dalton HR, et al. Cross-species infections of cultured cells by hepatitis E virus and discovery of an infectious virus-host recombinant. *Proc Natl Acad Sci U S A* (2011) 108(6):2438–43. doi:10.1073/pnas.1018878108
49. Tanaka T, Takahashi M, Kusano E, Okamoto H. Development and evaluation of an efficient cell-culture system for hepatitis E virus. *J Gen Virol* (2007) 88(Pt 3):903–11. doi:10.1099/vir.0.82535-0
50. Tanaka T, Takahashi M, Takahashi H, Ichiyama K, Hoshino Y, Nagashima S, et al. Development and characterization of a genotype 4 hepatitis E virus cell culture system using a HE-JF5/15F strain recovered from a fulminant hepatitis patient. *J Clin Microbiol* (2009) 47(6):1906–10. doi:10.1128/JCM.00629-09
51. Shukla P, Nguyen HT, Faulk K, Mather K, Torian U, Engle RE, et al. Adaptation of a genotype 3 hepatitis E virus to efficient growth in cell culture depends on an inserted human gene segment acquired by recombination. *J Virol* (2012) 86(10):5697–707. doi:10.1128/JVI.00146-12
52. Xia NS, Zhang J, Zheng YJ, Ge SX, Ye XZ, Ou SH. Transfusion of plasma from a blood donor induced hepatitis E in Rhesus monkey. *Vox Sang* (2004) 86(1):45–7. doi:10.1111/j.0042-9007.2004.00377.x
53. Sayed IM, Foquet L, Verhoye L, Abravanel F, Farhoudi A, Leroux-Roels G, et al. Transmission of hepatitis E virus infection to human-liver chimeric FRG mice using patient plasma. *Antiviral Res* (2017) 141:150–4. doi:10.1016/j.antiviral.2017.02.011
54. Sayed IM, Verhoye L, Cocquerel L, Abravanel F, Foquet L, Montpellier C, et al. Study of hepatitis E virus infection of genotype 1 and 3 in mice with humanised liver. *Gut* (2017) 66(5):920–9. doi:10.1136/gutjnl-2015-311109
55. Gallian P, Couchouron A, Dupont I, Fabra C, Piquet Y, Djoudi R, et al. Comparison of hepatitis E virus nucleic acid test screening platforms and RNA prevalence in French blood donors. *Transfusion* (2017) 57(1):223–4. doi:10.1111/trf.13889
56. Vollmer T, Knabbe C, Dreier J. Comparison of real-time PCR and antigen assays for detection of hepatitis E virus in blood donors. *J Clin Microbiol* (2014) 52(6):2150–6. doi:10.1128/JCM.03578-13
57. Vollmer T, Knabbe C, Dreier J. Knowledge is safety: the time is ripe for hepatitis E virus blood donor screening. *Transfus Med Hemother* (2016) 43(6):425–7. doi:10.1159/000450794

22

Early Fresh Frozen Plasma Transfusion: Is it Associated with Improved Outcomes of Patients With Sepsis?

Xiaoyi Qin[1†], Wei Zhang[2†], Xiaodan Zhu[3], Xiang Hu[4] and Wei Zhou[3]*

[1] Department of Hematology, The First Affiliated Hospital of Wenzhou Medical University, Wenzhou, China, [2] Department of Thoracic Surgery, The First Affiliated Hospital of Wenzhou Medical University, Wenzhou, China, [3] Department of Intensive Care Unit, The First Affiliated Hospital of Wenzhou Medical University, Wenzhou, China, [4] Department of Endocrine and Metabolic Diseases, The First Affiliated Hospital of Wenzhou Medical University, Wenzhou, China

***Correspondence:**
Wei Zhou
wyyyzw@yahoo.com

[†] These authors have contributed equally to this work

Background: So far, no study has investigated the effects of plasma transfusion in the patients with sepsis, especially in the terms of prognosis. Therefore, we aimed to explore the association of early fresh frozen plasma (FFP) transfusion with the outcomes of patients with sepsis.

Methods: We performed a cohort study using data extracted from the Medical Information Mart for Intensive Care III database (v1.4). External validation was obtained from the First Affiliated Hospital of Wenzhou Medical University, China. We adopted the Sepsis-3 criteria to extract the patients with sepsis and septic shock. The occurrence of transfusion during the first 3-days of intensive care unit (ICU) stay was regarded as early FFP transfusion. The primary outcome was 28-day mortality. We assessed the association of early FFP transfusion with the patient outcomes using a Cox regression analysis. Furthermore, we performed the sensitivity analysis, subset analysis, and external validation to verify the true strength of the results.

Results: After adjusting for the covariates in the three models, respectively, the significantly higher risk of death in the FFP transfusion group at 28-days [e.g., Model 2: hazard ratio (HR) = 1.361, P = 0.018, 95% CI = 1.054–1.756] and 90-days (e.g., Model 2: HR = 1.368, P = 0.005, 95% CI = 1.099–1.704) remained distinct. Contrarily, the mortality increased significantly with the increase of FFP transfusion volume. The outcomes of the patients with sepsis with hypocoagulable state after early FFP transfusion were not significantly improved. Similar results can also be found in the subset analysis of the septic shock cohort. The results of external validation exhibited good consistency.

Conclusions: Our study provides a new understanding of the rationale and effectiveness of FFP transfusion for the patients with sepsis. After recognizing the evidence of risk-benefit and cost-benefit, it is important to reduce the inappropriate use of FFP and avoid unnecessary adverse transfusion reactions.

Keywords: fresh frozen plasma, international normalized ratio, partial thromboplastin time, sepsis, septic shock

INTRODUCTION

Sepsis, a syndrome of pathophysiological abnormalities and severe organ dysfunction induced by infection, leads to high incidence and mortality rates worldwide (1–4). Since 2002, the Surviving Sepsis Campaign has made a highly successful international effort to decrease sepsis mortality by the therapeutic strategies of bundle elements (5). In its 2018 update, it is believed that the early effective fluid therapies with intravenous injection are crucial for the stabilization of sepsis-induced tissue hypoperfusion (6). The ideal fluid management in sepsis should improve euvolemia without causing edema, potentially by rebuilding the damaged endothelial glycocalyx layer and repairing the injured endothelium (7). The crystalloids are recommended as first-line therapy, however, the benefit following the administration of colloids compared with crystalloids in the patients with sepsis remains unclear (6–8).

Plasma, as a "super-colloid," is rich of proteins, such as albumin, coagulation factors, fibrin, immunoglobulins, antithrombin, protein C, and protein S (9). The studies regarding the effects of plasma transfusion in the patients with a critical illness are limited, and the conclusions have not reached an agreement. Much of what we know about the plasma-based fluid management comes from the studies performed in the setting of trauma. Early plasma transfusion instead of other blood products is associated with the decreased mortality in trauma patients (10, 11). In traditional clinical practice, the patients with critical illness who have abnormal coagulation may benefit from plasma transfusion at intensive care unit (ICU) admission. However, Dara SI et al. considered that the risk-benefit ratio of fresh frozen plasma (FFP) transfusion in the patients with critical illness with coagulopathy may not be favorable (12). This contradiction may attribute to the adverse effects accompanied by plasma transfusion in aspects of infections, immunomodulation, allergic reactions, circulatory overload, and citrate toxicity (13).

As no previous studies for reference, the effects of plasma transfusion in the patients with sepsis remain unknown. Therefore, we aimed to explore the potential relationship of early FFP transfusion with the outcomes of the patients with sepsis at ICU admission. Furthermore, we hypothesize that early FFP transfusion does not benefit the short-term survival of most patients with sepsis.

METHODS

Data Source

We performed a retrospective cohort study using data extracted from the Medical Information Mart for Intensive Care III (MIMIC III) database (v1.4) which integrated deidentified and comprehensive clinical data of the patients admitted to the Beth Israel Deaconess Medical Center (BIDMC) in Boston, Massachusetts, United States (14). MIMIC III database contains over 58,000 hospital admissions data for adult patients and neonates admitted to various critical care units between 2001 and 2012. The Institutional Review Board of the BIDMC (Boston, MA, USA) and Massachusetts Institute of Technology (Cambridge, MA, USA) have approved the use of MIMIC III database for authorized users. Wei Zhou was allowed to download data from the database, having completed the "Data or Specimens Only Research" course (record identity: 25222342).

External validation was collected from the First Affiliated Hospital of Wenzhou Medical University (Wenzhou, Zhejiang, China) after approval from the First Affiliated Hospital Ethics Committee.

The informed consents of all the patients were not required because the present study neither contained any protected health information nor impacted clinical care.

Study Cohort

A flowchart of the inclusion and exclusion procedure for the MIMIC III is depicted in **Figure 1**. We adopted the third international consensus definitions (Sepsis-3, a diagnosis flowchart is presented in **Supplementary Figure 1**) to extract the patients with sepsis and septic shock from the database (1). Based on the Sepsis-3 criteria, patients with suspected infection and evidence of organ dysfunction [Sequential Organ Failure Assessment (SOFA) score ≥ 2] were identified as the patients with sepsis (1). Suspected infection was defined as the concomitant administration of antibiotics and sampling of body fluid cultures (blood, urine, sputum, etc.) (1). In other words, if the culture was obtained, the antibiotic was required to be administered within 72 h, whereas if the antibiotic was first, the culture was required within 24 h (1). Moreover, we defined the period of suspected infection as ranging between 24 h before and 24 h after admission to an ICU. The patients in the CareVue and MetaVision information systems of MIMIC III were admitted before and after 2008, respectively. Only patient data stored in the MetaVision system were collected for analysis. Antibiotic prescription data were only available after 2002, thus, there was a fraction (1/7) of the CareVue patients who had missing data for the suspected infection definition. It was the simplest option for us to limit the cohort to the MetaVision system, because the resulting sample size was sufficient. Additionally, the exclusion criteria for the initial sepsis cohort were as follows: (1) repeat hospitalization at ICU, (2) aged 16 years or younger, and (3) current service relating to cardiac, vascular, or thoracic surgery. We assumed that these sub-populations had physiological abnormalities yet caused by the factors unrelated to sepsis. Furthermore, we excluded the patients who had incomplete covariate data for further multivariate analysis.

External validation data were collected between September 15, 2018 and December 31, 2020 according to the same inclusion and exclusion criteria. The main diagnosis of these patients clearly met the Sepsis-3 criteria within 24 h of ICU admission. The clinical outcomes were followed-up for 90-days after admission (13 patients were excluded due to loss to follow-up).

Abbreviations: APACHE II, Acute Physiology and Chronic Health Evaluation II; BIDMC, Beth Israel Deaconess Medical Center; CIs, confidence intervals; FFP, fresh frozen plasma; GCS, Glasgow coma scale; HRs, hazard ratios; ICU, intensive care unit; INR, international normalized ratio; IQRs, interquartile ranges; K–M, Kaplan–Meier; LOS, length of stay; MIMIC III, Medical Information Mart for Intensive Care III; ORs, odds ratios; PTT, partial thromboplastin time; SAPS II, Simplified Acute Physiology Score II; SOFA, Sequential Organ Failure Assessment; and TRALI, transfusion-related acute lung injury.

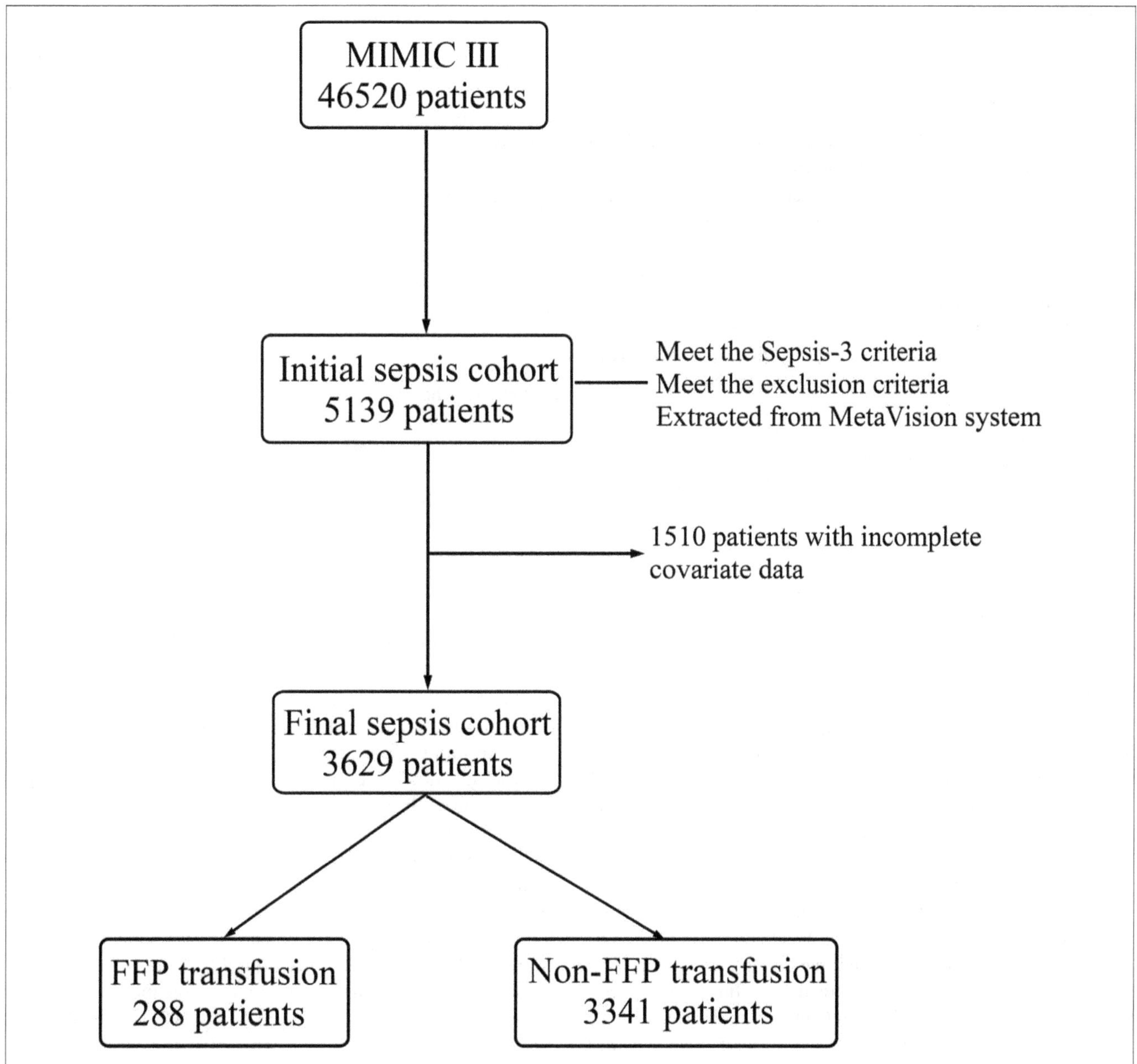

FIGURE 1 | The flowchart of the inclusion and exclusion procedure for the Medical Information Mart for Intensive Care III (MIMIC III) database. FFP, fresh frozen plasma; MIMIC III, Medical Information Mart for Intensive Care III.

Data Extraction

The data were extracted from MIMIC III and our hospital system, such as gender, age, laboratory data, vital statistics, comorbidities, ICU interventions, and hospital length of stay (LOS). The severity scores of illness, such as Simplified Acute Physiology Score II (SAPS II), Acute Physiology and Chronic Health Evaluation II (APACHE II), and SOFA were calculated on the basis of their predefined criteria (15–17). The mean values of laboratory data and vital statistics during the first 24 h of ICU stay were regarded as baseline data. The scores of Glasgow coma scale (GCS), SAPS II, APACHE II, and SOFA as well as the necessity to perform interventions with vasopressor and mechanical ventilation were evaluated during the first 24 h of ICU stay. Additionally, SAPS II and APACHE II were used for MIMIC III and the external validation data analysis, respectively.

Predictor and Outcome Variables

We recorded the FFP transfusion status of each patient during the first 3-days of their ICU stays. To minimize the potential bias, the values of international normalized ratio (INR) and partial thromboplastin time (PTT) were obtained before FFP transfusion.

The primary end point was 28-day mortality. The secondary end points were 90-day and in-hospital mortality. Mortality information in the MIMIC III was calculated based on the dates of admission and death obtained from the social security records.

Statistical Analysis

The Kolmogorov–Smirnov normality test was used to check the normality assumption for the numerical variables. Differences in the normally and non-normally distributed variables were compared using the unpaired Student's *t*-test and Wilcoxon's rank-sum test, respectively. Comparisons for the categorical variables were performed by Pearson's χ^2 test and Fisher's exact test. Normally distributed data were expressed as the means with SDs, and non-normally distributed data were expressed as the medians with inter-quartile ranges (IQRs). The categorical variables were expressed as frequencies with percentages.

We assessed the association of early FFP transfusion with survival in the patients with sepsis using the logistic regression and Kaplan–Meier (K–M) analysis. The results were presented in form of odds ratios (*OR*s) with 95% *CI*s and survival curve, respectively.

For the Cox regression analysis, three multivariate models were constructed as follows: Model 1, adjusting only for gender and age; Model 2, adjusting for gender, age, and scores of SAPS II (APACHE II for external validation) and SOFA; Model 3, adjusting for gender, age, laboratory data (white blood cell, platelet, hemoglobin, lactate, and creatinine), vital statistics (heart rate, mean blood pressure, respiration rate, temperature, pulse oxygen saturation, and glucose), scores of GCS, SOFA, and SAPS II (APACHE II for external validation), ICU interventions (vasopressor, mechanical ventilation, and renal replacement therapy), history of alcohol abuse, comorbidities, and hospital LOS. The hazard ratios (*HR*s) and 95% *CI*s were calculated for these models.

A sensitivity analysis was performed to further validate the effects of early FFP transfusion in the patients with sepsis with hypocoagulable and non-hypocoagulable state. Moreover, a subset analysis was performed for the patients with FFP transfusion (N = 288) to evaluate the relationship between the transfusion volume of FFP and survival. Subsequently, we performed an additional subset analysis to establish whether similar results also existed in the septic shock cohort (N = 625). Finally, external validation was introduced to verify whether similar results can be observed in the East Asian population.

A two-sided $P < 0.05$ was regarded as representing statistical significance. The statistical analyses were performed using the SPSS software 20.0 (SPSS, Chicago, IL, USA) and MedCalc software 19.0.5 (MedCalc, Ostend, Belgium).

RESULTS

Baseline Data of Study Cohort

A total of 3,629 patients with sepsis from the MIMIC-III database were included in final sepsis cohort (**Figure 1**). The baseline characteristics of final sepsis cohort are summarized in **Table 1**. The median transfusion volume in FFP transfusion group was 627 ml (IQR: 532–1,169 ml). Additionally, the baseline laboratory data and vital statistics for further multivariate analysis are shown in **Table 2**.

Comparison of the baseline characteristics of the initial sepsis cohort vs. final sepsis cohort is presented in **Supplementary Table 1**. Similar baseline data were found between the two cohorts.

Associations of Early FFP Transfusion With Primary and Secondary Outcomes

The rates of 28-, 90-day, and in-hospital mortality of the two groups were as follows: FFP transfusion group = 24.3, 32.6, and 22.2%, respectively, and non-FFP transfusion group = 14.7, 20.3, and 11.1%, respectively. For the univariate logistic regression analysis, the mortality of FFP transfusion group was significantly higher than the non-FFP transfusion group in 28-, 90-day, and in-hospital (OR = 1.859, $P < 0.001$, 95% CI = 1.397–2.474; OR = 1.907, $P < 0.001$, 95% CI = 1.470–2.474; and OR = 2.287, $P <$ 0.001, 95% CI = 1.698–3.081, respectively).

Moreover, based on the K–M survival analysis of 28- and 90-day, the patients of non-FFP transfusion conferred more favorable prognosis than those of FFP transfusion ($P < 0.001$, both) (**Figures 2A,B**).

Multivariate Analysis, Sensitivity Analysis, and Subset Analysis

In clinical practice, the patients with FFP transfusion are often more serious and accompanied by the coagulation abnormalities, thus, the multivariate analysis, sensitivity analysis, and subset analysis still need to be performed to verify the true intrinsic relationship on the premise of excluding potentially relevant bias.

The actual associations of FFP transfusion with 28- and 90-day mortality were evaluated by the Cox regression models. As shown in **Table 3**, after adjusting for the covariates of Model 1, Model 2, and Model 3, respectively, the significantly higher risk of death in the FFP transfusion group at 28 and 90-days remained distinct. Additionally, for the in-hospital mortality, a similar result can be found using a multivariate logistic regression analysis (Model 1: OR = 2.282, $P < 0.001$, 95% CI = 1.685–3.091; Model 2: OR = 1.887, $P < 0.001$, 95% CI = 1.366–2.606; and Model 3: OR = 1.899, $P < 0.001$, 95% CI = 1.350–2.672).

The sensitivity analysis on the basis of two different coagulation indexes was performed in our study. INR and PTT, representing exogenous and endogenous coagulation function, respectively, were divided into hypocoagulable and non-hypocoagulable state according to the upper limit of their normal range (18, 19). As presented in **Table 4**, after correcting for the same covariates (Model 2), the outcomes of the patients with sepsis with hypocoagulable state after early FFP transfusion were not significantly improved in the Cox regression models. Contrarily, for the patients with PTT $\leq$ 40, there was a statistically significant increasing trend for the patients with sepsis of early FFP transfusion in the risk of death at 28- and 90-days.

The distribution of transfusion volume in the FFP transfusion group (N = 288) during the first 3-days of ICU stay was as follows: the lowest tertile range from 220 to 567 ml; the

TABLE 1 | The baseline characteristics of study cohort.

Characteristics	Total (N = 3,629)	FFP transfusion (N = 288)	Non-FFP transfusion (N = 3,341)
Gender (men/women)	2,023/1,606	182/106	1,841/1,500**
Age (years)	66.6 (53.8–79.7)	68.4 (54.4–80.6)	66.4 (53.8–79.6)
≤30, *n* (%)	175 (4.8)	10 (3.5)	165 (4.9)
>30, ≤60, *n* (%)	1,132 (31.2)	87 (30.2)	1,045 (31.3)
>60, *n* (%)	2,322 (64.0)	191 (66.3)	2,131 (63.8)
Alcohol abuse, *n* (%)	388 (10.7)	41 (14.2)	347 (10.4)*
Culture specimen types			
Blood, *n* (%)	1,572 (43.3)	109 (37.8)	1,463 (43.8)
Lung, *n* (%)	122 (3.4)	8 (2.8)	114 (3.4)
Urinary system, *n* (%)	610 (16.8)	49 (17.0)	561 (16.8)
Gastrointestinal system, *n* (%)	11 (0.3)	0 (0)	11 (0.3)
Others, *n* (%)	1,314 (36.2)	122 (42.4)	1,192 (35.7)*
Culture positive, *n* (%)	476 (13.1)	46 (16.0)	430 (12.9)
Vasopressor (first 24 h), *n* (%)	1,082 (29.8)	101 (35.1)	981 (29.4)*
Mechanical ventilation (first 24 h), *n* (%)	1,884 (51.9)	177 (61.5)	1,707 (51.1)**
Renal replacement therapy, *n* (%)	173 (4.8)	27 (9.4)	146 (4.4)**
GCS score	15 (13–15)	15 (14–15)	15 (13–15)**
SOFA score	5 (3–6)	6 (4–7)	4 (3–6)**
SAPS II score	37.0 (30.0–46.0)	40.5 (34.0–50.0)	37.0 (29.0–46.0)**
Comorbidities			
Congestive heart failure, *n* (%)	850 (23.4)	72 (25.0)	778 (23.3)
Cardiac arrhythmias, *n* (%)	1,089 (30.0)	135 (46.9)	954 (28.6)**
Hypertension, *n* (%)	2,140 (59.0)	159 (55.2)	1,981 (59.3)
Chronic pulmonary, *n* (%)	788 (21.7)	55 (19.1)	733 (21.9)
Renal failure, *n* (%)	634 (17.5)	55 (19.1)	579 (17.3)
Liver disease, *n* (%)	347 (9.6)	57 (19.8)	290 (8.7)**
Solid tumor, *n* (%)	231 (6.4)	23 (8.0)	208 (6.2)
Diabetes, *n* (%)	1,043 (28.7)	78 (27.1)	965 (28.9)
Hospital LOS (days)	7.7 (4.9–12.7)	10.4 (6.2–16.5)	7.6 (4.8–12.4)**

**P-value < 0.05; **P-value < 0.01. The data were expressed as median (inter-quartile range) or frequency (percentage). FFP, fresh frozen plasma; GCS, Glasgow coma scale; LOS, length of stay; SAPS II, Simplified Acute Physiology Score II; SOFA, Sequential Organ Failure Assessment.*

medium tertile from 567 to 926 ml; the highest tertile from 926 to 8,148 ml. There seemed to be an increasing trend from the lowest tertile to the highest tertile in the risk of death at both 28-days (HR = 1.783, P = 0.055, 95% CI = 0.987–3.219) and 90-days (HR = 1.710, P = 0.035, 95% CI = 1.039–2.813) after correcting for the covariates of Model 2. Meanwhile, the survival curves of the three groups are presented in **Figures 3A,B**. The detailed distribution of FFP transfusion volume is shown in **Supplementary Figure 2**.

The comparison of baseline characteristics of septic shock cohort vs. sepsis cohort is summarized in **Supplementary Table 2**. There were significant differences between the septic shock cohort (N = 625) and sepsis cohort (N = 3,629) in the severity of disease (P < 0.001 for SOFA and SAPS II, both). For the subset analysis of septic shock cohort (**Supplementary Table 3**), early FFP transfusion was not associated with the improved 28- and 90-day survival, even in the hypocoagulable group. Similarly, no significant dose-effect relationship was found between the transfusion volume and prognosis.

External Validation

The baseline characteristics of the external validation cohort (N = 294) were presented in **Supplementary Tables 4, 5**. New data collected from our hospital also led to similar results (**Table 5**) as in the primary analysis, indicating that even in the hypocoagulable group, early FFP transfusion cannot improve the outcomes of patients with sepsis, even was unfavorable. Additionally, in the subset analysis of the septic shock cohort (**Supplementary Table 6**), early FFP transfusion was not associated with the improved 28- and 90-day survival. Contrarily, the mortality of high transfusion volume was higher than that of low transfusion volume.

DISCUSSION

The present study revealed that regardless of whether the patients were in hypocoagulable or non-hypocoagulable state, early FFP transfusion was not associated with improved survival of 28-, 90-day, and in-hospital for the patients with sepsis, was unfavorable. Contrarily, both 28- and 90-day mortality increased significantly with the increase of FFP transfusion volume. Additionally, for the subset analysis of septic shock, early FFP transfusion was not associated with the improved 28- and 90-day survival, even in the hypocoagulable group. Similarly, the results of external validation exhibited good consistency, which suggests the conclusions of our study have a certain generalization value.

TABLE 2 | The baseline laboratory data and vital statistics.

Parameters	FFP transfusion (N = 288)	Non-FFP transfusion (N = 3,341)
Laboratory data		
WBC (10^9/L)	11.3 (7.9–15.2)	11.6 (8.4–15.6)
Platelet (10^9/L)	166.3 (108.8–240.0)	209.7 (153.0–277.7)**
Hemoglobin (g/dL)	10.1 (9.0–11.5)	10.9 (9.6–12.3)**
Lactate (mmol/L)	2.2 (1.6–3.2)	1.8 (1.3–2.5)**
Creatinine (mg/dL)	1.1 (0.8–1.6)	1.0 (0.8–1.5)*
PTT (s)	34.1 (28.6–43.1)	28.3 (25.0–33.4)**
INR	1.8 (1.4–2.8)	1.2 (1.1–1.4)**
Vital statistics		
Heart rate (bpm)	89.2 (75.1–100.4)	87.2 (76.0–98.8)
Mean blood pressure (mmHg)	74.7 (69.8–82.9)	75.7 (69.5–83.3)
Respiration rate (times/min)	18.7 (16.4–21.6)	19.0 (16.6–22.1)
Temperature (°C)	36.7 (36.3–37.2)	36.8 (36.5–37.3)**
SpO_2 (%)	97.8 (96.2–99.1)	97.3 (95.9–98.6)**
Glucose (mg/dL)	138.2 (112.8–166.4)	133.3 (112.3–163.1)

**P-value < 0.05; **P-value < 0.01. The data were expressed as median (inter-quartile range). FFP, fresh frozen plasma; INR, international normalized ratio; PTT, partial thromboplastin time; SpO_2, pulse oxygen saturation; WBC, white blood cell.*

Sepsis, a syndrome of immense clinical importance, accounts for high incidence, high mortality, and high ICU admission rate in recent years (3, 20, 21). The latest Sepsis-3 definition, replacing the previous definitions of sepsis gradually, is defined as a life-threatening organ dysfunction caused by a dysregulated host response to infection (1, 22). Johnson et al. performed a comparative analysis of sepsis identification methods in the MIMIC III database (v1.4), indicating that Sepsis-3 criteria had several advantages over the previous methods as follows: (1) less susceptibility to the coding practices changes, (2) provision of temporal context because of extracting sepsis cohort by suspected infection with associated organ failure at a time point not by ICD-9 codes, and (3) more conform to the contemporary understanding of the pathophysiology of sepsis (23). Therefore, it is appropriate to extract the patients with sepsis from the MIMIC III database *via* Sepsis-3 criteria.

Early effective fluid management is a mainstay in the initial treatment of sepsis. The controversy for the effects of fluid therapies with colloids vs. crystalloids on mortality in the patients with sepsis has always attracted much attention. As lack of any clear benefit following the administration of colloids compared with crystalloids in the patients with sepsis, the crystalloids are still recommended as first-line therapy (6). However, a systematic review suggested that the patients with severe sepsis might benefit from the fluid therapies with albumin (24). The relevant study on sepsis concerning plasma involved in the fluid therapies has, to the best of our knowledge, not been previously reported.

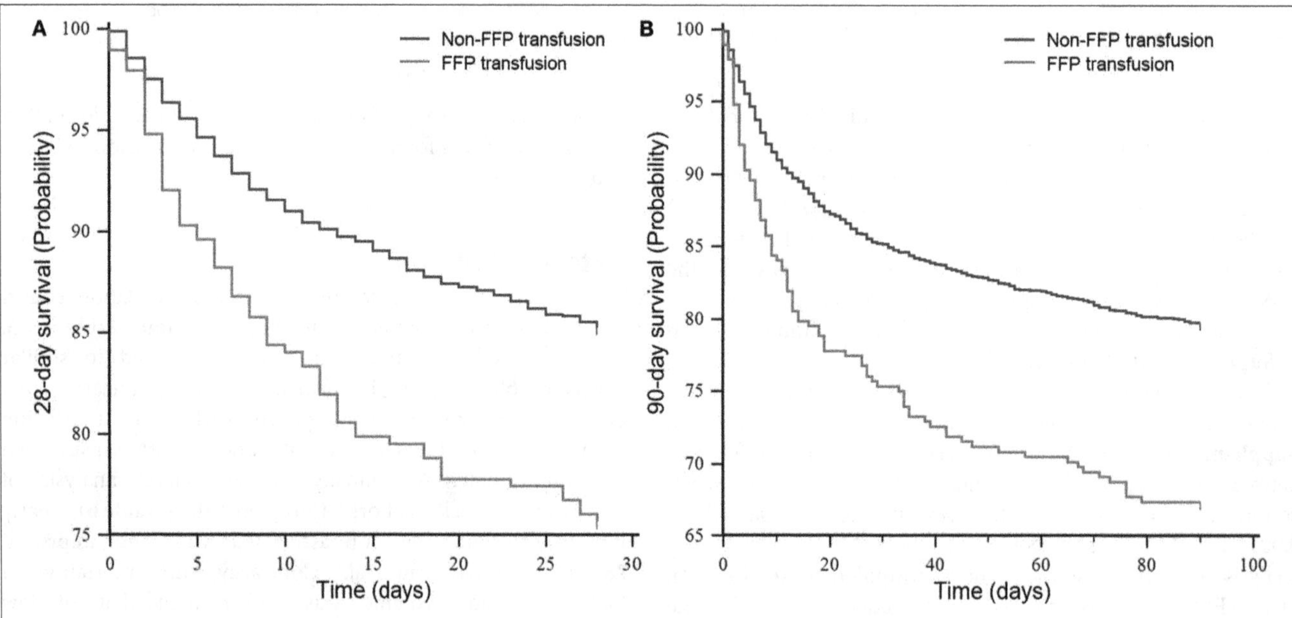

FIGURE 2 | The Kaplan–Meier survival analysis of sepsis cohort in the MIMIC III database. **(A)** 28-day survival curve and **(B)** 90-day survival curve. FFP, fresh frozen plasma; and MIMIC III, Medical Information Mart for Intensive Care III.

TABLE 3 | A multivariate Cox regression analysis of 28- and 90-day mortality.

Research variables	28-day mortality			90-day mortality		
	HR	95% CI	*P*-value	HR	95% CI	*P*-value
Model 1						
FFP transfusion vs. non-FFP transfusion	1.716	1.336–2.206	**<0.001**	1.692	1.363–2.100	**<0.001**
Model 2						
FFP transfusion vs. non-FFP transfusion	1.361	1.054–1.756	**0.018**	1.368	1.099–1.704	**0.005**
Model 3						
FFP transfusion vs. non-FFP transfusion	1.597	1.224–2.082	**0.001**	1.387	1.107–1.738	**0.004**

The significant P-value was indicated in bold. Model 1, adjusting for gender and age; Model 2, adjusting for gender, age, and scores of SAPS II and SOFA; Model 3, adjusting for all covariates. CI, confidence interval; FFP, fresh frozen plasma; HR, hazard ratio; SAPS II, Simplified Acute Physiology Score II; SOFA, Sequential Organ Failure Assessment.

TABLE 4 | The sensitivity analysis with INR and PTT by the Cox regression models.

Research subgroups	28-day mortality			90-day mortality		
	HR	95% CI	*P*-value	HR	95% CI	*P*-value
Non-hypocoagulable group (INR ≤ 1.20)*	1.000	0.371–2.693	0.999	1.494	0.739–3.021	0.264
Hypocoagulable group (INR > 1.20)*	1.264	0.960–1.664	0.095	1.188	0.936–1.509	0.157
Non-hypocoagulable group (PTT ≤ 40)*	1.373	1.013–1.862	**0.041**	1.336	1.027–1.736	**0.031**
Hypocoagulable group (PTT > 40)*	1.217	0.746–1.986	0.431	1.347	0.881–2.060	0.169

*The significant P-value was indicated in bold. *Adjusting for the covariates of Model 2. CI, confidence interval; HR, hazard ratio; INR, international normalized ratio; and PTT, partial thromboplastin time.*

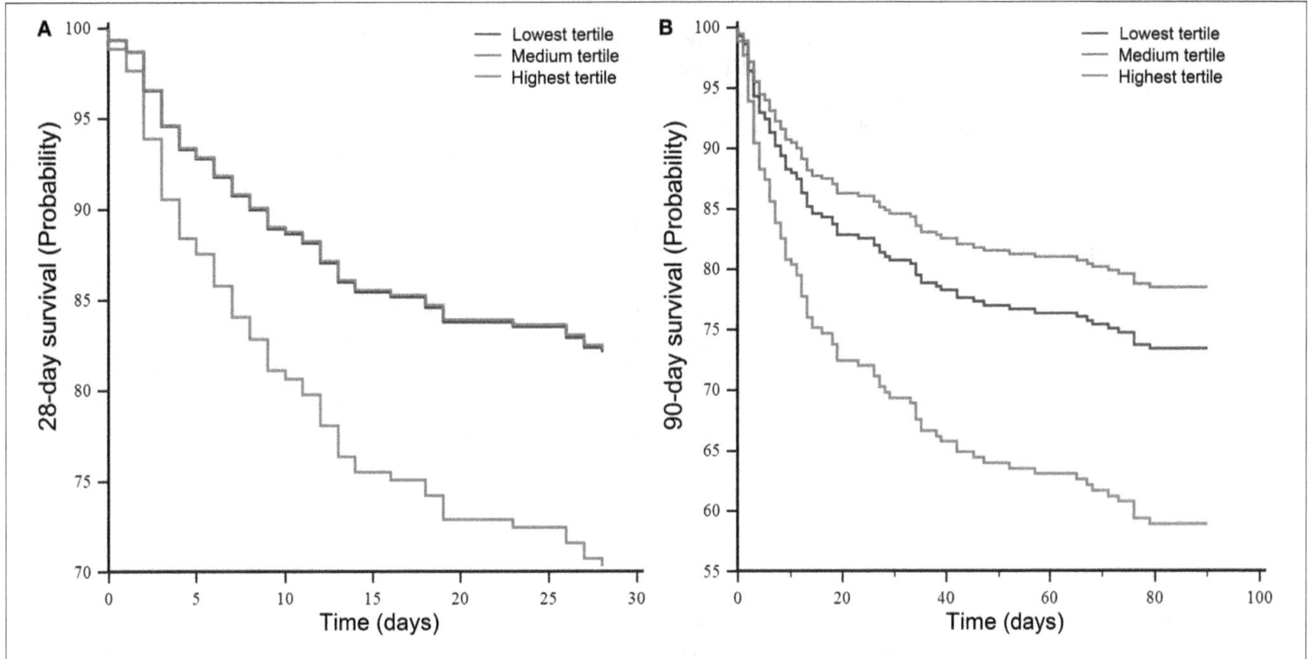

FIGURE 3 | The survival curves of Cox regression analysis for subset analysis in the MIMIC III database. **(A)** 28-day survival curve and **(B)** 90-day survival curve. MIMIC III, Medical Information Mart for Intensive Care III.

Plasma, a biological product containing the acellular portion of blood after centrifugation or by plasmapheresis, has important clinical effects, such as volume expansion, correction of abnormal coagulation tests, and transfusion-associated immunomodulation (13). The studies regarding the effects of plasma transfusion in the patients with a critical illness are limited, and the conclusions have not reached an agreement. Much of what we know about the effects of plasma transfusion

TABLE 5 | External validation with our hospital data.

Research variables	28-day mortality			90-day mortality		
	HR	95% CI	*P*-value	HR	95% CI	*P*-value
Model 1						
FFP transfusion vs. non-FFP transfusion	3.572	1.956–6.524	**<0.001**	2.758	1.690–4.500	**<0.001**
Model 2						
FFP transfusion vs. non-FFP transfusion	2.470	1.272–4.795	**0.008**	1.979	1.142–3.429	**0.015**
Model 3						
FFP transfusion vs. non-FFP transfusion	2.493	1.273–4.884	**0.008**	2.386	1.363–4.175	**0.002**
Sensitivity analysis with different coagulation indexes						
Non-hypocoagulable group (INR $\leq$ 1.20)*	1.313	0.175–9.856	0.791	0.793	0.172–3.658	0.767
Hypocoagulable group (INR > 1.20)*	1.931	0.905–4.119	0.089	1.608	0.853–3.030	0.142
Non-hypocoagulable group (PTT $\leq$ 40)*	2.775	0.617–12.472	0.183	2.748	0.805–9.379	0.107
Hypocoagulable group (PTT > 40)*	2.426	1.133–5.193	**0.023**	1.814	0.974–3.379	0.061
Subgroup analysis in FFP transfusion group (*N* = 174)						
Low transfusion volume vs. high transfusion volume*#	1.884	1.040–3.414	**0.037**	1.882	1.096–3.232	**0.022**

*The significant P-value was indicated in bold. *Adjusting for the covariates of Model 2. #Median as cutoff value. CI, confidence interval; FFP, fresh frozen plasma; HR, hazard ratio; INR, international normalized ratio; and PTT, partial thromboplastin time.*

come from the studies performed in the setting of trauma. With the deep understanding of trauma-induced coagulopathy, many studies advocated that early FFP transfusion of high ratio was associated with the improved survival in severe traumatic patients (10, 11, 25, 26). However, as to systemic meningococcal disease, a study by Busund et al. revealed that the use of FFP may negatively influence the outcomes (27). Similarly, in the children with critical illness, plasma transfusion seemed to be independently associated with an increased occurrence of new or progressive multiple organ dysfunction syndrome, nosocomial infections, prolonged length of stay, and risk of mortality (28, 29). Moreover, with regard to the rat and foal models of sepsis, several studies discovered that plasma transfusion was beneficial for the survival of septic animals (30, 31).

For the traditional clinical experience, the patients with critical illness with coagulation disorder may benefit from an early FFP transfusion, thus, it is worthy to verify this hypothesis by the setting of sensitivity analysis with different coagulation indexes. Obviously, early FFP transfusion cannot improve survival for the patients with sepsis with hypocoagulable state in our study. Similarly, Dara SI et al. study showed that the outcomes of the FFP transfusion group in the patients with critical illness with coagulopathy had no statistically significant improvement (12). Additionally, as failing to induce a more procoagulant state, Müller et al. did not advocate FFP transfusion in the non-bleeding patients with critical illness with coagulopathy (32). The prophylactic use of FFP before invasive procedures to correct abnormal INR or PTT is never shown to reduce bleeding, because there is no correlation between the coagulation tests and risk of bleeding (33, 34). These previous studies support our findings in a sense.

As to the septic shock, Nanna et al. study showed that ICU mortality, 30-day mortality, 90-day mortality, and 365-day mortality were comparable between the patients with FFP transfused and non-transfused patients (35), which was consistent with our results of subset analysis. Due to the lack of sufficient references and guidelines, the role of FFP in fluid therapy of septic shock remains to be further studied.

In trauma patients, plasma can decrease the edema-mediated and inflammatory-mediated complications which are the detrimental processes that contribute to the organ failure and increased mortality (36). Several studies hypothesized that plasma also had similar effects on sepsis, because sepsis produced trauma-like changes on the endothelial glycocalyx layer which was a matrix of membrane-bound glycoproteins and proteoglycans projecting from the luminal surface of endothelial cells (7). However, as no definitive data that state plasma mitigates endothelial injury in sepsis, it is too early to draw this conclusion. Contrarily, there may be factors in the donor plasma that are deleterious to the host. The passive transfusion of antileukocyte antibodies from the alloimmunized donors and biological response modifiers accumulated during the storage of cellular blood products lead to the development of transfusion-related acute lung injury (TRALI) (37). Several previous studies suggested that FFP transfusion for the patients with critical illness was associated with an increased risk of the development of TRALI, which was regarded as the most serious transfusion complication (37, 38). Moreover, FFP transfusion was associated with an increased risk of infection and systemic inflammatory response syndrome (39, 40), thus, the double strike for the patients with sepsis may not conducive to the recovery of inflammatory response. In addition to TRALI and infection, there are other adverse reactions with the FFP transfusion as follows: allergic reactions, febrile reactions, citrate toxicity, circulatory overload, graft vs. host disease, and inhibitors against deficient proteins (41–43). As we can imagine, the FFP transfusion may not conducive to survival on the patients with sepsis when the effects of adverse reactions play a dominant role. As lack of relevant studies, the exact mechanisms remain to be elucidated.

Our study has several limitations. First, there may be existing potential bias caused by the factors in the patients with FFP transfusion who tend to be more serious. Thus, we adjusted the severity scores of illness in Model 2 to eliminate the influence of confounding factors and make the research variables comparable. Second, our main study from MIMIC III, due to its retrospective design, was vulnerable to the selection bias as a result of the inclusion of only a single-center sample and the exclusion of patients with missing data. Additionally, there is no denying that the lack of records for the causes of FFP transfusion is a limitation in our study. This is a preliminary exploratory study, thus, further prospective studies are warranted to validate our findings *via* a randomized controlled trial with different intervention groups.

CONCLUSIONS

Through the data analyses of dual centers and dual populations, the present study uncovered for the first time that for the patients with sepsis with coagulopathy, early FFP transfusion cannot improve the outcomes and was unfavorable. Contrarily, the mortality increased significantly with the increase of FFP transfusion volume. Similar results can also be found in the subset analysis of the septic shock cohort.

Significantly, our study provides a new understanding of the rationale and effectiveness of FFP transfusion for the patients with sepsis in a different perspective. In the clinical practice, there may be two existing misunderstandings that the patients with sepsis can benefit from early FFP transfusion as follows: (1) FFP can be used as a volume replacement, and (2) FFP should be used to correct abnormal INR or PTT in the patients with non-bleeding who have no planned invasive procedures. After recognizing the evidence of risk-benefit and cost-benefit, it is important to reduce the inappropriate use of FFP and avoid unnecessary adverse transfusion reactions. However, it is too early to deny the role of plasma completely, further studies are warranted to explore the guidelines for optimizing the rational use of FFP in the patients with sepsis.

AUTHOR CONTRIBUTIONS

XQ and WZho conceived and designed this study. WZha, XZ, and XH helped with the collection and assembly of data. All the authors contributed toward data analysis, drafting, critically revising the paper, agreed to be accountable for all aspects of the work, and read and approved the final manuscript.

SUPPLEMENTARY MATERIAL

Supplementary Figure 1 | The diagnosis flowchart of Sepsis-3 criteria. *Vasopressors initiation (e.g., dopamine, norepinephrine, epinephrine, vasopressin, and phenylephrine). MAP, mean arterial pressure; qSOFA, quick Sequential Organ Failure Assessment; and SOFA, Sequential Organ Failure Assessment.

Supplementary Figure 2 | The detailed distribution of fresh frozen plasma (FFP) transfusion volume in the MIMIC III database. FFP, fresh frozen plasma and MIMIC III, Medical Information Mart for Intensive Care III.

Supplementary Table 1 | The baseline characteristics of final sepsis cohort and initial sepsis cohort.

Supplementary Table 2 | Comparison of the baseline characteristics of septic shock cohort vs. sepsis cohort.

Supplementary Table 3 | A subset analysis for septic shock cohort in the MIMIC III database.

Supplementary Table 4 | The baseline characteristics of external validation cohort.

Supplementary Table 5 | The baseline laboratory data and vital statistics of external validation cohort.

Supplementary Table 6 | A subset analysis for septic shock cohort with external validation.

REFERENCES

1. Singer M, Deutschman CS, Seymour CW, Shankar-Hari M, Annane D, Bauer M, et al. The third international consensus definitions for sepsis and septic shock (Sepsis-3). *JAMA.* (2016) 315:801–10. doi: 10.1001/jama.2016.0287
2. Angus DC, van der Poll T. Severe sepsis and septic shock. *N Engl J Med.* (2013) 369:840–51. doi: 10.1056/NEJMra1208623
3. Angus DC, Linde-Zwirble WT, Lidicker J, Clermont G, Carcillo J, Pinsky MR. Epidemiology of severe sepsis in the United States: analysis of incidence, outcome, and associated costs of care. *Crit Care Med.* (2001) 29:1303–10. doi: 10.1097/00003246-200107000-00002
4. Lagu T, Rothberg MB, Shieh MS, Pekow PS, Steingrub JS, Lindenauer PK. Hospitalizations, costs, and outcomes of severe sepsis in the United States 2003 to (2007). *Crit Care Med.* (2012) 40:754–61. doi: 10.1097/CCM.0b013e318232db65
5. Barochia AV, Cui X, Vitberg D, Suffredini AF, O'Grady NP, Banks SM, et al. Bundled care for septic shock: an analysis of clinical trials. *Crit Care Med.* (2010) 38:668–78. doi: 10.1097/CCM.0b013e3181cb0ddf
6. Levy MM, Evans LE, Rhodes A. The surviving sepsis campaign bundle: 2018. *Crit Care Med.* (2018) 46:997–1000. doi: 10.1097/CCM.0000000000003119
7. Chang R, Holcomb JB. Choice of fluid therapy in the initial management of sepsis, severe sepsis, and septic shock. *Shock.* (2016) 46:17–26. doi: 10.1097/SHK.0000000000000577
8. Levy MM, Rhodes A, Phillips GS, Townsend SR, Schorr CA, Beale R, et al. Surviving sepsis campaign: association between performance metrics and outcomes in a 7.5-year study. *Crit Care Med.* (2015) 43:3–12. doi: 10.1097/CCM.0000000000000723
9. Stanworth SJ, Hyde CJ, Murphy MF. Evidence for indications of fresh frozen plasma. *Transfus Clin Biol.* (2007) 14:551–6. doi: 10.1016/j.tracli.2008.03.008

10. Holcomb JB, del Junco DJ, Fox EE, Wade CE, Cohen MJ, Schreiber MA, et al. The prospective, observational, multicenter, major trauma transfusion (PROMMTT) study: comparative effectiveness of a time-varying treatment with competing risks. *JAMA Surg.* (2013) 148:127–36. doi: 10.1001/2013.jamasurg.387
11. Spinella PC, Perkins JG, Grathwohl KW, Beekley AC, Niles SE, McLaughlin DF, et al. Effect of plasma and red blood cell transfusions on survival in patients with combat related traumatic injuries. *J Trauma.* (2008) 64(2 Suppl.):S69–78. doi: 10.1097/TA.0b013e318160ba2f
12. Dara SI, Rana R, Afessa B, Moore SB, Gajic O. Fresh frozen plasma transfusion in critically ill medical patients with coagulopathy. *Crit Care Med.* (2005) 33:2667–71. doi: 10.1097/01.CCM.0000186745.53059.F0
13. Labarinas S, Arni D, Karam O. Plasma in the PICU: why and when should we transfuse? *Ann Intensive Care.* (2013) 3:16. doi: 10.1186/2110-5820-3-16
14. Johnson AE, Pollard TJ, Shen L, Lehman LW, Feng M, Ghassemi M, et al. MIMIC-III, a freely accessible critical care database. *Sci Data.* (2016) 3:160035. doi: 10.1038/sdata.2016.35
15. Auriant I, Vinatier I, Thaler F, Tourneur M, Loirat P. Simplified acute physiology score II for measuring severity of illness in intermediate care units. *Crit Care Med.* (1998) 26:1368–371. doi: 10.1097/00003246-199808000-00023
16. Knaus WA, Draper EA, Wagner DP, Zimmerman JE. APACHE II: a severity of disease classification system. *Crit Care Med.* (1985) 13:818–29. doi: 10.1097/00003246-198510000-00009
17. Ferreira FL, Bota DP, Bross A, Mélot C, Vincent JL. Serial evaluation of the SOFA score to predict outcome in critically ill patients. *JAMA.* (2001) 286:1754–8. doi: 10.1001/jama.286.14.1754
18. Tripathi MM, Egawa S, Wirth AG, Tshikudi DM, Van Cott EM, Nadkarni SK. Clinical evaluation of whole blood prothrombin time (PT) and international normalized ratio (INR) using a Laser Speckle Rheology sensor. *Sci Rep.* (2017) 7:9169. doi: 10.1038/s41598-017-08693-5
19. Oronsky B, Oronsky N, Cabrales P. Platelet inhibitory effects of the Phase 3 anticancer and normal tissue cytoprotective agent, RRx-001. *J Cell Mol Med.* (2018) 22:5076–5082. doi: 10.1111/jcmm.13791
20. Iwashyna TJ, Cooke CR, Wunsch H, Kahn JM. Population burden of long-term survivorship after severe sepsis in older Americans. *J Am Geriatr Soc.* (2012) 60:1070–7. doi: 10.1111/j.1532-5415.2012.03989.x
21. Gaieski DF, Edwards JM, Kallan MJ, Carr BG. Benchmarking the incidence and mortality of severe sepsis in the United States. *Crit Care Med.* (2013) 41:1167–74. doi: 10.1097/CCM.0b013e31827c09f8
22. Delano MJ, Ward PA. The immune system's role in sepsis progression, resolution, and long-term outcome. *Immunol Rev.* (2016) 274:330–53. doi: 10.1111/imr.12499
23. Johnson AEW, Aboab J, Raffa JD, Pollard TJ, Deliberato RO, Celi LA, et al. A Comparative Analysis of Sepsis Identification Methods in an Electronic Database. *Crit Care Med.* (2018) 46:494–9. doi: 10.1097/CCM.0000000000002965
24. Delaney AP, Dan A, McCaffrey J, Finfer S. The role of albumin as a resuscitation fluid for patients with sepsis: a systematic review and meta-analysis. *Crit Care Med.* (2011) 39:386–91. doi: 10.1097/CCM.0b013e3181ffe217
25. Chang R, Folkerson LE, Sloan D, Tomasek JS, Kitagawa RS, Choi HA, et al. Early plasma transfusion is associated with improved survival after isolated traumatic brain injury in patients with multifocal intracranial hemorrhage. *Surgery.* (2017) 161:538–45. doi: 10.1016/j.surg.2016.08.023
26. Maegele M, Lefering R, Paffrath T, Tjardes T, Simanski C, Bouillon B, et al. Red-blood-cell to plasma ratios transfused during massive transfusion are associated with mortality in severe multiple injury: a retrospective analysis from the Trauma Registry of the Deutsche Gesellschaft für Unfallchirurgie. *Vox Sang.* (2008) 95:112–9. doi: 10.1111/j.1423-0410.2008.01074.x
27. Busund R, Straume B, Revhaug A. Fatal course in severe meningococcemia: clinical predictors and effect of transfusion therapy. *Crit Care Med.* (1993) 21:1699–705. doi: 10.1097/00003246-199311000-00019
28. Karam O, Lacroix J, Robitaille N, Rimensberger PC, Tucci M. Association between plasma transfusions and clinical outcome in critically ill children: a prospective observational study. *Vox Sang.* (2013) 104:342–9. doi: 10.1111/vox.12009
29. Church GD, Matthay MA, Liu K, Milet M, Flori HR. Blood product transfusions and clinical outcomes in pediatric patients with acute lung injury. *Pediatr Crit Care Med.* (2009) 10:297–302. doi: 10.1097/PCC.0b013e3181988952
30. Chang R, Holcomb JB, Johansson PI, Pati S, Schreiber MA, Wade CE. Plasma resuscitation improved survival in a Cecal ligation and puncture rat model of sepsis. *Shock.* (2018) 49:53–61. doi: 10.1097/SHK.0000000000000918
31. McTaggart C, Penhale J, Raidala SL. Effect of plasma transfusion on neutrophil function in healthy and septic foals. *Aust Vet J.* (2005) 83:499–505. doi: 10.1111/j.1751-0813.2005.tb13304.x
32. Müller MC, Straat M, Meijers JC, Klinkspoor JH, de Jonge E, Arbous MS, et al. Fresh frozen plasma transfusion fails to influence the hemostatic balance in critically ill patients with a coagulopathy. *J Thromb Haemost.* (2015) 13:989–97. doi: 10.1111/jth.12908
33. Segal JB, Dzik WH, Transfusion Medicine/Hemostasis Clinical Trials Network. Paucity of studies to support that abnormal coagulation test results predict bleeding in the setting of invasive procedures: an evidence-based review. *Transfusion.* (2005). 45:1413–25. doi: 10.1111/j.1537-2995.2005.00546.x
34. Tinmouth A. Assessing the rationale and effectiveness of frozen plasma transfusions: an evidence-based review. *Hematol Oncol Clin North Am.* (2016) 30:561–72. doi: 10.1016/j.hoc.2016.01.003
35. Reiter N, Wesche N, Perner A. The majority of patients in septic shock are transfused with fresh-frozen plasma. *Dan Med J.* (2013) 60:A4606.
36. Watson JJ, Pati S, Schreiber MA. Plasma transfusion: history, current realities, and novel improvements. *Shock.* (2016) 46:468–79. doi: 10.1097/SHK.0000000000000663
37. Khan H, Belsher J, Yilmaz M, Afessa B, Winters JL, Moore SB, et al. Fresh-frozen plasma and platelet transfusions are associated with development of acute lung injury in critically ill medical patients. *Chest.* (2007) 131:1308–14. doi: 10.1378/chest.06-3048
38. van Stein D, Beckers EA, Sintnicolaas K, Porcelijn L, Danovic F, Wollersheim JA, et al. Transfusion-related acute lung injury reports in the Netherlands: an observational study. *Transfusion.* (2010) 50:213–20. doi: 10.1111/j.1537-2995.2009.02345.x
39. Sarani B, Dunkman WJ, Dean L, Sonnad S, Rohrbach JI, Gracias VH. Transfusion of fresh frozen plasma in critically ill surgical patients is associated with an increased risk of infection. *Crit Care Med.* (2008) 36:1114–8. doi: 10.1097/CCM.0b013e318168f89d
40. Mica L, Simmen H, Werner CM, Plecko M, Keller C, Wirth SH, et al. Fresh frozen plasma is permissive for systemic inflammatory response syndrome, infection, and sepsis in multiple-injured patients. *Am J Emerg Med.* (2016) 34:1480–5. doi: 10.1016/j.ajem.2016.04.041
41. O'Shaughnessy DF, Atterbury C, Bolton Maggs P, Murphy M, Thomas D, Yates S, et al. Guidelines for the use of fresh-frozen plasma, cryoprecipitate and cryosupernatant. *Br J Haematol.* (2004) 126:11–28. doi: 10.1111/j.1365-2141.2004.04972.x
42. United Kingdom Haemophelia Centre Doctors' Organization. Guidelines on the selection and use of therapeutic products to treat haemophilia and other hereditary bleeding disorders. *Haemophilia.* (2003). 9:1–23. doi: 10.1046/j.1365-2516.2003.00711.x
43. Liumbruno G, Bennardello F, Lattanzio A, Piccoli P, Rossetti G, Italian Society of Transfusion Medicine and Immunohaematology (SIMTI) Work Group. Recommendations for the transfusion of plasma and platelets. *Blood Transfus.* (2009) 7:132–50.

23

Establishment and Verification of a Perioperative Blood Transfusion Model After Posterior Lumbar Interbody Fusion: A Retrospective Study Based on Data From a Local Hospital

Bo Liu [1], Junpeng Pan [1], Hui Zong [2] and Zhijie Wang [1]*

[1] *Department of Spinal Surgery, The Affiliated Hospital of Qingdao University, Qingdao, China,* [2] *Department of Neurology, The People's Hospital of Qingyun, Dezhou, China*

Correspondence:
Zhijie Wang
simonwang1969@163.com

Objective: We aimed to analyze the related risk factors for blood transfusion and establish a blood transfusion risk model during the per-ioperative period of posterior lumbar interbody fusion (PLIF). It could provide a reference for clinical prevention and reduction of the risk of blood transfusion during the peri-operative period.

Methods: We retrospectively analyzed 4,378 patients who underwent PLIF in our hospital. According to whether they were transfused blood or not, patients were divided into the non-blood transfusion group and the blood transfusion group. We collected variables of each patient, including age, sex, BMI, current medical history, past medical history, surgical indications, surgical information, and preoperative routine blood testing. We randomly divide the whole population into training group and test group according to the ratio of 4:1. We used the multivariate regression analyses get the independent predictors in the training set. The nomogram was established based on these independent predictors. Then, we used the AUC, calibration curve and DCA to evaluate the nomogram. Finally, we verified the performance of the nomogram in the validation set.

Results: Three or more lumbar fusion segments, preoperative low hemoglobin, with hypertension, lower BMI, and elder people were risk factors for blood transfusion. For the training and validation sets, the AUCs of the nomogram were 0.881 (95% CI: 0.865–0.903) and 0.890 (95% CI: 0.773–0.905), respectively. The calibration curve shows that the nomogram is highly consistent with the actual observed results. The DCA shows that the nomogram has good clinical application value. The AUC of the nomogram is significantly larger than the AUCs of independent risk factors in the training and validation set.

Conclusion: Three or more lumbar fusion segments, preoperative low hemoglobin, with hypertension, lower BMI, and elder people are associated with blood transfusion during the peri-operative period. Based on these factors, we established a blood transfusion nomogram and verified that it can be used to assess the risk of blood transfusion after PLIF. It could help clinicians to make clinical decisions and reduce the incidence of peri-operative blood transfusion.

Keywords: posterior lumbar interbody fusion, blood transfusion, risk factors, nomogram, a retrospective study

INTRODUCTION

Posterior lumbar interbody fusion (PLIF) is a classic surgical method currently used by clinicians to treat lumbar degenerative diseases such as lumbar disc herniation, lumbar spinal stenosis, and lumbar spondylolisthesis (1). PLIF was reported to have a significant effect on relieving lumbar pain and improving radicular symptoms of the lower extremities. It can achieve good segmental fusion and fixation. In addition, it can completely restore the height of the intervertebral space to maintain the physiological curvature of the spine (2–4). However, PLIF is an open operation, during which the muscles on both sides of the spinous process need to be completely stripped. There are many blood vessels running in this area, and some areas of the blood vessels will inevitably be damaged during the operation (5).

The total blood loss during the peri-operative period is approximately 800–1,000 ml, and with the increase in the surgical segment, the blood loss during the peri-operative period also increases (6, 7). In clinical practice, the traditional method to solve severe per-ioperative anemia is allogeneic blood transfusion, which can quickly alleviate the condition and correct anemia (8, 9). However, it may bring about a series of problems, such as increased economic burden, iatrogenic infection, and postoperative complication rate (10). Especially for middle-aged and elderly patients during the peri-operative period, massive bleeding affects the heart, kidney, lung and other functions, leading to abnormal blood coagulation, incision infection, organ insufficiency and a series of complications (11, 12).

At present, nomograms are widely used in the prognosis and diagnosis of clinical medicine. In a nomogram, multiple risk factors can be combined to predict the probability of an outcome, and the results can be visualized. Nomogram is widely used in the diagnosis and prognosis of diseases. It can integrate multiple risk factors to make a comprehensive assessment of the risk of diseases, and visualize the results to make them easy to understand (13). After consulting the literature, we found that there are relatively few studies on the risk factors for blood transfusion during the peri-operative period of PLIF, and no researchers have established and verified the clinical prediction model of blood transfusion after PLIF. Therefore, this study aims to investigate the risk factors for postoperative blood transfusion and the incidence of blood transfusion in patients with PLIF for the treatment of lumbar degenerative diseases and to establish and verify a predictive nomogram of postoperative blood transfusion on this basis.

Abbreviations: PLIF, Posterior Lumbar Interbody Fusion; DCA, decision curve analysis; ROC, receiver operating characteristic; OR, odds ratio; AUC, area under the curve; CI, confidence interval; BMI, body mass index.

METHODS

Collection of Patients' Clinical Data

We retrospectively analyzed the clinical diagnosis and treatment data of patients who underwent PLIF. All of the patients underwent a standard posterior spinal fusion. This study was approved by the Ethics Committee of the Affiliated Hospital of Qingdao University. From January 2015 to December 2020, 5069 patients were in compliance with the requirements. Of these, 691 were excluded: 319 patients with incomplete clinical data such as blood routine training results; 247 were second revision surgery and were diagnosised of lumbar infectious diseases; 68 patients with severe complications within 3 days after the operation, such as spinal cord injury, renal or liver dysfunction; 57 used anti-coagulant and anti-platelet drugs within 15 days. Ultimately, 4,378 patients were included in this study. Although clinical blood transfusion events are still controversial, the criteria of the blood transfusion group in our hospital is that hemoglobin was <70 g/L or hemoglobin was <80 g/L, but patients had symptoms of anemia within 14 days.

We collected variables of each patient, included demographic data, past medical history, concomitant diseases, surgical indications, preoperative routine blood examination, intraoperative fusion segments. The fusion segments were defined as the segments number of lumbar interbody fusion, it was only PLIF without decompression at other levels. All data were collected independently from the hospital's medical record system by two surgeons, and any disputed data were modified with the consent of the two physicians who extracted the data. The surgical method was standard PLIF, and the surgeons were all senior chief physicians in charge. Each patient entered the clinical path for unified process management. We randomly divide the whole population into training group and test group according to the ratio of 4:1.

Statistical Analysis

All statistical analyses were performed in the R software (version 4.0.3, R Foundation for Statistical Computing, Austria). The normality of continuous variables was determined by Shapiro-Wilk training. Normally distributed data are represented by the Mean ± SD, non-normally distributed data are represented by the Quartiles and categorical data are represented by numbers or percentages. Univariate analysis was performed on the training set, the continuous variables were evaluated using Student's t-test or the Mann-Whitney U-test, while categorical variables were subjected to the chi-square test. Then, multivariate regression analysis was used on the training set to determine the independent predictors of blood transfusion after lumbar fusion. $P < 0.05$ (two-sided) was considered significant.

TABLE 1 | Comparison of demographic and preoperative data of the two groups of patients.

	Non-transfusion (*n* = 4,122)	Transfusion (*n* = 256)	$t/z/\chi^2$	*p*
Sex			−0.986	0.324
Female	2,136 (51.8)	124 (48.4)		
Male	1,986 (48.2)	132 (51.6)		
Age (years)			135.697	<0.001
<55	1,658 (40.2)	24 (9.4)		
55–65	1,183 (28.7)	70 (27.3)		
>65	1,281 (31.1)	162 (63.3)		
BMI (kg/m^2)	25.50 (23.30, 27.90)	24.20 (21.80, 26.72)	−5.995	<0.001
Comorbidities (%)				
Hypertension	1,392 (33.8)	110 (43.0)	−2.968	0.003
Diabetes mellitus	801 (19.4)	50 (19.5)	0.000	1.000
Coronary heart disease	571 (13.9)	43 (16.8)	−1.224	0.221
Cerebral thrombosis	33 (0.8)	2 (0.8)	0.000	1.000
Respiratory diseases	228 (5.5)	21 (8.2)	−1.650	0.099
Digestive system diseases	371 (9.0)	21 (8.2)	−0.321	0.748
Other	545 (13.2)	38 (14.8)	−0.646	0.518
Indications for surgery (%)			2.051	0.562
Lumbar disc herniation	1,776 (43.1)	115 (45.5)		
Spinal stenosis	1,170 (28.4)	71 (28.1)		
Lumbar spondylolisthesis	869 (21.1)	45 (17.8)		
Other	307 (7.4)	22 (8.6)		
Previous history (%)				
Surgical history	1,476 (35.8)	113 (44.1)	−2.612	0.009
Blood transfusion	106 (2.6)	4 (1.6)	−0.796	0.426
Allergies	80 (1.9)	3 (1.2)	−0.639	0.523
Smoking	681 (16.5)	37 (14.5)	−0.781	0.435
Alcohol	541 (13.1)	31 (12.1)	−0.372	0.710
ABO (%)			−1.296	0.195
A	1,206 (29.3)	62 (24.2)		
AB	446 (10.8)	32 (12.5)		
B	1,355 (32.9)	81 (31.6)		
O	1,115 (27.0)	81 (31.6)		
RH (%)			−0.451	0.652
Negative (−)	16 (0.4)	2 (0.8)		
Positive (+)	4,106 (99.6)	254 (99.2)		
Laboratory tests				
Hb	139.00 (129.00, 150.00)	128.00 (116.00, 138.00)	−11.166	<0.001
NRBC	5.02 (4.30, 5.65)	4.80 (4.17, 5.50)	−2.132	0.033
MCH	30.50 (29.50, 31.50)	30.60 (29.60, 31.83)	−2.108	0.035
MCHC	339.00 (332.00, 346.00)	339.00 (331.00, 346.25)	−0.020	0.984
MCV	89.80 (87.10, 92.40)	90.10 (87.60, 93.62)	−2.366	0.018

(Continued)

TABLE 1 | Continued

	Non-transfusion (*n* = 4,122)	Transfusion (*n* = 256)	$t/z/\chi^2$	*p*
WBC	6.16 (5.16, 7.51)	5.94 (5.08, 6.98)	−2.308	0.021
PLT	131.00 (96.00, 171.00)	133.50 (97.75, 165.00)	−0.429	0.668
Decompression Fusion Segment			407.256	<0.001
1	1,695 (41.1)	36 (14.1)		
2	1,815 (44.0)	55 (21.5)		
≥3	612 (14.8)	165 (64.5)		

Meaningful variables of logistics multifactor regression analysis were included in R solfware, and a nomogram was constructed. The AUC of the ROC curve was used to illustrate the predictive ability of the model. The calibration curve is an image comparison between the predicted risk and the patient's true risk. The closer the predicted risk is to the standard curve, the better the compliance of the model. The decision curve analysis method was used to evaluate the net benefit and the effectiveness of the nomogram. Finally, in the training and validation sets, the independent nomogram and each meaningful variable subgroup were analyzed and compared, and the nomogram and the ROC curve of each independent predictor were generated to compare the predictive ability.

RESULTS

Demographic Characteristics of the Patients

From January 2015 to December 2020, a total of 4,378 patients underwent lumbar fusion in the Affiliated Hospital of Qingdao University, of whom 256 patients had blood transfusions during the peri-operative period, and the blood transfusion rate during the perioperative period was 5.8%. **Table 1** demonstrates the baseline characteristics. There was no significant difference between the two groups ($P > 0.05$). This shows that there is comparability between the two. Among them, there were 2,118 males and 2,260 females. The average age of the patients was 56.73 ± 14.11 years, and the average body mass index (BMI) was 25.64 ± 3.63 kg/m^2. Among these patients, there were 1,731 patients with 1 fusion segment, 1,870 patients with two fusion segments, and 777 patients with three or more fusion segments.

Independent Risk Factors for Blood Transfusion in Training Set

In the training set, 205 patients received blood transfusion within 14 days after lumbar fusion, and the incidence of postoperative blood transfusion was 5.85%. The multivariate regression analysis showed that three or more lumbar fusion segments, preoperative low hemoglobin, with hypertension,

TABLE 2 | Univariate and multivariate logistic analyses for risk factors of blood transfusion.

	Univariable			Multivariable		
	OR	**95%CI**	***P***	**OR**	**95%CI**	***p***
Sex						
Female	–	–	–			
Male	1.179	0.889–1.564	0.252			
Age	1.094	1.078–1.111	<0.001	1.082	1.065–1.099	<0.001
BMI	0.862	0.825–0.900	<0.001	0.855	0.813–0.899	<0.001
Comorbidities						
Hypertension	1.366	1.025–1.820	0.033	1.427	1.028–1.982	0.034
Diabetes mellitus	0.975	0.681–1.397	0.892			
Coronary heart disease	1.410	0.978–2.034	0.065			
Cerebral thrombosis	0.534	0.073–3.927	0.538			
Digestive system diseases	1.449	0.851–2.466	0.172			
Respiratory diseases	0.890	0.534–1.483	0.655			
Other	1.073	0.715–1.609	0.734			
Indications for surgery						
Lumbar disc herniation	0.918	0.421–2.004	0.830			
Lumbar spinal stenosis	0.975	0.56–1.699	0.930			
Lumbar spondylolisthesis	1.184	0.665–2.111	0.566			
Previous history						
Surgical history	1.628	1.227–2.162	0.001			
Blood transfusion	0.548	0.172–1.746	0.309			
Allergies	0.240	0.033–1.736	0.158			
Smoking	0.960	0.654–1.409	0.836			
Alcohol	0.875	0.565–1.355	0.549			
ABO						
A	–	–	–			
AB	1.400	0.858–2.283	0.178			
B	1.148	0.785–1.679	0.475			
O	1.419	0.970–2.074	0.071			
RH						
Negative	–	–	–			
Positive	0.340	0.075–1.543	0.162			
Laboratory tests						
Hb	0.960	0.953–0.967	<0.001	0.981	0.972–0.989	<0.001
NRBC	0.809	0.703–0.931	0.003			
MCH	1.064	0.991–1.143	0.088			
MCHC	1.001	0.989–1.012	0.902			
MCV	1.037	1.008–1.067	0.012			
WBC	0.919	0.853–0.990	0.027			
PLT	1.000	0.998–1.002	0.910			
Decompression Fusion Segment						
1	–	–	–	–	–	–
2	1.565	0.971–2.523	0.066	1.473	0.892–2.433	0.130
≥3	12.889	8.466–19.624	<0.001	12.438	7.893–19.600	<0.001

lower BMI, and elder people were independent predictors of blood transfusion after PLIF (**Table 2**). Among them, the AUC of the three or more fusion segments ROC in the training set was 0.745, and the corresponding AUC of the validation set was 0.758. In addition, the AUC of age in the training set was 0.773, while the corresponding AUC in the validation set was 0.778. Age and three or more fusion segments were the main influencing factors of the model, indicating that these two parameters have the greatest impact on the model.

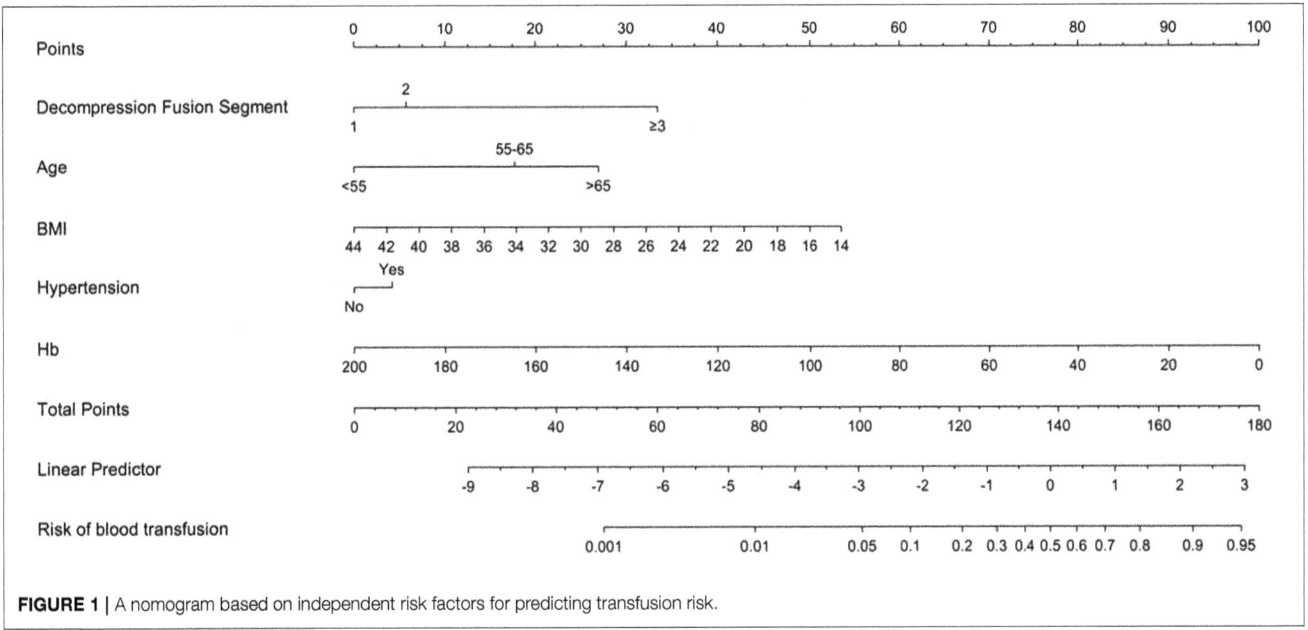

FIGURE 1 | A nomogram based on independent risk factors for predicting transfusion risk.

Development and Validation of the Nomogram

We used five independent predictors to build a nomogram (**Figure 1**). For example, one patient in the clinic, with three or more fusion segments on PLIF, aged over 65 years, BMI is 18 kg/m^2, hypertension history, and the preoperative hemoglobin was 100 g/L, We calculated the score of each single index, and then, the single item scores could be added together, Total score is 35 + 27.5 + 45 + 5 + 50 = 162.5 points. The probability of perioperative blood transfusion is as high as 85%. In the training set, the AUC of our nomogram was 0.881 (95% CI = 0.853–0.910, $p < 0.001$) (**Figure 2A**), showing good accuracy in predicting the risk of blood transfusion in patients after lumbar fusion. The calibration curve shows that there is good agreement between the predicted and observed results in terms of the probability of blood transfusion (**Figure 2B**). Furthermore, DCA shows that there is a net benefit to using this nomogram to predict postoperative blood transfusion if the patient and physician threshold probability is <72% (**Figure 2C**).

A total of 876 patients were included in the training set, and 51 patients received blood transfusion within 14 days after lumbar fusion. In the training set, the AUC of the nomogram blood transfusion probability prediction model was 0.890 (95% CI = 0.848–0.932, $p < 0.001$) (**Figure 2D**), and the calibration curve showed that the prediction of blood transfusion probability was in good agreement with the observation (**Figure 2E**). In addition, the DCA proved that if the threshold probability of patients and doctors is <62%, using a nomogram to predict postoperative blood transfusion has a net benefit (**Figure 2F**).

Evaluation the Predictability of Nomogram

By comparing the ROC curve of the nomogram with the ROCs of other independent risk factors, the results showed that the AUC of the nomogram blood transfusion risk predictor was significantly higher than that of the blood transfusion risk predictor of patients after PLIF ($P < 0.001$) (**Figure 3A**). Similar to the training set, the AUC was also significantly higher than the AUC of each independent predictor in the validation set ($P < 0.001$) (**Figure 3B**).

DISCUSSION

Spine surgery has a long operation time and large associated wounds, especially when dealing with cancellous bone with abundant blood supply, and it is often accompanied by obvious peri-operative bleeding, usually requiring multiple blood transfusions (14). As an important strategy for the treatment of anemia, allogeneic blood transfusion is extremely important to ensure the safety of patients after surgery. The reported incidence of peri-operative blood transfusion is quite different. The incidence in our study was ~3%, which is lower than the 11–18% reported abroad (15, 16) and far lower than the 32.6% reported in China (17). Wong et al. (18) found that the injection of tran-examic acid can effectively reduce the blood loss and blood transfusion rate after PLIF without causing pulmonary embolism and venous thrombosis of the lower extremities.

After reviewing previous relevant literature, we found that Wang et al. (17) concluded that preoperative low hemoglobin, fusion stage, long operation time, and high total intraoperative blood loss are risk factors for blood transfusion. However, the sample size in this model was relatively small, the blood transfusion rate was ~30% higher, and there was no distinction between the training group and the validation group to verify the effectiveness and accuracy of the model. White et al. (19) also found that female sex, age ≥65 years, long-segment fixation and fusion, surgical fixation to the pelvis, and other factors can increase the risk of massive blood loss during surgery. Butler et al. (20) showed that increasing age, ASA grading of multilevel

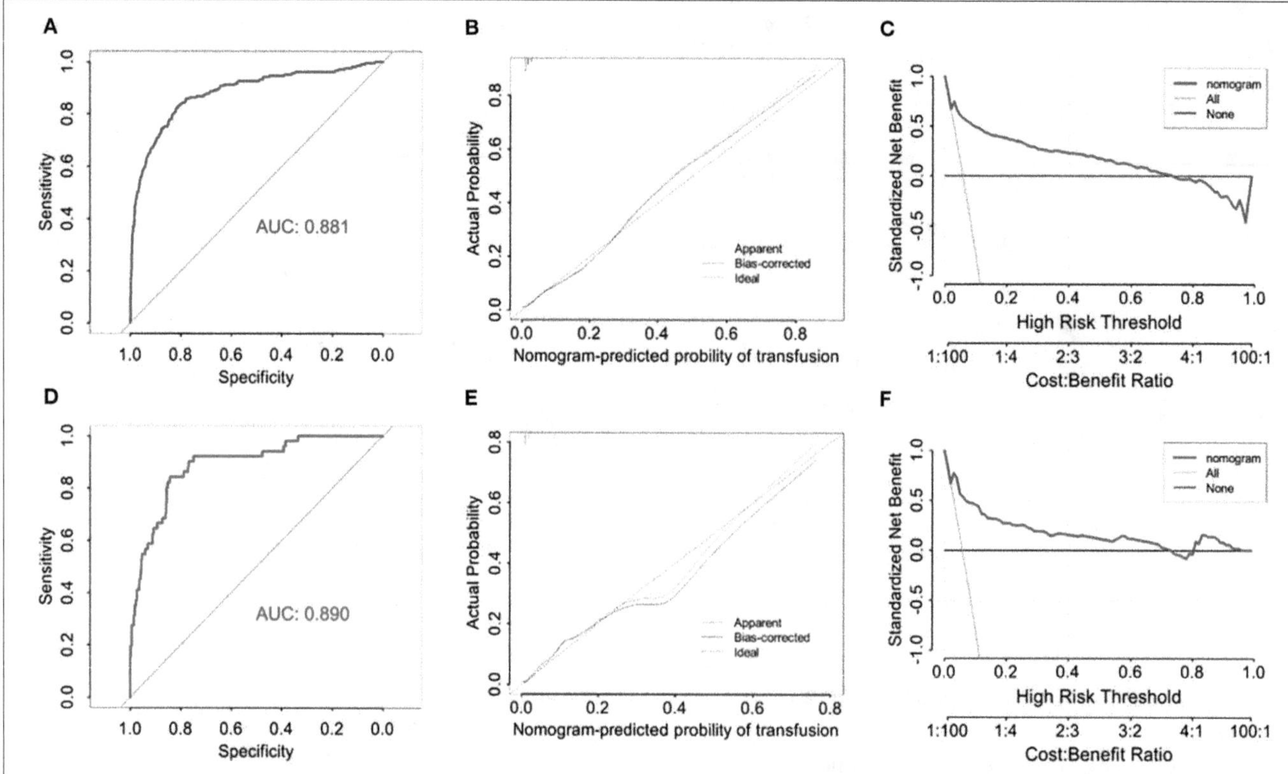

FIGURE 2 | (A) ROC curve in training set to evaluate prediction accuracy; **(B)** decision curve analysis in training set; **(C)** calibration curve in training set; **(D)** ROC curve in test set to evaluate prediction accuracy; **(E)** decision curve analysis in test set; **(F)** calibration curve in test set.

FIGURE 3 | Comparison of the predictive power of different indicators and nomogram plots for transfusion risk in training **(A)** and test datasets **(B)**.

surgery, and prolonged operation time were risk factors affecting lumbar fusion, but neither of them established a predictive model for postoperative blood transfusion. The results of our study show that ≥3 lumbar fusion segments, preoperative low hemoglobin, a history of hypertension, low BMI, and advanced age are risk factors for blood transfusion. This is consistent with domestic and foreign studies on some independent risk factors and establishes and verifies the risk model of blood transfusion after PLIF.

This study found that three or more fusion segments was a risk factor affecting peri-operative blood transfusion. The increase in inter-vertebral fusion segments means an increase in the number of inter-vertebral disc removals. It is often necessary to scrape the endplate cartilage of the upper and lower vertebral bodies of the inserted segments before inserting the inter-vertebral fusion cage. At the same time, it is necessary to extensively strip the paravertebral muscles and soft tissues during the operation to insert the pedicle screws and decompress the spinal canal, which will increase intraoperative bleeding. Morcos et al. (15) also found that multi-segment fusion was an independent risk factor for perioperative blood transfusion, and the blood transfusion rate was 6 times higher. More decompressed and fused segments mean a longer operation time. Many studies have found that the operation time and the number of fusion segments were important predictors of blood transfusion. The probability of blood transfusion increases by 4.2% for every additional hour of operation time. The probability of peri-operative blood transfusion for each additional fusion segment increases by 6 times (16, 21, 22). Aoude et al. (23) showed that the operation time and blood loss were related to an increase in the fusion segments. Therefore, the operation time can be reduced by reducing intra-operative fusion, thereby reducing the risk of peri-operative blood transfusion.

It is worth noting that lower hemoglobin before surgery can also increase the blood transfusion rate of patients during the perioperative period. The lower the red blood cell count, hemoglobin, and hematocrit of the patient before surgery, the poorer their ability to compensate for bleeding during surgery, and the higher the probability that blood transfusions will be required during the peri-operative period. Research by Myers et al. (24) showed that patients with lumbar fusion with preoperative anemia have a higher postoperative infection rate and blood transfusion rate and a longer postoperative hospital stay. In a large-sample retrospective study, Wu et al. (25) showed that preoperative HCT ≤39% was associated with an increase in the 30-day postoperative mortality rate. In addition, Carson et al. (26) showed that when Hb ≤ 80 g/L, with every 10 g/L decrease, the risk of death increased by 2.5-fold. Rasouli et al. (27) believed that when preoperative Hb ≤ 100 g/L, the perioperative infection rate increased significantly (~4.23%), the preoperative hemoglobin content was 110–130 g/L, and the postoperative infection rate was significantly reduced (~0.84%). Early identification and correction of preoperative anemia patients is of great significance. We can infuse concentrated red blood cells in advance to supplement hemoglobin to normal levels. Otherwise, patients in the perioperative period are prone to anemia, leading to related complications in multiple organs of the human body, increasing the risk of surgical incision infection, prolonging the hospital stay, and increasing the risk of death.

Older age is one of the risk factors that affect peri-operative blood transfusion. Rasouli et al. (27) showed that age ≥50 years was an independent risk factor for increased blood transfusion risk in the 13,170 patients undergoing lumbar fusion surgery. Yoshihara and Yoneoka (28) showed that middle-aged and elderly patients were more likely to receive allogeneic blood transfusions than middle-aged and young patients. Similarly, Hu et al. (29) collected clinical data from more than 4,000 patients who underwent total knee arthroplasty in the Affiliated Hospital of Qingdao University and found that advanced age was an independent predictor of peri-operative blood transfusion. The older the patient's age is, the worse the hematopoietic function, and the greater the decreases in the lifespan and function of red blood cells. Coupled with the decline of the digestive function of elderly patients, these changes will lead to deficiencies in hematopoietic materials such as iron and vitamins. These findings suggest that once elderly patients undergo lumbar spine surgery, the hematopoietic system cannot replenish blood cells in a short period of time, leading to varying degrees of anemia during the perioperative period. This requires rapid allogeneic blood transfusion treatment.

Patients with lower BMI have relatively low body weight and a relatively low blood volume. The same absolute amount of bleeding leads to an increase in the bleeding score of the patient, and anemia is more likely to occur during the perioperative period. In patients with a low BMI, the proportion of the spine relative to the whole body is relatively large, which may lead to an increase in bleeding scores during spinal surgery (30). The risk of peri-operative blood transfusion in patients with hypertension accompanied by disease is higher than that in patients without hypertension. The author believes that this may be related to changes in the patients' cardiovascular systems caused by hypertension. These patients also have the habit of taking oral anti-hypertensive drugs and anticoagulants such as aspirin. Moreover, these patients are older and have vascular sclerosis, hyalinosis, decreases in capillary contraction and blood clotting abilities, and more intra-operative bleeding (31). Perioperative blood pressure control is not ideal, and the amounts of bleeding and drainage are higher than those in healthy patients.

Our research has some limitations. First, as this is a retrospective study, some data are missing or incomplete, and the conclusions of this study need to be further demonstrated in prospective randomized controlled studies. Second, the sample size of this study was not large enough, and the patient variables were not all included. Furthermore, patients diagnosed with spinal tumors, infection, tuberculosis, trauma fractures, and spinal deformities were excluded from this study. Considering that these groups are more prone to anemia during the perioperative period, it will be necessary to further collect data on patients with these diseases. In addition, postoperative complications such as pneumonia, urinary tract infection, and deep vein thrombosis of the lower extremities were not included. The analysis of the correlations between these complications and blood transfusion is difficult. Our study only included patients from a single medical center; a multicenter study with a large sample size will be required to confirm the results.

CONCLUSION

Three or more lumbar fusion segments, preoperative low hemoglobin, with hypertension, lower BMI, and elder people are associated with blood transfusion during the perioperative period. Based on these factors, we established a blood transfusion nomogram and verified that it can be used to assess the risk of blood transfusion after PLIF. It could help clinicians to make clinical decisions and reduce the incidence of perioperative blood transfusion.

AUTHOR CONTRIBUTIONS

BL performed the data analysis. BL and JP wrote the manuscript. BL, HZ, and ZW contributed to the manuscript revise. JP and HZ contributed to literature search and data extraction. BL and ZW conceived and designed the study. All authors contributed to the article and approved the submitted version.

REFERENCES

1. Mobbs RJ, Phan K, Malham G, Seex K, Rao PJ. Lumbar interbody fusion: techniques, indications and comparison of interbody fusion options including PLIF, TLIF, MI-TLIF, OLIF/ATP, LLIF and ALIF. *J Spine Surg.* (2015) 1:2–18. doi: 10.3978/j.issn.2414-469X.2015.10.05
2. Ekman P, Moller H, Tullberg T, Neumann P, Hedlund R. Posterior lumbar interbody fusion versus posterolateral fusion in adult isthmic spondylolisthesis. *Spine.* (2007) 32:2178–83. doi: 10.1097/BRS.0b013e31814b1bd8
3. Luo J, Cao K, Yu T, Li L, Huang S, Gong M, et al. Comparison of posterior lumbar interbody fusion versus posterolateral fusion for the treatment of isthmic spondylolisthesis. *Clin Spine Surg.* (2017) 30:E915–22. doi: 10.1097/BSD.0000000000000297
4. de Kunder SL, van Kuijk S, Rijkers K, Caelers I, van Hemert W, de Bie RA, et al. Transforaminal lumbar interbody fusion (TLIF) versus posterior lumbar interbody fusion (PLIF) in lumbar spondylolisthesis: a systematic review and meta-analysis. *Spine J.* (2017) 17:1712–21. doi: 10.1016/j.spinee.2017.06.018
5. Elgafy H, Bransford RJ, McGuire RA, Dettori JR, Fischer D. Blood loss in major spine surgery: are there effective measures to decrease massive hemorrhage in major spine fusion surgery? *Spine.* (2010) 35(9 Suppl.):S47–56. doi: 10.1097/BRS.0b013e3181d833f6
6. Xu D, Ren Z, Chen X, Zhuang Q, Hui S, Sheng L, et al. The further exploration of hidden blood loss in posterior lumbar fusion surgery. *Orthop Traumatol Surg Res.* (2017) 103:527–30. doi: 10.1016/j.otsr.2017.01.011
7. Ren Z, Li S, Sheng L, Zhuang Q, Li Z, Xu D, et al. Topical use of tranexamic acid can effectively decrease hidden blood loss during posterior lumbar spinal fusion surgery: a retrospective study. *Medicine.* (2017) 96:e8233. doi: 10.1097/MD.0000000000008233
8. Carson JL, Stanworth SJ, Roubinian N, Fergusson DA, Triulzi D, Doree C, et al. Transfusion thresholds and other strategies for guiding allogeneic red blood cell transfusion. *Cochrane Database Syst Rev.* (2016) 10:D2042. doi: 10.1002/14651858.CD002042.pub4
9. Mueller MM, Van Remoortel H, Meybohm P, Aranko K, Aubron C, Burger R, et al. Patient blood management: recommendations from the 2018 Frankfurt Consensus Conference. *JAMA.* (2019) 321:983–97. doi: 10.1001/jama.2019.0554
10. Carson JL, Carless PA, Hebert PC. Transfusion thresholds and other strategies for guiding allogeneic red blood cell transfusion. *Cochrane Database Syst Rev.* (2012) 10:CD002042. doi: 10.1002/14651858.CD002042.pub3
11. Jang SY, Cha YH, Yoo JI, Oh T, Kim JT, Park CH, et al. Blood transfusion for elderly patients with hip fracture: a nationwide cohort study. *J Korean Med Sci.* (2020) 35:e313. doi: 10.3346/jkms.2020.35.e313
12. Loftus TJ, Brakenridge SC, Murphy TW, Nguyen LL, Moore FA, Efron PA, et al. Anemia and blood transfusion in elderly trauma patients. *J Surg Res.* (2018) 229:288–93. doi: 10.1016/j.jss.2018.04.021
13. Lubelski D, Feghali J, Nowacki AS, Alentado VJ, Planchard R, Abdullah KG, et al. Patient-specific prediction model for clinical and quality-of-life outcomes after lumbar spine surgery. *J Surg Res.* (2021) 1–9. doi: 10.3171/2020.8.SPINE20577
14. Kushioka J, Yamashita T, Okuda S, Maeno T, Matsumoto T, Yamasaki R, et al. High-dose tranexamic acid reduces intraoperative and postoperative blood loss in posterior lumbar interbody fusion. *J Neurosurg Spine.* (2017) 26:363–7. doi: 10.3171/2016.8.SPINE16528
15. Morcos MW, Jiang F, McIntosh G, Johnson M, Christie S, Wai E, et al. Predictors of blood transfusion in posterior lumbar spinal fusion: a Canadian spine outcome and research network study. *Spine.* (2018) 43:E35–9. doi: 10.1097/BRS.0000000000002115
16. Basques BA, Anandasivam NS, Webb ML, Samuel AM, Lukasiewicz AM, Bohl DD, et al. Risk factors for blood transfusion with primary posterior lumbar fusion. *Spine.* (2015) 40:1792–7. doi: 10.1097/BRS.0000000000001047
17. Wang H, Wang K, Lv B, Xu H, Jiang W, Zhao J, et al. Establishment and assessment of a nomogram for predicting blood transfusion risk in posterior lumbar spinal fusion. *J Orthop Surg Res.* (2021) 16:39. doi: 10.1186/s13018-020-02053-2
18. Wong J, El BH, Rampersaud YR, Lewis S, Ahn H, De Silva Y, et al. Tranexamic acid reduces perioperative blood loss in adult patients having spinal fusion surgery. *Anesth Analg.* (2008) 107:1479–86. doi: 10.1213/ane.0b013e3181831e44
19. White S, Cheung ZB, Ye I, Phan K, Xu J, Dowdell J, et al. Risk factors for perioperative blood transfusions in adult spinal deformity surgery. *World Neurosurg.* (2018) 115:e731–7. doi: 10.1016/j.wneu.2018.04.152
20. Butler JS, Burke JP, Dolan RT, Fitzpatrick P, O'Byrne JM, McCormack D, et al. Risk analysis of blood transfusion requirements in emergency and elective spinal surgery. *Eur Spine J.* (2011) 20:753–8. doi: 10.1007/s00586-010-1500-0
21. Zheng F, Cammisa FJ, Sandhu HS, Girardi FP, Khan SN. Factors predicting hospital stay, operative time, blood loss, and transfusion in patients undergoing revision posterior lumbar spine decompression, fusion, and segmental instrumentation. *Spine.* (2002) 27:818–24. doi: 10.1097/00007632-200204150-00008
22. Nuttall GA, Horlocker TT, Santrach PJ, Oliver WJ, Dekutoski MB, Bryant S. Predictors of blood transfusions in spinal instrumentation and fusion surgery. *Spine.* (2000) 25:596–601. doi: 10.1097/00007632-200003010-00010
23. Aoude A, Nooh A, Fortin M, Aldebeyan S, Jarzem P, Ouellet J, et al. Incidence, predictors, and postoperative complications of blood transfusion in thoracic and lumbar fusion surgery: an analysis of 13,695 patients from the American College of Surgeons National Surgical Quality Improvement Program Database. *Global Spine J.* (2016) 6:756–64. doi: 10.1055/s-0036-1580736
24. Myers E, O'Grady P, Dolan AM. The influence of preclinical anaemia on outcome following total hip replacement. *Arch Orthop Trauma Surg.* (2004) 124:699–701. doi: 10.1007/s00402-004-0754-6
25. Wu WC, Schifftner TL, Henderson WG, Eaton CB, Poses RM, Uttley G, et al. Preoperative hematocrit levels and postoperative outcomes in older patients undergoing noncardiac surgery. *JAMA.* (2007) 297:2481–8. doi: 10.1001/jama.297.22.2481

26. Carson JL, Noveck H, Berlin JA, Gould SA. Mortality and morbidity in patients with very low postoperative Hb levels who decline blood transfusion. *Transfusion.* (2002) 42:812–8. doi: 10.1046/j.1537-2995.2002.00123.x
27. Rasouli MR, Restrepo C, Maltenfort MG, Purtill JJ, Parvizi J. Risk factors for surgical site infection following total joint arthroplasty. *J Bone Joint Surg Am.* (2014) 96:e158. doi: 10.2106/JBJS.M.01363
28. Yoshihara H, Yoneoka D. Predictors of allogeneic blood transfusion in spinal fusion in the United States, 2004-2009. *Spine.* (2014) 39:304–10. doi: 10.1097/BRS.0000000000000123
29. Hu C, Wang YH, Shen R, Liu C, Sun K, Ye L, et al. Development and validation of a nomogram to predict perioperative blood transfusion in patients undergoing total knee arthroplasty. *BMC Musculoskelet Disord.* (2020) 21:315. doi: 10.1186/s12891-020-03328-9
30. Jain A, Sponseller PD, Newton PO, Shah SA, Cahill PJ, Njoku DB, et al. Smaller body size increases the percentage of blood volume lost during posterior spinal arthrodesis. *J Bone Joint Surg Am.* (2015) 97:507–11. doi: 10.2106/JBJS.N.01104
31. Lei F, Li Z, He W, Tian X, Zheng L, Kang J, et al. Hidden blood loss and the risk factors after posterior lumbar fusion surgery: a retrospective study. *Medicine.* (2020) 99:e20103. doi: 10.1097/MD.0000000000020103

24

Early Blood Transfusion After Kidney Transplantation Does Not Lead to dnDSA Development: The BloodIm Study

Thomas Jouve[1,2]**, Johan Noble*[1,2]*, Hamza Naciri-Bennani*[1]*, Céline Dard*[3]*, Dominique Masson*[3]*, Gaëlle Fiard*[2,4]*, Paolo Malvezzi*[1] *and Lionel Rostaing*[1,2]

[1] *Nephrology, Hemodialysis, Apheresis and Kidney Transplantation Department, University Hospital Grenoble, Grenoble, France,* [2] *Faculty of Health, Univ. Grenoble Alpes, Grenoble, France,* [3] *Human Leukocyte Antigen (HLA) Laboratory, Etablissement Français du Sang (EFS), La Tronche, France,* [4] *Urology and Kidney Transplantation Department, University Hospital Grenoble, Grenoble, France*

Correspondence:
Thomas Jouve
tjouve@chu-grenoble.fr

Outcomes after kidney transplantation are largely driven by the development of *de novo* donor-specific antibodies (dnDSA), which may be triggered by blood transfusion. In this single-center study, we investigated the link between early blood transfusion and dnDSA development in a mainly anti-thymocyte globulin (ATG)-induced kidney-transplant cohort. We retrospectively included all recipients of a kidney transplant performed between 2004 and 2015, provided they had >3 months graft survival. DSA screening was evaluated with a Luminex assay (Immucor). Early blood transfusion (EBT) was defined as the transfusion of at least one red blood-cell unit over the first 3 months post-transplantation, with an exhaustive report of transfusion. Patients received either anti-thymocyte globulins (ATG) or basiliximab induction, plus tacrolimus and mycophenolic acid maintenance immunosuppression. A total of 1088 patients received a transplant between 2004 and 2015 in our center, of which 981 satisfied our inclusion criteria. EBT was required for 292 patients (29.7%). Most patients received ATG induction (86.1%); the others received basiliximab induction (13.4%). dnDSA-free graft survival (dnDSA-GS) at 1-year post-transplantation was similar between EBT+ (2.4%) and EBT- (3.0%) patients (chi-squared p=0.73). There was no significant association between EBT and dnDSA-GS (univariate Cox's regression, HR=0.88, p=0.556). In multivariate Cox's regression, adjusting for potential confounders (showing a univariate association with dnDSA development), early transfusion remained not associated with dnDSA-GS (HR 0.76, p=0.449). However, dnDSA-GS was associated with pretransplantation HLA sensitization (HR=2.25, p=0.004), hemoglobin >10 g/dL (HR=0.39, p=0.029) and the number of HLA mismatches (HR=1.26, p=0.05). Recipient's age, tacrolimus and mycophenolic-acid exposures, and graft rank were not associated with dnDSA-GS. Early blood transfusion did not induce dnDSAs in our cohort of ATG-induced patients, but low hemoglobin level was associated with dnDSAs-GS. This suggests a protective effect of ATG induction therapy on preventing dnDSA development at an initial stage post-transplantation.

Keywords: kidney transplantation, induction treatment, blood transfusion, HLA sensitization, anti-thymocyte globulin (ATG)

INTRODUCTION

Outcomes after kidney transplantation have improved over the last 70 years. However, long-term graft survival remains limited by chronic antibody-mediated rejection (cABMR) (1, 2), treatment adherence, and toxicities related to immunosuppression (especially calcineurin Inhibitors [CNIs]) (3-6). The development of *de novo* donor-specific antibodies (dnDSA) is one of the main hurdles that limits long-term graft survival.

Prevention of dnDSA development is of utmost importance due to the lack of an efficient treatment to limit DSA antibody-related allograft injuries (7-9). Educating patients to adhere to their immunosuppressive drugs is a cornerstone for dnDSA prevention. In addition, an optimal immunosuppressive strategy must be sought.

The usual sensitizing events, before or following transplantation, are blood-product transfusions (e.g., red blood cells [RBC]), pregnancy, or any history of solid-organ transplantation. RBC transfusion is frequently given to chronic kidney-disease patients, especially early after kidney transplantation in this setting of acute renal injury and due to the potential blood loss associated with surgical procedures. Avoidance of early post-kidney transplant RBC transfusion using erythropoiesis-stimulating agents (ESAs) is a goal even though we do not really know if ESAs are very efficient in that setting.

Among the sensitizing events after kidney transplantation, early RBC transfusion was shown to induce dnDSA development (10, 11). The study by Ferrandiz et al. considered transfusion performed in the first-year post-transplantation: they found transfusion was a risk factor for DSA formation and antibody-mediated rejection11. A specific analysis of sensitization against RBC donors was performed by Hassan et al.: they reported a higher rate of DSA development in post-kidney transplantation recipients that had undergone a transfusion, regardless of the transfusion chronology (i.e., early and/or late transfusion events) (12). However, data are scarce from this setting, and the impact of sensitizing events is highly dependent on the type of immunosuppressive regimen. Low adherence and therefore low exposure to tacrolimus induces higher rates of DSAs (1, 2). The impact of the induction strategy has not been estimated in previous studies. A depleting compared to a non-depleting induction therapy may play an important role in dnDSA development (13, 14).

In this study, we investigated the effect of early (within 3 months post-transplantation) blood transfusion (EBT) on dnDSA-free kidney-allograft survival (dnDSA-GS) in a retrospective cohort of kidney recipients that received (mainly) depleting anti-thymocyte globulins (ATG) as the induction therapy.

PATIENTS AND METHODS

All patients that received a kidney between January 1st 2004 and June 30th 2015 in our university hospital were considered for inclusion in this study. Luminex ® HLA antibody data were gathered from all patients: indeed, Luminex screening was initiated in 2004 in our center. A minimum graft survival of 90 days was required for inclusion to avoid early competitive risks. The threshold for anti-HLA alloantibody positivity was set at a 1000 mean fluorescence intensity (MFI), using the Immucor platform.

RBC transfusion data were obtained from the regional blood bank, which registered all transfusion events, thereby providing a full picture (every single RBC unit was delivered by the regional blood bank, ensuring no missing data). The policy for RBC transfusion was mainly based on hemoglobin levels and the presence of a heart disease: the hemoglobin threshold for transfusion was 8 g/dl in heart disease-free patients, and 10 g/dl in patients with a hearth disease. All transfused RBC were leukodepleted using a leukodepletion filter fixed on collection devices. Quality controls were randomly performed to ensure that the residual leucocyte count was below 1x10*6/RBC unit. The volume of each packed RBC unit was 230-300 mL. The RBC were not irradiated excepted for the patient with deep immunosuppression or with hematological malignancy.Hemoglobin and tacrolimus trough levels were recorded from every available blood test (at least a monthly follow-up, more frequently as clinically advised). Drug prescriptions were evaluated at M3, M6, M12, and then annually. Luminex screening for HLA antibody data was performed at the time of transplantation, at 3- and 6-months post-transplantation, then annually, and also if there was an acute kidney event, with identification whenever the screening was positive.

Regarding post-transplant immunosuppression, all the recipients received an induction therapy based either on ATG or basiliximab. Patients receiving a first kidney transplant, at low allosensitization risk and/or high infection/cancer risks, were treated with basiliximab. Maintenance immunosuppression was based on tacrolimus, mycophenolic acid (MPA), and prednisone. Trough levels of tacrolimus were between 7 and 10 ng/mL during the first 3 months post-transplantation and thereafter between 4.5-6 ng/ml. Patients were usually weaned off steroids after 3 months except in cases of IgA nephropathy or pretransplant HLA sensitization, or if the surveillance kidney-allograft biopsy (performed at month 3 post-transplantation) showed borderline changes or subclinical acute rejection. Cytomegalovirus (CMV) and Pneumocystis jirovecii prophylaxes were based on valganciclovir (900mg/d, adapted to eGFR, given for 3 to 6 months according to the CMV donor/recipient serostatus), and sulfamethoxazole-trimethoprim given at 800/160 mg every other day for 6 months (adapted to eGFR as well), respectively.

Kaplan–Meier curves and Cox's proportional-hazard regression analyses were used to assess dnDSA-free graft survival (dnDSA-GS). We also performed a subanalysis among patients without any HLA sensitization before transplantation to assess anti-HLA antibody development, regardless of their target, and the predictors of these HLA antibodies. Covariates possibly evolving over time after transplantation were considered as time-dependent covariates in the different Cox's models (e.g., medication dosages, tacrolimus trough levels, hemoglobin). In order to evaluate possible confusion factors, we systematically included EBT in the multivariate analysis, despite its absence of association with dnDSA development. Schoenfeld's residuals were tested to evaluate departure from the proportionality assumption, i.e., to test the stability of the regression coefficients over time. The Wilcoxon test was used to make a comparison between two groups for continuous covariates. The chi-squared test was used to compare discrete covariates between two groups. All analyses were performed using the R statistical software.

The study was conducted according to the guidelines of the Declaration of Helsinki and approved by CNIL (French National committee for data protection; approval number 1987785v0). The biobank collection number is BRIF BB-0033-00069. The patients provided their written informed consent to participate in this study. No potentially identifiable human images or data is presented in this study.

The raw data supporting the conclusions of this article will be made available by the authors, without undue reservation.

RESULTS

Between 2004 and 2015, a total of 1088 kidney transplantations were performed in our center. Following exclusion criteria (i.e.: patients with a pre-transplantation DSA, or with graft survival of less than 90 days), the study cohort comprised 981 kidney-transplant recipients (49 [5%] patients lost their graft before 3 months, 59 [6%] had either a pre-transplantation DSA or no clear HLA antibody profile before transplantation). Median follow-up time was 9.07 years (IQ 6.57–12.2).

The induction therapy was based on ATG for 845 patients (86.1%) and basiliximab for 132 patients (13.4%). Information regarding induction therapy was missing for 4 patients (0.04%). Maintenance immunosuppression was based on tacrolimus, mycophenolate mofetil, and prednisone. The median trough tacrolimus level was 9.4 ng/mL (1st Q. 7.8, 3rd Q 11.3) over the first 3 months and 5.8 ng/mL (1st Q 5.3, 3rd Q 6.35) thereafter. The median dose of mycophenolate mofetil prescribed was 1 g per day. Patients were usually weaned off steroids after 3 months except in cases of IgA nephropathy, pretransplant HLA sensitization, or where a surveillance kidney-allograft biopsy performed at month 3 post-transplantation showed borderline changes or subclinical acute rejection. The median duration of steroid prescription was 175.5 (1st Q. 97, 3rd Q 643) days. A total of 155 patients (16%) remained on steroids at the time of last follow-up.

Demographic characteristics and potential confounders are detailed in **Table 1**. Patients in the early blood-transfusion

TABLE 1 | Comparative demographics and potential confounders between transfusion groups.

	Early RBC - (*N*=689)	Early RBC + (*N*=292)	Total (*N*=981)	*p*-value
Recipient's age, yrs	50.02 (14.71)	55.86 (12.80)	51.76 (14.42)	<0.001
Recipient's gender, female	243 (35.3%)	130 (44.5%)	373 (38.0%)	0.006
Graft rank	0.22 (0.48)	0.24 (0.51)	0.22 (0.49)	0.779
Time on dialysis, yrs	3.99 (4.89)	4.58 (4.42)	4.18 (4.75)	<0.001
Pretransplantation HLA sensitization	157 (22.8%)	85 (29.1%)	242 (24.7%)	0.036
Donor type				<0.001
- DCD	22 (3.2%)	8 (2.7%)	30 (3.1%)	
- BD	566 (82.1%)	276 (94.5%)	842 (85.8%)	
- LD	101 (14.7%)	8 (2.7%)	109 (11.1%)	
ATG induction, yes	582 (84.7%)	263 (90.7%)	845 (86.1%)	0.014
Cold ischemia time, min	909.76 (503.41)	1112.12 (466.43)	970.06 (501.08)	<0.001
dnDSA	85 (12.3%)	29 (9.9%)	114 (11.6%)	0.282
Nbr. of post-transplantation transfusion	0.23 (1.07)	2.94 (3.63)	1.03 (2.50)	<0.001
Nbr. of HLA mismatches	5.46 (0.93)	5.33 (0.86)	5.42 (0.91)	0.043
eGFR at M3 post-KTx, mL/min/1.73m^2	58.34 (21.86)	52.44 (22.00)	56.62 (22.05)	<0.001
BPAR up to 1-year post-KTx.	21 (3.0%)	10 (3.4%)	31 (3.2%)	0.758
Follow-up time, yrs	9.63 (3.63)	8.48 (4.47)	9.28 (3.93)	<0.001

RBC, red blood-cell transfusion; yrs, years; HLA, human leukocyte antigen; dnDSA, de novo donor-specific alloantibody; DCD, donation after circulatory death; BD, brain dead; LD, living donor; eGFR, estimated glomerular-filtration rate; M, month; BPAR, biopsy-proven acute rejection; KTx, kidney transplantation.
The p-values are from chi-squared tests or Wilcoxon tests depending on type of data.
HLA mismatch numbers are based on a 2-digits level for A, B, DR, DQ.

(EBT+) group were more fragile: i.e., they were older, had longer cold ischemia time, and lower M3 estimated glomerular-filtration rates (eGFR) than patients in the EBT- group. There was no significant association with the initial nephropathy (chi-squared test p=0.079), but a trend toward more diabetic and hypertensive nephropathies (i.e., comorbid patients) in the EBT group. Also, early blood transfusion was more often performed in the ATG group than in the basiliximab group (31.1% in the ATG group, 20.5% in the basiliximab group, Fisher exact test p=0.014). The median hemoglobin level triggering the blood transfusion was 8.3 g/dl [1st Q 7.9, 3rd Q 9.7]. Overall, there were 86 [1st Q 60, 3rd Q 112] hemoglobin measurements available per patient over their post-transplantation follow-up, with a median value of 12.8 g/dl (standard deviation 1.77 g/dl).

Among the 981 patients, 292 (29.7%) received at least one RBC transfusion within the first 3 months post-transplantation. A total of 114 patients (11.6%) developed a *de novo* DSA (dnDSA): 19 patients (1.9%) developed a class 1 dnDSA, 83 (8.5%) a class 2 dnDSA, and 12 (1.2%) developed dnDSAs against both classes. **Table 2** describes the characteristics of the immunodominant DSAs for all targets encountered in at least two different patients.

Over the follow-up period, there were 213 death-censored graft losses, i.e., 21.7%. As expected, there was a clear relationship between graft loss (death-censored) and dnDSA development (p<0.001). Demographic characteristics and potential confounders of patients with and without a dnDSA are detailed in **Table 3**.

Donor-Specific Antibody Development (DSA)

The number of dnDSAs detected up to 1-year post-transplantation was not associated with EBT: 21 (3.0%) patients developed a dnDSA in the EBT- group vs. 7 (2.4%) in the EBT+ group (p=0.73). When we also took the value of median hemoglobin between 3- and 6-months post-transplantation into account (in a multivariate logistic regression model, adjusting for early transfusion and median hemoglobin over this 3-month period), the effect of early transfusion remained non-significant (OR=0.58, p=0.295), as well as the effect of median hemoglobin (OR=0.85 for each 1 g/dL increase, p=0.255).

Among the 933 patients with an available 1-year transfusion history (i.e., up to one year after transplantation), 292 patients received at least one unit of RBC with the same result: i.e., transfusion during the first-year post-transplantation did not induce a higher rate of DSA development (HR 0.89, p=0.607). Most transfusions took place within the first 3 months: only 10

TABLE 2 | Description of immunodominant DSAs identified in the cohort.

iDSA	Min MFI	Max MFI	Number of patients	Number of sera
DQ2	410	19,348	14	27
DQ7	851	17,860	12	32
DQ3	1551	17,176	10	15
DQ5	1233	20,480	10	16
DQ6	319	16,436	9	26
DR4	1187	11,745	5	9
A24	659	4886	4	6
DQ4	1031	15,596	4	13
DQ9	253	1461	4	5
A1	964	11,232	3	3
DQ8	1585	10,223	3	11
DR53	1546	17,004	3	8
A2	4664	4664	2	2
C7	756	11,911	2	9
DP2	598	2755	2	3
DQ1	1060	11,932	2	2
DQA3	1362	3700	2	5
DR1	4169	10,590	2	5
DR15	3659	21,320	2	2

MFI, mean fluorescence intensity; DSA, donor-specific alloantibody; iDSA, immunodominant DSA.
Minimum and maximum values of the immunodominant DSA are shown, together with the number of patients developing the corresponding DSA. The number of different sera containing the DSA is also shown.

TABLE 3 | Description of the dnDSA⁻ and dnDSA⁺ groups.

	No dnDSA (*N*=867)	dnDSA⁺ (*N*=114)	Total (*N*=981)	*p*-value
Recipient's age, yrs	52.19 (14.30)	48.49 (14.95)	51.76 (14.42)	0.014
Recipient's gender, F	330 (38.1%)	43 (37.7%)	373 (38.0%)	0.943
Graft rank	0.21 (0.47)	0.34 (0.58)	0.22 (0.49)	0.004
Time on dialysis, yrs	4.02 (4.59)	5.27 (5.68)	4.18 (4.75)	0.033
Pretransplantation HLA sensitization	193 (22.3%)	49 (43.0%)	242 (24.7%)	<0.001
Donor type				0.103
- DCD	29 (3.3%)	1 (0.9%)	30 (3.1%)	
- BD	737 (85.0%)	105 (92.1%)	842 (85.8%)	
- LD	101 (11.6%)	8 (7.0%)	109 (11.1%)	
Cold ischemia time, min	962.03 (502.99)	1031.04 (484.08)	970.06 (501.08)	0.234
Nbr. of HLA mismatches	5.40 (0.89)	5.59 (1.05)	5.42 (0.91)	0.250
Early transfusion	263 (30.3%)	29 (25.4%)	292 (29.8%)	0.282
eGFR at M3 post-KTx, mL/min/1.73m^2	56.59 (22.09)	56.86 (21.85)	56.62 (22.05)	0.929
BPAR up to 1 year post-KTx.	25 (2.9%)	6 (5.3%)	31 (3.2%)	0.172
Follow-up time, days	9.28 (3.92)	9.35 (4.08)	9.28 (3.93)	0.831

yrs, year; F, female; dnDSA, de novo donor-specific alloantibody; HLA, human leukocyte antigen; DCD, donation after circulatory death; BD, brain dead: LD, living donor; eGFR, estimated glomerular-filtration rate; M, month; KTx, kidney transplantation; BPAR, biopsy-proven acute rejection.
The p-values are from chi-squared tests or Wilcoxon tests depending on the type of data.
HLA mismatch numbers are based on a 2-digits level for A, B, DR, DQ.

patients received a transfusion between month-3 and 1-year post-transplantation.

The association between dnDSAs (over the whole follow-up period) and EBT was not significant: 85 (12.33%) patients not receiving any RBCs over the first 3 months developed a DSA compared to 29 (9.9%) patients that did receive at least one transfusion of RBCs over the first 3 months (chi-squared, p=0.33). The dnDSA onset time was 2.77 years in the EBT- group [1st Q 1.02, 3rd Q 5.45] VS 4.73 years in the EBT+ group [1st Q 1.1, 3rd Q 6.79] (Wilcoxon p=0.511). In the EBT- group, 11 patients (12.5%) developed a class 1 DSA, 66 (75%) developed a class 2 DSA and 11 (12.5%) developed both class 1 and class 2 DSAs. In the EBT+ group, 9 (33%) patients developed a class 1 DSA, 17 (63%) developed a class 2 DSA and 1 patient developed both class 1 and class 2 DSAs.

The effect of EBT on overall dnDSA-free death-censored graft survival (dnDSA-GS, i.e., up to and beyond 1 year) was not significant (HR=0.88, p=0.556). The Kaplan–Meier survival curves, depending on EBT, are shown in **Figure 1**. Significant univariate predictors (p-value threshold of 0.1) for dnDSA development were recipient's age (HR=0.99 for each increase of 1 year, p=0.062), pre-transplantation HLA sensitization (HR=2.57, p<0.001), HLA mismatch number between donor and recipient (HR=1.27, p=0.02), tacrolimus trough levels (HR=0.88 for each increment of 1 µg/L of tacrolimus trough level, p=0.027), hemoglobin level > 10 g/dl (HR=0.33, p=0.006), graft rank (HR=1.60 for each previous kidney transplant, p=0.003), and the C/D ratio of tacrolimus (HR=1.66 for a C/D ratio <1.05, p=0.036). Non-significant predictors were recipient gender, donor type, donor age, induction strategy (ATG vs. basiliximab), MPA dose, and month-3 post-transplantation eGFR. Visual trends are provided in **Supplementary Figure 1**, showing the dnDSA-free survival curves between the 4 EBT x induction groups.

In the multivariate Cox's regression model that retained all significant univariate covariates (with a p=0.1 threshold for inclusion), EBT was not associated with dnDSA-GS (HR=0.76, p=0.449). Pre-transplantation HLA sensitization was clearly associated with dnDSA-GS (HR=2.25, p=0.004) as well as hemoglobin levels (HR=0.39 for hemoglobin of >10 g/dL, p=0.029) and the number of HLA mismatches (HR=1.26 per HLA mismatch, p=0.05). However, recipient's age, a low C/D ratio (<1.05), tacrolimus dose, MPA dose, and graft rank were no longer significant, as represented in **Figure 2**. The interaction between early transfusion and pre-transplantation HLA sensitization was not significant either, showing no synergistic effect of EBT and pretransplant HLA sensitization. **Table 4** summarizes the DSA-free survival analyses. The effect of hemoglobin did not change with time at post-transplantation in our model: the influence of hemoglobin on dnDSA-free survival was stable over time (Schoenfeld residual test, p=0.92). On the other hand, the effect of EBT changed over time (Schoenfeld residual test, p=0.026), from protective to deleterious at around 5 years post-transplantation. This suggests that factors associated with the risk of transfusion are later associated with the risk of dnDSA.

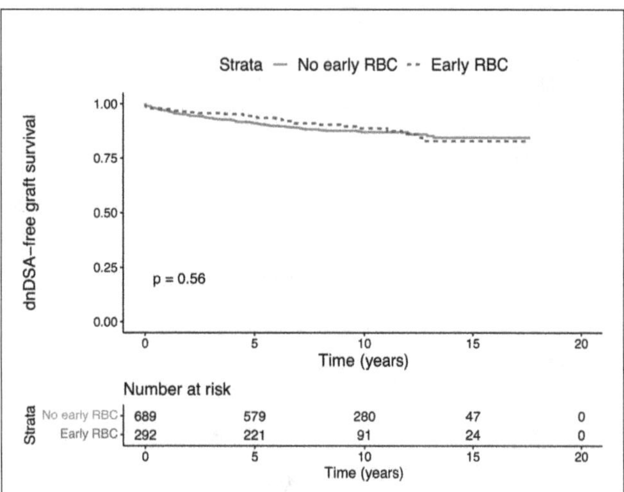

FIGURE 1 | Kaplan–Meier survival analysis of early (within 3 months post-transplantation) red blood-cell transfusion on dnDSA-free graft survival. The given p-value stands for the log-rank test.

To further investigate this hypothesis, we investigated the effect of late (> 1-year post-transplantation) transfusion events on dnDSA-free survival. There were only 37 patients receiving a late transfusion in our cohort, among which only 5 developed a dnDSA. Adjusting a Cox model with both EBT and late transfusion as predictors, we find non-significant yet opposite effects of EBT and late transfusion, in terms of HR (HR for EBT 0.81, p=0.36; HR for late transfusion 1.59, p=0.131). This also suggests a detrimental effect of late transfusion VS EBT.

HLA Antibody Development (HSA)

We also focused on HLA antibodies, regardless of the HLA target, referred to as HLA-specific antibodies (HSA). For this analysis, we focused on the cohort of 739 patients without any pretransplantation HLA sensitization. The raw association between EBT and overall development of HSA (regardless of the time post-transplantation) was not significant: 115 (21.6%) in the EBT- group developed HSA, whereas 50 (24.2%) patients in the EBT+ group developed HSA (chi-square, p=0.519).

Early transfusion was not a significant predictor of HSA-free death-censored graft survival either (HR=1.25, p=0.188). Factors univariately associated with HSA-free death-censored graft survival were recipient's age (protective, HR=0.99 for each increase of 1 year, p=0.06), male gender (protective, HR=0.72, p=0.04), the number of serologic donor/recipient HLA mismatches (HR=1.19, p=0.046), hemoglobin level > 10g/dl (protective, HR=0.43, p=0.056), and graft rank (HR=3.06 for each previous kidney transplant, p<0.001). ATG induction, month-3 eGFR, donor type and donor age, tacrolimus or MPA doses were not significantly associated with HSA-free death-censored graft survival. **Table 4** summarizes the HSA-free survival analysis. There again, visual trends are provided in **Supplementary Figure 2**, showing the dnDSA-free survival curves between the 4 EBT x induction groups.

In the multivariate analysis, adjusting for EBT and all previously mentioned significant factors, only recipient's age (HR=0.98, p=0.013), hemoglobin level (HR=0.41, p=0.044) and

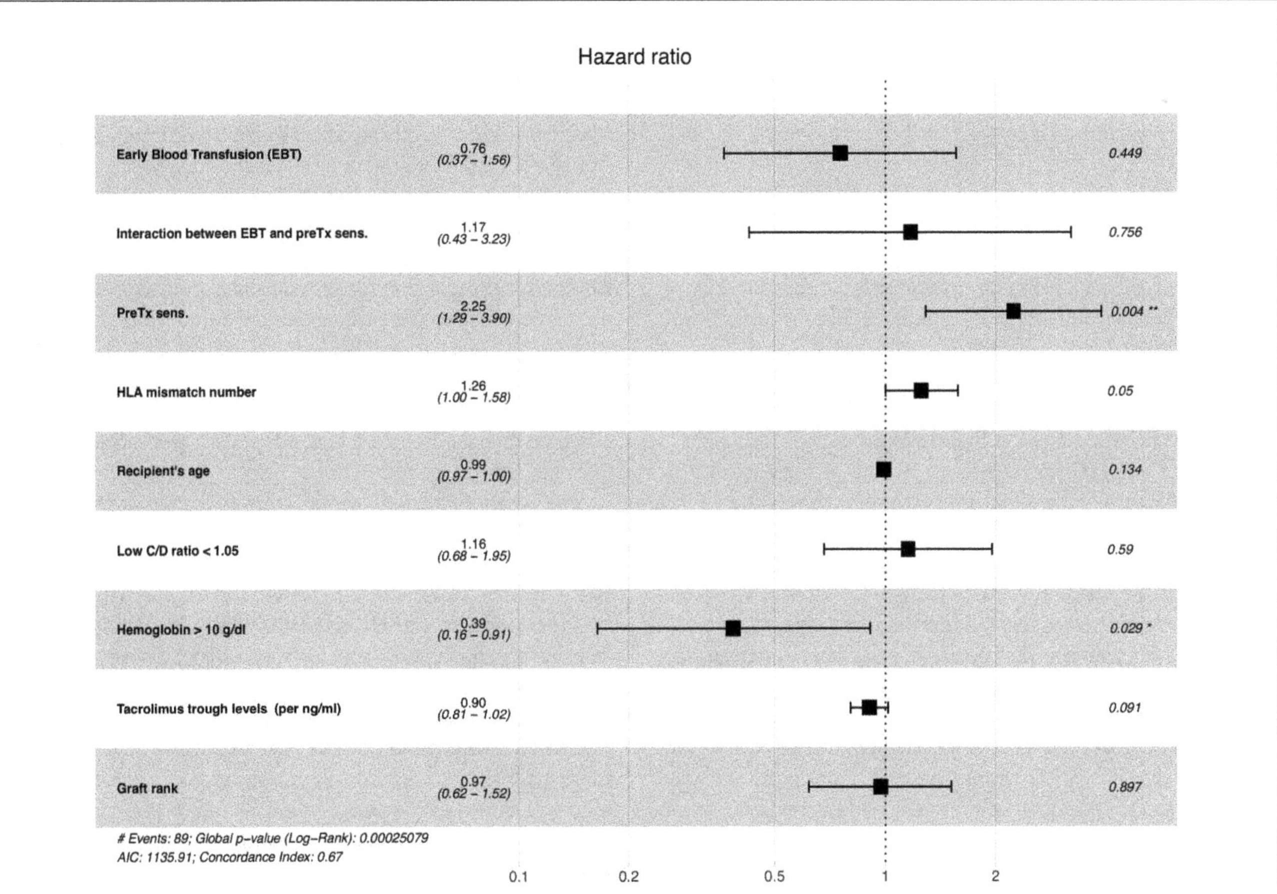

FIGURE 2 | Multivariate Cox's survival model predicting the occurrence of a dnDSA, based on significant univariate predictors of dnDSAs. PreTx = pre-transplantation; sens. = HLA sensitization (presence of anti-HLA antibody); C/D ratio = Tacrolimus concentration-to-dose ratio. Time-varying covariates were considered as such in this multivariate Cox model *p < 0.05, **p < 0.01.

TABLE 4 | Survival analysis for DSA: univariate and multivariate models, hazard ratios (*p*-values).

	HSA		DSA	
Covariate	***Univariate***	***Multivariate***	***Univariate***	***Multivariate***
Pretransplantation HLA sensitization	NA	NA	2.57 (p<0.001)	2.25 (p=0.004)
Early transfusion (ref=no)	1.25 (p=0.188)	1.27 (p=0.259)	0.88 (p=0.556)	0.76 (p=0.449)
Interaction between pretr. HLA sensitization and EBT	NA	NA	NA	1.17 (p=0.756)
Number of HLA mismatches (per each HLA MM)	1.19 (p=0.046)	1.13 (p=0.247)	1.27 (p=0.02)	1.26 (p=0.050)
ATG induction (ref=basiliximab)	0.95 (p=0.822)	-	1.24 (p=0.455)	-
Age (year)	0.99 (p=0.06)	0.98 (p=0.013)	0.99 (p=0.062)	0.99 (p=0.134)
Gender (ref=F)	0.72 (p=0.037)	0.93 (p=0.706)	1.03 (p=0.866)	-
Donor age > median donor age (52 years)	0.88 (p=0.398)	-	1.07 (p=0.734)	-
Month-3 GFR < 30 ml/min/1.73m^2	0.82 (p=0.559)	-	0.97 (p=0.933)	-
Donor type (ref=DCD, VS LV)	0.78 (p=0.323)	-	0.58 (p=0.137)	-
Tacrolimus C/D ratio (ref>1.05)	1.35 (p=0.216)	-	1.66 (p=0.036)	1.16 (p=0.590)
Tacrolimus trough level (per 1 µg/L)	1.06 (p=0.155)	-	0.88 (p=0.027)	0.90 (p=0.091)
Hemoglobin (>10g/dl)	0.43 (p=0.056)	0.41 (p=0.045)	0.33 (p=0.006)	0.39 (p=0.029)
MPA dose (per 1 g increase)	1.25 (p=0.307)	-	1.22 (p=0.464)	-
Graft rank (for each previous transplant)	3.06 (p<0.001)	2.13 (p=0.006)	1.60 (p=0.003)	0.97 (p=0.897)

DSA, donor-specific alloantibody; HSA, HLA-specific antibody; NA, not applicable; ATG, antithymocyte globulins; HLA, human leukocyte antigen; MM, mismatch; yrs, years; F, female; eGFR, estimated glomerular-filtration rate; DCD, donation after circulatory death; LD, living donor; MPA, mycophenolic acid.

graft rank (HR=2.13 per each previous transplant, p=0.006 were associated with dhHSA graft survival. Both age and hemoglobin were protective (increased age or increased hemoglobin were associated with better dnHSA-free allograft survival). These results are detailed in **Table 4**.

DISCUSSION

Development of a *de novo* DSA is a major threat for kidney-transplant recipients. Early post-transplant RBC transfusions, a potentially sensitizing procedure, are a potential trigger for dnDSA formation. In this study, we show that kidney transplant recipients receiving RBC transfusions within the first three months post-transplantation are not at higher risk of dnDSA formation.

Our data suggest that anemia < 10 g/dl is a risk factor for dnDSA, while early transfusion events (up to 3 months and up to 1 year) are not associated with dnDSA development. Since our maintenance immunosuppressive regimen does not change over time (except for tacrolimus exposure, which is not a significant multivariate predictor of dnDSA development), we suggest that ATG induction creates a time window of at least 3-months post-transplantation, within which transfusion is not deleterious in terms of HLA sensitization. While we adjusted our analysis on covariates that were different between ATG-treated patients and basiliximab-treated patients (recipient's age, gender and donor type), it should be noted that a confusion factor cannot be ruled out since there was a clear indication bias for the induction therapy.

The detrimental effect of hemoglobin levels, in terms of dnDSA, can be interpreted in at least two ways. A low hemoglobin level might be associated with a higher rate of RBC transfusions, leading to more DSA, at least beyond the protection of ATG; or hemoglobin levels are a surrogate of some allosensitization risk, e.g., anemic patients undergo more inflammatory events, leading to more allosensitization.

In the study by Ferrandiz et al. (11), early (within 1-year post-transplantation) RBC transfusion was associated with an increased rate of dnDSAs, as well as more antibody-mediated rejections. However, in their study, patients mainly received basiliximab as the induction therapy. The differences observed in head-to-head comparison of 1-year dnDSA-free survival between the cohort of Ferrandiz et al. and our cohort can be explained by the different induction strategies, the rest of the immunosuppressive strategy being very similar. We hypothesize that ATG induction prevented the potentially sensitizing effect of early post-transplant blood transfusions. While the effect of induction was not a significant predictor in our analysis, the small proportion of basiliximab-induced patients leads to a low power to detect an effect of induction.

In the study by Hassan et al. (12), sensitization against a shared HLA antigen between a RBC donor and the kidney transplant was detrimental: there were more DSAs and worse overall kidney-transplant survival. In their study, ~60% of RBC transfusions were performed in the first-year post-transplantation and 40% of transfusions were performed beyond 1 year. Induction drugs used were mostly depleting. However, late RBC transfusions (i.e., >1-year post-transplantation) may impact on DSA development beyond the protective effect of a depleting induction. A more rigorous analysis would demand considering transfusion events as a time-varying covariate to decipher the intricate effects of the type of induction therapy and RBC transfusion. Indeed, the former may prevent the detrimental HLA sensitizing effect of the latter. In our analysis, we considered hemoglobin as a time-dependent covariate, and show that a low hemoglobin < 10 g/dl is indeed a risk factor for dnDSA development.

This role of ATG induction is all the more important because a RBC transfusion is frequently required after transplantation. In our center, despite the early and frequent use of erythropoiesis-stimulating agents, more than a quarter of our patients require an early RBC transfusion. It is therefore important to evaluate the impact of such RBC transfusions: different immunosuppressive regimens may prevent DSA development even when an early RBC transfusion is required.

The major limitation of our study is that it is retrospective. However, its major strengths are that i) it is very homogeneous, i.e., ATG induction, and tacrolimus plus mycophenolic acid were used as the maintenance therapy, ii) we precisely and timely monitored for the presence of anti-HLA alloantibodies using Luminex at pre- and post-transplantation, and iii) we had an exhaustive record of transfusion occurences (however, without blood donor HLA typing). Our focus on pre-transplantation DSA-free patients precludes any conclusion on the post-transfusion rebound of pre-existing DSAs. This specific investigation is not possible in our cohort of mostly pre-transplantation DSA-free patients (since we did not have a desensitization program until 2017). However, it would be very interesting to focus on these specific pre-existing DSAs, as their evolution over time post-transplantation might be different from that of dnDSAs.

CONCLUSION

Our results suggest that a RBC transfusion may be safely given to kidney-transplant recipients in the early post-transplantation period (first 3 months) provided that they receive an ATG-based induction therapy. This result, although apparently at variance with previous studies, reinforces the importance of considering the type of induction therapy used when evaluating allosensitization.

ETHICS STATEMENT

The studies involving human participants were reviewed and approved by CNIL (French National committee for data protection) - approval number 1987785v0. The patients/participants provided their written informed consent to participate in this study.

AUTHOR CONTRIBUTIONS

TJ designed the study, collected the data, performed the statistical analysis and wrote the manuscript. DM and CD checked the blood transfusion data at the blood bank and performed assessment of dn DSA tests. GF is the leader of the kidney transplant surgery team. TJ, JN, HN, and PM took care of patients within the immediate post-transplant period. Finally, LR designed the study, supervised the manuscript and edited it. All authors contributed to the article and approved the submitted version.

ACKNOWLEDGMENTS

We thank the EFS Biobank team for their help in collecting the transfusion data, especially Ms Sabine Noviant, as well as Claudine Giroud Lathuile, Sophie Anselme Martin, and Sandrine Fournel. We also thank our research team, especially Mathilde Bugnazet, Farida Imerzoukene and David Tartry.

REFERENCES

1. Sellarés J, de Freitas DG, Mengel M, Reeve J, Einecke G, Sis B, et al. Understanding the Causes of Kidney Transplant Failure: The Dominant Role of Antibody-Mediated Rejection and Nonadherence. *Am J Transplant* (2012) 12:388–99. doi: 10.1111/j.1600-6143.2011.03840.x
2. Wiebe C, Nevins TE, Robiner WN, Thomas W, Matas AJ, Nickerson PW. The Synergistic Effect of Class II HLA Epitope-Mismatch and Nonadherence on Acute Rejection and Graft Survival. *Am J Transplant* (2015) 15:2197–202. doi: 10.1111/ajt.13341
3. Nankivell BJ, Borrows RJ, Fung CL-S, O'Connell PJ, Allen RDM, Chapman JR. The Natural History of Chronic Allograft Nephropathy. *N Engl J Med* (2003) 349:2326–33. doi: 10.1056/NEJMoa020009
4. Nankivell BJ, P'Ng CH, O'Connell PJ, Chapman JR. Calcineurin Inhibitor Nephrotoxicity Through the Lens of Longitudinal Histology: Comparison of Cyclosporine and Tacrolimus Eras. *Transplantation* (2016) 100:1723–31. doi: 10.1097/TP.0000000000001243
5. Naesens M, Kuypers DRJ, Sarwal M. Calcineurin Inhibitor Nephrotoxicity. *Clin J Am Soc Nephrol* (2009) 4:481–508. doi: 10.2215/CJN.04800908
6. Naesens M, Lerut E. Calcineurin Inhibitor Nephrotoxicity in the Era of Antibody-Mediated Rejection. *Transplantation* (2016) 100:1599–600. doi: 10.1097/TP.0000000000001244
7. Eskandary F, Regele H, Baumann L, Bond G, Kozakowski N, Warhmann M, et al. A Randomized Trial of Bortezomib in Late Antibody-Mediated Kidney Transplant Rejection. *J Am Soc Nephrol* (2018) 29:591–605. doi: 10.1681/ASN.2017070818
8. Wan SS, Ying TD, Wyburn K, Roberts DM, Wyld M, Chadban SJ. The Treatment of Antibody-Mediated Rejection in Kidney Transplantation: An Updated Systematic Review and Meta-Analysis. *Transplantation* (2018) 102:557–68. doi: 10.1097/TP.0000000000002049
9. Böhmig GA, Eskandary F, Doberer K, Halloran PF. The Therapeutic Challenge of Late Antibody-Mediated Kidney Allograft Rejection. *Transpl Int* (2019) 32:775–88. doi: 10.1111/tri.13436
10. Fidler S, Swaminathan P, Lim W, Ferrari P, Witt C, Christiansen F, et al. Peri-Operative Third Party Red Blood Cell Transfusion in Renal Transplantation and the Risk of Antibody-Mediated Rejection and Graft Loss. *Transpl Immunol* (2013) 29:22–7. doi: 10.1016/j.trim.2013.09.008
11. Ferrandiz I, Congy-Jolivet N, Del Bello A, Debiol B, Trébern-Launay K, Esposito L, et al. Impact of Early Blood Transfusion After Kidney Transplantation on the Incidence of Donor-Specific Anti-HLA Antibodies. *Am J Transplant* (2016) 16:2661–9. doi: 10.1111/ajt.13795
12. Hassan S, Regan F, Brown C, Harmer A, Anderson H, Beckwith N, et al. Shared Alloimmune Responses Against Blood and Transplant Donors Result in Adverse Clinical Outcomes Following Blood Transfusion Post–Renal Transplantation. *Am J Transplant* (2019) 19:1720–9. doi: 10.1111/ajt.15233
13. Augustine JJ, Poggio ED, Heeger PS, Hricik DE. Preferential Benefit of Antibody Induction Therapy in Kidney Recipients With High Pretransplant Frequencies of Donor-Reactive Interferon-Gamma Enzyme-Linked Immunosorbent Spots. *Transplantation* (2008) 86:529–34. doi: 10.1097/TP.0b013e31818046db
14. Zecher D, Bach C, Staudner C, Böger CA, Bergler T, Banas B, et al. Characteristics of Donor-Specific Anti-HLA Antibodies and Outcome in Renal Transplant Patients Treated With a Standardized Induction Regimen. *Nephrol Dial Transplant* (2017) 32:730–7. doi: 10.1093/ndt/gfw445

25

Comparison of Different Blood Transfusion Methods in Patients Undergoing Cesarean Section

*Fei Guo†, Heshan Tang† and Xiaoqiang Wei**

Department of Blood Transfusion, The First Affiliated Hospital of Naval Military Medical University, Shanghai, China

***Correspondence:**
Xiaoqiang Wei
Weixiaoqiang1998@smmu.edu.cn

†These authors share first authorship

Purpose: To compare the effect of allogeneic transfusion and acute normovolemic hemodilution (ANH) autologous transfusion in patients undergoing cesarean section.

Methods: Patients who underwent cesarean section and received blood transfusion therapy from February 2019 to July 2021 in our hospital were observed and divided into the allogeneic group (n = 55) who received allogeneic transfusion therapy and the autologous group (n = 55) who received ANH autologous transfusion therapy according to the mode of transfusion. Observations included vital signs [heart rate (HR), mean arterial pressure (MAP), stroke volume variation (SVV)], blood routine [red blood cells (RBC), platelets (PLT), hematocrit (HCT), hemoglobin (Hb)], T-cell subsets ($CD4^+$, $CD8^+$, $CD4^+/CD8^+$), immunoglobulins (IgA, IgM, IgG), inflammatory factors [C-reactive protein (CRP), tumor necrosis factor (TNF)-α, interleukin (IL)-6], and adverse effects were counted in both groups.

Results: There was no statistical significance in the intra-group and inter-group comparisons of HR, MAP, and SVV between the two groups before transfusion and transfusion for 10 min ($P > 0.05$). 5d after operation, the RBC, PLT, HCT, and Hb of the allogeneic group were lower than those before operation, and the autologous group was higher than that of the allogeneic group ($P < 0.05$). 5d after operation, the CRP, TNF-α, and IL-6 of the allogeneic group were higher than those before operation, and the autologous group was lower than that of the allogeneic group ($P < 0.05$). 5d after operation, the $CD4^+$, $CD4^+/CD8^+$ of the allogeneic group were lower than before operation, and the $CD8^+$ was higher than before operation. The $CD4^+$ and $CD4^+/CD8^+$ of the autologous group were higher than that of the allogeneic group, and $CD8^+$ was lower than that of the allogeneic group ($P < 0.05$). 5d after operation, the IgA, IgG, and IgM of the allogeneic group were lower than those before operation, and the autologous group was higher than that of the allogeneic group ($P < 0.05$). During blood transfusion, there was no significant difference in the adverse reaction rate between the two groups ($P > 0.05$).

Conclusion: Both allogeneic transfusion and ANH autologous transfusion have little effect on the vital signs of patients undergoing cesarean section, but ANH autologous transfusion is more helpful to the stability of blood routine, T-cell subsets, immunoglobulin, and inflammation levels after surgery, which is a safe and effective way of blood transfusion.

Keywords: cesarean section, allogeneic transfusion, acute normovolemic hemodilution, autologous transfusion, application effect

INTRODUCTION

Cesarean section is an important midwifery procedure in the field of obstetrics. It is suitable for cases where the fetus cannot be delivered from the vagina normally, such as cephalopelvic error, birth canal abnormalities, fetal distress, fetal position error, umbilical cord prolapse, history of cesarean section, multiple births, etc. (1, 2). Placenta praevia and placental abruption are common complications of cesarean section, which can exacerbate the incidence of perinatal hemorrhage in cesarean section, and the incidence is much higher than that of natural delivery, therefore, in obstetric surgery, the blood transfusion rate of cesarean section 0.77% is higher than natural delivery 0.23% (3, 4). Preoperative blood preparation is an important preoperative preparation for cesarean section. It can effectively reduce the risk of disseminated intravascular coagulation (DIC), shock and even death in patients with cesarean section bleeding. Therefore, it is beneficial to improve the uterine retention rate and survival rate of pregnant women. For patients with large blood loss during cesarean section, urgent blood transfusion is often required in clinic, currently, allogeneic blood transfusion is mainly used, but it is associated with postoperative infection, immunosuppression and a poor prognosis (5). Acute normovolemic hemodilutio (ANH) autologous transfusion is an autologous blood transfusion method in which autologous blood is drawn preoperatively and supplemented with an equal volume of crystal or colloidal fluid, and the patient's blood loss is combined during the operation to return the autologous blood (6).

The acute normovolemic hemodilutio (ANH) autologous transfusion is a form of autotransfusion in which autologous blood is drawn preoperatively and replenished with an equal volume of crystalloid or colloidal fluid, and then returned autologous blood intraoperatively according to the amount of blood lost by the patient (6). It can effectively reduce the hematocrit (HCT), reduce the loss of blood elements during bleeding, improve the body's tolerance after hemodilution, and shorten the time of ischemia and hypoxia in patients through blood dilution, which is a blood conservation technique that can reduce the risk of anesthesia and surgery and provide fresh

TABLE 1 | Comparison of patients' general conditions (n, $M \pm SD$, %).

Indexs	Allogeneic group (n = 55)	Autologous group (n = 55)	t/χ^2 value	P value
Age (years old)	28.02 ± 3.11	28.76 ± 2.98	1.274	0.205
Gestational week (weeks)	36.54 ± 0.59	36.62 ± 0.61	0.699	0.486
Body mass index (kg/cm^2)	26.85 ± 3.24	27.03 ± 3.26	0.290	0.772
Operative time (h)	1.57 ± 0.83	1.61 ± 0.79	0.259	0.796
Blood loss (mL)	953.25 ± 26.01	956.24 ± 25.47	0.609	0.544
Number of outputs (times)			0.147	0.702
1	24 (43.64)	26 (47.27)		
≥2	31 (56.36)	29 (52.73)		
History of cesarean section (cases)			0.042	0.838
No	37 (67.27)	38 (69.09)		
Yes	18 (32.73)	17 (30.91)		
ASA classification (cases)			0.146	0.702
II	28 (50.91)	30 (54.55)		
III	27 (49.09)	25 (45.45)		
Maternity status (cases)			0.326	0.955
Placenta previa	38 (69.09)	39 (70.91)		
Placental abruption	5 (9.09)	4 (7.27)		
Placental implantation	3 (5.46)	4 (7.27)		
Others	9 (16.36)	8 (14.55)		

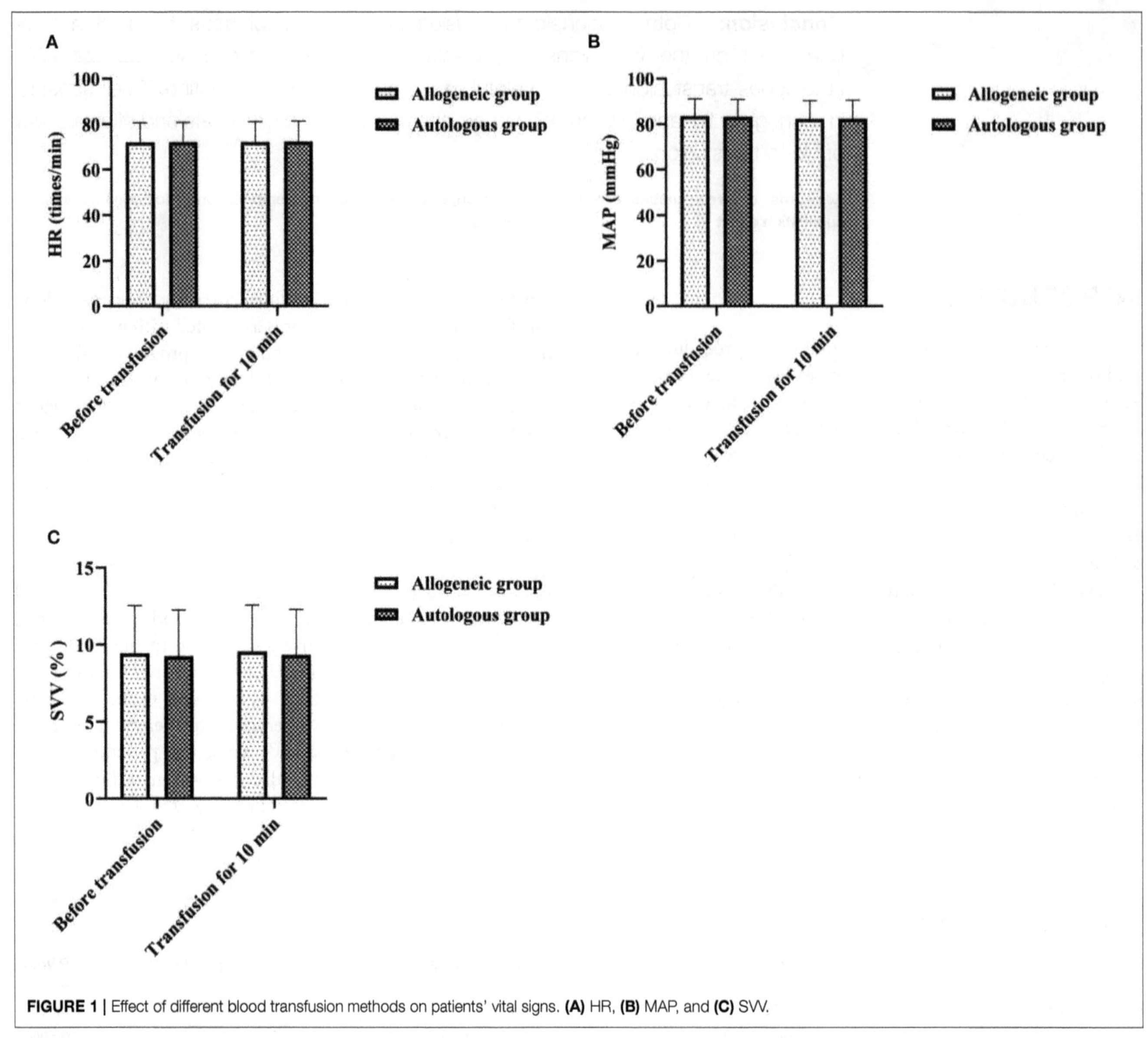

FIGURE 1 | Effect of different blood transfusion methods on patients' vital signs. **(A)** HR, **(B)** MAP, and **(C)** SVV.

whole blood to the patient (7). It has been widely used in major surgeries such as orthopedics, oncology and neurosurgery, but there are very few applications and related reports in the field of obstetrics (8, 9). This study compares the application effect of allogeneic transfusion and ANH autologous transfusion in patients undergoing cesarean section, aiming to explore the effectiveness and safety of ANH autologous transfusion in patients undergoing cesarean section.

MATERIALS AND METHODS

Research Object

Patients who underwent cesarean section and received blood transfusion from February 2019 to July 2021 in our hospital were used as observation subjects. Inclusion criteria: age 20–35 years old; proposed cesarean section; American Society of Anesthesiologists (ASA) classification II–III (10); normal liver and kidney function, normal cardiopulmonary function; normal four items before transfusion; normal coagulation function; preoperative platelet (PLT) $> 100\times10^9$/L, HCT $> 33\%$, hemoglobin (Hb) > 110 g/L (11); patients or her family had signed the informed consent. Exclusion criteria: people undergoing allogeneic and autologous transfusion at the same time; people who had a history of heart disease or tumor disease; people who had a history of neurological or psychiatric disease; people with immune system diseases; people with systemic acute and chronic infections; People with cognitive and communication impairments. They were divided into the allogeneic group ($n = 55$) receiving allogeneic transfusion therapy and the autologous group ($n = 55$) receiving ANH autologous transfusion therapy according to the mode of blood transfusion. There was no significant difference between the two groups in terms of age, gestational weeks and other general conditions,

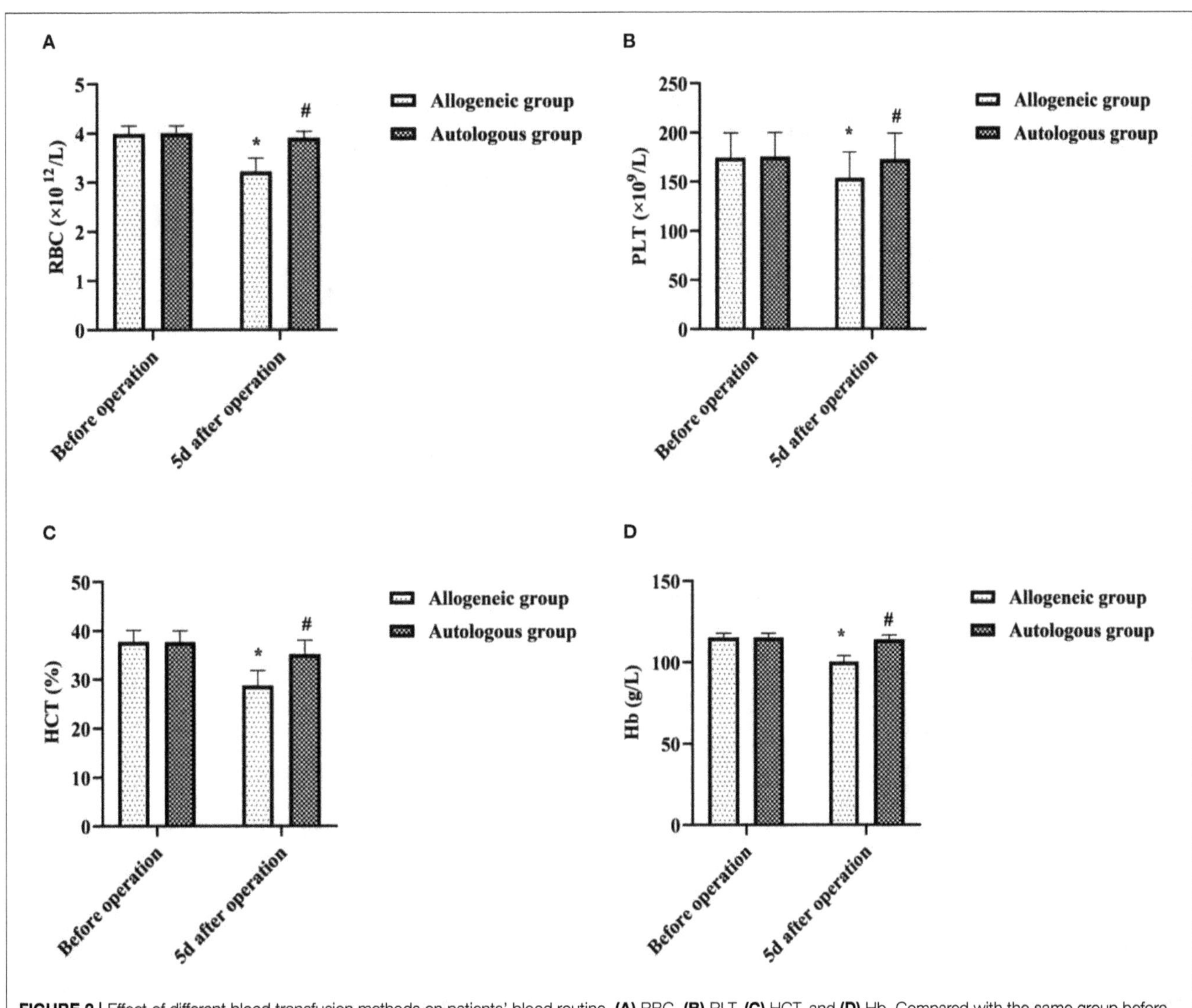

FIGURE 2 | Effect of different blood transfusion methods on patients' blood routine. **(A)** RBC, **(B)** PLT, **(C)** HCT, and **(D)** Hb. Compared with the same group before operation, $^{*}P < 0.05$; compared with allogeneic group 5d after operation, $^{\#}P < 0.05$.

which were comparable, which were comparable ($P > 0.05$) (**Table 1**).

Research Methods

Patients in both groups underwent cesarean section and general anesthesia was induced intraoperatively. On this basis, the allogeneic group received allogeneic transfusion therapy, i.e., when HCT < 24% or Hb < 80 g/L, stock blood was taken for transfusion perfusion according to the amount of blood lost by the patient. The autologous group received ANH autologous transfusion therapy, i.e., radial artery and right internal jugular vein puncture placement were performed after induction of anesthesia and before the start of surgery. Preoperatively, according to the patient's intraoperative bleeding prediction, the CZK-IB microcomputer liquid sampling controller (purchased from Zhengzhou Feilong Medical Equipment Co., Ltd.) was used to collect 300–420 mL of autologous blood through the radial artery and stored in a blood storage bag and treated with light shielding and freshness. An equal volume of 6% hydroxyethyl starch (HES) 130/0.4 (purchased from Shandong Hualu Pharmaceutical Co., Ltd., approval number H37022757) was then infused *via* the internal jugular vein. autologous blood was transfused at the end of the main intraoperative step or when the bleeding volume was ≥ 1,000 mL or Hb was ≤100 g/L.

Observation Index

(1) Vital signs: heart rate (HR), mean arterial pressure (MAP), and stroke volume variation (SVV) were monitored before transfusion and transfusion for 10 min by a PICCO monitor (purchased from Beijing Shimao Medical Equipment Trading Co., Ltd.).

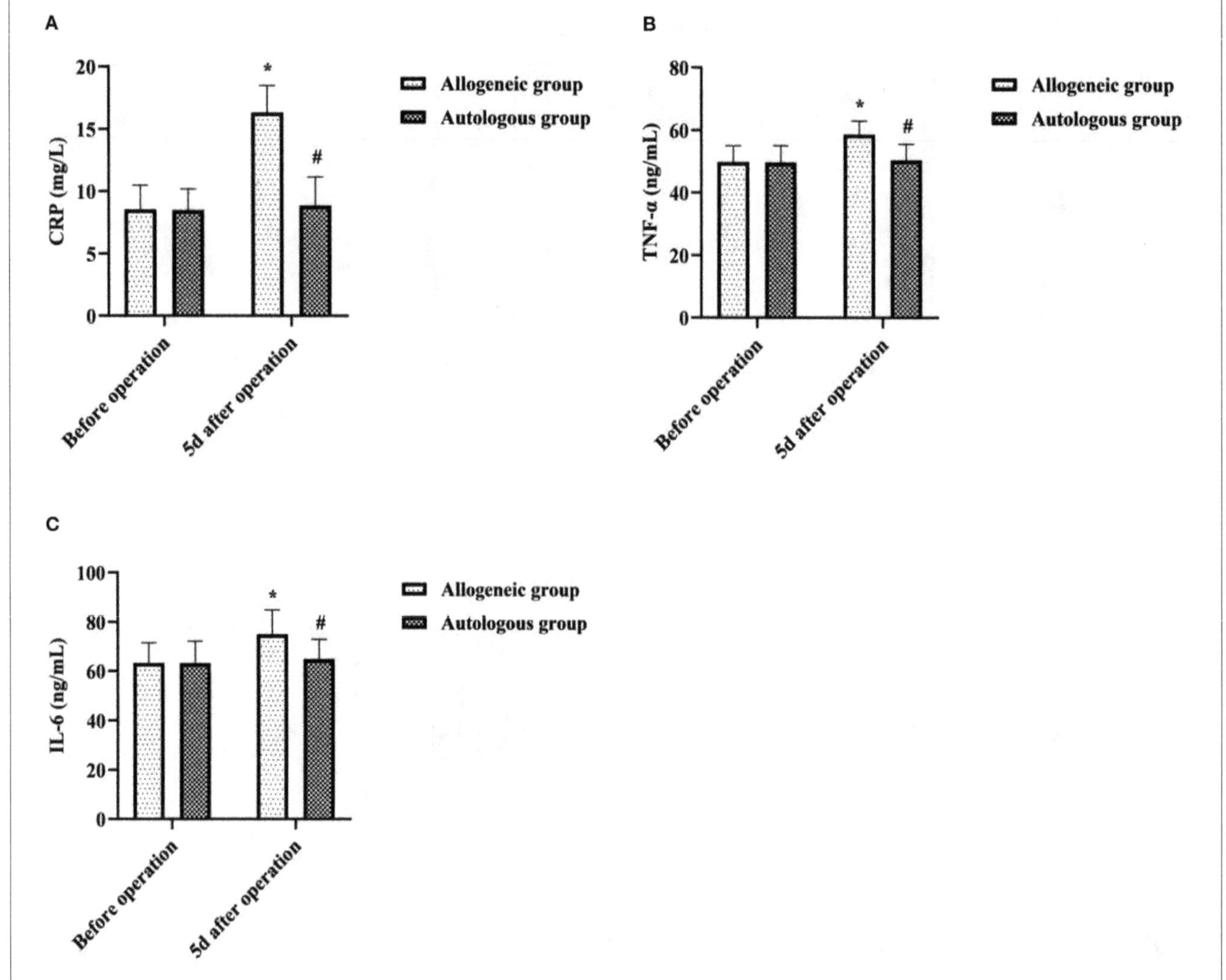

FIGURE 3 | Effect of different blood transfusion methods on patients' inflammatory factors. **(A)** CRP, **(B)** **TNF-α**, and **(C)** IL-6. Compared with the same group before operation, *$P < 0.05$; compared with allogeneic group 5d after operation, #$P < 0.05$.

(2) Blood routine: The red blood cell (RBC), PLT, HCT and Hb levels were measured before and 5 d after surgery by MAXM automatic hematology analyzer (purchased from Beckman Coulter, Inc.).

(3) T-cell subsets: The $CD4^+$, $CD8^+$, $CD4^+/CD8^+$ levels were measured before and 5 d after surgery by a Cytomics FC500 flow cytometer (purchased from Beckman Coulter, Inc.).

(4) Immunoglobulins: The IgA, IgM, and IgG levels were measured before and 5 d after surgery by enzyme-linked immunosorbent assay (The kit was purchased from Roche).

(5) Inflammatory factors: C-reactive protein (CRP), tumor necrosis factor (TNF)-α and interleukin (IL)-6 levels were measured before and 5 d after surgery by enzyme-linked immunosorbent assay (The kit was purchased from Shanghai Sange Biotechnology Co., Ltd.).

(6) Adverse reaction rate: Allergy, fever, hemolysis and other adverse reactions occurred during blood transfusion in the two groups were counted.

Statistical Methods

SPSS 22.0 software was applied, and the measurement data were expressed as mean ± standard deviation ($M \pm SD$) and compared by t-test. Count data were expressed as ratio, and the χ^2 test was used for comparison. $P < 0.05$ was considered statistically significant.

RESULTS

Effect of Different Blood Transfusion Methods on Patients' Vital Signs

There was no statistical significance in the intra-group and inter-group comparisons of HR, MAP, and SVV between the two

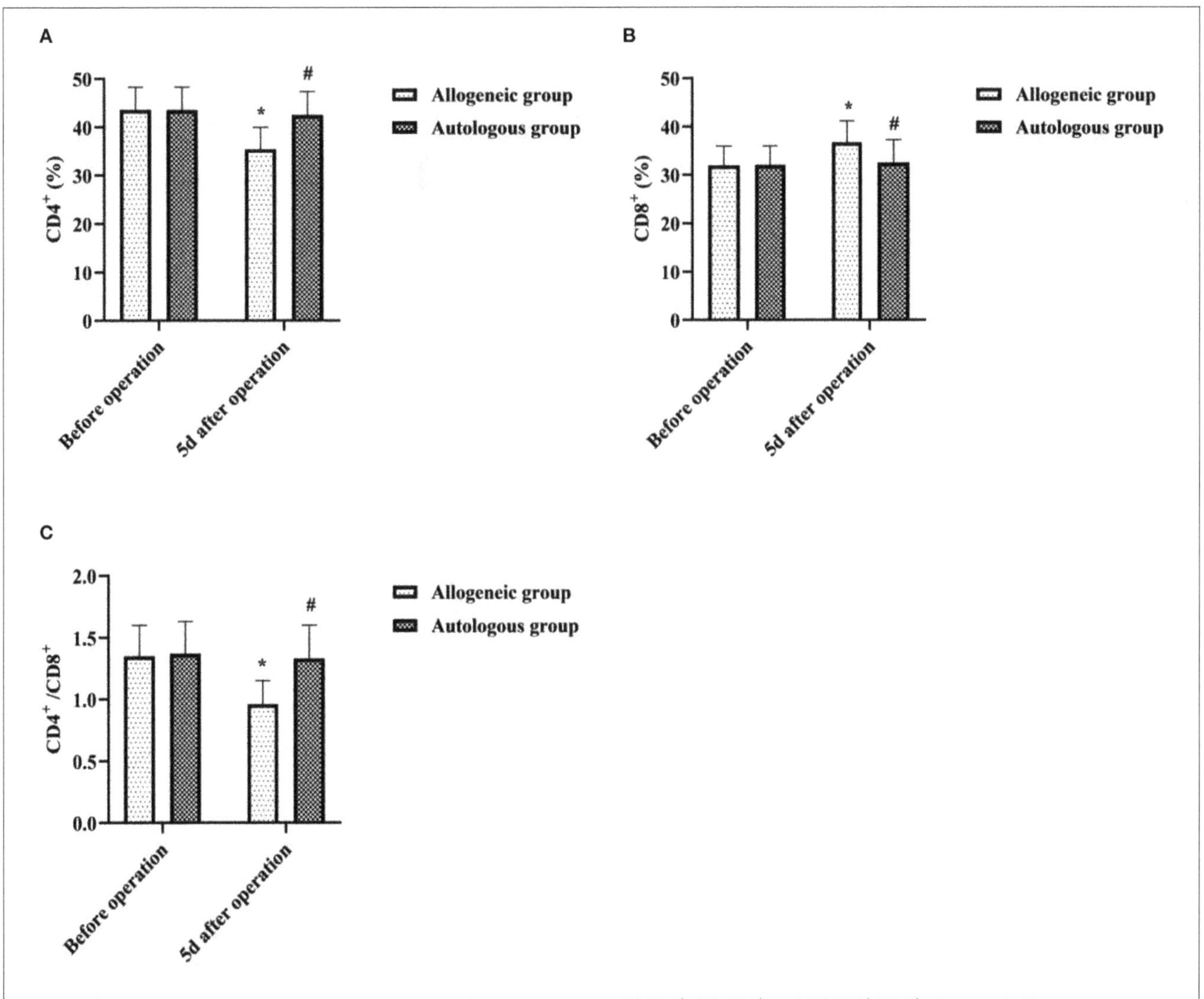

FIGURE 4 | Effect of different blood transfusion methods on patients' T-cell subsets. **(A)** $CD4^+$, **(B)** $CD8^+$, and **(C)** $CD4^+/CD8^+$. Compared with the same group before operation, *$P < 0.05$; compared with allogeneic group 5d after operation, #$P < 0.05$.

groups before transfusion and transfusion for 10 min ($P > 0.05$) (**Figure 1**).

Effect of Different Blood Transfusion Methods on Patients' Blood Routine

5d after operation, the RBC, PLT, HCT, and Hb of the allogeneic group were lower than those before operation, and the autologous group was higher than that of the allogeneic group ($P < 0.05$) (**Figure 2**).

Effect of Different Blood Transfusion Methods on Patients' Inflammatory Factors

5d after operation, the CRP, TNF-α, and IL-6 of the allogeneic group were higher than those before operation, and the autologous group was lower than that of the allogeneic group ($P < 0.05$) (**Figure 3**).

Effect of Different Blood Transfusion Methods on Patients' T-Cell Subsets

5d after operation, the $CD4^+$, $CD4^+/CD8^+$ of the allogeneic group were lower than before operation, and the $CD8^+$ was higher than before operation. The $CD4^+$ and $CD4^+/CD8^+$ of the autologous group were higher than that of the allogeneic group, and $CD8^+$ was lower than that of the allogeneic group ($P < 0.05$) (**Figure 4**).

Effect of Different Blood Transfusion Methods on Patients' Immunoglobulins

5d after operation, the IgA, IgG, and IgM of the allogeneic group were lower than those before operation, and the autologous group was higher than that of the allogeneic group ($P < 0.05$) (**Figure 5**).

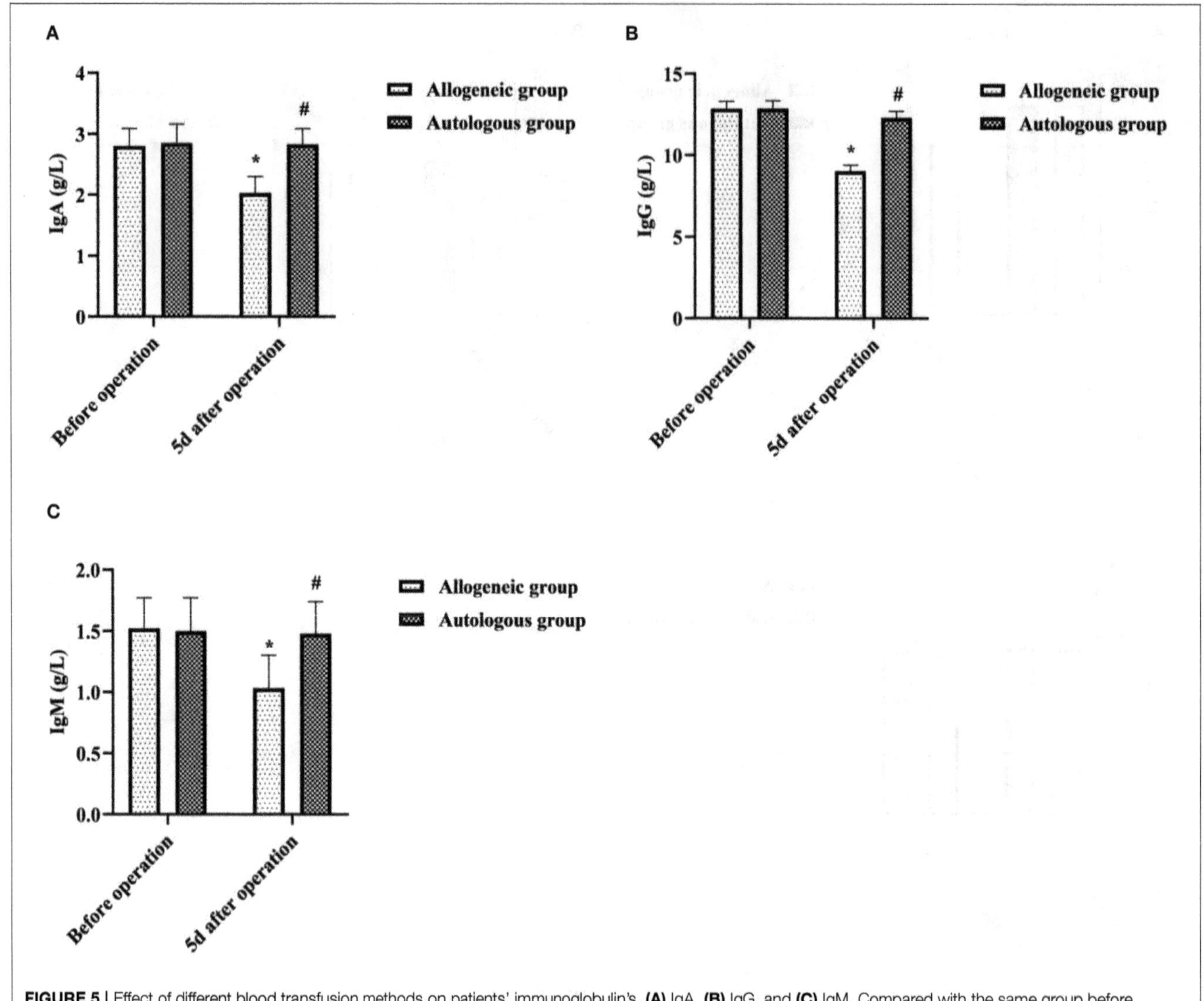

FIGURE 5 | Effect of different blood transfusion methods on patients' immunoglobulin's. **(A)** IgA, **(B)** IgG, and **(C)** IgM. Compared with the same group before operation, $^{*}P < 0.05$; compared with allogeneic group 5d after operation, $^{\#}P < 0.05$.

Adverse Reaction Rate of Different Blood Transfusion Methods

During blood transfusion, there was no significant difference in the adverse reaction rate between the two groups ($P > 0.05$) (**Table 2**).

DISCUSSION

In recent years, due to social factors such as late marriage and late childbirth, and second child policy, the number of advanced maternal age and scarred uterus re-pregnancy in China has been increasing, and the cesarean delivery rate has also increased, and in some areas it has exceeded 50% (12). It is reported that cesarean section patients are prone to severe bleeding that is not easy to control during the perinatal period, which is one of the main reasons for the poor prognosis or even death of mothers and babies (13). So, timely, reasonable, and adequate blood transfusion treatment is of great significance for suppressing perinatal hemorrhage and ensuring the safety of mothers and babies. Allogeneic transfusion is the main method at present, but it has been plagued by problems such as tight blood source and many adverse reactions of blood transfusion. It has been reported that ANH autologous transfusion may be superior to allogeneic blood transfusion in terms of blood safety (14). However, this blood transfusion method uses exogenous fluid for dilution, and whether the blood transfusion will affect the vital signs, immune function, and inflammation levels of patients undergoing cesarean section is still unknown. This study provided a comparative analysis in this regard.

It has been suggested that blood volume increases in women after pregnancy and that ANH autologous transfusion can achieve a reduction in blood viscosity, increase blood oxygen uptake, reduce cardiac burden, and protect the myocardium through preoperative blood sampling and dilution (15). In this

TABLE 2 | Adverse reaction rate of different blood transfusion methods (*n*, %).

Group	Allergy	Fever	Hemolysis	Others	Total
Allogeneic group ($n = 55$)	1 (1.82)	2 (3.64)	1 (1.82)	3 (5.45)	7 (12.73)
Autosomal group ($n = 55$)	1 (1.82)	1 (1.82)	0 (0.00)	2 (3.64)	4 (7.28)
χ^2 value					0.909
P value					0.340

study, there was no statistical significance in the intra-group and inter-group comparisons of HR, MAP, and SVV between the two groups before transfusion and transfusion for 10 min ($P > 0.05$). It showed that ANH autologous transfusion helps to maintain hemodynamic stability in patients undergoing cesarean section. To analyze the reasons, HES, as an artificial colloidal fluid with large molecular weight, has the pharmacological properties of being unable to penetrate the vessel wall, long intravascular retention time, and good effect of maintaining plasma colloidal osmotic pressure (16). Therefore, compared with isotonic crystalloids, it can achieve hemodynamic stability with less dosage and faster effect, and is one of the most commonly used resuscitation fluids in hemorrhagic shock. Surgery may result in loss of tangible components of blood, and allogeneic transfusions may result in destruction of blood components due to the long storage time of blood. In this study, 5d after operation, the RBC, PLT, HCT, and Hb of the allogeneic group were lower than those before operation, and the autologous group was higher than that of the allogeneic group ($P < 0.05$). It was suggested that ANH autologous transfusion is an effective way to improve hematoprotection and prevent the development of postoperative anemia. Analyze the reasons. Compared with allogeneic blood transfusion, ANH autologous blood transfusion is performed by drawing autologous blood before surgery and returning it to the patient during surgery, which not only reduces the loss of red blood cells and platelets during surgery, but also has a short storage time and does not require refrigeration, so the blood components are less damaged, which facilitates the patient's postoperative recovery. CRP, TNF-α, and IL-6 are all key cytokines that initiate inflammatory or immune responses when the body perceives inflammatory stimuli such as trauma (17, 18). In this study, 5d after operation, the CRP, TNF-α, and IL-6 of the allogeneic group were higher than those before operation, and the autologous group was lower than that of the allogeneic group ($P < 0.05$). It was suggested that allogeneic transfusion can lead to varying degrees of inflammatory response in patients undergoing cesarean section, whereas ANH autologous transfusion has a mild effect on the level of inflammation in patients. This may be related to the fact that the blood dilution of ANH autotransfusion reduces concentrations of cortisol and catecholamines in plasma, and that the blood released out of the body after hemodilution is not involved in the acute phase response.

As an immunogenic and reactogenic substance, blood can be accompanied by a series of adverse reactions involving immune regulation in the process of blood transfusion therapy, mainly manifested as immunosuppression (19). Both T-cell subsets and immunoglobulins are important indicators to assess the immune function of the body, with the former playing a central regulatory role in cellular immunity and the latter being closely related to humoral immunity undertaken by B cells (20, 21). When allogeneic blood enters the human body as foreign protein antigen, the differentiation of T lymphocytes into $CD4^+$ cells is inhibited, cytotoxic T lymphocytes ($CD8^+$ T cells) are activated, and then the proportion of $CD4^+/CD8^+$ is unbalanced, resulting in abnormal immune function. In this study, 5d after operation, the $CD4^+$, $CD4^+/CD8^+$, IgA, IgG and IgM of the allogeneic group were lower than before operation, and the $CD8^+$ was higher than before operation. The $CD4^+$, $CD4^+/CD8^+$, IgA, IgG and IgM of the autologous group were higher than that of the allogeneic group, and $CD8^+$ was lower than that of the allogeneic group ($P < 0.05$). It indicated that allogeneic transfusion can cause a decrease in immune function in the recipient, while ANH autologous transfusion has less effect on immune function in patients undergoing cesarean section. Analysis of the causes may be related to a decrease in the immune function of red blood cells due to the long storage time of the stock blood used for allogeneic transfusion. Numerous studies (22–24) have shown that the erythrocyte system has some immune functions that cannot be replaced by other immune cells, namely, reducing free radical damage, scavenging immune complexes, and participating in immune defense. Under normal circumstances, stock blood used for allogeneic transfusion can be stored at a constant temperature of 4°C for 2–3 weeks. However, the longer the storage time, the more serious the deformation and aging of RBCs, the gradual decrease of RBC-C3b receptor activity, the excessive accumulation of related metabolites, the increase of immune complexes, and finally the impaired immune function of RBCs (25). In contrast, autologous blood of ANH autologous transfusion has a short retention time outside the body and does not require refrigeration, has few changes in red blood cells and their associated metabolites, and is free of alloantigens and proteins, and has few white blood cell fragments, thus causing minimal suppression of the immune system. The results of this study also showed that the incidence of adverse transfusion reactions such as allergy, fever, and hemolysis was slightly lower in the autologous group than in the allogeneic group ($P > 0.05$). It can be seen that ANH autologous transfusion is safer and will not increase the incidence of adverse blood transfusion reactions.

CONCLUSION

Through the comparative analysis of the above results, we found that both allogeneic and ANH autologous transfusion had little effect on the vital signs of patients undergoing cesarean section, but ANH autologous transfusion was more helpful in stabilizing the postoperative blood routine, *T*-cell subpopulation, immunoglobulin, and inflammation levels, and was a safe and effective way of blood transfusion. It is worth noting that although ANH autologous transfusion is a safe and effective way of blood transfusion, it can not completely replace allogeneic blood transfusion. Some studies

(26) pointed out that when high-dose HES is used, due to the dilution effect, it may cause dose-related abnormal blood coagulation and decrease of HCT. Therefore, when the body has massive bleeding and the amount of recovered blood is also large, RBC, PLT and coagulation factors need to be supplemented at the same time in order to avoid serious coagulation dysfunction. The specific blood transfusion method should also depend on the specific situation of the patient.

ETHICS STATEMENT

The studies involving human participants were reviewed and approved by the Ethics Committee of the First Affiliated Hospital of Naval Military Medical University. The patients/participants provided their written informed consent to participate in this study.

AUTHOR CONTRIBUTIONS

FG and HT are responsible for the design of the study and manuscript writing. XW is the instructor of the entire study, responsible for the inclusion of cases, and data statistics. All authors contributed to the article and approved the submitted version.

REFERENCES

1. Yapca OE, Topdagi YE, Al RA. Fetus delivery time in extraperitoneal versus transperitoneal cesarean section: a randomized trial. *J Matern Fetal Neonatal Med.* (2020) 33:657–63. doi: 10.1080/14767058.2018.1499718
2. Zou YQ, Chen XX, Feng Y. Clinical study on perinatal outcomes of 80 cases with unicornuate uterus pregnancy. *Zhonghua Fu Chan Ke Za Zhi.* (2020) 55:510–5. doi: 10.3760/cma.j.cn112141-20200107-00019
3. Hulse W, Bahr TM, Morris DS, Richards DS, Ilstrup SJ, Christensen RD. Emergency-release blood transfusions after postpartum hemorrhage at the Intermountain Healthcare hospitals. *Transfusion.* (2020) 60:1418–23. doi: 10.1111/trf.15903
4. Lecarpentier E, Gris JC, Cochery-Nouvellon E, Mercier E, Abbas H, Thadhani R, et al. Urinary placental growth factor for prediction of placental adverse outcomes in high-risk pregnancies. *Obstet Gynecol.* (2019) 134:1326–32. doi: 10.1097/AOG.0000000000003547
5. Wright GP, Wolf AM, Waldherr TL, Ritz-Holland D, Laney ED, Chapman HA, et al. Preoperative tranexamic acid does not reduce transfusion rates in major oncologic surgery: Results of a randomized, double-blind, and placebo-controlled trial. *J Surg Oncol.* (2020) 122:1037–42. doi: 10.1002/jso.26142
6. Terai A, Terada N, Yoshimura K, Ichioka K, Ueda N, Utsunomiya N, et al. Use of acute normovolemic hemodilution in patients undergoing radical prostatectomy. *Urology.* (2005) 65:1152–6. doi: 10.1016/j.urology.2004.12.034
7. Bennett J, Haynes S, Torella F, Grainger H, McCollum C. Acute normovolemic hemodilution in moderate blood loss surgery: a randomized controlled trial. *Transfusion.* (2006) 46:1097–103. doi: 10.1111/j.1537-2995.2006.00857.x
8. Iwase Y, Kohjitani A, Tohya A, Sugiyama K. Preoperative autologous blood donation and acute normovolemic hemodilution affect intraoperative blood loss during sagittal split ramus osteotomy. *Transfus Apher Sci.* (2012) 46:245–51. doi: 10.1016/j.transci.2012.03.014
9. Oppitz PP, Stefani MA. Acute normovolemic hemodilution is safe in neurosurgery. *World Neurosurg.* (2010) 79:719–24. doi: 10.1016/j.wneu.2012.02.041
10. Irlbeck T, Zwißler B, Bauer A. ASA-Klassifikation : Wandel im Laufe der Zeit und Darstellung in der Literatur [ASA classification : transition in the course of time and depiction in the literature]. *Anaesthesist.* (2017) 66:5–10. doi: 10.1007/s00101-016-0246-4
11. Akinlusi FM, Rabiu KA, Durojaiye IA, Adewunmi AA, Ottun TA, Oshodi YA. Cesarean delivery-related blood transfusion: correlates in a tertiary hospital in Southwest Nigeria. *BMC Pregnancy Childbirth.* (2018) 18:24. doi: 10.1186/s12884-017-1643-7
12. Su Y, Heitner J, Yuan C, Si Y, Wang D, Zhou Z, et al. Effect of a text messaging-based educational intervention on cesarean section rates among pregnant women in china: quasirandomized controlled trial. *JMIR Mhealth Uhealth.* (2020) 8:e19953. doi: 10.2196/19953
13. Khanal V, Karkee R, Lee AH, Binns CW. Adverse obstetric symptoms and rural-urban difference in cesarean delivery in Rupandehi district, Western Nepal: a cohort study. *Reprod Health.* (2016) 13:17. doi: 10.1186/s12978-016-0128-x
14. Sarkanović ML, Gvozdenović L, Savić D, Ilić MP, Jovanović G. Autologous blood transfusion in total knee replacement surgery. *Vojnosanit Pregl.* (2013) 70:274–8. doi: 10.2298/VSP1303274L
15. van der Post JA, van Buul BJ, Hart AA, van Heerikhuize JJ, Pesman G, Legros JJ, et al. Vasopressin and oxytocin levels during normal pregnancy: effects of chronic dietary sodium restriction. *J Endocrinol.* (1997) 152:345–54. doi: 10.1677/joe.0.1520345
16. Duncan AE, Jia Y, Soltesz E, Leung S, Yilmaz HO, Mao G, et al. Effect of 6% hydroxyethyl starch 130/0.4 on kidney and haemostatic function in cardiac surgical patients: a randomized controlled trial. *Anaesthesia.* (2020) 75:1180–90. doi: 10.1111/anae.14994
17. Li K, Xu Y, Hu Y, Liu Y, Chen X, Zhou Y. Effect of enteral immunonutrition on immune, inflammatory markers and nutritional status in gastric cancer patients undergoing gastrectomy: a randomized double-blinded controlled trial. *J Invest Surg.* (2020) 33:950–9. doi: 10.1080/08941939.2019.1569736
18. Nelson KA, Aldea GS, Warner P, Latchman Y, Gunasekera D, Tamir A, et al. Transfusion-related immunomodulation: gamma irradiation alters the effects of leukoreduction on alloimmunization. *Transfusion.* (2019) 59:3396–404. doi: 10.1111/trf.15555
19. Arasaratnam RJ, Tzannou I, Gray T, Aguayo-Hiraldo PI, Kuvalekar M, Naik S, et al. Dynamics of virus-specific T cell immunity in pediatric liver transplant recipients. *Am J Transplant.* (2018) 18:2238–49. doi: 10.1111/ajt.14967
20. Longbrake EE, Mao-Draayer Y, Cascione M, Zielinski T, Bame E, Brassat D, et al. Dimethyl fumarate treatment shifts the immune environment toward an anti-inflammatory cell profile while maintaining protective humoral immunity. *Mult Scler.* (2021) 27:883–94. doi: 10.1177/1352458520937282
21. Li H, Zhang XS. Impacts of moxibustion on erythrocyte immune function and T-lymphocyte subsets in athletes. *Zhongguo Zhen Jiu.* (2013) 33:415–8.
22. Evers D, Middelburg RA, de Haas M, Zalpuri S, de Vooght KM, van de Kerkhof D, et al. Red-blood-cell alloimmunisation in relation to antigens' exposure and their immunogenicity: a cohort study. *Lancet Haematol.* (2016) 3:e284–92. doi: 10.1016/S2352-3026(16)30019-9
23. Wang S, Gao G, He Y, Li Q, Li Z, Tong G. Amidation-Modified Apelin-13 regulates ppary and perilipin to inhibit adipogenic differentiation and promote lipolysis. *Bioinorg Chem Appl.* (2021) 2021:3594630. doi: 10.1155/2021/3594630

Permissions

All chapters in this book were first published by Frontiers; hereby published with permission under the Creative Commons Attribution License or equivalent. Every chapter published in this book has been scrutinized by our experts. Their significance has been extensively debated. The topics covered herein carry significant findings which will fuel the growth of the discipline. They may even be implemented as practical applications or may be referred to as a beginning point for another development.

The contributors of this book come from diverse backgrounds, making this book a truly international effort. This book will bring forth new frontiers with its revolutionizing research information and detailed analysis of the nascent developments around the world.

We would like to thank all the contributing authors for lending their expertise to make the book truly unique. They have played a crucial role in the development of this book. Without their invaluable contributions this book wouldn't have been possible. They have made vital efforts to compile up to date information on the varied aspects of this subject to make this book a valuable addition to the collection of many professionals and students.

This book was conceptualized with the vision of imparting up-to-date information and advanced data in this field. To ensure the same, a matchless editorial board was set up. Every individual on the board went through rigorous rounds of assessment to prove their worth. After which they invested a large part of their time researching and compiling the most relevant data for our readers.

The editorial board has been involved in producing this book since its inception. They have spent rigorous hours researching and exploring the diverse topics which have resulted in the successful publishing of this book. They have passed on their knowledge of decades through this book. To expedite this challenging task, the publisher supported the team at every step. A small team of assistant editors was also appointed to further simplify the editing procedure and attain best results for the readers.

Apart from the editorial board, the designing team has also invested a significant amount of their time in understanding the subject and creating the most relevant covers. They scrutinized every image to scout for the most suitable representation of the subject and create an appropriate cover for the book.

The publishing team has been an ardent support to the editorial, designing and production team. Their endless efforts to recruit the best for this project, has resulted in the accomplishment of this book. They are a veteran in the field of academics and their pool of knowledge is as vast as their experience in printing. Their expertise and guidance has proved useful at every step. Their uncompromising quality standards have made this book an exceptional effort. Their encouragement from time to time has been an inspiration for everyone.

The publisher and the editorial board hope that this book will prove to be a valuable piece of knowledge for researchers, students, practitioners and scholars across the globe.

List of Contributors

Rob C. Roach and Kirk C. Hansen
Department of Biochemistry and Molecular Genetics, University of Colorado Denver - Anschutz Medical Campus, Aurora, CO, United States

Kaiqi Sun, Alexander Q. Wen and Yang Xia
University of Texas Houston - McGovern Medical School, Houston, TX, United States

Tatsuro Yoshida and Andrew Dunham
New Health Sciences Inc., Boston, MA, United States

Edward Y. Wen
University of Texas Houston - McGovern Medical School, Houston, TX, United States
University of California Berkeley, Berkeley, CA, United States

Hara T. Georgatzakou
Department of Biology, School of Science, National and Kapodistrian University of Athens, Athens, Greece

Federica Gevi and Sara Rinalducci
Department of Ecological and Biological Sciences, University of Tuscia, Viterbo, Italy

Lello Zolla
Department of Science and Technology for Agriculture, Forestry, Nature and Energy, University of Tuscia, Viterbo, Italy

Anastasios G. Kriebardis
Department of Medical Laboratories, Faculty of Health and Caring Professions, Technological and Educational Institute of Athens, Athens, Greece

Julie A. Reisz, Travis Nemkov and Angelo D'Alessandro
Department of Biochemistry and Molecular Genetics, School of Medicine, University of Colorado, Aurora, CO, United States

Vassilis L. Tzounakas, Issidora S. Papassideri and Marianna H. Antonelou
Department of Biology, School of Science, National and Kapodistrian University of Athens, Athens, Greece

Artemis I. Voulgaridou
"Apostle Paul" Educational Institution, Thessaloniki, Greece

Stefano Barell
Division of Haematology and Central Haematology Laboratory, CHUV, Lausanne University Hospital, University of Lausanne, Lausanne, Switzerland

Lorenzo Alberio
Division of Haematology and Central Haematology Laboratory, CHUV, Lausanne University Hospital, University of Lausanne, Lausanne, Switzerland
Faculté de Biologie et Médecine, UNIL, University of Lausanne, Lausanne, Switzerland

Caroline Le Van Kim and Yves Colin
Biologie Intégrée du Globule Rouge UMR_S1134, Institut National de la Santé et de la Recherche Médicale, Université Paris Diderot, Sorbonne Paris Cité, Université de La Réunion, Université des Antilles, Paris, France
Institut National de la Transfusion Sanguine, Paris, France
Laboratoire d'Excellence GR-Ex, Paris, France

Michael Dussiot
Laboratoire d'Excellence GR-Ex, Paris, France
Laboratory of Cellular and Molecular Mechanisms of Hematological Disorders and Therapeutic Implications U1163, Centre National de la Recherche Scientifique ERL 8254, Institut National de la Santé et de la Recherche Médicale, Université Paris Descartes, Sorbonne Paris Cité, Paris, France

Elisabeth Farcy
Université Paris Descartes, Paris, France

Sylvain Monnier
Institut Curie, Centre National de la Recherche Scientifique, UMR 144, PSL Research University, Paris, France

Olivier Hermine
Laboratoire d'Excellence GR-Ex, Paris, France
Université Paris Descartes, Paris, France
Laboratory of Cellular and Molecular Mechanisms of Hematological Disorders and Therapeutic Implications U1163, Centre National de la Recherche Scientifique ERL 8254, Institut National de la Santé et de la Recherche Médicale, Université Paris Descartes, Sorbonne Paris Cité, Paris, France
Assistance Publique des Hôpitaux de Paris, Paris, France

Matthieu Piel
Institut Curie, Centre National de la Recherche Scientifique, UMR 144, PSL Research University, Paris, France
Institut Pierre-Gilles de Gennes, PSL Research University, Paris, France

Chaker Aloui, Hind Hamzeh-Cognasse and Philippe Berthelot
GIMAP-EA3064, Université de Lyon, Saint-Étienne, France

Caroline Sut, Sofiane Tariket, Sandrine Laradi and Fabrice Cognasse
GIMAP-EA3064, Université de Lyon, Saint-Étienne, France
Etablissement Français du Sang, Auvergne-Rhône-Alpes, Saint-Etienne, France

Cécile Aubron
Médecine Intensive Réanimation, Centre Hospitalier Régionale et Universitaire de Brest, Université de Bretagne Occidentale, Brest, France

Andreas Greinacher
Institute for Immunology and Transfusion Medicine, University of Greifswald, Greifswald, Germany

Pascal Amireault
Biologie Intégrée du Globule Rouge UMR_S1134, INSERM, Univ. Paris Diderot, Sorbonne Paris Cité, Univ. de la Réunion, Univ. des Antilles, Paris, France
Institut National de la Transfusion Sanguine, Paris, France
Laboratoire d'Excellence GR-Ex, Paris, France
Laboratory of Cellular and Molecular Mechanisms of Hematological Disorders and Therapeutic Implications U1163/CNRS ERL 8254, INSERM, CNRS, Univ Paris Descartes, Sorbonne Paris Cité, Paris, France

Camille Roussel
Biologie Intégrée du Globule Rouge UMR_S1134, INSERM, Univ. Paris Diderot, Sorbonne Paris Cité, Univ. de la Réunion, Univ. des Antilles, Paris, France
Institut National de la Transfusion Sanguine, Paris, France
Laboratoire d'Excellence GR-Ex, Paris, France
Laboratory of Cellular and Molecular Mechanisms of Hematological Disorders and Therapeutic Implications U1163/CNRS ERL 8254, INSERM, CNRS, Univ Paris Descartes, Sorbonne Paris Cité, Paris, France
Université Paris Descartes, Paris, France

Mart P. Janssen
Department of Transfusion Technology Assessment, Sanquin Research, Amsterdam, Netherlands

Pierre A. Buffet
Biologie Intégrée du Globule Rouge UMR_S1134, INSERM, Univ. Paris Diderot, Sorbonne Paris Cité, Univ. de la Réunion, Univ. des Antilles, Paris, France
Institut National de la Transfusion Sanguine, Paris, France
Laboratoire d'Excellence GR-Ex, Paris, France
Université Paris Descartes, Paris, France
Assistance publique des hôpitaux de Paris, Paris, France

Joost H. J. van Sambeeck
Department of Transfusion Technology Assessment, Sanquin Research, Amsterdam, Netherlands
Center for Healthcare Operations Improvement and Research, University of Twente, Enschede, Netherlands

Katja van den Hurk, Anne van Dongen and Puck D. de Wit
Department of Donor Studies, Sanquin Research, Amsterdam, Netherlands

Jessie Luken
Sanquin Diagnostic Services, Amsterdam, Netherlands

Barbera Veldhuisen
Sanquin Diagnostic Services, Amsterdam, Netherlands
Sanquin Research and Landsteiner Laboratory, Department of Experimental Immunohematology, Academic Medical Center, University of Amsterdam, Amsterdam, Netherlands

C. Ellen van der Schoot and Henk Schonewille
Sanquin Research and Landsteiner Laboratory, Department of Experimental Immunohematology, Academic Medical Center, University of Amsterdam, Amsterdam, Netherlands

Maria M. W. Koopman
Department of Transfusion Medicine, Sanquin Blood Bank, Amsterdam, Netherlands

Marian G. J. van Kraaij
Department of Transfusion Medicine, Sanquin Blood Bank, Amsterdam, Netherlands
Department of Donor Affairs, Sanquin Blood Bank, Amsterdam, Netherlands
Department of Clinical Transfusion Research, Sanquin Research, Amsterdam, Netherlands

Wim L. A. M. de Kort
Department of Donor Studies, Sanquin Research, Amsterdam, Netherlands
Department of Social Medicine, Academic Medical Center, Amsterdam, Netherlands

José Eduardo Levi
Hospital Israelita Albert Einstein, São Paulo, Brazil

Antoine Haddad
Department of Clinical Pathology and Blood Banking, Sacré-Coeur Hospital, Lebanese University, Beirut, Lebanon
EA3064, Faculty of Medicine of Saint-Etienne, University of Lyon, Saint-Etienne, France

Tarek Bou Assi
Department of Laboratory Medicine, Psychiatric Hospital of the Cross, Jal El Dib, Lebanon
Department of Laboratory Medicine and Blood Banking, Saint Joseph Hospital, Dora, Lebanon

Olivier Garraud
EA3064, Faculty of Medicine of Saint-Etienne, University of Lyon, Saint-Etienne, France
Institut National de la Transfusion Sanguine, Paris, France

David Juhl and Holger Hennig
Institute of Transfusion Medicine, University Hospital of Schleswig-Holstein, Lübeck, Germany

Victor J. Drew, Ching-Li Tseng and Thierry Burnouf
International PhD Program of Biomedical Engineering, College of Biomedical Engineering, Taipei Medical University, Taipei, Taiwan
College of Biomedical Engineering, Graduate Institute of Biomedical Materials and Tissue Engineering, Taipei Medical University, Taipei, Taiwan

Jerard Seghatchian
Independent Researcher, London, United Kingdom

Stefan Handtke, Andreas Greinacher and Thomas Thiele
Institut für Immunologie und Transfusionsmedizin, Greifswald, Germany

Leif Steil
Interfakultäres Institut für Funktionelle Genomforschung, Greifswald, Germany

Giel J. C. G. M. Bosman
Department of Biochemistry, Radboud University Nijmegen Medical Centre, Nijmegen, Netherlands

Jean-Daniel Tissot
Transfusion Interrégionale CRS, Epalinges, Switzerland
Faculty of Biology and Medicine, University of Lausanne, Lausanne, Switzerland

Peter Schubert and Dana V. Devine
Canadian Blood Services, Vancouver, BC, Canada
Centre for Blood Research, University of British Columbia, Vancouver, BC, Canada

Lacey Johnson
Research and Development, Australian Red Cross Blood Service, Sydney, NSW, Australia

Denese C. Marks
Research and Development, Australian Red Cross Blood Service, Sydney, NSW, Australia
Sydney Medical School, The University of Sydney, Sydney, NSW, Australia

Axel Seltsam
German Red Cross Blood Service NSTOB, Institute Springe, Springe, Germany

Catherine Strassel, Christian Gachet and François Lanza
Université de Strasbourg, INSERM, EFS Grand Est, BPPS UMR-S 1255, FMTS, Strasbourg, France

Daniel Candotti and Syria Laperche
Department of Blood-Transmitted Pathogens, National Transfusion Infectious Risk Reference Laboratory, National Institute of Blood Transfusion, Paris, France

Philippe Gillet and Esther Neijens
Service du Sang, Belgian Red-Cross, Suarlée, Belgium

Jens Dreier, Cornelius Knabbe and Tanja Vollmer
Institut für Laboratoriums- und Transfusionsmedizin, Herz- und Diabeteszentrum Nordrhein-Westfalen, Universitätsklinik der Ruhr-Universität Bochum, Bad Oeynhausen, Germany

Xiaoyi Qin
Department of Hematology, The First Affiliated Hospital of Wenzhou Medical University, Wenzhou, China

Wei Zhang
Department of Thoracic Surgery, The First Affiliated Hospital of Wenzhou Medical University, Wenzhou, China

Xiaodan Zhu and Wei Zhou
Department of Intensive Care Unit, The First Affiliated Hospital of Wenzhou Medical University, Wenzhou, China

Xiang Hu
Department of Endocrine and Metabolic Diseases, The First Affiliated Hospital of Wenzhou Medical University, Wenzhou, China

Bo Liu, Junpeng Pan and Zhijie Wang
Department of Spinal Surgery, The Affiliated Hospital of Qingdao University, Qingdao, China

Hui Zong
Department of Neurology, The People's Hospital of Qingyun, Dezhou, China

Hamza Naciri-Bennani and Paolo Malvezzi
Nephrology, Hemodialysis, Apheresis and Kidney Transplantation Department, University Hospital Grenoble, Grenoble, France

Thomas Jouve, Johan Noble and Lionel Rostaing
Nephrology, Hemodialysis, Apheresis and Kidney Transplantation Department, University Hospital Grenoble, Grenoble, France
Faculty of Health, Univ. Grenoble Alpes, Grenoble, France

Céline Dard and Dominique Masson
Human Leukocyte Antigen (HLA) Laboratory, Etablissement Français du Sang (EFS), La Tronche, France

Gaëlle Fiard
Urology and Kidney Transplantation Department, University Hospital Grenoble, Grenoble, France

Fei Guo, Heshan Tang and Xiaoqiang Wei
Department of Blood Transfusion, The First Affiliated Hospital of Naval Military Medical University, Shanghai, China

Index

Printed in the USA
CPSIA information can be obtained
at www.ICGtesting.com
JSHW051551051023
49754JS00005B/39